Handbook of
The Biology of Aging

D1568177

The Handbooks of Aging
Consisting of Three Volumes

Critical comprehensive reviews of
research knowledge, theories, concepts, and issues

Editor-in-Chief
James E. Birren

Handbook of the Biology of Aging
Edited by Edward L. Schneider and John W. Rowe

Handbook of the Psychology of Aging
Edited by James E. Birren and K. Warner Schaie

Handbook of Aging and the Social Sciences
Edited by Robert H. Binstock and Linda K. George

Handbook of
The Biology of Aging
Fourth Edition

Editors
Edward L. Schneider and John W. Rowe

Volume Associate Editors
Thomas E. Johnson, Nikki J. Holbrook,
and John H. Morrison

Academic Press
San Diego   New York   Boston   London   Sydney   Tokyo   Toronto

Cover photograph: Images © 1995 PhotoDisc, Inc.

This book is printed on acid-free paper. ∞

Copyright © 1996, 1990, 1985, 1977 by ACADEMIC PRESS, INC.

All Rights Reserved.
No part of this publication may be reproduced or transmitted in any form or by any
means, electronic or mechanical, including photocopy, recording, or any information
storage and retrieval system, without permission in writing from the publisher.

Academic Press, Inc.
A Division of Harcourt Brace & Company
525 B Street, Suite 1900, San Diego, California 92101-4495

United Kingdom Edition published by
Academic Press Limited
24-28 Oval Road, London NW1 7DX

Library of Congress Cataloging-in-Publication Data

The handbook of the biology of aging / edited by Edward L. Schneider,
   John W. Rowe; volume associate editors, Thomas E. Johnson, Nikki J.
   Holbrook, John H. Morrison. -- 4th ed.
          p.   cm. -- (The handbooks of aging)
   Includes bibliographical references and index.
   ISBN 0-12-627873-3 (pbk: alk. paper)
   1. Aging--Physiological aspects--Handbooks, manuals, etc.
   I. Schneider, Edward L.   II. Rowe, John W. (John Wallis), date.
   III. Series.
   QP86.H35 1996
   574.3'72--dc20   95-33705
                                                                     CIP

DISCARDED

PRINTED IN THE UNITED STATES OF AMERICA
96   97   98   99   00   01   QW   9   8   7   6   5   4   3   2   1

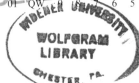
WIDENER UNIVERSITY
WOLFGRAM LIBRARY
CHESTER, PA.

Contents

Part One
Introduction
Edited by Edward L. Schneider and John W. Rowe

Part Two
Genetic Analyses
Edited by Thomas E. Johnson

Part Three
Molecular and Cellular Biology
Edited by Nikki J. Holbrook

Part Four
Neurobiology
Edited by John H. Morrison

Part Five
Physiology, Endocrinology, and Nutrition
Edited by John W. Rowe and Edward L. Schneider

Contributors

Numbers in parentheses indicate the pages on which the authors' contributions begin.

Marilyn S. Albert (217), Departments of Psychiatry and Neurology, Harvard Medical School, Massachusetts General Hospital, Cambridge, Massachusetts 02138

Steven N. Austad (3), Department of Biological Sciences, University of Idaho, Moscow, Idaho 83843

Michele F. Bellantoni (415), Johns Hopkins University School of Medicine, Baltimore, Maryland 21224

Marc R. Blackman (415), Division of Endocrinology and Metabolism, General Clinical Research Center, Johns Hopkins Bayview Medical Center, Baltimore, Maryland 21224

Jeffrey B. Blumberg (393), Jean Mayer USDA Human Nutrition Research Center on Aging, Tufts University, Boston, Massachusetts 02111

Judith Campisi (121), Department of Cancer Biology, Life Sciences Division, Lawrence Berkeley Laboratory, University of California, Berkeley, California 94720

Carl W. Cotman (283), Institute for Brain Aging and Dementia, University of California, Irvine, Irvine, California 92717

Donald R. Dengel (331), Ann Arbor VA Medical Center, GRECC (11G), Ann Arbor, Michigan 48105

Goberdhan Dimri (121), Department of Cancer Biology, Life Sciences Division, Lawrence Berkeley Laboratory, University of California, Berkeley, California 94720

Dariush Elahi (23), GRECC (18), VAMC, Baltimore, Maryland 21201

Charles Filburn (197), Laboratory of Biological Chemistry, National Institute on Aging, Baltimore, Maryland 21224

Caleb E. Finch (299), Andrus Gerontology Center and, Department of Biological Sciences, University of Southern California, Los Angeles, California 90089

James E. Fleming (73), Institute of Molecular Medical Sciences, Palo Alto, California 94306

Andrew P. Goldberg (330), Division of Gerontology, School of Medicine, University of Maryland, Baltimore, Maryland 21201; and Geriatrics Research Education Clinical Center, Baltimore VA Medical Center, Baltimore, Maryland 21201

Juan J. Guiamét (93), Instituto de Fisiologia Vegetal, Universidad Nacional de La Plata, CC327 1900 La Plata, Argentina

James M. Hagberg (331), Preventive Cardiology, University of Pittsburgh, Pittsburgh, Pennsylvania 15260

Eiji Hara (121), Imperial Cancer Research Fund, Molecular Oncology Laboratory, London WC2A 3PX, United Kingdom

S. Michal Jazwinski (39), Department of Biochemistry and Molecular Biology and LSU Center on Aging, Louisiana State University Medical Center, New Orleans, Louisiana 70112

Steven A. Johnson (299), Cortex Pharmaceuticals, Inc., Irvine, California 92718

David T. Kuninger (149), Department of Human Biological Chemistry & Genetics, University of Texas Medical Branch, Galveston, Texas 77550

Rodney L. Levine (183), Laboratory of Biochemistry, National Heart, Lung, and Blood Institute, National Institutes of Heath, Bethesda, Maryland 20892

Gordon J. Lithgow (55), Biological Gerontology Group, The School of Biological Sciences, The University of Manchester, Manchester M13 9PT, England

Li Liu (149), Department of Human Biological Chemistry & Genetics, University of Texas Medical Branch, Galveston, Texas 77550

Marjorie Luckey (431), OB/GYN and Reproductive Science, Mt. Sinai Medical Center, New York, New York 10029

Diane Meier (431), Mt. Sinai Medical Center, New York, New York 10029

Richard A. Miller (355), Department of Pathology, Institute of Gerontology Geriatrics Center and DVA Medical Center, University of Michigan School of Medicine, Ann Arbor, Michigan 48109

Charles V. Mobbs (233), Fishberg Center for Neurobiology, and Department of Geriatrics, Mt. Sinai School of Medicine, New York, New York 10029

Mark B. Moss (217), Department of Anatomy and Neurobiology and Department of Neurology, Boston University School of Medicine, Boston, Massachusetts 02215

Denis C. Muller (23), Gerontology Research Center, National Institute on Aging, Baltimore, Maryland 21224

Carolyn Murray (431), Mt. Sinai Medical Center, New York, New York 10029

Schawne Neeper (283), Institute for Brain Aging and Dementia, University of California, Irvine, Irvine, California 92717

Larry D. Noodén (93), Biology Department, University of Michigan, Ann Arbor, Michigan 48109

John Papaconstantinou (149), Department of Human Biological Chemistry & Genetics, University of Texas Medical Branch, Galveston, Texas 77550

Erika Randerath (197), Division of Toxicology, Department of Pharmacology, Baylor College of Medicine, Houston, Texas 77030

Kurt Randerath (197), Division of Toxicology, Department of Pharmacology, Baylor College of Medicine, Houston, Texas 77030

Peter D. Reisner (149), Department of Human Biological Chemistry & Genetics, University of Texas Medical Branch, Galveston, Texas 77550

Michael R. Rose (73), Department of Ecology and Evolutionary Biology, University of California, Irvine, California 92717

John W. Rowe (23), Mt. Sinai Medical Center, New York, New York 10029

Richard L. Sprott (3), National Institute on Aging, National Institutes of Health, Bethesda, Maryland 20892

Earl R. Stadtman (183), Laboratory of Biochemistry, National Heart, Lung, and Blood Institute, National Institutes of Heath, Bethesda, Maryland 20892

Foreword

This volume is one of three handbooks on aging now in their fourth editions: *Handbook of the Biology of Aging, Handbook of the Psychology of Aging,* and *Handbook of Aging and Social Sciences.* Their publication reflects a dramatic expansion of research on aging with an accompanying acceleration in the publication rate of information.

The handbooks are being used by research personnel, graduate students, and professionals for efficient access to contemporary research literature on aging. It is gratifying to see the subject matter of aging becoming a mainstream topic in the scientific disciplines and professions. The editors are pleased to provide these volumes that reflect advances in research findings, theory, and concepts that will guide further research as well as efforts to improve the well-being of older persons.

Stimulation of research on aging by government and private foundation sponsorship is a major factor in the growth of publications. There has also been an expansion of teaching in the universities and colleges of related subject matter. Furthermore, the growth of professional services to older persons has brought about an increasing interest in the knowledge base for organizing services in the health professions, social welfare, and design of institutions serving the elderly.

Aging is one of the most complex topics to challenge modern science and it is difficult to put all of the relevant information in one volume. For this reason, we have focused on three sources of influence on aging: the biological, the psychological, and the social. Human aging is an ecological phenomenon reflecting the influences of genetics, physical and social environments, and the organization of individual behavior. In the early 20th century, infectious diseases contributed highly to mortality and left residual effects expressed as later-life disabilities. Given the ecological character of aging, it is expected that there will continue to be drifts in the amount of variance contributed from different sources.

These volumes can be used to trace pathways through a large volume of scientific information about particular aspects of aging. Not all of the topics covered in early editions appear in the present volumes. It is suggested that readers also consult earlier volumes, not only for historical background, but for information on topics that developed earlier in methods and findings.

I thank the editors of the individual volumes for their cooperation and efforts: Robert H. Binstock, Linda K. George, John W. Rowe, K. Warner Schale, and Edward L. Schneider. I also thank the associate editors: Ronald Abeles, Margaret Gatz, Nikki Holbrook, Thomas Johnson, Victor W.

Marshall, John H. Morrison, George C. Myers, Timothy A. Salthouse, and James H. Schulz.

I express my appreciation to Nikki Fine, the editor at Academic Press whose cooperation facilitated the publication of the handbooks.

James E. Birren

Preface

Since the publication of the first edition of the *Handbook of the Biology of Aging* in 1978, there has been a virtual explosion of research in the field of aging. Whether you measure the budget of the National Institute on Aging, the number of investigators in the field, the number of publications, or the references in the lay press, the intensity of aging research has increased exponentially during this period. In a field that has developed so impressively over the past two decades, it is impossible to cover all the potential areas of aging research. Therefore, the fourth edition of the *Handbook of the Biology of Aging* continues the tradition of earlier editions in presenting an overview of critical areas of biomedical research on aging. In this edition, we have focused primarily on basic biological research on aging and left most of the clinical aging research areas to textbooks in the field of geriatrics.

We begin with critical chapters on the use of animal models and human subjects for aging research. Both chapters update and expand material presented in previous editions. We feel that these chapters are invaluable guides to both new and established investigators as they pursue aging research. With the increased interest in in-vertebrate models for aging research, we have devoted a section to the genetic analyses of a number of model systems that have displayed great potential. The section includes chapters on yeast and filamentous fungi, *Caenorhabditis elegans*, drosophila, and plants.

Few areas have witnessed as great a growth in knowledge as cellular and molecular biology over the past five years. This is reflected in substantial increases in our knowledge of the molecular and cellular biology of aging. The progress in these fields is amply demonstrated in the chapters on replicative senescence, protein modifications, and gene expression, which, although covered in the last edition, are composed of almost entirely new material. The final chapter in this section, on DNA alterations with aging, explores the exciting new discoveries in mitochondrial DNA damage with aging.

Research on the neurobiology of aging has also progressed at an extraordinary rate since the last edition of the *Handbook*. As a result, four chapters in the current edition reflect the astonishing pace of advances in our understanding of the aging brain. The *Handbook* is concluded by a series of chapters on broad areas of interest to aging research. The chapters on immunology, nutrition, and exercise are important updates of similar chapters in the previous edition of the *Handbook*, and there are new chapters on menopause and on the musculoskeletal system.

This edition of the *Handbook* was a collaborative effort and a large share of the credit for the quality of this edition goes to the Associate Editors, Drs. Nikki J. Holbrook, Thomas E. Johnson, and John H. Morrison, who devoted considerable time and effort to reviewing and revising these chapters. As with our previous editions we thank our colleagues who served as outside reviewers: Drs. Norman Klinman, Alice Liu, Kelvin J. A. Davies, Arlen Richardson, Anthony B. Bleecker, William Orr, Helmut Bertrand, Shin Murakami, Pamela Larsen, Simon Melow, Jim Cortsinger, Robert Schmookler-Reis, Dariush Elahi, Marilyn Albert, Kenneth Minniker, Catherine Devons, and John Morrison.

Edward L. Schneider
John W. Rowe

About the Editors

Edward L. Schneider

Dr. Schneider is Executive Director of the Ethel Percy Andrus Gerontology Center and Dean of the Leonard Davis School of Gerontology at the University of Southern California. Dr. Schneider became the first William and Sylvia Kugel Professor of Gerontology in 1989. He is Professor of Medicine at the USC School of Medicine and Adjunct Professor of Biology at the University Park Campus, USC. He also is Scientific Director of the Buck Center for Research on Aging, Novato, California. Before coming to the University of Southern California in 1986, Dr. Schneider spent 14 years at the National Institute on Aging (NIA). He was head of the laboratory that studied genetic aspects of aging. Before becoming Deputy Director of the NIA, Dr. Schneider was Associate Director for Biomedical Research and Clinical Medicine and Chief of the Laboratory of Molecular Genetics at the Gerontology Research Center of NIA. Dr. Schneider has served on the faculties of Johns Hopkins University, Georgetown University, and the University of Colorado's School of Medicine. While in Colorado, Dr. Schneider was Director of the Davis Institute on Aging and founder of the Colorado Gerontology Society. Dr. Schneider is a Fellow of the Gerontological Society of America and member of the American Society for Clinical Investigation, as well as past president of the Begg Honor Society. He has been the recipient of many honors, including Alpha Omega Alpha, the Roche Award, Boston University's Distinguished Alumnus Award, and the Sigma Xi Distinguished Lecturer Award. Frequently asked to speak, Dr. Schneider was named the Archibald Watson Lecturer at the annual scientific meetings of the Royal Australasian College of Physicians and the Jacobsen Lecturer for the Faculty of Medicine at the University of Newcastle upon Tyne. In addition to serving on editorial and advisory boards for a number of publications, Dr. Schneider has written more than 150 articles and has edited 12 books. Dr. Schneider is best known for the breadth of his aging interests, ranging from molecular genetics to policy issues.

John W. Rowe

Dr. Rowe is President of the Mount Sinai School of Medicine and The Mount Sinai Hospital in New York City, where he also serves as Professor of Medicine and as Professor of Geriatrics and Adult Development. Mount Sinai is one of the nation's largest academic health science centers. Before joining Mount Sinai in 1988, Dr. Rowe was Professor of Medicine and the founding director of the Division on Aging at Harvard Medical School and Chief of Gerontology at Boston's Beth Israel Hospital. He has authored over 200 scientific publications, mostly on the basic biology and physiology of the aging process, and a leading textbook of geriatric medicine. His major research interests include the physiological changes that occur with normal aging in regulation of homeostatic systems involved in the maintenance of blood pressure and the volume and composition of the extracellular fluid. His clinical research has focused on the mechanisms and natural history of geriatric syndromes, including delirium and postprandial hypotension. Most recently, Dr. Rowe has articulated the concept of "Successful Aging." As Director of the MacArthur Foundation Research Network on Successful Aging, he and his colleagues have designed and conducted a systematic series of studies that elucidate the factors and characteristics that permit older persons to function well. Dr. Rowe has received many honors and awards for his basic and clinical research and his work in health care policy, particularly regarding care of the elderly. He has served on and chaired many national and regional panels on these issues. He has been president of the Gerontological Society of America and the American Federation for Aging Research. He has served on the Board of Governors of the American Board of Internal Medicine, is a member of the Institute of Medicine of the national Academy of Sciences, and is on the Board of Directors of the New York Academy of Medicine.

Thomas E. Johnson

Dr. Johnson is Associate Professor for Behavioral Genetics at the University of Col-

orado at Boulder, where he teachers and conducts research on the genetics of aging and of alcoholism. He is widely recognized as "the major player" in the field of the genetics of aging. Among numerous other awards, he is the 1993 recipient of the Busse Research Award for Biomedical Gerontology, presented at the International Association for Gerontology meeting in Budapest, Hungary. Dr. Johnson is a member of Biological and Clinical Aging: An Initial Review Group of the NIA, is on the Board of Managing Editors for *Mutation Research DNAging*, and is Associate Editor for both *Experimental Gerontology* and *Journals of Gerontology, Biological Sciences*. He received the 1995 Nathan Shock Award for the Gerontology Research Center and has been elected Chair for the Gordon Conference on the Biology of Aging in 1997. A major part of his work continues to focus on the genetic basis of the aging processes, primarily in *C. elegans*.

Nikki J. Holbrook

Dr. Holbrook is an Investigator at the National Institute on Aging, where she serves as Chief of the Research Section on Gene Expression and Aging within the Laboratory of Cellular and Molecular Biology. She is a member of a number of scientific societies, including the American Association for Advancement of Science, American Society for Biochemistry and Molecular Biology, and Gerontological Society of America. Her laboratory research focuses on molecular and cellular responses to stress and the importance of these defenses to the aging process. Specific areas of interest include the regulation and function of heat shock protein expression and signal transduction pathways controlling cellular response to genotoxic stress. Dr. Holbrook is internationally recognized for her contributions in these areas, both in the aging arena as well as the general scientific community. Author of over 100 scholarly articles, she has served as a consultant–reviewer for a host of journals, granting agencies, and private organizations.

John H. Morrison

Dr. Morrison is the Willard T. C. Johnson Research Professor of Geriatrics and Adult Development (Neurobiology of Aging) and Professor and Co-Director of the Fishberg Research Center for Neurobiology at the Mount Sinai School of Medicine. Dr. Morrison received his B.A. degree from Johns Hopkins University and his Ph.D. in Neuroscience from the Department of Cell Biology and Anatomy at Johns Hopkins University School of Medicine. He then went on to a postdoctoral fellowship with Dr. Floyd Bloom, in the A. V. Davis Center for Behavioral Neurobiology at the Salk Institute in La Jolla, California. Throughout his training and career as an independent scientist, Dr. Morrison's research has remained focused on the cellular and neurochemical organization of cerebral cortex. His interest in the basic organization of cerebral cortex led Dr. Morrison to carry out a series of detailed investigations of the cellular pathology of Alzheimer's disease and other neurodegenerative disorders. More recently, he has also focused on sublethal age-related changes in cortical circuits that might form the basis of selective vulnerability. He has published approximately 150 articles which reflect his dual interests in basic neurobiology of cerebral cortex and human neuropathology. Dr. Morrison is on the editorial board of several international journals, has served on N.I.H. study sections, and is on numerous advisory boards, including the Board of Directors for The American Federation for Aging Research (AFAR). In addition, Dr. Morrison has received several awards, including the Moore Award (1992) for the best paper on Clinicopathologic correlation at the annual meeting of the American Association of Neuropathologists and a Faculty Scholar Award from the Alzheimer's Disease and Related Disorders Association. In addition, Dr. Morrison was the RSL Visiting Professor of Geriatric Medicine in Australia in 1993, as well as the Smith, Kline and French Visiting Professor of Neuroscience in Australia in 1985. Dr. Morrison's research continues to focus on molecular and cellular determinants of selective vulnerability in age-related disorders, particularly in respect to glutamate receptors.

Part One

Introduction

Edited by
Edward L. Schneider and John W. Rowe

One
_____

Animal Models for Aging Research

Richard L. Sprott and Steven N. Austad

I. Introduction

Experimental research into the fundamental mechanisms of aging cannot be carried out on humans; consequently, animal models are used in their stead. Scientific investigators therefore routinely need to choose appropriate animal models. The choices they make may be critical to the success of their research and its acceptance by other investigators. While great strides have been made in providing information about the characteristics of commonly available animal models, there is room for significant improvement in the particular species available and in providing information about them. Most investigators, unfortunately, still pick their animal model for convenience rather than for scientific suitability. However, the most convenient model may not be the best. Model selection should be a logical process in which the species, sex or sexes used, and genetic configuration of the study population are chosen carefully with the ultimate goal of the research in mind.

Therefore, whatever the source of the models, the most important aspect of the choice is that it be well-informed. The fact that the National Institute on Aging (NIA) has made some models readily available has increased information about these models, but at the same time has narrowed the research base. If the readily available species and genotypes are not really suitable for the purposes of the research, then investigators have a genuine obligation to find more suitable models. To assist in clarifying aspects of animal model selection, we will briefly review the history of animal model development in aging research and specify some principles of model selection.

II. History of Animal Model Development in Aging Research

The development of the fruit fly, *Drosophila* spp., for use in experimental genetic studies early in this century naturally led to its adoption for aging research as well (Northrop, 1917; Pearl & Parker, 1921). By the 1930s the *Drosophila* experiments had demonstrated that there were clear genetic influences on aging and longevity and that environmental factors such as

Handbook of the Biology of Aging, Fourth Edition
Copyright © 1996 Academic Press, Inc. All rights of reproduction in any form reserved.

crowding, temperature, and food availability could substantially affect aging as well. The manipulation of senescence by nutritional means ultimately was extended to a variety of other invertebrates, such as water fleas (Ingle, Wood, & Banta, 1937) and cockroaches (Haydak, 1953).

The development of animal models for aging research had its origins in the work of McCay in the 1930s (McCay, Crowell, & Maynard, 1935; McCay, Maynard, Sperling, & Barnes, 1939). McCay's pioneering research on the effects of caloric restriction (CR) had little impact on gerontology for nearly 50 years. Along with the rapid growth of interest in the "young" science of gerontology, which followed the creation of NIA in 1975, came a rediscovery of the potential importance of McCay's work. Any manipulation that could reliably increase life span by 35% had to be important.

A series of papers by Ross (1961, 1976, 1978; Ross & Bras, 1971, 1973) provided details about the effects of CR on growth, tumor incidence, and longevity. While these observations offered important suggestions about possible mechanisms for the CR effect on longevity, they also dampened interest in some quarters. The possibility that CR "merely" eliminated or postponed disease and had no "real" effect on basic aging processes led many gerontologists to assume that research in this area would not be fruitful. The question of disease is important and underlies many assumptions and decisions about the utility of animal models for gerontological research. This issue and related questions about "appropriate" and "optimum" environments have generated a great deal of heat and much less light over the 2 decades since the founding of NIA.

The rapid growth of aging research in the late 1960s and early 1970s was both a contributor to and a beneficiary of the creation of NIA. Even before the institute was created it was evident to the scientists planning its research agenda, and to the community of scientists that would be expected to carry out that agenda, that a reliable supply of useful animal models would be a critical component of research development.

The initial discussions about how to provide models for research and which models to provide were spirited. Some investigators championed their favorite model (rat, mouse, rabbit, armadillo, etc.) as the "best" model for the field, and, indeed, some advisors to the NIA believed that an ideal model suitable for all aspects of aging research existed or could be created. Most investigators in the field, however, understood that there could be no single "ideal" model. If aging is the result of diverse processes, then diverse models would be needed to study those processes. Further, much of the research agenda of gerontology is disease-related. Here too, a variety of models is required.

The developmental process that gerontology went through, and in which it is still involved, is essentially the same process that each investigator must carry out while choosing the model, or models, best suited for a particular research problem. Most animal models for aging research are intended to mimic some aspects of human physiology, function, or behavior. The primary advantage of an animal model is that it can be used to obtain observations or try manipulations that are not possible in the primary system. The major disadvantage is that results obtained with a model may not generalize to the system of primary interest. Models, therefore, are inherently neither good nor bad; they are simply more or less useful depending upon the question being asked. Finch (1990) and Rose (1991) review in depth a number of issues related to the use of animal models.

III. Logic of Model Selection

In general, model selection will depend upon three criteria: (1) specificity, or the direct investigation of specific aging mechanisms that are presumably analogous to mechanisms in humans; (2) generality, or usefulness in assessing the scope of previously identified mechanisms; and (3) feasibility, or the logistic ease and cost effectiveness associated with the use of particular species or strains, compatible with either criterion (1) or (2).

The concept of specificity is a straightforward one and means simply that a given animal model exhibits a trait of particular interest. Since virtually all animals age, it could be argued that any species would satisfy this criterion. Thus by default, feasibility would become the overriding concern in the choice of an animal model. This argument is, in fact, the rationale for the nearly exclusive use of laboratory rodents in aging research. An unspoken assumption behind the use of rodents is that rapidly aging animals, such as most rodents, are similar to slowly aging species, such as humans, with respect to the mechanisms involved. They simply do everything faster. This assumption has never been validated, but we know that there are certain similarities, as well as substantial differences, in the manner in which different mammals age. For instance, humans, laboratory rodents, and all mammals for which there is sufficient information develop a variety of types of cancer as they age. On the other hand, common laboratory rodents do not get benign prostatic hyperplasia, Parkinson's or Alzheimer's type neuropathologies, or coronary or cerebral infarcts due to artherosclerotic lesions histologically similar to humans (i.e., consisting of focal accumulations of lipids, complex carbohydrates, blood products, fibrous tissue, and calcium deposits) (National Academy of Sciences, 1981).

A second aspect of specificity is that a useful experimental strategy for isolating specific mechanisms of aging is to compare two populations that are as similar as possible except in their rate of aging. This logic is why gerontologists have been so attracted to the CR paradigm of aging

research—the animals are genetically identical and differ only in the environment to which they have been exposed. Similar logic was behind Sacher and Hart's (1978) suggestion that insight into the mechanisms of aging might be revealed by comparing aspects of *Mus domesticus* with its 2- to 3-year life span and a species of *Peromyscus* with a 6- to 8-year life span. This comparative approach represents a reasonable genetic complement to the environmental CR paradigm. It is important to note, however, that detailed knowledge of the evolutionary relationships between study species is essential for a comparative genetic approach. We now know, for instance, that *Mus* and *Peromyscus* are not particularly close relatives within the rodents and that their 30 million years of separation (Brownell, 1983) is several times longer than that now thought to separate *Mus* and *Rattus*. Many closer mouse relatives such as *Apodemus* (Old World wood mice), *Acomys* (spiny mice), and several genera of gerbils are better suited than *Peromyscus* for this type of comparison (Catzeflis, Dickerman, Michaux, & Kirsch, 1993). All of these animals have reported maximum life spans considerably longer (5–9 years) than that of *Mus* (Austad, unpublished data).

An ideal comparison for isolating specific genetic mechanisms of aging would be between two populations within a species that age at different rates. Such a procedure has the substantial advantage that populations within a species are genetically more similar than different species (i.e., fewer uncontrolled variables to deal with). This experimental strategy has been followed to very promising effects using artificial selection in *Drosophila* (Rose, 1984a; Luckinbill, Arking, Clare, Cirocco, & Buck, 1984) and the screening of mutants in the nematode *Caenorhabditis elegans* (Johnson, 1987). Finch's *Longevity Senescence, and the Genome* (1990) is a masterful exposition of all of the issues relevant to this discussion.

The second criterion, that of generality, concerns whether findings from one species or strain are applicable to others. A central question in gerontology today, for instance, is whether the age-retarding properties of CR apply to humans, as well as to laboratory rodents. Assessment of the generality suggested by phenomena observed in animal models requires thorough knowledge of the phylogeny, that is, evolutionary history, between extant models and any other target species, such as humans (Austad, 1993). Generality is maximized when study species that are alike in other relevant characteristics are distantly related in evolutionary time.

For answering the direct question of the applicability of mechanisms of aging identified in animal models, an alternative to the assessment of overall generality would be to investigate the mechanism in a species as closely related to humans as is feasibly possible. Most primates are too expensive and long-lived to permit extensive experimental investigations of aging, but we will identify several species of small lemuroid primates for which this may not be true.

Third, feasibility simply means that, all other things being equal, an animal model should be as inexpensive, readily available, and well-characterized with respect to husbandry, physiology, genetics, and pathology as possible. This is the sole traditional consideration for much aging research, and it is an important consideration.

A consideration in addition to the species or populations chosen is the genetic structure of that population. Researchers working with laboratory rodents have their choice of inbred strains (where all individuals are genetically identical and homozygous at all loci), F_1 hybrids between strains (individuals are genetically identical, but heterozygous at many loci), or outbred varieties (individuals are genetically different and heterozygous at many loci).

The advantage of using genetically identical individuals is that experiments can be repeated at different times and places without concern for the effects of different genetic backgrounds. Also, genetic similarity allows heterochronic organ transplants (i.e., the transplantation of organs from individuals of one age into individuals of another age), a demonstrably useful technique for assessing the effects of the aging of certain organs on other physiological parameters (Felicio, Nelson, Gosden, & Finch, 1983).

The advantage of using F_1 hybrids is that the genetic background is as highly replicable as in single strains, but in addition F_1 hybrids are often phenotypically more uniform than individual strains, suggesting that heterozygosity leads to greater developmental stability (Phelan & Austad, 1994). Also, heterozygous animals may show some fundamental differences from completely homozygous ones. For instance, Cohen, Cutler, and Roth (1987) found that, unlike inbred mice, populations of two outbred species of *Peromyscus* showed accelerated rates of wound healing with age. Also, Rose (1984b) demonstrated that a negative correlation between fecundity and longevity could be reversed by 10 generations of inbreeding in *Drosophila.*

Outbred animals do not have a replicable genetic background that can be duplicated in studies at various times and places. However, such populations are useful for the assessment of whether research results observed in genetically uniform populations are generalizable with respect to genetic background. In addition, such populations are useful for directionally selecting for certain traits or for asking whether certain pathologies have a heritable component. Thus, each genetic configuration has its own advantages.

In light of these principles of animal model selection, we now consider existing widely available models, as well as nontraditional species that might be fruitfully developed to meet certain criteria of particular relevance to aging research.

IV. Models Available from the National Institute on Aging

A. Rodents

McCay's research on CR in rats fore-shadowed several issues of importance to gerontology. As a nutritionist, not a genet-icist, McCay's (McCay, Crowell, & May-nard, 1935) first full report of the effect of CR on life span described his subjects only as "white rats." It took many years for ger-ontologists to appreciate the importance of complete characterization of animal models so that research potentially could be replicated and extended. Not until the publication of *Mammalian Models for Re-search on Aging* by the National Academy of Sciences (NAS, 1981) was there any gen-eral survey of available animals and their genetic composition, disease susceptibil-ity, and recommended husbandry. That publication set a new standard for animal model use in gerontological research.

After several years of research on the ef-fects of CR on the growth and longevity of white rats, McCay became interested in the differences in pathology seen in *ad libitum*-fed and CR animals (McCay, Ellis, Barnes, Smith, & Sperling, 1939). He noted a lower incidence of tumors in CR ani-mals. This observation was not systemat-ically explored until Ross's research (Ross & Bras, 1971). In the 1939 paper, McCay also appears to have begun to suspect that individual colonies of rats might differ in their life expectancies. He noted that "limited observations indicate that our stock colony of rats suffers from a high in-cidence of lung disease when about one year of age . . . from the few observations published elsewhere and from our dissec-tion of rats from other sources, it seems that this is general." By the time Ross (1961) began his studies, careful investiga-tors like Ross described the stock of their animals, their source, and their husbandry in some detail. A decade later Russell pro-vided a clear rationale for the use of genet-ically defined animals, characterized the

mouse models then available, and intro-duced the issue of specific genotype–environment interactions into the discus-sion of model suitability for aging research (Russell, 1972).

In the mid-1970s, the NIA established colonies of aged rats and mice for use in gerontological research. The choices made at that time and that were modified over the next 5 years largely settled the issues of which species (rats and mice) and with-in species which stocks and strains would be most commonly used (Table I). The spe-cific choices and some consequences of those choices are discussed in more detail in a review of the history of the develop-ment of animal models at NIA (Sprott, 1991).

Once the basic choices about species and genotypes were made, attention turned to questions of housing and hus-bandry. McCay's concern about lung dis-ease in his colony in the 1930s could still have been voiced with regard to one dis-ease or another in almost any laboratory 40 years later. The technology needed to create barriers against many pathogens at a cost that was feasible for large vivaria emerged in the late 1970s. Discussions about the relationship between aging and disease acquired increased salience as it became possible to exclude many com-mon rodent diseases from colonies of aged animals. At the animal model level at least, aging and disease were deemed to be separable, and the field opted for barrier-reared animal models (Sprott, 1991). Im-provements in housing and disease pre-vention in the past 25 years have led to a near doubling of median and maximum life spans for the commonly used rat and mouse models (Sprott, 1993).

At the same time that debates about ge-notype and housing were being resolved, questions about appropriate diet arose. The 1981 NAS report noted the "dearth of information about the most suitable nutri-tional regimens for aging rodents and oth-er species." Most diets available for labora-tory rodents in 1980 were developed for

Table I
Rodents Available from the National Institute on Aging

Species	Genotype	Diet
Mouse (*Mus domesticus*)	C57BL/6NNia	*Ad libitum*
	C57BL/6NNia	60% *Ad libitum*
	B6D2F$_1$Nia	*Ad libitum*
	B6D2F$_1$Nia	60% *Ad libitum*
	BALB/cJNia	*Ad libitum*
	DBA/2JNia	*Ad libitum*
	CBA/JNia	*Ad libitum*
	B6C3F$_1$Nia	*Ad libitum*
	CB6F$_1$Nia	*Ad libitum*
	Swiss Webster	*Ad libitum*
Rat (*Rattus norvegicus*)	F344NNia	*Ad libitum*
	F344NNia	60% *Ad libitum*
	BN/RijNia	*Ad libitum*
	BN/RijNia	60% *Ad libitum*
	F344 × BNF$_1$Nia	*Ad libitum*
	F344 × BNF$_1$Nia	60% *Ad libitum*

the production of vigorous, healthy animals that reproduced efficiently. Diets to maximize life span were nonexistent. The situation has not changed much since. One of the reasons CR may be so effective in increasing longevity in these animals may be that the diets developed to maximize the reproduction of young animals are deleterious later in life.

The characteristics of existing mammalian models are very well described in Masoro's excellent chapter in the previous edition of this volume (Masoro, 1990). Masoro describes rodents (including house mice, field mice, rats, hamsters, and gerbils), carnivores (including cats and dogs), and nonhuman primates. Little has changed since that time except for the expansion of NIA's colonies to include calorically restricted C57BL6/NNia, DBA/2NNIA, B6D2NNIA, and B6C3F1 mice and F344, BN, and F344xBN rats, in collaboration with The National Center for Toxicological Research (NCTR). Figures 1–7 from the NIA/NCTR biomarker colonies show mortality curves for these animals, while Tables IIa and IIb give the median and maximal life spans (calculated by the mean of

the last decile of survivors) of animals in these colonies.

Several points are worth emphasizing

Table II
Life Spans

	Male		Female	
	Ad lib.	Restr.	*Ad lib.*	Restr.
a. Median life span (weeks)				
Mouse				
B6D2F1	138	187	128	168
DBA/2N	88	104	77	117
B6C3F1	140	191	131	180
C57BL/6N	120	138	116	145
Rat				
BN	129	153	133	168
F344BNF1	145	175	137	187
F-344	103	125	116	132
b. Maximal life span (weeks)				
Mouse				
B6D2F1	180	215	163	207
DBA2/N	130	144	130	148
B6C3F1	180	221	164	208
C57BL/6N	150	178	147	174
Rat				
BN	158	190	163	194
F344BNF1	174	214	168	227
F-344	124	161	148	171

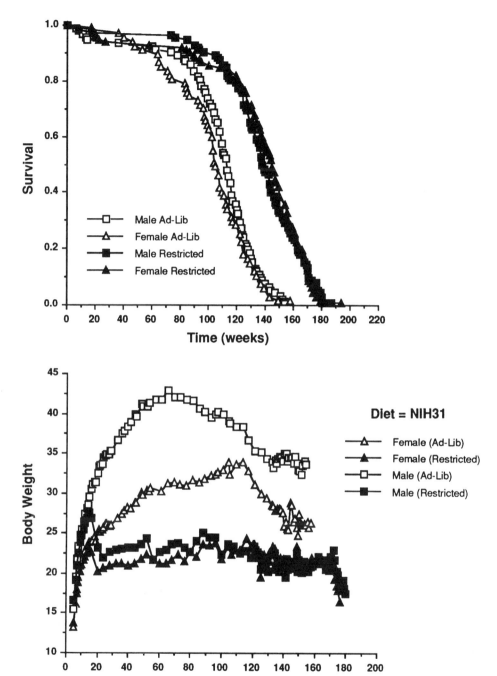

Figure 1. Probability of survival and mean body weight for C57BL6 mice in the NIA/NCTR biomarkers of aging colony. All mice were fed an NIH31 autoclavable diet. Animals were housed one per side in modified polycarbonate cages, which allowed visual and olfactory contact between pairs of animals but prevented physical contact.

10   Sprott and Austad

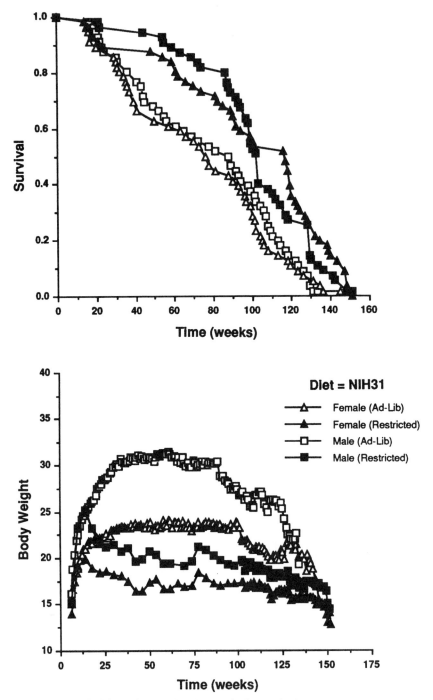

Figure 2. Probability of survival and mean body weight for DBA mice in the NIA/
NCTR biomarkers of aging colony.

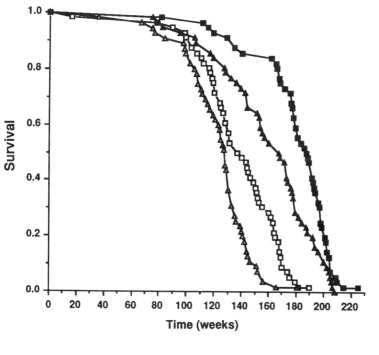

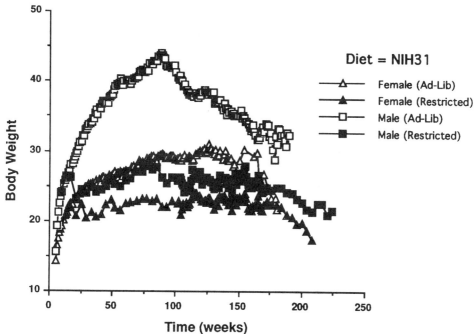

Figure 3. Probability of survival and mean body weight for B6D2F1 mice in the NIA/NCTR biomarkers of aging colony.

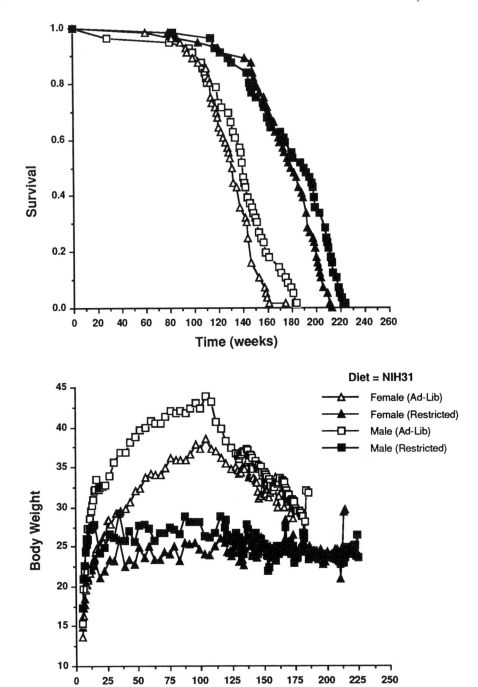

Figure 4. Probability of survival and mean body weight for B6C3F1 mice in the NIA/NCTR biomarkers of aging colony.

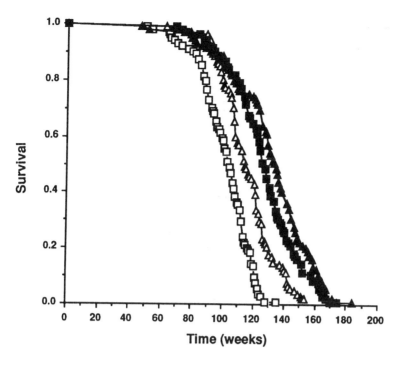

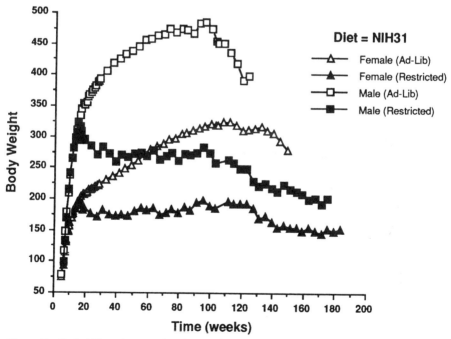

Figure 5. Probability of survival and mean body weight for F344 rats in the NIA/NCTR biomarkers of aging colony.

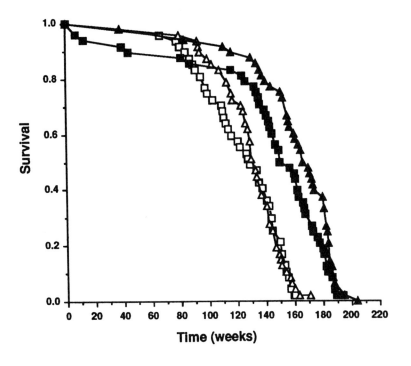

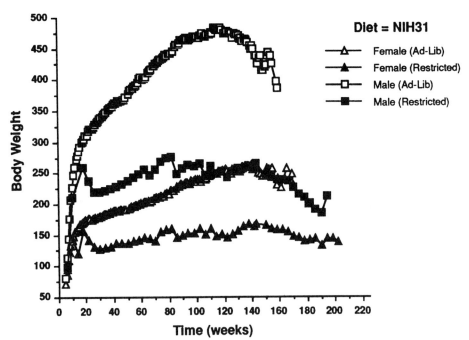

Figure 6. Probability of survival and mean body weight for Brown-Norway rats in the NIA/NCTR biomarkers of aging colony.

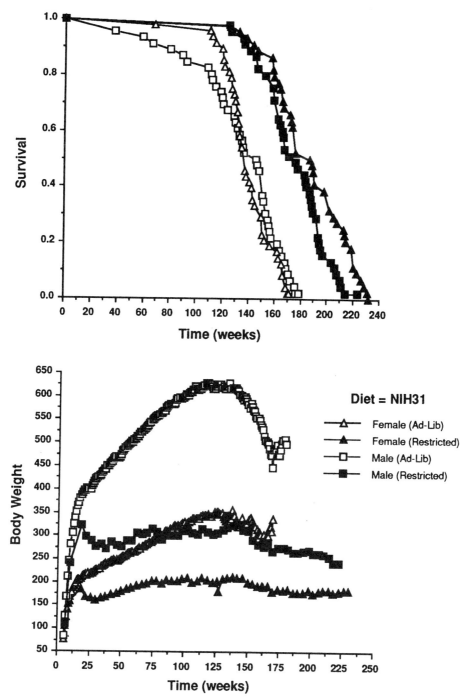

Figure 7. Probability of survival and mean body weight for F344xBN rats in the NIA/NCTR biomarkers of aging colony.

from these data. First, caloric restriction extends life in all genotypes of both species. Second, even though the F_1 hybrid strains are considerably longer lived than either parental strain, the life extension effect of caloric restriction is not ameliorated. Finally, there are no consistent differences between the sexes in their survival response to caloric restriction.

In the same chapter, Masoro discussed the relevance of CR to some common rodent pathologies. This can be illustrated by the pathological analysis of the NIA/NCTR's biomarker colonies, which have demonstrated decreased incidence of common pathologies such as pituitary tumors in F-344 rats (Thurman, Bucci, Hart, & Turturro, 1994) and delays in the age-associated incidence of others, such as mononuclear cell leukemia (Turturro & Hart, 1994) as well as delays in the age-associated incidences of common neoplasias in mice (Bronson & Lipman, 1991; Sheldon, Bucci, Blackwell, & Turturro, 1995). The need to develop a diet or diets that maximize longevity along with *ad libitum* feeding has been obvious for at least 25 years. This again can be illustrated by the experience of the biomarker colonies, in which C57BL/6 mice consuming the same total calorie intake *ad libitum* with different diets have different growth curves, with the relatively higher fat diet resulting in decreased survival (Turturro & Hart, 1992). That the problem still exists is, in our opinion, more the result of a lack of effort than a reflection of the difficulty of the task.

Ross's careful studies of the impact of CR on growth (Ross, Lustbader, & Bras, 1976), tumor prevalence (Ross & Bras, 1973), and longevity (Ross, 1976) focused attention on another approach to "optimize" diet. Subsequent research by Masoro (1988), Weindruch (1985), and Walford (Walford, Liu, Gerbase-Delima, Mathies & Smith, 1974; Walford, Harris, & Weindruch, 1987) produced great interest in the CR paradigm. The use of CR as the standard maintenance regimen was suggested by Masoro (1990). Interest in this topic has grown to such an extent that the International Life Sciences Institute (ILSI) organized a conference to discuss whether the CR condition should become the standard maintenance condition for all toxicity and carcinogenicity testing. The conference proceedings provide a thorough review of the relevant literature, current practices, and recommendations for the future (Hart, Robertson, & Neuman, 1995). Aged, calorically restricted mice and rats are now available from NIA-supported colonies in the same manner as *ad libitum*-fed rodents (Table I). With additional use, it is likely that CR animals will become the model of choice for investigators concerned about disease incidence or about modeling late life events. It seems likely that some real attention will be paid to the diet issue in the near future, and the development of better diets for aging rodents clearly should be a research priority.

We also expect that the development of additional mammalian models using "classical" genetic techniques is likely to culminate with the development of colonies of rodents (most probably mice) that are genetically selected for long life. Selection for longer and shorter life spans, in the absence of disease, could produce useful resources for the identification of specific genes with significant effects on longevity, and these new genotypes would then be useful for a broad range of research problems.

It seems to us that the next generation of rodent models is likely to be more specifically targeted. The emergence of techniques to produce transgenic animals undoubtedly will revolutionize animal model development. Initial methods for creating transgenic mice involved the introduction of the DNA of interest (the transgene) into the pronuclei of fertilized mouse oocytes or into embryonic stem (ES) cells, with the resulting random integration of various numbers of copies of the injected DNA into a single site on the mouse chromosome. Where fertilized oocytes are used, the integrated DNA can be passed on to succeeding generations. Where ES cells are used, cells are screened for the presence of the transgene, and positive cells are microinjected into blastocysts to produce chimeric mice, which can be mated with wild-type animals to create heterozygous offspring that carry the transgene. The result of such methodology is to create animals with altered gene dosage for the gene in question (Epstein, Avraham, Lovett, Smith, Elroy-Stein, Rotman, Bry, & Groner, 1987). By varying the regulatory region attached to the gene in question it is also possible to obtain regulated expression of a transgene (Ornitz, Palmiter, Hammer, Brinster, Swift, & MacDonald, 1985). Capecchi (1989) has described methods for selecting homologous recombination between an incoming transgene and the resident chromosomal gene. Where this methodology works (since it appears that homologous recombination cannot be obtained with all genes), it is possible to obtain mice carrying null mutations in a gene of interest (e.g., van Deursen, Heerschap, Oerlemans, Ruitenbeek, Jap, ter Laak, & Wieringa, 1993).

B. Nonhuman Primates

Nonhuman primates are generally expensive to obtain and keep, have life spans ranging from 20 to more than 60 years, and have less thoroughly developed husbandry than laboratory rodents. Consequently, they are difficult to perform experimental aging studies on. Nevertheless, it is critical that some aging research proceed using primates, because it is the only way to assess the probability that phenomena discovered in rodents, or other mammals more distantly related to humans than the other primates, are likely to apply to humans as well. In line with this reasoning,

there are two primate studies in progress, both focusing primarily on rhesus macaques (Macaca mulatta), addressing whether caloric restriction retards aging in primates (Cutler, Davis, Ingram, & Roth, 1992; Roth, Blackman, Ingram, Lane, Ball, & Cutler, 1993; Kemnitz, Weindruch, Roecker, Crawford, Kaufman, & Ershler, 1993). Because the rhesus life span is 40 years or more, whether caloric restriction retards again in primates as well as rodents is not likely to be known for some time yet, unless a shorter lived primate model is developed (see the following).

The National Institute on Aging maintains approximately 300 rhesus macaques, ranging in age from approximately 18 to 35 years, for aging research. Many of these monkeys were captured from the wild, so birthdates were estimated. The colonies are dispersed over four Regional Primate Research Centers and are available for both noninvasive and invasive studies (Masoro, 1990; Hazzard, personal communication, 1994).

V. Models Worthy of Development

A. Small Marsupials

One sensible route to quickly and easily assess the generality of aging phenomena discovered in rodents would be to develop a short-lived marsupial model. The advantage of marsupials is that even though there is considerable disagreement about the phylogenetic relations between most orders of mammals, taxonomic opinion unanimously supports an early separation between marsupials and the placental mammals, such as rodents and primates, of at least 100 million years (Eisenberg, 1981). Therefore, any phenomena found in both rodents and marsupials are likely to be very general mammalian phenomena.

The marsupial order consists of approximately 250 species occupying a variety of terrestrial habitats (Lee & Cockburn, 1985), and some species are already commonly used in the laboratory in Australia (Tyndale-Biscoe & Renfree, 1987).

An increasingly popular laboratory marsupial elsewhere is *Monodelphis domestica*, the Brazilian gray short-tailed opossum, which could easily be adopted for aging studies. *M. domestica* weighs 80–150 g, reaches sexual maturity at age 4–5 months, has litters of 5–12 offspring four times per year in captivity, lives 3–4 years, and has a reasonably well developed husbandry. Reproduction ceases in females by about 2 years of age (Fadem, Trupin, Maliniak, VandeBerg, & Hayssen, 1982; VandeBerg, 1983; Trupin, 1991; Stonerook & Harder, 1992). More than 100 papers have been published in medically oriented journals on *M. domestica* since 1990, including some on topics of interest to gerontologists such as the identification and sequencing of a mutationally activated K-ras oncogene (Kusewitt, Kelly, Sabourin, & Ley, 1993), the occurrence of several types of spontaneous tumors (Kusewitt, Applegate, Bucana, & Ley, 1990; Kuehl-Kovarik, Ackermann, Hanson, & Jacobson, 1994), and alterations of serum lipoprotein profiles under differing diets (Rainwater & VandeBerg, 1992). The ease of maintenance and obvious suitability for a variety of experimental purposes make this species seem especially promising as a marsupial aging model.

Marsupial mouse equivalents may also be found among the 40-odd species of the didelphid genus *Marmosa*, an omnivorous group that is roughly the same size as a mouse. These species reach sexual maturity in 6–9 months, have litters of 7–9, and live 1–3 years in captivity (Nowak, 1991). Some species breed year-round.

B. Small Primates

As already mentioned, there would be enormous advantages to developing a small, relatively short lived and consequently more feasible primate model because of the necessity to determine whether aging phenomena observed in rodents also occur in primates, especially humans. Current primate models are expensive to maintain, long-lived, and slow to sexually mature and produce only one offspring every few years even during their optimum reproductive years. Therefore, the cost of developing large colonies of these models specifically dedicated to aging research is prohibitive. Even if such colonies were developed, their long life spans make many types of aging research impossibly slow.

Fortunately, there are a number of primate species for which these disadvantages are somewhat mitigated, especially among the strepsirhine primates (lemurs and lorisoids). Although the phylogeny of primates is contentious (see Martin, 1990), there is no disagreement that the strepsirhines are true primates. They are estimated to have diverged from the rest of the living primates between 50 and 90 million years ago (in contrast with the 30–40 million year estimates for the divergence of humans and Old World monkeys, such as rhesus) (Sarich & Cronin, 1976; Martin, 1990).

The advantages for aging research represented by some of the strepsirhines are the following: (1) they are small, 80–300 g; (2) they are relatively short lived for a primate, 12–18 years typically; and (3) they mature rapidly (generally less than 1 year) and frequently produce twins. These traits together suggest that they would be vastly more productive in captivity than the larger, Old World primates, and aging studies would not take several decades.

One species that seems especially promising for aging research is the mouse lemur, *Microcebus murinus*. This species weighs 80–100 g and is omnivorous and nocturnal. Females become sexually mature in less than 1 year and commonly have two or three offspring per year thereafter. A current field study finds that their longevity in nature is 1–3 years (J. Schmid, personal communication, 1994) and in captivity individuals live 8–12 years. At an advanced age, mouse lemurs show signs of senescence such as fur whitening, blindness due to lens opacity, and the development of tumors, and there is even a report of brain lesions similar to Alzheimer's lesions in humans accompanied by a range of behavioral changes (Bons, Mestre, & Petter, 1992). In conditions of reduced temperature and shortened day length, mouse lemurs enter a semitorpid state where activity and metabolic rate are reduced and sexual activity ceases (Perret & Schilling, 1993). A number of primate facilities and zoos throughout the world keep mouse lemurs without difficulty, and a research colony in France has been in existence since 1953 (Bons, Mestre, & Petter, 1992).

A second species that might be assessed as an aging model is the lesser bush baby (*Galago senegalensis*). This species weighs about 180–300 g, eats insects and tree gum in nature, and is also nocturnal. Females have reached sexual maturity in less than 7 months, twins are born in about half of all births, and there can be two litters per year. The maximum recorded life span is 16.5 years (Nowak, 1991). This species does not enter torpor (W. Hess, personal communication, 1994) and has been bred successfully in a number of zoos and primate centers around the world (International Zoo Yearbook, 1990). There have been no published reports of age-related changes in bush baby appearance or physiology.

C. Small Birds

One type of model that is completely lacking in aging research is one that is more successful than mammals generally, or humans in particular, at managing some of life's destructive processes, such as oxidative and nonenzymatic glycation damage (Holmes & Austad, 1995). Birds are ideal models for exactly this purpose, however,

and many species are manageably short-lived, are inexpensive to maintain, and have a well-developed husbandry from centuries of domestication.

Most bird species are dramatically longer lived than mammals of equal body size (Lindstedt & Calder, 1976). In fact, the shortest lived known bird is the 90-g Japanese quail, *Coturnix coturnix*, which lives 7–8 years in captivity (Puigcerver, Gallego, Rodrigues-Teijeiro, & Senar, 1992)—considerably longer than laboratory rodents, opossums, or a large number of other mammalian species. Such longevity is particularly surprising because avian metabolic rates are as much as 2–2.5 times as high as those of similar-sized mammals, presumably exposing them to a higher rate of free oxygen radical production and consequent accelerated tissue damage (Harman, 1956; Del Maestro, 1980). In addition, they exhibit blood sugar levels that are typically 2–4 times as high as those of mammals along with a comparatively elevated body temperature (about 3°C higher than mammals), factors which should accelerate the formation of advanced Maillard products, now hypothesized to be involved in aging-related tissue degeneration as well (Cerami, 1985; Monnier, 1990; Monnier, Sell, Ramanakoppa, & Miyata, 1991). A hypothesis even suggests that aging is largely a consequence of the synergistic relationship between free radical damage and the formation of advanced Maillard products (Kristal & Yu, 1992).

Among specific bird species that would bear investigating as new aging models would be the domestic canary (*Serinus canarius*), a 20-g species with a very well known husbandry, considerable previous use in neurobiological laboratory research (e.g., Nottebohm & Nottebohm, 1978; Nottebohm, Nottebohm, Crane, & Wingfield, 1987), and a maximum reported longevity of 24 years (Altman & Dittmer, 1962). Also of interest might be the cockatiel (*Nymphicus hollandicus*), a somewhat larger (80 g) psittacine, which has also been domesticated for many years, has a well-understood husbandry, and routinely lives into its teens. In addition, both of these species have a variety of genetic strains available from breeders. These species are not closely related to one another and would make excellent mutual controls for generality.

VI. Summary

As should now be apparent, aging research requires considerable thought devoted to the determination of which animal model is most appropriate for specific research questions and methodologies. Fortunately, a relatively straightforward logic of model selection is available for aiding in the choice process. Researchers also need to be aware of the variety of models already available to the research community, so that they can make an informed choice before beginning a project. The National Institute on Aging supports a spectrum of rat and mouse genotypes that are well-suited for the investigation of aging mechanisms in short-lived mammals and also supports colonies of aged thesus monkeys.

It should also be obvious that sole reliance on rat and mouse genotypes for the investigation of general aging processes is not a wise policy. Long-lived animals may have distinctive processes at work, so that the range of relevant processes for rodents may not be identical to that for humans and other primates. The addition of several judiciously chosen species to the armamentarium of animal models will go a long way toward allowing insight into the generality of processes discovered in rodents and may even identify mechanisms of life extension that are nonexistent in traditional models.

A healthy, vigorous animal model research program clearly is gerontology's best insurance against producing a body of research with an overly narrow focus and with questionable relevance to an understanding of human health and function.

References

Altman P. L., & Dittmer, D. S. (1962). *Growth.* Washington, DC: Federation of the American Society of Experimental Biology.

Austad, S. N. (1993). The comparative perspective and choice of animal models in aging research. *Aging, Clinical and Experimental Research, 5,* 259–267.

Bons, N., Mestre, N., & Petter, A. (1992). Senile plaques and neurofibrillary changes in the brain of an aged lemurian primate. *Neurobiology of Aging, 13,* 99–105.

Bronson, R. T., & Lipman, R. D. (1991). Reduction in rate of occurrence of age related lesions in dietary restricted laboratory mice. *Growth, Development, & Aging, 55,* 169–184.

Brownell, E. (1983). DNA/DNA hybridization studies of muroid rodents: symmetry and rates of molecular evolution. *Evolution, 37,* 1034–1051.

Capecchi, M. R. (1989). Altering the genome by homologous recombination. *Science, 244,* 1288–1292.

Catzeflis, F. M., Dickerman, A. W., Michaux, J., & Kirsch, J. A. W. (1993). DNA hybridization and rodent phylogeny. In F. S. Szalay, M. J. Novacek, & M. C. McKenna (Eds.), *Mammal Phylogeny* (Vol. 2, pp. 159–172). New York: Springer-Verlag.

Cerami, A. (1985). Hypothesis: glucose as a mediator of aging. *Journal of the American Geriatric Society, 33,* 626–634.

Cohen, B. J., Cutler, R. G., & Roth, G. S. (1987). Accelerated wound repair in old deer mice (*Peromyscus maniculatus*) and white-footed mice (*Peromyscus leucopus*). *Journals of Gerontology, 42,* 302–307.

Cutler, R. G., Davis, B. J., Ingram, D. K., & Roth, G. S. (1992). Plasma concentrations of glucose, insulin and percent glycosylated hemoglobin are unaltered by food restriction in thesus and squirrel monkeys. *Journals of Gerontology, 47,* B9–B12.

Del Maestro, R. F. (1980). An approach to free

radicals in medicine and biology. *Acta Physiologica Scandinavica, 492,* 153–168.

Eisenberg, J. F. (1981). *The Mammalian Radiations.* Chicago: University of Chicago Press.

Epstein, C. J., Avraham, K. B., Lovett, M., Smith, S., Elroy-Stein, O., Rotman, G., Bry, C., & Groner, Y. (1987). Transgenic mice with increased Cu/Zn-superoxide dismutase activity: animal model of dosage effects in Down syndrome. *Proceedings of the National Academy of Sciences of the United States of America, 84,* 8044–8048.

Fadem, B. H., Trupin, G. L., Maliniak, E., VandeBerg, J. L., & Hayssen, V. (1982). Care and breeding of the gray, short-tailed opossum (*Monodephis domestica*). *Laboratory Animal Science, 32,* 405–409.

Felicio, L. S., Nelson, J. F., Gosden, R. G., & Finch, C. E. (1983). Restoration of ovulatory cycles by young ovarian grafts in aging mice: potentiation by long-term ovariectomy decreases with age. *Proceedings of the National Academy of Sciences of the United States of America, 80,* 6076–6080.

Finch, C. E. (1990). *Longevity, Senescence, and the Genome.* Chicago: University of Chicago Press.

Harman, D. (1956). Aging: a theory based on free radical and radiation chemistry. *Journals of Gerontology, 11,* 289–300.

Hart, R. W., Robertson, R. T., & Neuman, D. A. (Eds.) (1995). *Dietary Restriction: Implications for the Design and Interpretation of Toxicity and Carcinogenicity Studies.* Washington, DC: International Life Sciences Institute.

Haydak, M. H. (1953). Influence of the protein level of the diet on the longevity of cockroaches. *Annals of the Entomological Society of America, 46,* 547–560.

Holmes, D. J., & Austad, S. N. (1995). Birds as animal models for the comparative biology of aging: a prospectus. *Journals of Gerontology, 50,* B59–B66.

Ingle, I., Wood, T. R., & Banta, A. M. (1937). A study of longevity, growth, reproduction and heart rate in *Daphnia longispina* as influenced by limitations in quantity of food. *Journal of Experimental Zoology, 76,* 325–352.

International Zoo Yearbook (1990). Species of wild animals bred in captivity during 1988–1989 and multiple generations captive births. *International Zoo Yearbook, 29,* 425–443.

Johnson, T. E. (1987). Aging can be genetically dissected into component processes using long-lived lines of *Caenorhabditis elegans. Proceedings of the National Academy of Sciences of the United States of America 84,* 3777–3781.

Kemnitz, J. W., Weindruch, R., Roecker, E. B., Crawford, K., Kaufman, P. L., & Ershler, W. B. (1993). Dietary restriction of adult thesus monkeys: design, methodology, and preliminary findings from the first year of study. *Journals of Gerontology, 48,* B17–B26.

Kristal, B. S., & Yu, B. P. (1992). An emerging hypothesis: synergistic inductions of aging of free radicals and Maillard reactions. *Journals of Gerontology, 47,* B107–114.

Kuehl-Kovarik, M. C., Ackermann, M. R., Hanson, D. L., & Jacobson, C. D. (1994). Spontaneous pituitary adenomas in the Brazilian gray short-tailed opossum (*Monodelphis domestica*). *Veterinary Pathology, 31,* 377–379.

Kusewitt, D. F., Applegate, L. A., Bucana, C. D., & Ley, R. D. (1990). Naturally occurring malignant melanoma in the South American opossum (*Monodelphis domestica*). *Veterinary Pathology, 27,* 66–68.

Kusewitt, D. F., Kelly, G., Sabourin, C. L., & Ley, R. D. (1993). Characterization of the K-ras gene of the marsupial *Monodelphis domestica. DNA Sequence, 4,* 37–42.

Lee, A. K., & Cockburn, A. (1985). *The Evolutionary Ecology of Marsupials.* Cambridge, UK: Cambridge University Press.

Lindstedt, S. L., & Calder, W. A. (1976). Body size and longevity in birds. *Condor, 78,* 91–94.

Luckinbill, L. S., Arking, R., Clare, M. J., Cirocco, W. C., & Buck, S. A. (1984). Selection for delayed senescence in *Drosophila melanogaster. Evolution, 38,* 996–1003.

Martin, R. D. (1990). *Primate Origins and Evolution.* Princeton, NJ: Princeton University Press.

Masoro, E. J. (1988). Food restriction in rodents: an evaluation of its role in the study of aging. *Journal of Gerontology, 43,* B59–B64.

Masoro, E. J. (1990). Animal models in aging research. In E. L. Schneider & J. W. Rowe

(Eds.), *Handbook of the Biology of Aging* (pp. 72–94). New York: Academic Press.

McCay, C. M., Crowell, M. F., & Maynard, L. A. (1935). The effects of retarded growth upon the length of life span and upon the ultimate body size. *Journal of Nutrition, 10,* 63–79.

McCay, C. M., Ellis, G. H., Barnes, L. L., Smith, C. A. H., & Sperling, G. (1939). Chemical and pathological changes in aging and after retarded growth. *Journal of Nutrition, 18,* 15–25.

McCay, C. M., Maynard, L. A., Sperling, G., & Barnes, L. L. (1939). Retarded growth, life span, ultimate body size and age changes in the albino rat after feeding diets restricted in calories. *Journal of Nutrition, 18,* 1–13.

Monnier, V. M. (1990). Minireview. Non-enzymatic glycosylation, the Maillard reaction and the aging process. *Journals of Gerontology, 45,* B105–111.

Monnier, V. M., Sell, D. R., Ramanakoppa, H. N., & Miyata, S. (1991). Mechanisms of protection against damage mediated by the Maillard reaction in aging. *Gerontology, 37,* 152–165.

National Academy of Sciences. (1981). *Mammalian Models for Research on Aging.* Washington, DC: National Academy Press.

Northrop, J. H. (1917). The effect of prolongation of the period of growth on the total duration of life. *Journal of Biological Chemistry, 32,* 123–126.

Nottebohm, F., & Nottebohm, M. (1978). Relationship between song repertoire and age in the canary, *Serinus canaria. Zeitschrift für Tierpsychologie, 46,* 298–305.

Nottebohm, F., Nottebohm, M., Crane, L., & Wingfield, J. (1987). Seasonal changes in gonadal hormone levels of adult male canaries and their relation to song. *Behavioral Neurobiology, 27,* 197–211.

Nowak, R. M. (1991). *Mammals of the World* (5th ed., Vol. I). Baltimore: John Hopkins University Press.

Ornitz, D. M., Palmiter, R. D., Hammer, R. E., Brinster, R. L., Swift, G. H., & MacDonald, R. J. (1985). Specific expression of an elastase-human growth hormone fusion gene in pancreatic acinar cells of transgenic mice. *Nature, 313,* 600–602.

Pearl, R., & Parker, S. L. (1921). Experimental studies on the duration of life. 1. Introductory discussion of the duration of life in Drosophila. *American Naturalist, 55,* 481–509.

Perret, M., & Schilling, A. (1993). Response to short photoperiod and spontaneous sexual recrudescence in the lesser mouse lemur: role of olfactory bulb removal. *Journal of Endocrinology, 137,* 511–518.

Phelan, J. P., & Austad, S. N. (1994). Selecting animal models of human aging: inbred strains often exhibit less biological uniformity than F_1 hybrids. *Journals of Gerontology, 49,* B1–B11.

Puigcerver, M., Gallego, S., Rodrigues-Teijeiro, J. D., & Senar, J. C. (1992). Survival and mean life span of the quail *Coturnix c. coturnix. Bird Study, 39,* 120–123.

Rainwater, D. L., & VandeBerg, J. L. (1992). Dramatic differences in lipoprotein composition among gray short-tailed opossums (*Monodelphis domestica*) fed a high cholesterol/saturated fat diet. *Biochimica et Biophysica Acta, 1126,* 159–166.

Rose, M. R. (1984a). Laboratory evolution of postponed senescence in *Drosophila melanogaster. Evolution, 38,* 1004–1010.

Rose, M. R. (1984b). Genetic covariation in *Drosophila* life history: untangling the data. *American Naturalist, 123,* 565–569.

Rose, M. R. (1991). *Evolutionary Biology of Aging.* New York: Oxford University Press.

Ross, M. H. (1961). Length of life and nutrition in the rat. *Journal of Nutrition, 75,* 197–210.

Ross, M. H. (1976). Nutrition and longevity in experimental animals. In M. Winick (Ed.), *Nutrition and Aging* (pp. 43–57). New York: John Wiley & Sons.

Ross, M. H. (1978). Nutritional regulation of longevity. In J. A. Behnke, C. E. Finch, & G. B. Moment (Eds.), *The Biology of Aging* (pp. 173–189). New York: Plenum.

Ross, M. H., & Bras, G. (1971). Lasting influence of early caloric restriction on prevalence of neoplasms in the rat. *Journal of the National Cancer Institute, 47,* 1095–1113.

Ross, M. H., & Bras, G. (1973). Influence of protein under- and overnutrition on spontaneous tumor prevalence in the rat. *Journal of Nutrition, 103,* 944–963.

Ross, M. H., Lustbader, E., & Bras, G. (1976). Dietary practices and growth responses as predictors of longevity. *Nature, 262,* 548–553.

Roth, G. S., Blackman, M. R., Ingram, D. K., Lane, M. A., Ball, S. S., & Cutler, R. G. (1993). Age-related changes in androgen levels of rhesus monkeys subjected to diet restriction. *Endocrine Journal, 1,* 227–234.

Russell, E. S. (1972). Genetic considerations in the selection of rodent species and strains for research in aging. In D. C. Gibson (Ed.), *Development of the Rodent as a Model System of Aging* (DHEW Publication No. NIH 72–121, pp. 33–53). Washington, DC: U.S. Government Printing Office.

Sacher, G. A., & Hart, R. W. (1978). Longevity, aging and comparative cellular and molecular biology of the house mouse, *Mus musculus,* and the white-footed mouse, *Peromyscus leucopus.* In D. Bergsma & D. E. Harrison (Eds.), *Genetic Effects on Aging* (pp. 71–96). New York: Liss.

Sarich, V. M., & Cronin, J. E. (1976). Molecular systematics of the primates. In M. Goodman & R. E. Tashian (Eds.), *Molecular Anthropology* (pp. 141–170). New York: Plenum Press.

Sheldon, W., Bucci, T., Blackwell, B., & Turturro, A. (1995). Effect of ad libitum feeding and forty percent food restriction on body weight, longevity, and neoplasia in B6C3F1, C57B16 and B6D2F1 mice. In R. Hart, D. Neuman, & R. Robertson (Eds.), *Dietary Restriction: Implications for the Design and Interpretation of Toxicity and Carcinogenicity Studies.* Washington, DC: ILSI Press

Sprott, R. L. (1991). Development of animal models of aging at the National Institute on Aging. *Neurobiology of Aging, 12,* 635–638.

Sprott, R. L. (1993). Mouse and rat genotype choices. *Aging, Clinical and Experimental Research, 5,* 249–252.

Stonerook, M. J., & Harder, J. D. (1992). Sexual maturation in female gray short-tailed opossums, *Monodelphis domestica,* is dependent upon male stimuli. *Biology of Reproduction, 46,* 290–294.

Thurman, J. D., Bucci, T., Hart, R., & Turturro, A. (1994). Survival, body weight, and sponta- neous neoplasms in ad libitum fed and di- etary restricted Fisher 344 rats. *Toxicologic Pathology, 22,* 1–9.

Trupin, G. L. (1991). Care and breeding of the gray, short-tailed opossum (*Monodelphis domestica*). *Laboratory Animal Science, 41,* 96.

Turturro, A., & Hart, R. (1992). Dietary alter- ation in the rate of cancer and aging. *Experimental Gerontology, 27,* 583–592.

Turturro, A., & Hart, R. (1994). Modulation of toxicity by diet; Implications for response at low-level exposures. In E. Calabrese (Ed.), *Biological Effects of Low Level Exposures: Dose Response Relationships* (pp. 143–152). Boca Raton, FL: Lewis Publishers.

Tyndale-Biscoe, H., & Renfree, M. (1987). *Reproduction Physiology of Marsupials.* Cambridge, UK: Cambridge University Press.

VandeBerg, J. A. (1983). The grey short-tailed opossum: a new laboratory animal. *Institute of Laboratory Animal Research News, 26,* 9–12.

van Deursen, J., Heerschap, A., Oerlemans, F., Ruitenbeek, W., Jap, P., ter Laak, H., & Wieringa, B. (1993). Skeletal muscles of mice deficient in muscle creatine kinase lack burst activity. *Cell, 74,* 621–633.

Walford, R. L., Liu, R. K., Gerbase-Delima, M., Mathies, M., & Smith, G. S. (1974). Long term dietary restriction and immune function in mice: response to sheep red blood cells and to mitogenic agents. *Mechanisms of Aging & Development, 2,* 447–451.

Walford, R. L., Harris, S. B., & Weindruch, R. (1987). Dietary restriction and aging: histori- cal phases, mechanisms and current direc- tions. *Journal of Nutrition, 117,* 1650–1654.

Weindruch, R. H. (1985). Aging in rodents fed restricted diets. *Journal of the American Geriatric Society, 33,* 125–132.

Two

Design, Conduct, and Analysis
of Human Aging Research

Dariush Elahi, Denis C. Muller, and John W. Rowe

I. Introduction

The study of normal human aging can have many goals, but the most important from the general society's point of view are to develop strategies to prevent or minimize the handicaps of old age and to find better therapeutic approaches to major geriatric disabilities. These goals require increased understanding at the mechanistic level of the aging process in all its manifestations. It is not sufficient merely to document differences between young and old subjects or to reach obvious conclusions. Aging, per se, may be a surrogate for unknown mechanisms that are the true reasons behind the decline in function. For example, on average, glucose tolerance declines across the age span, but detrimental changes in lifestyle (increased adiposity, physical inactivity) partially explain this decline. In the future, the decline in glucose tolerance with age may be fully explained by differences in the molecular pathway of glucose metabolism.

As interest in, and support for, gerontological research increases, there is a need to recognize the methodological issues inherent in the study of human aging and to review the difficulties and pitfalls that

have been discovered from experience. This chapter will discuss these issues and will focus on clinical (i.e., *in vivo* human) studies, followed by some comments on *in vitro* studies with human tissues. The interested reader is referred to previous reviews of this topic (Andres, 1981; Birren, 1959; Minaker & Rowe, 1986; Rowe, 1977; Shock, 1984; Williamson & Milne, 1978).

II. Methodological Issues in Clinical Studies

In clinical studies on aging, special attention must be paid to study design, subject selection and characterization, and the clinical relevance of the aging changes studied.

A. Study Design: Cross-Sectional and Longitudinal Studies

Clinical gerontological studies can be designed by subject in two general ways: cross-sectional and longitudinal. In cross-sectional studies, groups of individuals at various ages are observed at one time and age-related differences are sought. In lon-

Handbook of the Biology of Aging, Fourth Edition
Copyright © 1996 Academic Press, Inc. All rights of reproduction in any form reserved.

gitudinal studies, serial prospective measurements are obtained for one group of subjects at specified intervals, and slopes of these variables are determined as a function of age for each individual. Since the human life span is so long, most longitudinal studies follow subjects in several age cohorts throughout the adult age range concurrently. Thus, slopes for different age cohorts can be compared. These longitudinal studies have the added benefit of showing "time" effects due to secular or environmental changes affecting specific cohorts or all cohorts, effects that are distinguishable from "age" effects. Examples of such changes might be the introduction of widespread use of antibiotics, fluoridation of water supplies, addition of vitamin D to milk, and major political–economic upheavals such as the Great Depression.

Cross-sectional studies must be interpreted with caution because there are several ways in which they may not give an accurate picture of age-related changes. One problem in the design of comparisons of old subjects with very young subjects (often college students) is the common misconception of the human life cycle. It is often assumed that the growth and development phase ends before the age of 20 followed by a prolonged plateau, during which the variable under study is stable, and then, at approximately the age of 60 years, there is the onset of a fairly rapid decline. However, most variables that have been found to change with age peak between the ages of 20 and 30 years and then gradually decline. On the other hand, expediency often dictates the comparison of old with very young subjects, because this allows for statistically significant differences to be obtained more readily. Although studies over three or four age groups are more desirable, they can be very expensive to perform.

Other variants of cross-sectional studies have been proposed, and they include cross-sequential and time series analyses. In the former, the participants are all members of the same birth cohort, but different subsets of individuals are measured at two or more different time periods. In the latter variant, the participants from different birth cohorts are measured and compared at the same age. The interested reader is referred to a review by Costa and McCrae (1995).

B. Selective Mortality

Another caveat in the interpretation of cross-sectional studies is that older subjects represent a sample of biologically superior survivors from a cohort that may have experienced extensive mortality. If the variable under study is related to survival, either because it is a risk factor or because it has a protective effect, cross-sectional studies will seem to show age-related differences that do not exist. This effect, called selective mortality, is shown in Fig. 1. The figure concerns an imaginary

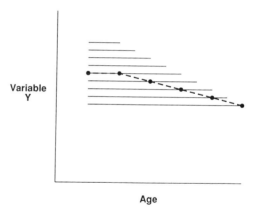

Figure 1. Effect of selective mortality on age trends in cross-sectional data. Each horizontal line represents measurements of a variable Y in one group of subjects over a number of years. The population has been stratified into nine groups on the basis of their levels of Y. Higher values of the variable Y are associated with increased risk of mortality (e.g., cholesterol level). In this hypothetical example, the level of Y remains constant in any individual subject. The circles represent mean values of Y in the surviving subjects in a cross-sectional study and show an apparent decline with age, which actually results from a progressive loss of subjects with higher levels of Y in older age groups.

study of the influence of age on the mean value of the variable Y, a risk factor that is found at widely varying levels in the population, but does not change with age in any given individual. The population can be stratified into nine levels of factor Y. Since Y is related to survival, individuals with high levels will have shortened life spans, and individuals with low levels will have longer life spans. In a cross-sectional study, values for the young subjects will be similar in both mean and variance. The older cohorts, however, have lost their members with the highest values, and thus their mean values are less, with lower variances. This trend continues with advancing age, and the cross-sectional results wrongly suggest that Y declines with age. This serious methodological error can be avoided with the use of a prospective longitudinal study design, in which each subject is followed over time and the rate of change of each variable is calculated for each subject and for each age group followed. An effect similar to selective mortality may be introduced in cross-sectional studies by any cause of variation in follow-up that is related to the level of the variable under study.

C. Drawbacks of Longitudinal Studies

While longitudinal studies avoid these problems of cross-sectional studies, longitudinal studies can also have major drawbacks, including the need to observe a stable population over a long period. Also, when subjects return at regular intervals and become increasingly familiar with the testing environment, a "stress" effect may introduce error into serial measurements.

Table I, from the Framingham Study, shows an example of this effect. The researchers set out to determine the influence of age on blood pressure and the impact of high blood pressure on morbidity from heart disease. Systolic and diastolic blood pressures at the first seven biennial examinations are depicted for a population

Table I
Stress Effects in a Longitudinal Study[a]

Examination no.[b]	Blood pressure (mm Hg)	
	Systolic	Diastolic
1	133.2	84.6
2	129.6	82.4
3	128.2	81.5
4	130.1	82.6
5	131.9	83.2
6	133.9	84.3
7	135.2	85.1

[a]Source: data from Gordan and Shurtleff (1973).
[b]Examinations were at 2-year intervals, and analysis included only subjects present for all examinations to exclude the impact of differential follow-up.

that had completed all seven examinations, thus removing the possibility of selective mortality or differential follow-up. At the first visit, the averages were 133 mm Hg systolic and 85 mm Hg diastolic. Surprisingly, the second visit averages showed lower pressures, 129 mm systolic and 82 mm diastolic. At the third visit, blood pressure averages were still lower, 128 and 81 mm. After 6 years of measurement at great expense, the researchers found that blood pressure declined with age—an unlikely conclusion, since blood pressure rose on subsequent visits. The initial decrease was attributed to the "stress" effect—the stress of the testing environment had an effect on blood pressure that dominated any age effect until the subjects became accustomed to the tests. Four years passed before the first useful data for calculating blood pressure slopes as a function of age were collected. In retrospect, more frequent measurements should have been done in the beginning to accustom participants to the testing environment. If one ignored the "stress" effect and calculated slopes using all the data, the slopes would be much less steep than those reflecting the actual effect of age.

Additionally, in survival analyses, where risk factors are measured at entry into a study and the participants are then followed to a specific event (mortality, disease incidence) or until the end of the study, it has been suggested that taking only one measurement underestimates the true risk (Peto, 1976; MacMahon *et al.*, 1990). A second measurement of the risk factor within a short time period can ameliorate the "regression–dilution bias."

Another serious drawback of longitudinal studies is their sensitivity to alterations in methods of measurement. Subtle changes in laboratory techniques over several years may introduce "laboratory drifts" that are difficult to separate from age-related changes. Methodological improvements (increased sensitivity, specificity, and ease of operation) often are not introduced in order to maintain equivalency of the measured variable. We believe that this is not justified. However, a new, improved technique should only be introduced if appropriate precautions are followed. This necessitates exhaustive measurement of suitable "control" samples over the physiological range of values obtained by the prior measurement method. This will allow for correction from the old measurements if necessary.

D. Changes in Populations

It is important to remember that longitudinal differences may be due to temporal changes in populations rather than to aging, that is, due to changes that affect all age groups. The origins of these temporal changes may be quite diverse, including educational, nutritional, environmental, and other influences that can result in misleading data regarding the possible effects of age. An example of such a change is the decrease in intake of cholesterol and increase in intake of polyunsaturated fatty acids in the American population over the last 30 years. Elahi *et al.* (1983) have devised an age–time matrix for presenting variables followed over a longitudinal study (in their case, intake of different

nutrients). By using this matrix, data can easily be followed by time, by age, and by cohort and can be analyzed in three perspectives: cross-sectional, longitudinal, and "time series." If a pure aging effect is present, both cross-sectional and longitudinal slopes of changes in the dependent variable will be significant, but the time series (i.e., temporal changes) slope should be flat. If only cohort or time series effects are operating, other combinations of slopes will be significant. A detailed discussion and the limitations of this approach, which is particularly applicable to studies where many subjects and variables are being followed longitudinally, are presented elsewhere (Elahi *et al.*, 1983).

E. Planning a Longitudinal Study

The major elements in a longitudinal study are the size of the samples, the frequency of measurements, and the duration of the study. Clearly, a variable that changes dramatically with age and is easily measured with great accuracy need only be tested a few times before age-related changes are well-defined. On the other hand, variables that change slowly with age and are difficult to measure accurately require frequent observations over a long period of time. Schlesselman (1973) has reviewed the quantitative and statistical issues in the design of longitudinal studies. Appropriate strategies for each variable can be estimated once reliable cross-sectional data or limited longitudinal data are available.

F. Interpreting the Data of a
     Longitudinal Study

The data from the usual cohort-grouped longitudinal study are likely to fall into one pattern or a combination of six patterns. These are diagrammed in Fig. 2, in which the value of a measured variable is plotted on the *y*-axis and the subject's age

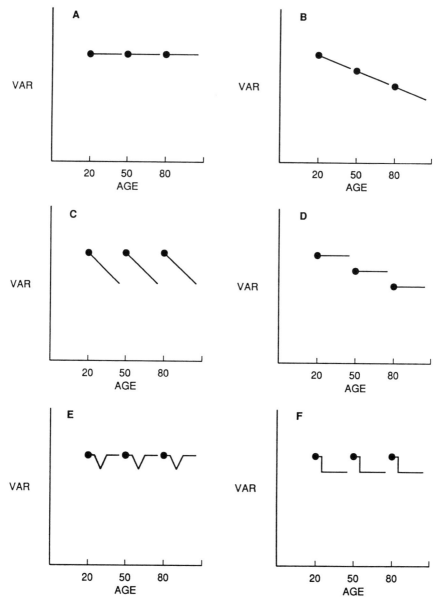

Figure 2.   Paradigms of data patterns from cohort-grouped longitudinal studies. Measurements of variable Y are plotted against subjects' age X: (A) no change in the variable with age; (B) decrease (or increase) in the variable with age; (C) secular (temporal) change affecting all cohorts equally; (D) cohort change affecting each cohort to a different extent; (E) methodological change—one time only; (F) methodological change—continuous over time. See the text for a discussion of these patterns. (Modified from R. Andres, personal communication.)

is slotted on the x-axis. The patterns can be characterized as showing

(a) no change of the variable with age,
(b) decrease (or increase) of the variable with age,
(c) secular (temporal) change effecting all cohorts equally,
(d) cohort change affecting each cohort to a different extent,
(e) methodological change—one time only, and
(f) methodological change—continuing over time.

The data from a cross-sectional study can be characterized similarly. Careful study of the data and proper checks should be made to ensure that changes or differences ascribed to an aging effect are not due to secular, cohort, or methodological changes.

Concerning methodological changes, several techniques are available that can identify their magnitude and duration. Once identified, either these values can be excluded from further analyses or the bias can be computed and the measurements corrected.

The first method involves quantification to the relationship between the measurement and time. When sufficient measurements are available for each participant, linear regression can show the average change in the measurement over time. In the upper panel of Fig. 3, serial measurements of variable Y are obtained on three individuals over the same time period. Each individual has a regression line computed, and a residual value (actual value of the measurement minus the predicted value from the regression line) is obtained for each measurement. The lower panel of Fig. 3 shows the mean of the residuals for each time period for the three individuals. Significant deviation from a value of zero indicates methodological drift for that time period.

Another technique for detecting methodological drift in a variable with time involves the computation of a mean and standard deviation (Y, SD) of the variable over the entire duration of the study, as well as the means of the same variable over discrete time periods (Y_i). Two caveats of this technique are that the participants were tested at random, that is, no temporal separation in the testing of young and old participants, obese and lean subjects, etc., and that there were a sufficient number of participants overall, as well as at each of the time intervals, to detect a significant methodological difference. For each time period, the difference between Y and Y_i is computed and this difference is compared to the SD of the mean of the entire study. In essence the test to be applied to the data by this technique is that differences between the mean values at discrete time intervals and the overall mean experience are not large enough to result in a major misclassification due to methodological error. The question then is how to define "major misclassification." We have based this decision on one of the standard techniques for assigning subjects to quantitative categories: the use of the quintile classification scheme, where subjects in quintile 1 (Q1) are composed of those in the lowest 20% of the population, Q5 those in the highest 20%, and so forth. An individual subject can easily be misclassified from one quintile to the neighboring quintile by the slightest methodological error if the experimental value falls very close to one of the cut points. Thus, when one deals with classification based on cutpoints, a quintile misclassification of some participants is inevitable. Our definition then of a methodological error that is "major" is one that could result in a two quintile misclassification (a subject who correctly belongs in Q2 is, by error, assigned to Q4, for example). By using the common statistical table that defines the area under the normal curve, we computed that a methodological error in a specific time interval that was *not* greater than one-half of the standard deviation of the distribution of

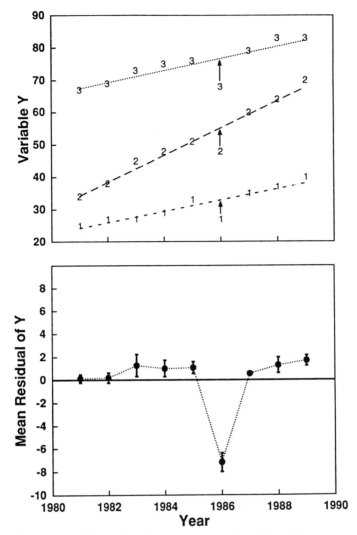

Figure 3. Technique for detecting methodological or "laboratory" drift. Variable Y values for three individuals (1, 2, 3) are plotted as a function of time in the upper panel. Linear regression lines are plotted showing the average change in variable Y with time for the three individuals. Arrows represent the residual values for selected measurements (the difference between the actual value and the predicted value from the regression line). The lower panel shows the means of the residuals for the three individuals with respect to time. Error bars are SEM. (Modified from R. Andres, personal communication.)

results in the total study could *not* cause a misclassification of greater than one quintile. This, then, is a rule for the use of this technique.

It should also be appreciated that a repeated observation with an adequate separation of time is all that is theoretically necessary for a longitudinal study. However, even accounting for the test effect described earlier ("stress", learning, etc.), two points are not sufficient to describe the change. For example, the change in

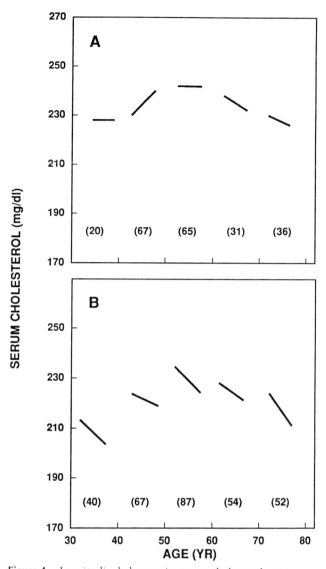

Figure 4. Longitudinal changes in serum cholesterol concentration. Longitudinal results are represented by line segments that indicate the mean slope of changes in serum cholesterol for each age decade. Each line is drawn with the midpoint at the cholesterol mean, with the length along the abscissa representing the mean time span over which the longitudinal data were collected. The upper panel (A) presents the longitudinal change during the period prior to the drop in cholesterol (1963–1971). The lower panel (B) presents the longitudinal change that occurred during the period in which cholesterol levels fell off (1969–1977). The number of subjects used to compute each mean slope is given in parentheses (Hershcopf et al., 1982)

serum cholesterol levels from the period 1963–1977 was examined in the Baltimore Longitudinal Study of Aging (Hershcopf *et al.*, 1982). Only cholesterol measurements from participants who were not on medications did not have specific diseases that would influence cholesterol levels were included in the analyses. The participant's change in serum cholesterol with age was characterized by the slope of a linear regression line computed from three or more "normal" cholesterol measurements. The participants were grouped into age decades by the mean age of their cholesterol measurements, and the individual slopes of each age decade were then averaged. This mean slope represents the change in cholesterol for each decade and is displayed graphically as line segments (Fig. 4). The mean cholesterol is the midpoint of the line segment, and the length along the abscissa represents the mean time span over which longitudinal data were collected for that decade. During the two time periods shown in the figure, there was a change in serum cholesterol that could be attributed to both aging and a secular effect. If this longitudinal study was carried out only when subjects were in their third decade and again when they were in their eighth decade (two point analysis), no significant changes would have been observed (Fig. 4A). Furthermore, a two point analysis would not be sensitive and could not detect a temporal or time series effect where all cohorts display a drop in their cholesterol levels (Fig. 4B).

G. Subject Selection and Characterization

Subject selection and characterization are crucial to the conduct and evaluation of a clinical gerontological study. In the past, geriatric studies were often flawed by major differences in the general health of the subjects being studied. Not infrequently, medical students or healthy hospital employees constituted the young group, while the old group was composed of residents of long-term care facilities or, in some cases, patients in acute care hospitals and clinics. Although these individuals were generally screened to exclude those with an abnormality of the particular organ system under study, they were often disabled or multiply impaired and were suboptimal for a study of the physiological concomitants of normal aging. In such studies, differences between young and old individuals were a complex mixture of disease-related and age-related effects, and the studies failed to provide insight into the normal aging process.

A new phase in gerontological research was pioneered by Shock (1984) in the Baltimore Longitudinal Study of Aging at the National Institute on Aging, in which investigators carefully scrutinized study subjects in an effort to avoid, to whatever degree possible, contamination from disease. However, careful attention to the exclusion of diseased individuals and those taking medications, informally called "cleaning up" the physiological data, also entails risk. One must be aware that intensive screening of the population may result in a select group of elderly "superperformers," whose data do not reflect the influence of age-related changes. For instance, in attempting to exclude diabetics, one might adopt criteria by which individuals with a 2-hr postprandial blood glucose level greater than 140 mg/dl would be excluded. Since carbohydrate tolerance is well-known to decline with age in nondiabetics, the application of this uniform criterion to all age groups would result in an increasingly stringent selection procedure with advancing age. The marked changes in carbohydrate tolerance with age would result in only a small fraction on individuals in the eighth or ninth decade of life qualifying for the study. Similarly, since systolic blood pressure increases with age, a strong selection effect would be introduced in studies excluding all individuals with systolic blood pressure over 130 mm Hg. In these examples, generally accepted age-adjusted criteria for normality are available and might be applied as a screening technique. However, such guidelines are lacking for most variables.

Investigators embarking on gerontological studies should also be aware that differences in habits, such as the use of alcohol, caffeine, or tobacco, might introduce apparent age effects by modifying an individual's metabolism. Other variables can have a major impact on gerontological studies: antecedent diet, activity and exercise status, body composition (including not just increased adiposity but also fat distribution), and psychosocial and socioeconomic factors. In addition, the genetic heterogeneity of human subjects and the increasing variability of parameters with aging may make it difficult to define standards of normality to compare the old to the young. A reasonable approach would entail avoiding the presence of overt clinical disease or the administration of medications and carefully describing the study population and the selection criteria applied to all age groups.

An additional approach would be to include individuals from across the adult age range rather than just young and old adults. Such a strategy provides not only insight into the status on old individuals but also some view of the change in the variable during the life cycle. Since most age-related changes in physiological variables have been found to be linear, the finding of a marked change in middle age or late middle age suggests the presence of an underlying disease process.

A practical caution that should be mentioned is that it may be difficult to recruit sufficient numbers of appropriate older subjects for clinical studies, particularly more intensive ones, and this difficulty often proves to be the limiting factor in carrying out a study.

It should be reemphasized that subject selection will heavily influence the results of clinical as well as social–psychological gerontological studies and that extrapolation from any given study with only a handful of subjects must be done with great caution. Random sampling, the length of separation between examinations, and the generalizability of the results of other populations are other issues that pertain to subject selection. The interested reader is referred to a detailed examination of these issues in the review by Nesselroade (1988). The only studies that are specifically designed to be representative of the American population are the HANES (National Health and Nutrition Examination Surveys) studies, undertaken periodically by the National Center for Health Statistics; these are not longitudinal studies. An example of the use of data gathered in the HANES studies, estimating the prevalence of diabetes and impaired glucose tolerance in the U.S. population from ages 20 to 74 years, and the potential biases in extrapolating from the data are summarized in a paper by Harris *et al.*, (1987).

H. Clinical Relevance of Aging Changes

Even if one finds a change with age in carefully screened, "normal" subjects, it is important to understand that normality does not necessarily mean harmlessness. If healthy old individuals perform less well on glucose tolerance tests than young individuals, that does not imply that the carbohydrate intolerance and the underlying insulin resistance and elevated insulin levels of the elderly, which is "normal" for their age, are harmless. That conclusion would require a study of another dependent variable—for example, cardiovascular complications or death—since it may be that among normal 80-year-olds those with the worst carbohydrate tolerance are actually at greater risk from these complications. Likewise, although systolic blood pressure increases "normally" with age, that does not mean it is harmless.

Advancing age is a risk factor for disease and death. Just because one defines some age-related changes as normative, one must not overlook their potential adverse effects.

On the other hand, it is important clinically to know which changes occur as a function of normal aging and which do not. There are systems in which no change occurs as a function of age, and these need to be identified. Too frequently, physicians unfamiliar with normal aging will dismiss a clinically significant finding as being due to normal age-related changes. As an example, hematocrit does not change with normal aging; thus, "anemia of old age" is not a meaningful diagnosis.

There are also subjects who have minimal changes with aging, even in their seventies. These individuals with "successful aging" can be contrasted with the majority of the population with "usual aging," who, while generally healthy, exhibit impairments when their physiological systems are stressed. Identification and comparison of subjects showing "successful aging" with those showing "usual aging" may allow one to delineate factors leading to the former that might be generally applicable to the population. These important issues have been discussed in detail (Rowe & Kahn, 1987).

III. Methodological Issues in Studies with Human Tissues

In vitro studies with human tissues can be done with controls and interventions that are not possible in clinical studies. While the methodological issues in clinical studies are also relevant to *in vitro* studies, there are other problems that need to be considered in the latter studies. Issues arising in the use of animal models for aging research are discussed in Chapter 1 of this volume.

A. Size of Changes with Aging

Many changes in measured parameters with aging are modest, on the order of 30–50%, and thus much smaller than the changes usually studied in other *in vitro* biochemical and cellular studies. With changes of such small magnitude, one must either measure samples from a large number of subjects or have very precise measurements to be sure that one is detecting a real change. At the subcellular and molecular levels, it may be very difficult to elucidate the mechanisms of such small changes with currently available techniques.

B. Changes Due to Factors Other Than Aging

It may not be easy to ensure that one is studying an aging change rather than a change due to disease, genetic, dietary, or environmental factors. Human genetic heterogeneity may give rise to substantial variation in measured parameters in tissue samples, and this large variation may obscure aging changes. One should also be aware of how tissues have been handled prior to delivery for investigation, since this can have a substantial effect on the quality of the tissues.

C. Isolated Cells and Tissues

Studies with isolated cells and tissues may also suffer from a major difficulty in interpretation. Usually, with aging, there are an increase in extracellular matrix material and increased cross-linking of this material. If one sees aging effects in isolated tissues or cells, one must ask whether these effects are really intrinsic to the tissue of interest or just due to more disruption of the tissue in its isolation. If one studies cells grown *in vitro*, one must ask whether the differences one might find between cells from young and old subjects are primary differences or due to differential adaptation to artificial culture conditions, which can, among other things, lead to differences in cell cycling stage that can profoundly influence results.

IV. Conclusions

Ideally, in studying an aging change in humans, one would like to precisely quantitate a change, study the detailed mechanism of the change, pinpoint effector agents causing the change, and show that one can produce the change by appropriate manipulation of the mechanism or effector agents. One would also like to demonstrate that the change progresses with age would hope that its study will lead to insights into, and better treatments for, age-related disabilities. Although a vast descriptive catalog of changes with human aging has been assembled, investigators have begun to approach these further goals. The exciting and accelerating developments in the study of the neurobiology of aging show the potential of these approaches for the future. Finally, it must be stressed that one cannot hope to understand the mechanism of aging changes without first having a clear picture of normal function. Advances in the study of human aging are obviously dependent on advances in biomedical research as a whole.

References

Andres, R. (1981). Problems in the study of human aging. In R. T. Schimke (Ed.), *Biological Mechanisms of Aging* (NIH Publ. No. 81–2194, pp. 696–700). Washington, DC: U.S. Government Printing Office.

Birren, J. E. (1959). Principles of research on aging. In J. E. Birren (Ed.), *Handbook of Aging and the Individual. Psychological and Biological Aspects* (pp. 3–42). Chicago: University of Chicago Press.

Costa, P. T., & McCrae, R. R. (1995). Design and analysis of aging studies. In E. J. Masaro (Ed.), *Handbook of Physiology: Physiology of Aging* (pp. 25–36). New York: Oxford University Press.

Elahi, V. K., Elahi, D., Andres, R., Tobin, J. D., Butler, M. G., & Norris, A. H. (1983). A longitudinal study of nutritional uptake in men. *Journal of Gerontology, 38,* 162–180.

Gordan, J., & Shurtleff, D. (1973). In W. B. Kannel & T. Gordon (Eds.), *The Framingham Study: An Epidemiological Investigation of Cardiovascular Disease* (NIH Publ. No. 74–478). Washington, DC: U.S. Government Printing Office.

Harris, M. I., Hadden, W. C., Knowler, W. C., & Bennett, P. H. (1987). Prevalence of diabetes and impaired glucose tolerance and plasma glucose levels in U.S. population aged 20–74 yr. *Diabetes, 36,* 523–534.

Hershcopf, R. J., Elahi, D., Andres, R., Baldwin, H. L., Raizes, G. S., Schocken, D. D., & Tobin, J. D. (1982). Longitudinal changes in serum cholesterol in man: an epidemiologic search for an etiology. *Journal of Chronic Diseases, 35,* 101–114.

MacMahon, S., Peto, R., Cutler, J., Collins, R., Sorlie, P., Neaton, J., Abbott, R., Godwin, J., Dyer, A., & Stamler, J. (1990). Epidemiology. Blood pressure, stroke, and coronary heart disease. Part 1, prolonged differences in blood pressure: prospective observational studies corrected for regression dilution bias. *Lancet, 335,* 765–774.

Minaker, K. L., & Rowe, J. W. (1986). Methodological issues in clinical research in the aging reproductive system. In L. Mastroianni, Jr., & C. A. Paulsen (Eds.), *Aging, Reproduction, and the Climacteric* (pp. 35–44). New York: Plenum.

Nesselroade, J. R. (1988). Sampling and generalizability: adult development and aging research issues examined within the general methodological framework of selection. In K. W. Schaie, R. T. Campbell, W. Meredith, & S. C. Rawlings (Eds.), *Methodological Issues in Aging Research* (pp. 13–42). New York: Springer.

Peto, R. (1976). Two properties of multiple regression analysis; and regression to the mean (and regression from the mean). In C. M. Fletcher, R. Peto, C. M. Tinker, & F. E. Spezier (Eds.), *The Natural History of Chronic Bronchitis and Emphysema. An Eight Year Study of Early Chronic Obstructive Lung*

Disease in Working Men in London (pp. 218–223). Oxford: Oxford University Press.

Rogusa, D. (1988). Myths about longitudinal research. In K. W. Schaie, R. T. Campbell, W. Meredith, & S. C. Rawlings (Eds.), *Methodological Issues in Aging Research* (pp. 171–209). New York: Springer.

Rowe, J. W. (1977). Clinical research on aging: Strategies and directions. *New England Journal of Medicine, 297*, 1332–1336.

Rowe, J. W., & Kahn, R. L. (1987). Human aging: usual and successful. *Science, 237,* 143–149.

Schlesselman, J. J. (1973). Planning a longitudinal study. I. Sample size determination. II. Frequency of measurement and study duration. *Journal of Chronic Diseases, 26,* 553–570.

Shock, N. W. (Ed.) (1984). *Normal Human Aging: The Baltimore Longitudinal Study of Aging* (NIH Publ. No. 84–2450, pp. 5–18). Washington, DC: U.S. Government Printing Office.

Williamson, J., & Milne, J. S. (1978). Research methods in aging. In J. C. Brocklehurst (Ed.), *Textbook of Geriatric Medicine and Gerontology* (2nd ed., pp. 807–814). Edinburgh, Scotland: Churchill Livingstone.

Part Two

Genetic Analyses

Edited by
Thomas E. Johnson

Three
<hr>

Longevity-Assurance Genes and Mitochondrial DNA Alterations: Yeast and Filamentous Fungi

S. Michal Jazwinski

I. Fungal Models in Aging Research

Research on fungal aging was not reviewed in the previous edition of this Handbook. Thus, this chapter will seek to bring the reader up to date on current research and to provide the background necessary to fully appreciate its significance. The reader might legitimately ask: Why focus on fungi? I hope that by the end of this chapter this question is answered to satisfaction. Let me preempt a bit by stating that the filamentous fungi and yeasts represent excellent genetic systems. They are exceedingly useful if the focus of the research is genetic. In addition, there is reason to suspect that these organisms have something to offer for a more general understanding of the aging process. Although certain biochemical and physiological aspects of aging have been addressed in fungi, my focus will be primarily genetic in this chapter.

It is curious that the two fungal models for aging complement each other so beautifully. The filamentous fungi present a mitochondrial etiology of aging while yeast presents a nuclear etiology, so to speak. The proximal mechanisms of

senescence in the former involve mitochondrial DNA alterations. In yeast, the proximal mechanisms are not entirely clear, but nuclear genes are clearly implicated. Thus, the filamentous fungi may present a window on the mitochondrial DNA alterations that have been found in tissues from aging humans, and they may ultimately provide a system suitable for examining the importance of mitochondrial dysfunction in aging. Yeasts, on the other hand, are more likely to allow access to the nuclear genes that play a role in determining longevity and to the homeostatic processes they specify, such as stress responses.

Before proceeding to a more detailed analysis of gerontological research on the premier fungal models, I would like to dispose of two issues. The first concerns other fungal models. Apart from the studies on *Podospora*, *Neurospora*, and *Saccharomyces*, literature on aging in several other fungal species exists. Table I provides a brief summary of fungal gerontology. The acellular slime mold *Didymium iridis* displays a progressive reduction in growth and movement with time prior to death. Plasmodial fragmentation occurs, and these smaller individuals degenerate into

Handbook of the Biology of Aging, Fourth Edition
Copyright © 1996 Academic Press, Inc. All rights of reproduction in any form reserved.

Table I
Fungal Models for the Study of the Genetics of Aging

Fungus	Etiology of Senescence	References
Didymium iridis	Polyploidization	Clark and Mulleavy (1982)
Physarum polycephalum	Increase in nuclear DNA content	McCullough *et al.* (1973)
Podospora curvicola	Excision and amplification of mtDNA[a] sequences	Bockelmann and Esser (1986)
Podospora anserina	Excision and amplification of mtDNA sequences	Stahl *et al.* (1978, 1980); Cummings *et al.* (1979)
Neurospora intermedia: Kalilo strain	Integration of a linear DNA plasmid into mtDNA	Bertrand *et al.* (1986)
Neurospora crassa: Mauriceville and Varkud strains	Integration of circular DNA plasmids into mtDNA	Akins *et al.* (1986)
Maranhar strain	Integration of a linear DNA plasmid into mtDNA	Bertrand and Griffiths (1989)
Saccharomyces cerevisiae	Activity of nuclear genes	Jazwinski (1993); D'mello *et al.* (1994); Sun *et al.* (1994)

[a]mtDNA, mitochondrial DNA.

spheroids (Lott & Clark, 1980). Prior to death, there is an increase in the frequency of large, polyploid nuclei (Clark & Hakim, 1980a; Clark & Mulleavy, 1982). Studies with heterokaryons and heteroplasmons have demonstrated that the senescent phenotype is dominant in that it is determined by the older parent nucleus (Clark & Hakim, 1980b). Indeed, the implication was that the nuclei carry the aging factor, and nuclear sieving studies suggested that these were the polyploid nuclei (Clark & Hakim, 1980a). Life span was not determined directly by the sexual reproductive system but varied from one strain to another, implying genetic control (Clark, 1984). *Physarum polycephalum*, a true slime mold, also exhibits increases in nuclear DNA content that are correlated with senescence (McCullough *et al.*, 1973); however, the aging phenomenon is not as well-studied in this fungus.

Several other fungi exhibit cycles of "stop and start" growth that are associated with a variety of manifestations of aging. These fungi are listed in Table I. In all of the examples shown, the senescent phenotype appears to be cytoplasmically determined and involves aberrant processes that impact mitochondrial DNA. Our discussion will be limited to *Podospora anserina* and *Neurospora* among the filamentous fungi, because the phenomenon has been studied in these most extensively.

It is important to mention the extensive analysis of conidial aging in *Neurospora crassa* (Munkres, 1984). These vegetative spores exhibit a finite life span. Survival of conidia has been dissected genetically. One view might be that conidia present a good model for the aging of postmitotic cells. I personally feel that these spores are a developmental form associated with survival under inhospitable conditions. The general relevance to aging therefore is not clear.

II. Total Reproductive Effort as a Measure of Life Span

A. Senescence in Filamentous Fungi: Mycelial Length

1. Podospora anserina

Wild strains of this filamentous fungus exhibit a reduction in growth rate upon prolonged vegetative propagation on solid medium (Rizet, 1953). Attendant pigmentation changes are followed by mycelial death. This contrasts with the related species *Podospora curvicola*, which shows alternate periods of growth and no growth similar to the stopper mutants of *Neurospora crassa* (Bockelmann & Esser, 1986). Detailed studies in *Podospora anserina* have clearly demonstrated that senescence is determined by particulate factors in the cytoplasm of senescing mycelia, which increase in concentration as hyphal growth progresses (Marcou, 1961; Smith & Rubenstein, 1973a,b). Mycelial life span is under the control of both nuclear and cytoplasmic genetic factors (Tudzynski & Esser, 1979). This life span is measured by the length attained by the mycelium before it senesces and dies. It can also be measured as the time between the inception of mycelial elongation and its cessation. Senescence is associated with mitochondrial DNA rearrangements and the accumulation of new DNA species in the mitochondria.

2. Neurospora crassa and Neurospora intermedia

Some strains of *Neurospora crassa* and *Neurospora intermedia* display a senescent phenotype that expresses itself as the termination of vegetative growth during serial subculture or growth cessation of the mycelium. Thus, longevity can be measured in culture passage number, mycelial length, or chronological time (reviewed by Griffiths, 1992). Senescence is associated with progressive mitochondrial disability (Akins *et al.*, 1986), a lethal or at least sublethal consequence in this obligate aerobe. The phenomenology is similar to that of *Podospora* senescence. The capacity for senescence is inherited maternally. Senescence entails rearrangements of the mitochondrial genome. Nonsenescing strains do not display these rearrangements. Furthermore, strains that recover from a slow growth deficit lose them.

B. Aging of Yeasts: Number of Buds Produced

1. Saccharomyces cerevisiae

Yeasts possess a limited life span, as measured by the total number of progeny produced by an individual cell (Mortimer & Johnston, 1959). This unicellular eukaryote divides asymmetrically by budding, allowing a distinction between the parent cell (mother) and its progeny (buds or daughters). The last two or three divisions the mother undergoes take an extremely long time to complete (Mortimer & Johnston, 1959). This likely reflects the process of dying. Ultimately, the cell stops dividing, becomes less refractile, and ultimately lyses. Yeast aging has been reviewed (Jazwinski, 1993).

The actual processes underlying death are not known; however, it is clear that yeasts undergo a variety of morphological and physiological changes as they age (Table II). These changes include an increase in generation time, the interval between two consecutive buddings (Egilmez & Jazwinski, 1989), and an increase in cell size (Bartholomew & Mittwer, 1953; Mortimer & Johnston, 1959; Johnson & Lu, 1975; Egilmez *et al.*, 1990). Thus, the longer the cell life span, as measured by the number of cell divisions, the longer the chronological life span will be. In addition, the total metabolic effort must be greater when the life span is longer, given the additional cellular mass that must be produced. It is necessary to follow individual yeast cells microscopically to determine their life spans. Thus, it is more accurate to measure life span by the number of cell divisions, rather than chronologically. Generation time is very dependent on incubation temperature, reinforcing the choice of number of generations rather than duration of life span as the metric.

The budding process marks the mother cell with a permanent bud scar. It was initially suggested that exhaustion of bud sites on the cell surface or reduction in the ratio of metabolically active surface to cell

Table II
Age-Dependent Changes in Yeast Morphology and Physiology

Phenotype	Change	References
Cell size	Increase	Bartholomew and Mittwer (1953); Mortimer and Johnston (1959); Johnson and Lu (1975); Egilmez et al. (1990)
Cell shape	Altered	Chen and Jazwinski (unpublished results)
Granular appearance		Mortimer and Johnston (1959)
Surface wrinkles		Mortimer and Johnston (1959); Muller (1971)
Loss of turgor		Muller (1971)
Cell fragility (prior to death)	None	Egilmez et al. (1990)
Cell lysis		Mortimer and Johnston (1959)
Bud scar number	Increase	Barton (1950); Bartholomew and Mittwer (1953); Beran et al. (1967); Egilmez et al. (1990)
Cell wall chitin	Increase	Egilmez et al. (1990)
Vacuole size	Increase	Egilmez et al. (1990)
Generation (cell cycle) time	Increase	Mortimer and Johnston (1959); Egilmez and Jazwinski (1989)
Response to pheromones (haploids)	None	Muller (1985)
Mating ability (haploids)	Decrease	Muller (1985)
Sporulation ability (diploids)	Increase	Sando et al. (1973)
Cessation of division at G_1/S boundary of cell cycle (putative)		Egilmez and Jazwinski (1989)
Senescence factor		Egilmez and Jazwinski (1989)
Mutability of mtDNA	Decrease	James et al. (1975)
UV resistance	Increase[a]	Kale and Jazwinski (unpublished results)
Ty1 transposon mobility	None	Pinswasdi and Jazwinski (unpublished results)
Telomere length	None	D'mello and Jazwinski (1991)
Specific gene expression	Altered	Egilmez et al. (1989)
rRNA levels	Increase	Kale and Jazwinski (unpublished results); Motizuki and Tsurugi (1992)
Cellular rRNA concentration	Decrease	Kale and Jazwinski (unpublished results); Motizuki and Tsurugi (1992)
Protein synthesis	Decrease	Motizuki and Tsurugi (1992)
Ribosome activity, polysome recruitment	Decrease	Motizuki and Tsurugi (1992)

[a]Bimodal, increase through middle age followed by decrease.

volume due to the accumulation of bud scars is the cause of yeast aging (Mortimer & Johnston, 1959). This etiology of aging in yeasts is not likely (Table III). A mitochondrial source of yeast aging also is not persuasive. Mitochondrial mutations do not accumulate during yeast aging (Muller, 1971). Furthermore, the life spans of spontaneous and induced mitochondrial mutants are not significantly different from that of the parent strain (Muller & Wolf, 1978). Indeed, the mutability of cells resulting in respiration deficiency decreases with age (James et al., 1975). Finally, the life span of a wild-type strain does not differ significantly whether the cells are grown on medium in which they are forced to respire or on medium in which they can produce energy by fermentation (Egilmez et al., 1990). It also does not ap-

Table III
Bud Scars Do Not Determine Yeast Longevity

Evidence/Rationale	References
Less than 50% of possible sites for scars are ever occupied	Bartholomew and Mittwer (1953); Mortimer and Johnston (1959)
Cell wall expands more than necessary to oblige a bud scar at each cell division	Beran et al. (1967); Johnson and Lu (1975)
Bud scars can overlap	Bartholomew and Mittwer (1953)
Live spans of individual cells of a given strain vary; mean and maximum life spans of different strains also vary	Jazwinski (1990a,b)
Overexpression of certain genes extends longevity without affecting bud scars	Chen et al. (1990); Jazwinski (1993); Sun et al. (1994)
Adaptive increases in surface to volume ratio are not the rule during evolution over about 300 generations in a chemostat	Adams et al. (1985)
Isogenic strains of increasing ploidy (and size) up to tetraploid do not differ in life span	Muller (1971); Franklin and Jazwinski (unpublished results)
The large daughters of older mothers do not differ in life expectancy from the small daughters of younger mothers	Pinswasdi and Jazwinski (unpublished results); Egilmez and Jazwinski (1989); Johnston (1966)
Ethanol increases yeast life span without affecting bud scars	Muller et al. (1980)
Induced deposition of chitin, the major component of the bud scar, does not curtail life span	Egilmez and Jazwinski (1989)
Yeasts display the Lansing effect,[a] which cannot be mediated by the bud scar	Hogel and Muller (personal communication)
Transmission of the mother cell effect on generation time within a lineage cannot be mediated by the bud scar	Egilmez and Jazwinski (1989)
Life span of zygote reflects that of the older parent, even though the number of bud scars per unit of cell surface is smaller than in the parents	Muller (1985)
Overexpression of v-Ha-RAS at moderate levels increases life span irrespective of the increase in cell size	Chen et al. (1990)
LAG1 mutant that displays increased longevity does not differ in size from its isogenic parent	D'mello et al. (1994)

[a]In the case of yeasts, this refers to the extinction of a lineage through the continuous selection of the final daughters produced during the life span.

pear that the frequency with which the yeast transposon Ty1 becomes mobilized increases very dramatically with age (Pinswasdi and Jazwinski, unpublished). Thus, this most frequent mode of spontaneous mutation, leading to adaptive changes in yeast populations (Adams & Oeller, 1986), does not appear to be a major determinant of aging.

C. Correlates with Invertebrates

It is rather obvious, particularly in yeasts, that there is a strict association between life span and reproduction in fungi. This is regardless of the fact that life span can be measured chronologically. At first blush, this would seem to distinguish these organisms from invertebrates such as nematodes and fruit flies, which are popular models in aging research, not to mention mammals. I believe this distinction to be superficial and only one of degree. In fact, fruit flies continue to reproduce well into old age. Much of the mycelium of filamentous fungi becomes postmitotic, in similarity to the soma of nematodes and fruit flies. There is some connection between reproductive effort and longevity throughout the animal kingdom (Rose, 1991). I would therefore consider fungi, and especially yeasts, to represent one end of the scale. On this scale, yeasts would represent an organism in which there is no real post-reproductive life span as such. Reproduction is the raison d'etre of yeasts. In higher organisms, this may cease to be the driving force that it is in yeasts, but the capability for reproduction frequently remains throughout the life span, especially in males.

D. Correlates with Tissue Culture Fibroblasts

A strong superficial similarity exists between aging in the fungi and limited population doubling potential of normal cells in culture (Hayflick limit) (Goldstein, 1990). The number of cellular divisions seems to be the determining factor in either case. Other similarities are also discernible. Fibroblasts display an increase in size and cell cycle time with age. In the last few years, it has been shown that normal cells from several species suffer telomere attrition with replicative age (reviewed by Broccoli and Cooke, 1993). This telomere reduction does not occur in germ cells. In contrast, *Saccharomyces cerevisiae* (D'mello & Jazwinski, 1991) and *Podospora anserina* (H. Osiewacz, personal communication) do not display telomere shortening with age. The yeast cell is the organism. Individual somatic cells of metazoans do not "care" about the propagation of the species, while individual yeast cells, most obviously, have a "vested interest" in it. This would preclude tel-

omere shortening in the latter, because it would lead to the extinction of the yeast population, more strictly the clone or pedigree. Under normal conditions, the yeast population is immortal, even though individuals are not. When telomere shortening is induced artificially by mutation of the *EST1* gene, the entire yeast population dies (Lundblad & Szostak, 1989). Yeast may provide a good model for the aging of stem cells however, especially since they divide asymmetrically, providing a clear distinction of the progenitor compartment.

E. Cellular or Clonal Senescence versus Single-Cell or Organismal Senescence

The comparisons of fungal aging and aging of invertebrates and aging in tissue culture provide us with an important distinction. Cellular or clonal senescence can be defined as the demise in time of an entire population or clone of cells. On the other hand, organismal senescence does not lead to the extinction of the population, even when the organism is unicellular. In cases in which the distinction between cell and organism may not be immediately obvious from the morphological vantage point, a molecular analysis of the state of the telomeres may be informative. I would predict that stem cells will prove to be the exception to the rule that telomere attrition can discriminate between unicellular organisms and individual somatic cells of multicellular organisms. The theoretical significance of this fact has been discussed previously (Jazwinski, 1993).

III. Mitochondrial DNA Alterations

A. Excision and Amplification of Mitochondrial DNA Sequences in *Podospora*

A circular DNA species derived from mitochondrial DNA, called α-senDNA or plDNA, has been associated with the onset of senescence (Stahl *et al.*, 1978, 1980; Cummings *et al.*, 1979; Jamet-Vierny *et al.*, 1980; Belcour *et al.*, 1981). In young mycelia, this DNA is an integral part of the mitochondrial genome. It is derived from an intron in the cytochrome oxidase subunit I gene (COI or oxi3) (Wright *et al.*, 1982; Osiewacz & Esser, 1984; Cummings *et al.*, 1985). The α-senDNA is only the most prevalent of several mitochondrially derived circular DNAs associated with *Podospora* senescence (Wright *et al.*, 1982; Cummings *et al.*, 1985). Fig. 1 depicts the *Podpospora anserina* mitochondrial genome and the location of the regions of the DNA that are the origin of the most frequently encountered amplified circular DNAs in senescent mycelia. The precise manner in which the mitochondrial DNA is released and amplified is not clear. An interesting possibility is that it occurs via an RNA intermediate (Osiewacz & Esser, 1984). An open reading frame in α-senDNA could encode a protein homologous to reverse transcriptases (Michel & Lang, 1985). Such an activity has been identified in crude extracts from middle-aged *Podospora* (Steinhilber & Cummings, 1986). Additional evidence in support of the retrotransposition of α-senDNA has been presented (Sainsard-Chanet *et al.*, 1993).

The liberation and amplification of the mitochondrially derived, circular DNAs are crucial in the development of the senescent phenotype. The concomitant rearrangements in the mitochondrial genome result in widespread deletions of essential regions, leading to mitochondrial dysfunction. This loss of function could manifest itself not only as a deficit in energy production but also by enhanced

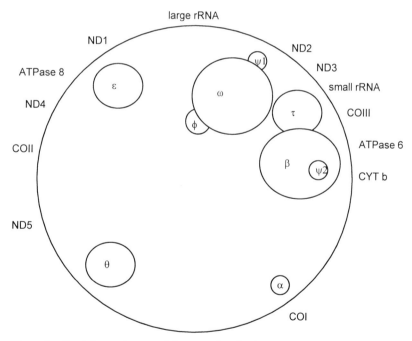

Figure 1. Partial genetic map of the mitochondrial genome of *Podospora anserina* race s. The genetic distances are not exactly to scale. The approximate, relative size of most of the known senDNAs is indicated by the smaller circles (or portions of circles) inside the largest circle representing the mitochondrial genome. The location of these circles along the map indicates approximately the region of the mitochondrial genome from which they are derived. The greek letters within the circles are the designated names of the corresponding senDNAs.

production of aberrant products of oxygen metabolism, such as the superoxide free radical. The crucial role of α-senDNA in these events is evidenced by the fact that release or subsequent amplification is restricted in long-lived mutants of *Podospora anserina* (reviewed by Osiewacz and Hermanns, 1992). For example, in the mutant AL2, which shows a 10-fold increase in longevity, a mutation in the mitochondrial DNA results in a rearrangement of the DNA and delayed amplification of α-senDNA (Osiewacz *et al.*, 1989). The expression of longevity in AL2 appears to be associated with the presence of linear DNA in the mitochondrion (Hermanns *et al.*, 1994).

One of the consequences of senescence in *Podospora anserina* is the loss of mitochondrial function (Belcour & Begel, 1978; Tudzynski & Esser, 1979; Belcour *et al.*, 1982). This is a lethal event in this obligate aerobe and could readily be the consequence of α-senDNA amplification. This DNA might integrate into nuclear or mitochondrial DNA to disrupt the expression of genes whose products are located in the mitochondrion. Although there was a report that α-senDNA integrated into nuclear DNA (Wright & Cummings, 1983), this has not subsequently been detected (Koll, 1986). A more attractive possibility is that α-senDNA has a selective replication advantage over intact mitochondrial DNA and that it progressively overtakes the mitochondrial genome as the major circular DNA species in the mitochondria. Indeed, senescent mycelia contain α-senDNA almost exclusively (Wright & Cummings, 1983). This situation resembles that found in petite yeasts. In any case, the mobility of the COI intron and its integration into mitochondrial DNA with the resulting increase in recombinogenic activity might be viewed as the first step in the disintegration of the mitochondrial genome (Osiewacz, 1992). Experimental evidence has been obtained in support of the first step in such a series of events (Sellem

et al., 1993). It is interesting that the senescence phenomenon does not occur in liquid culture. The speculation has been made that these growth conditions exert pressure for the maintenance of the intact mitochondrial genome (Turker & Cummings, 1987).

B. Integration of Plasmid DNA into Mitochondrial DNA in *Neurospora*

Most wild-type strains of *Neurospora* do not display any symptoms of aging, even after prolonged cultivation. Mutants were selected from strains possessing two circular mitochondrial DNA plasmids, called Mauriceville (3.6 kb) and Varkud (3.8 kb), by repeated serial passage (Akins *et al.*, 1986). These mutants contain variant plasmids that are suppressive to mitochondrial DNA. At 37°C, the mutants displayed alternating periods of growth and no growth, called start and stop. They are called stopper mutants. In the nonsenescing wild type, the plasmids are present exclusively as free molecules, while in the mutants the plasmids become integrated in the mitochondrial DNA during senescence. This appears to result in the instability of the mitochondrial genome, leading to deletions and insertions in the DNA (Akins *et al.*, 1986). The integration of the plasmids appears to occur via an RNA intermediate in a retrotransposition process, and it has been demonstrated that the plasmids code for a reverse transcriptase (Kuiper & Lambowitz, 1988). Superficially, this situation resembles that found in *Podospora*, with the difference that the plasmids are not originally derived from the mitochondrial genome.

In addition to the circular plasmids mentioned earlier, certain wild isolates of *Neurospora* contain linear DNA plasmids in their mitochondria that are not normal constituents of mitochondrial DNA (Bertrand *et al.*, 1986; Bertrand & Griffiths, 1989). In *N. intermedia*, the plasmid is called Kalilo (9.0 kb) and in *N. crassa* it is Maranhar (7.2 kb). The plasmids contain inverted long terminal repeats (LTRs), and they have open reading frames for both DNA and RNA polymerase activities. The plasmids are absent from nonsenescing strains. During the senescence of strains containing these plasmids, they become integrated in the mitochondrial genome at various positions (Bertrand *et al.*, 1985, 1986). This leads to inactivation of the targeted genes and DNA instabilities characteristic of transposable elements (Nevers *et al.*, 1986). The defective mitochondrial DNA molecules become suppressive, that is, they become the predominant species in the mitochondrial DNA population. The molecular events surrounding the eventual debilitation of the mitochondrial genome during senescence are quite diverse in filamentous fungi, particularly in *Neurospora.* Only the highlights are discussed here to illustrate the basic principles.

C. Nuclear Genes Affecting Mitochondrial DNA Stability

1. Podospora

Both mitochondrial and nuclear mutants that display postponed senescence or immortality have been isolated. The *mex* and *ex* mutants are mitochondrially based. *mex-1* lacks the 2.6-kb α-senDNA sequence in the mitochondrial genome (Vierny *et al.*, 1982). Several longevity mutants have been isolated that possess a novel family of very small circular DNAs derived from the mitochondrial genome (Turker *et al.*, 1987a). Five different excision sites in mitochondrial DNA were identified, and they were correlated with the presence of direct repeats and palindromes. TS1 is a mutant that becomes senescent and possesses α-senDNA at 34°C, while neither senescing nor showing the presence of this DNA at 27°C (Turker *et al.*, 1987b). Several nuclear mutations

have been isolated on the basis of resulting morphological peculiarities. These mutants act synergistically to yield an immortal phenotype. They include *i*, *gr*, and *viv* (reviewed by Esser and Tudzynski, 1980). The *gr* gene has been cloned and its partial sequence determined (H. Osiewacz, personal communication). High-fidelity mutants in the EF-1α-encoding gene have been shown to possess drastically increased longevity (Silar & Picard, 1994).

2. Neurospora

A natural death nuclear mutant of *Neurospora crassa* has been isolated (Seidel-Rogol *et al.*, 1989). The mutant, called *nd*, displays a decreased life span. Reduced stability of the mitochondrial genome is encountered in this mutant. It appears that the wild-type gene product is responsible for the maintenance of intact mitochondrial DNA. In fact, increased levels of recombination were detected in the mitochondrial DNA of the mutant (Bertand *et al.*, 1993).

IV. Identification of Longevity-Assurance Genes in Yeast

A. Differential Gene Expression During the Life Span

The increase in generation time during the yeast life span was mentioned earlier. Surprisingly, daughters mimic their mothers with regard to this parameter, but after a few cell divisions they begin multiplying at a rate characteristic of young cells (Egilmez & Jazwinski, 1989). This suggested that there might be differences in the activity of certain genes with age. A differential hybridization screen was developed to clone such genes, and it proved successful (Egilmez *et al.*, 1989). A total of 14 genes have been cloned in this fashion. One of the genes identified in this way that has been characterized in some detail is called *Lag1* (D'mello *et al.*, 1994). This is a novel gene. By using the opposite approach of analyzing candidate longevity genes for differential expression, we have shown that the yeast *ras* protooncogene homologues *RAS1* and *RAS2* are also differentially expressed (Sun *et al.*, 1994). The identification of genes that are expressed in an age-dependent fashion is but one of the genetic approaches to aging.

B. *LAG1*

The *LAG1* gene codes for a 411 amino acid protein that is predicted to be an integral membrane protein (D'mello *et al.*, 1994). The apparent molecular weight of the Lag1 protein translated *in vitro* is consistent with this assignment (Royals and Jazwinski, unpublished). A null mutation in *LAG1* created by the deletion of about 70% of the open reading frame results in a 50% increase in mean and maximum life spans of the yeasts (D'mello *et al.*, 1994). Thus, the gene plays a role in determining

yeast longevity. The action of *LAG1* is complicated, however. Truncation of the gene from the 5' end, resulting in a product about one-half the size of the wild-type protein, creates a dominant mutation that increases longevity (Fig. 2). This suggests that the C-terminal domain of the protein has a life maintenance function and that the N-terminal domain attenuates its effect. Thus, when *LAG1* is present, its activity determines yeast longevity. When *LAG1* is absent, another gene or gene hierarchy takes over in this capacity. The two domains of Lag1 would appear to function as a homeostatic device in yeast longevity, maintaining a balance between life extension and attenuation, but clearly is not the only such device present in the yeast cell.

3. The *RAS* Genes

The yeast *RAS* genes are highly pleiotropic, and they function to integrate cell growth and cell division (Broach & Deschenes, 1990). In some way they sense the nutritional status of the cell, and the nor-

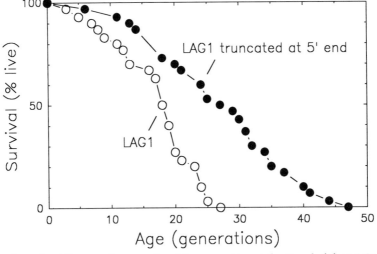

Figure 2. Life span of yeast cells with a truncation at the 5' end of the *LAG1* gene. Life spans of individual cells were determined on rich medium. The mean life span of cells with a truncated *LAG1* gene was 27 generations, whereas the mean life span of cells with the intact, wild-type gene was 17 generations (*p* ≪ 0.0001). Corresponding maximum life spans were 47 and 27 generations, respectively.

mal function of these genes is required by yeasts to resist a variety of stressful environmental conditions. In *Saccharomyces cerevisiae*, the *RAS* genes function by stimulating the activity of adenylate cyclase; however, *RAS1*, in particular, has been implicated in another signal transduction pathway, which involves inositol phospholipid turnover. Only one of the two *RAS* genes needs to be present for yeasts to grow normally, although some differences in the expression of *RAS1* and *RAS2* have been detected under different growth conditions. Given the central position of the *RAS* genes in yeast cellular regulation, it was only natural to examine the possibility that they may be implicated in yeast longevity. It should be kept in mind that the mammalian *ras* genes are not only implicated in cancer in their mutated oncogenic form but also play important roles in organismal development, not to mention normal cell cycling (Barbacid, 1987).

The overexpression of *RAS2* in transgenic yeasts resulted in an approximately 30% extension in the mean and maximum life spans (Sun *et al.*, 1994), which is somewhat less than that observed previously with the activated allele (Chen *et al.*, 1990). The disruption of the gene attenuated the life span as expected, indicating that *RAS2* is involved in determining yeast longevity. The results of genetic manipulation of *RAS1* were quite different (Sun *et al.*, 1994). Overexpression of the transgene had no effect on longevity. In contrast, deletion of the gene resulted in a marked extension of life span. Thus, *RAS1* plays a role in establishing the yeast life span. This is the first clear-cut example of a functional difference between the two *RAS* genes in yeast. Perhaps the two genes function as a homeostatic device in yeast longevity, much like the N- and C-terminal domains of Lag1 appear to.

RAS1 and *RAS2*, like *LAG1*, can be considered "genes of youth." The expression of both *RAS* genes declines with age, as determined at the mRNA and protein lev-
els (Sun *et al.*, 1994). One possibility is that once the expression of the *RAS* genes diminishes, other genes become limiting for longevity. Overexpression of *RAS2* has a rejuvenating effect on the yeasts: they continue dividing at the rapid rate characteristic of young cells well into old age (Sun *et al.*, 1994).

The biochemical function of *RAS* in determining yeast longevity is not yet clear; however, some clues are available. An extensive genetic and pharmacological dissection clearly indicates that stimulation of the cAMP pathway is not sufficient to result in life extension by *RAS* (Sun *et al.*, 1994). Overexpression of a *RAS2* mutated in its effector domain, the region of the protein that is involved in the interaction with adenyl cyclase, is as effective as the wild type in promoting yeast longevity (Sun *et al.*, 1994). Thus, the cAMP pathway is not even necessary for life extension. The results suggest that another pathway must be operative. The possibility arises that this may be a MAP kinase pathway, in analogy to the function of *ras* in higher cells (Johnson & Vaillancourt, 1994). In fact, some evidence exists that the cAMP pathway may be inhibitory in life maintenance (Sun *et al.*, 1994), opening the possibility of cross-talk between pathways. The studies on *RAS* demonstrate the significance of signal transduction in aging.

V. Perspectives

A. Nuclear–Mitochondrial Interactions in Aging

As discussed earlier, several nuclear mutants that affect longevity have been identified in *Podospora* and *Neurospora*. In one case, the gene has been cloned. The cloning of *gr* from *Podospora* is a most important development, because it foretells a deeper understanding of the processes underlying the "disintegration" of the mitochondrial genome with age. This is likely to be a complex phenomenon, because senescence in *Podospora anserina* appears to be polygenic (Silliker & Cummings, 1990). The proximal mechanisms leading to senescence are clear at the molecular level in this organism, at least in their outlines. The cloning of nuclear genes involved in this phenomenon is likely to provide important insight into nuclear–mitochondrial interactions in senescence that may be more generally applicable.

The premature death phenotype associated with the congruence of two nuclear genes in *Podospora* results in a site-specific deletion in mitochondrial DNA (Belcour *et al.*, 1991). This phenotype is reminiscent of the mitochondrial DNA deletions in brain and heart that occur in humans during aging (Cortopassi & Arnheim, 1990). Such mitochondrial deletions and mutations have been termed "the tip of the iceberg," and they may be a harbinger of widely spread deficiencies in mitochondrial function during aging. It is worth pointing out, however, that alterations in mitochondrial DNA are not the only means by which mitochondrial function may be compromised during aging. Studies in *Drosophila* indicate that a coordinate down regulation of both nuclear and mitochondrial genes that code for mitochondrial proteins may exist as a function of age (Calleja *et al.*, 1993). Thus, an understanding of the interaction of the nucleus and the mitochondrion may be a key element in deciphering the aging process.

The importance of nuclear genes in the maintenance of the mitochondrial genome has been demonstrated in yeast (Chen *et al.*, 1993). As mentioned earlier, similar evidence has been obtained in *Podospora* (Belcour *et al.*, 1991). Also, in *Neurospora crassa*, the existence of nuclear genes that lend stability to the mitochondrial genome has been adduced (Bertrand *et al.*, 1993). Unlike the *Podospora* mutants mentioned earlier, mutants in these nuclear genes render the

mitochondrial DNA less stable. The recombination events observed in the *Neurospora* mutant closely resembled those found in human mitochondrial deletions that occur in neuro-myopathies. It should be kept in mind, however, that there are marked distinctions between the mitochondrial genomes of humans and fungi. Fungal mitochondrial DNA possesses introns, in addition to more' subtle differences. Nevertheless, the filamentous fungi present a unique opportunity to examine the role of the mitochondrion in aging, inasmuch as this aspect of the aging process is accentuated in these organisms.

B. Interface with the Environment in Aging

There is no need to emphasize the importance of the mutual interaction of the genome and the environment in aging. Any phenotype, including longevity, expresses itself in such an interaction. The genetics of aging in *Saccharomyces cerevisiae* is beginning to give us the first glimmers of understanding of this interaction at the molecular level. The genetic analysis of the role of the *RAS* genes in yeast longevity indicates the fundamental role of signal transduction. As alluded to earlier, it also implicates the importance of resistance to environmental stress, including nutritional status, in aging. It is possible that Lag1, as a transmembrane protein, constitutes the interface with the environment.

Further evidence for the significance of the interface with the environment comes from an analysis of the resistance of yeasts to an environmental stress they normally encounter, ultraviolet light (Kale and Jazwinski, submitted). The resistance of yeasts to UV increases with age, through about eight generations, and then plummets. This is not true for another DNA-damaging agent, ethyl methanesulfonate, to which they are not normally exposed. Resistance to EMS declines monotonically with age. It is curious that the expression of the "genes of youth," such as *LAG1*, *RAS1*, and *RAS2*, decreases and plateaus about the time UV resistance reaches its zenith. I believe this suggests that active life maintenance processes are operative through middle age (about eight generations), after which the organism simply coasts on whatever life maintenance reserves it still has available. This proposal, and certainly the interface with the environment, should have general significance in aging.

C. Glucose Balance and Metabolism in Aging

The yeast *Saccharomyces cerevisiae* devotes a lot of its physiological attention to energy metabolism, in particular to carbohydrate utilization (Gancedo & Serrano, 1989). Glucose is the preferred carbohydrate. Yeasts do not employ endocrine signals to regulate glucose utilization. The sugar itself is the signal. The *RAS* genes are involved in sensing and transducing the glucose signal in a yet undetermined manner (Broach & Deschenes, 1990). Given the importance of *RAS* in both glucose metabolism and longevity, one would conclude that glucose balance plays a significant role in yeast aging. It is provocative to imagine that yeasts could serve as a model for obtaining a better understanding of the role of glucose balance in organismal aging in mammals, where significant departures from homeostasis occur during aging (Florini & Mangiacapra, 1990).

Acknowledgments

The work from the author's laboratory was supported by grants from the National Institute on Aging of the National Institutes of Health (U.S.P.H.S.).

References

Adams, J., & Oeller, P. W. (1986). Structure of evolving populations of *Saccharomyces cere-visiae:* Adaptive changes are frequently associated with sequence alterations involving mobile elements belonging to the Ty family. *Proceedings of the National Academy of Sciences of the United States of America, 83,* 7124–7127.

Adams, J., Pacquin, C., Oeller, P. W., & Lee, L. (1985). Physiological characterization of adaptive clones in evolving populations of the yeast, *Saccharomyces cerevisiae. Genetics, 110,* 173–185.

Akins, R. A., Kelley, R. L., & Lambowitz, A. M. (1986). Mitochondrial plasmids of *Neurospora:* Integration into mitochondrial DNA and evidence for reverse transcription in mitochondria. *Cell, 47,* 505–516.

Barbacid, M. (1987). *ras* genes. *Annual Reviews in Biochemistry, 56,* 779–827.

Bartholomew, J. W., & Mittwer, T. (1953). Demonstration of yeast bud scars with the electron microscope. *Journal of Bacteriology, 65,* 272–275.

Barton, A. A. (1950). Some aspects of cell division in *Saccharomyces cerevisiae. Journal of General Microbiology, 4,* 84–87.

Belcour, L. & Begel, O. (1978). Lethal mitochondrial genotypes in *Podospora anserina:* A model of senescence. *Molecular & General Genetics, 163,* 113–124.

Belcour, L., Begel, O., Mosse, M. O., & Vierny, C. (1981). Mitochondrial DNA amplification in senescent cultures of *Podospora anserina. Current Genetics, 3,* 13–21.

Belcour, L., Begal, O., Keller, A. M., & Vierny, C. (1982). Does senescence in *Podospora anserina* result from instability of the mitochondrial genome? In P. P. Slonimski, P. Borst, & G. Attardi (Eds.), *Mitochondrial Genes* (pp. 415–422). Cold Spring Harbor, NY: Cold Spring Harbor Laboratory Press.

Beran, K., Malek, I., Streiblova, E., & Lieblova, J. (1967). The distribution of the relative age of cells in yeast populations. In E. O. Powell, C. G. T. Evans, R. E. Strange & D. W. Tempest (Eds), *Microbial Physiology and Continuous Culture* (pp. 57–67). London: Her Majesty's Stationery Office.

Bertrand, H., & Griffiths, A. J. F. (1989). Linear plasmids that integrate into mitochondrial DNA in *Neurospora. Genome, 31,* 155–159.

Bertrand, H., Chen, B. S. S., & Griffiths, A. J. F. (1985). Insertion of a foreign nucleotide sequence into mitochondrial DNA causes senescence in *Neurospora intermedia. Cell, 41,* 877–884.

Bertrand, H., Griffiths, A. J. F., Court, D. A., & Cheng, C. K. (1986). An extrachromosomal plasmid is the etiological precursor of kalDNA insertion sequences in the mitochondrial chromosome of senescent *Neurospora. Cell,* 47, 829–837.

Bertrand, H., Wu, Q., & Seidel-Rogol, B. L. (1993). Hyperactive recombination in the mitochondrial DNA of the natural death nuclear mutant of *Neurospora crassa. Molecular and Cellular Biology,* 13, 6778–6788.

Bockelmann, B., & Esser, K. (1986). Plasmids of mitochondrial origin in senescent mycelia of *Podospora curvicola. Current Genetics,* 10, 803–810.

Broach, J. R., & Deschenes, R. J. (1990). The function of *RAS* gene in *Saccharomyces cerevisiae. Advances in Cancer Research,* 54, 79–139.

Broccoli, D., & Cooke, H. (1993). Aging, healing, and the metabolism of telomeres. *American Journal of Human Genetics,* 52, 657–660.

Calleja, M., Pena, P., Ugalde, C., Ferreiro, C. Marco, R., & Garesse, R. (1993). Mitochondrial DNA remains intact during *Drosophila* aging, but the levels of mitochondrial transcripts are significantly reduced. *Journal of Biological Chemistry,* 268, 18891–18897.

Chen, J. B., Sun, J., & Jazwinski, S. M. (1990). Prolongation of the yeast life span by the v-Ha-*RAS* oncogene. *Molecular Microbiology,* 4, 2081–2086.

Chen, X.-J., Guan, M.-X., & Clark-Walker, G. D. (1993). MHM101, a nuclear gene involved in maintenance of the mitochondrial genome in *Saccharomyces cerevisiae. Nucleic Acids Research,* 21, 3473–3477.

Clark, J. (1984). Lifespans and senescence in six slime molds. *Mycologia,* 76, 366–368.

Clark, J., & Hakim, R. (1980a). Nuclear sieving of *Didymium iridis* plasmodia. *Experimental Mycology,* 4, 17–22.

Clark, J., & Hakim, R. (1980b). Aging of plasmodial heterokaryons in *Didymium iridis. Molecular & General Genetics,* 178, 419–422.

Clark, J., & Mulleavy, P. (1982). The effects of polyploidy on lifespan of *Didymium iridis. Experimental Mycology,* 6, 71–76.

Cortopassi, G. A., & Arnheim, N. (1990). Detection of a specific mitochondrial DNA deletion in tissues of older humans. *Nucleic Acids Research,* 18, 6927–6933.

Cummings, D. J., Belcour, L., & Grandchamp, C. (1979). Mitochondrial DNA from *Podospora anserina.* II. Properties of mutant DNA and multimeric circular DNA from senescent cultures. *Molecular & General Genetics,* 171, 239–250.

Cummings, D. J., MacNiel, I. A., Domenico, J. & Matsura, E. T. (1985). Excision-amplification of mitochondrial DNA during senescence in *Podospora anserina.* DNA sequence analysis of three unique 'plasmids.' *Journal of Molecular Biology,* 185, 659–680.

D'mello, N. P., & Jazwinski, S. M. (1991). Telomere length constancy during aging of *Saccharomyces cerevisiae. Journal of Bacteriology,* 173, 6709–6713.

D'mello, N. P., Childress, A. M., Franklin, D. S., Kale, S. P., Pinswasdi, C., & Jazwinski, S. M. (1994). Cloning and characterization of *LAG1,* a longevity-assurance gene in yeast. *Journal of Biological Chemistry,* 269, 15451–15459.

Egilmez, N. K., & Jazwinski, S. M. (1989). Evidence for the involvement of a cytoplasmic factor in the aging of the yeast *Saccharomyces cerevisiae. Journal of Bacteriology,* 171, 37–42.

Egilmez, N. K., Chen, J. B., & Jazwinski, S. M. (1989). Specific alterations in transcript prevalence during the yeast life span. *Journal of Biological Chemistry,* 264, 14312–14317.

Egilmez, N. K., Chen, J. B., & Jazwinski, S. M. (1990). Preparation and partial characterization of old yeast cells. *Journal of Gerontology,* 45, B9–17.

Esser, K., & Tudzynski, P. (1980). Senescence in fungi. In K. V. Thimann (Ed.), *Senescence in Plants* (pp. 63–67). Boca Raton, FL: CRC Press.

Florini, J. R., & Mangiacapra, F. J. (1990). Problems in design and interpretation of aging studies: Illustration by reports on hormone secretion and actions. In M. Rothstein (Ed.), *Review of Biological Research in Aging* (Vol. 4, pp. 231–241). New York: Wiley-Liss.

Gancedo, C., & Serrano, R. (1989). Energy-yielding metabolism. In A. H. Rose & J. S. Harrison (Ed.), *The Yeasts* (Vol. 3, 2nd ed., pp. 205–259). San Diego: Academic Press.

Goldstein, S. (1990). Replicative senescence:

The human fibroblast comes of age. *Science, 249,* 1129–1133.

Griffiths, A. J. F. (1992). Fungal senescence. *Annual Review of Genetics, 26,* 351–357.

Hermanns, J., Asseburg, A., & Osiewacz, H. D. (1994). Evidence for a life span-prolonging effect of a linear plasmid in a longevity mutant of *Podospora anserina. Molecular & General Genetics, 243,* 297–307.

James, A. P., Johnson, B. F., Inhaber, E. R., & Gridgeman, N. T. (1975). A kinetic analysis of spontaneous ρ- mutations in yeast. *Mutation Research, 30,* 199–208.

Jamet-Vierny, C., Begel, O., & Belcour, L. (1980). Senescence in *Podospora anserina:* Amplification of a mitochondrial DNA sequence. *Cell, 21,* 189–194.

Jazwinski, S. M. (1990a). Aging and senescence of the budding yeast *Saccharomyces cerevisiae. Molecular Microbiology, 4,* 337–343.

Jazwinski, S. M. (1990b). An experimental system for the molecular analysis of the aging process: The budding yeast *Saccharomyces cerevisiae. Journal of Gerontology, 45,* B68–74.

Jazwinski, S. M. (1993). The genetics of aging in the yeast *Saccharomyces cerevisiae. Genetica, 91,* 35–51.

Johnson, B. F., & Lu, C. (1975). Morphometric analysis of yeast cells IV. Increase of the cylindrical diameter of *Schizosaccharomyces pombe* during the cell cycle. *Experimental Cell Research, 95,* 154–158.

Johnson, G. L., & Vaillancourt, R. R. (1994). Sequential protein kinase reactions controlling cell growth and differentiation. *Current Opinion in Cell Biology, 6,* 230–238.

Johnston, J. R. (1966). Reproductive capacity and mode of death of yeast cells. *Antonie van Leeuwenhoek, 32,* 94–98.

Koll, F. (1986). Does nuclear integration of mitochondrial sequences occur during senescence in *Podospora!* *Nature, 324,* 597–599.

Kuiper, M. T. R., & Lambowitz, A. M. (1988). A novel transcription activity associated with mitochondrial plasmids of *Neurospora. Cell, 55,* 693–704.

Lott, T., & Clark, J. (1980). Plasmodial senescence in the acellular slime mold *Didymium iridis. Experimental Cell Research, 128,* 455–458.

Lundblad, V., & Szostak, J. W. (1989). A mutant with a defect in telomere elongation leads to senescence in yeast. *Cell, 57,* 633–643.

Marcou, D. (1961). Notion de longevite et nature cytoplasmique du determinant de la senescence chez quelque champignons. *Annales des Sciences Naturelles, Botanique et Biologie Vegetale, 12,* 653–764.

McCullough, C. H. R., Cooke, D. J., Foxon, J. L., Sudbery, P. E., & Grant, W. D. (1973). Nuclear DNA content and senescence in *Physarum polycephalum. Nature, 245,* 263–265.

Michel, F., & Lang, B. F. (1985). Mitochondrial class II introns encode proteins related to the reverse transcriptase of retroviruses. *Nature, 316,* 641–643.

Mortimer, R. K., & Johnston, J. R. (1959). Life span of individual yeast cells. *Nature, 183,* 1751–1752.

Motizuki, M., & Tsurugi, K. (1992). The effect of aging on protein synthesis in the yeast *Saccharomyces cerevisiae. Mechanisms of Ageing and Development, 64,* 235–245.

Muller, I. (1971). Experiments on ageing in single cells of *Saccharomyces cerevisiae. Archiv fur Mikrobiologie, 77,* 20–25.

Muller, I. (1985). Parental age and the life-span of zygotes of *Saccharomyces cerevisiae. Antonie van Leeuwenhoek, 51,* 1–10.

Muller, I., & Wolf, F. (1978). A correlation between shortened life span and UV-sensitivity in some strains of *Saccharomyces cerevisiae. Molecular & General Genetics, 160,* 231–234.

Muller, I., Zimmermann, M., Becker, D., & Flomer, M. (1980). Calendar life span versus budding life span of *Saccharomyces cerevisiae. Mechanisms of Ageing and Development, 12,* 47–52.

Munkres, K. D. (1984). Dominance and complementation relationships of conidial longevity mutants of *Neurospora crassa. Mechanisms of Ageing and Development, 25,* 79–89.

Nevers, P., Shepherd, N. S., & Saedler, H. (1986). Plant transposable elements. *Advances in Botanical Research, 12,* 103–203.

Osiewacz, H. D. (1992). The genetic control of aging in the ascomycete *Podospora anserina.* In R. Zwilling & C. Balduini (Eds.), *Biology of Aging* (pp. 153–164). Berlin: Springer Verlag.

Osiewacz, H. D., & Esser, K. (1984). The mitochondrial plasmid of *Podospora anserina:* a mobile intron of a mitochondrial gene. *Current Genetics, 8,* 299–305.

Osiewacz, H. D., & Hermanns, J. (1992). The role of mitochondrial DNA rearrangements in aging and human diseases. *Aging/Clinical and Experimental Research, 4,* 273–286.

Osiewacz, H. D., Hermanns, J., Marcou, D., Triffi, M., & Esser, K. (1989). Mitochondrial DNA rearrangements are correlated with a delayed amplification of the mobile intron (plDNA) in a long-lived mutant of *Podospora anserina. Mutation Research, 219,* 9–15.

Rizet, G. (1953). Sur l'impossibilite d'obtenir la multiplication vegetative ininterrompue et illimite de l'ascomycete *Podospora anserina. Comptes Rendus de l'Academie des Sciences Paris, 237,* 838–855.

Rose, M. R. (1991). *Evolutionary Biology of Aging.* New York: Oxford University Press.

Sainsard-Chanet, A., Begel, O., & Belcour, L. (1993). DNA deletion of mitochondrial introns is correlated with the process of senescence in *Podospora anserina. Journal of Molecular Biology, 234,* 1–7.

Sando, N., Maeda, M., Endo, T., Oka, R., & Hayashibe, M. (1973). Induction of meiosis and sporulation in differently aged cells of *Saccharomyces cerevisiae. Journal of General and Applied Microbiology, 19,* 359–373.

Seidel-Rogol, B. L., King, J., & Bertrand, H. (1989). Unstable mitochondrial DNA in natural-death nuclear mutants of *Neurospora crassa. Molecular and Cellular Biology, 9,* 4259–4264.

Sellem, C. H., Lecellier, G., & Belcour, L. (1993). Transposition of a group II intron. *Nature, 366,* 176–178.

Silar, P., & Picard, M. (1994). Increased longevity of EF-1 alpha high-fidelity mutants in *Podospora anserina. Journal of Molecular Biology, 235,* 231–236.

Silliker, M. E., & Cummings, D. J. (1990). Genetic and molecular analysis of a long-lived strain of *Podospora anserina. Genetics, 125,* 775–781.

Smith, J. R., & Rubenstein, I. (1973a). The development of 'senescence' in *Podospora anserina. Journal of General Microbiology, 76,* 283–296.

Smith, J. R., & Rubenstein, I. (1973b). Cytoplasmic inheritance of the timing of 'senescence' in *Podospora anserina. Journal of General Microbiology, 76,* 297–304.

Stahl, U., Lemke, P. A., Tudzynski, P., Kuck, U., & Esser, K. (1978). Evidence for plasmid like DNA in a filamentous fungus, the asomycete *Podospora anserina. Molecular & General Genetics, 162,* 341–343.

Stahl, U., Kuck, U., Tudzynski, P., & Esser, K. (1980). Characterization and cloning of plasmid like DNA of the ascomycete *Podospora anserina. Molecular & General Genetics, 178,* 639–646.

Steinhilber, W., & Cummings, D. J. (1986). A DNA polymerase activity with characteristics of a reverse transcriptase in *Podospora anserina. Current Genetics, 10,* 389–392.

Sun, J., Kale, S. P., Childress, A. M., Pinswasdi, C., & Jazwinski, S. M. (1994). Divergent roles of *RAS1* and *RAS2* in yeast longevity. *Journal of Biological Chemistry, 269,* 18638–18645.

Tudzynski, P., & Esser, K. (1979). Chromosomal and extrachromosomal control of senescence in the ascomycete *Podospora anserina. Molecular & General Genetics, 173,* 71–84.

Turker, M. S., & Cummings, D. J. (1987). *Podospora anserina* does not senesce when serially passaged in liquid culture. *Journal of Bacteriology, 169,* 454–460.

Turker, M. S., Domenico, J. M., & Cummings, D. J. (1987a). A novel family of mitochondrial plasmids associated with longevity mutants of *Podospora anserina. Journal of Biological Chemistry, 262,* 2250–2255.

Turker, M. S., Nelson, J. G., & Cummings, D. J. (1987b). A *Podospora anserina* longevity mutant with a temperature-sensitive phenotype for senescence. *Molecular and Cellular Biology, 7,* 3199–3204.

Vierny, C., Keller, A. M., Begel, O., & Belcour, L. (1982). A sequence of mitochondrial DNA is associated with the onset of senescence in a fungus. *Nature, 297,* 157–159.

Wright, R. M., & Cummings, D. J. (1983). Integration of mitochondrial gene sequences within the nuclear genome during senescence in a fungus. *Nature, 302,* 86–88.

Wright, R. M., Horrum, M. A., & Cummings, D. J. (1982). Are mitochondrial structural genes selectively amplified during senescence in *Podospora anserina? Cell, 29,* 505–515.

Four

Molecular Genetics of *Caenorhabditis elegans* Aging

Gordon J. Lithgow

I. Introduction

If a model system is to return its investment, then it must yield findings likely to be of significance to the general gerontological researcher. *Caenorhabditis elegans* has been proposed as an excellent model system for the genetic dissection of aging processes and life-span determination. We expect to identify life-span-limiting genes, define the physiological consequences of expression of these genes, test specific aging hypotheses, and provide coherent models of aging in mammals. Invertebrate systems are unique; life-span-limiting genes can be defined by mutation and those genes manipulated and reintroduced to allow causation to be established. This chapter will attempt to critically assess whether the worm system has fulfilled (or is likely to fulfill) these expectations. I will concentrate on recently published material and recommend the reader to consult previous reviews for a more detailed appraisal of the biology and genetics of *C. elegans* aging (Russell & Jacobson, 1984; Johnson, 1984, 1988, 1990b, 1993; Klass & Johnson, 1985; Johnson & Lithgow, 1992; Wood & Johnson, 1994). I will exclude descriptions

of age-related changes and biomarkers (Hosono, 1978b; Hosono, Sato, Aizawa, & Mitsui, 1980; Bolanowski, Russell, & Jacobson, 1981; Davis, Anderson, & Dusenbery, 1982; Bolanowski, Jacobson, & Russell, 1983; Klass, Nguyen, & Dechavigny, 1983; Johnson, 1984, 1987, 1990b; Johnson & McCaffrey, 1985; Meheus & Vanfleteren, 1986; Meheus, Van Beeumen, Coomans, & Vanfleteren, 1987; Johnson, Conley, & Keller, 1988; Sarkis, Ashcom, Hawdon, & Jacobson, 1988; Johnson & Lithgow, 1992; Egilmez & Shmookler Reis, 1994; Fabian & Johnson, 1994; Lithgow, White, Hinerfeld, & Johnson, 1994; Duhon & Johnson, 1995), except when considering specific mechanisms of aging.

Perhaps the most significant aspect of the nematode model is that mutation of any one of a number genes, including *age-1*, *daf-2*, *daf-23*, *rad-8*, and *spe-26*, extends the adult nematode life span. Whether these mutations extend life span by similar physiological processes is unknown. In addition to the study of single gene mutations, quantitative trait loci (QTL) maps of life span have been produced, biomarkers of aging recorded, age-specific gene expression described, the ef-

Handbook of the Biology of Aging, Fourth Edition
Copyright © 1996 Academic Press, Inc. All rights of reproduction in any form reserved.

fects of temperature, nutrition, oxygen pressure, and ionizing and nonionizing radiation on life span reported, and large-scale demographic studies undertaken. As a result of this activity, we may begin to consider the nature of life-span-limiting processes.

A crucial issue now arising is whether model systems such as *C. elegans* and *Drosophila* can reveal aging mechanisms that are applicable to human life span and age-related diseases. Although outside the scope of this chapter, we can approach this issue by comparing our conclusions with those arising from other systems.

A. Basic *C. elegans* Biology

C. elegans was chosen by Brenner to shed light on complex problems in developmental and neurological biology (Brenner, 1974, 1988). Work on this system has generated over 1000 publications, a complete description of the cell lineage, and an essentially complete physical map of the six chromosomes. Moreover, some 1200 genetic loci have been identified (Durbin & Thierry-Mieg, 1991). This nematode is a nonparasitic, hermaphroditic, soil metazoan which, conveniently for geneticists, produces a spontaneously occurring male. At 1.2 mm in length, the animal can be cultured in large numbers on agar plates or in liquid culture while feeding on *Escherichia coli* (monoxenic culture). Axenic culture, in which the worms are maintained in a complex medium, has also been employed in a number of aging studies (Croll, Smith, & Zuckerman, 1977; Vanfleteren, 1980).

B. The Genome and Generation of Transgenic Nematodes

The haploid genome of *C. elegans* is approximately 100 megabases (Mb), 36% G+C (Sulston & Brenner, 1974), and is estimated to encode almost 18,000 genes (Emmons, 1988; Wilson, Ainscough, An-

derson, *et al.*, 1994). A largely complete physical map has been available since 1992 (Coulson, Waterston, Kiff, Sulston, & Kohara, 1988; Coulson, Kozono, Lutterbach, Shownkeen, Sulston, & Waterston, 1991). By the end of 1998, the *C. elegans* genome should be sequenced and will provide a boost for the cloning of genes that influence complex traits such as life span. The sequencing of 2.2 Mb of the *C. elegans* genome has yielded some 483 putative genes (Wilson, Ainscough, Anderson, *et al.*, 1994). One-third of these genes were similar to previously identified genes with known functions in other organisms (Wilson, Ainscough, Anderson, *et al.*, 1994). Sequencing of cDNA libraries constructed from mixed-age worm mRNA has generated 1517 expressed-sequence-tagged (EST) clones (Waterston, Martin, Craxton, *et al.*, 1992), with 30% of the clones showing similarity to previously identified genes. In a second study of cDNA clones, 585 ESTs were obtained with 18 homologues of human genes identified (McCombie, Adams, Kelley, *et al.*, 1992).

Orr and Sohal (1994) have powerfully demonstrated with *Drosophila* that transgenics can be used to directly test mechanistic theories of aging. This approach ushers in a new era in gerontological research in which the causal relationship between physiological processes and longevity can be established. Homologues of genes implicated in the aging of other invertebrates and in the replicative senescence of cells can now be readily obtained in *C. elegans*. The extensive availability of cloned genes should result in *C. elegans* being used as a "test bed" for candidate genes from other systems.

The availability of genes that may influence longevity is not in question. If we wish to test the effects of individual genes or suites of genes on life span, however, a number of factors place the study of transgenic nematodes at a disadvantage. *C. elegans* is transformed by microinjection of

DNA into the distal gonad of young adults (Kimble, Hodgkin, Smith, & Smith, 1982; Stinchcomb, Shaw, Carr, & Hirsh, 1985). Trangenic F_1 animals are commonly identified by the inclusion of DNA encoding the dominant mutant allele for *rol-6* (Mello, Kramer, Stinchcomb, & Ambros, 1991) This allele causes a distinctive behavioral alteration, such that the worm moves in a circle with a rolling motion. In the transgenic worms, the transgene is carried as a multicopy, extrachromosomal array. Chromosomal integration is stimulated by exposure to γ irradiation. The first problem for transgenic studies is the lack of control of transgene copy number (Stinchcomb, Shaw, Carr, & Hirsh, 1985; Fire, Kondo, & Waterston, 1990), and without integration the transgenic worms display mosaicism due to mitotic loss. The second problem is that the transgene inserts at the homologous chromosomal sites at very low frequency (Fire, 1986). As a consequence of both of these problems, expression of transgenes may be different from expression from the normal locus and, therefore, may have unpredictable effects on life span. A preliminary study of the effects of transgene expression on life span has been carried out (Johnson, Tedesco, & Lithgow, 1993) and highlights some of the potential problems. In this study, a number of transgenic lines were established to complement the *fer-15* fertility defect. Strains containing *fer-15* were injected with a cosmid previously shown to detect a mutation-specific restriction fragment length polymorphism (RFLP). Although the cosmid DNA partially complemented the fertility defect, it also had an unexpected effect on life span: when the cosmid array was integrated, a much more effective complementation of *fer-15* was achieved, but life span was now shortened. The authors concluded that misappropriate expression from the transgenic arrays may be detrimental to life span.

If we are to utilize *C. elegans* to establish the genetic causality of aging, then the effects on life span of inappropriate gene expression must be a concern. However, some studies of genes of developmental interest indicate that correct expression of a transgene can occur: Blumenthal and co-workers (Spieth, MacMorris, Broverman, Greenspoon, & Blumenthal, 1988) looked at four independent transgenic lines that were selected on the basis of fertility and viability as homozygotes. Expression of the transgene was examined in detail in two of these lines and was shown to be sex-, tissue-, and stage-specific. In addition, rare homologous recombination events may be screened for (Broverman, MacMorris, & Blumenthal, 1993).

It would be desirable to control transgene expression with an inducible promoter that initiates transcription at distinct ages. A number of inducible promoters have been used to study *C. elegans* developmental processes, but they are unsuitable for aging studies. For example, the *hsp 16* transcriptional promoter requires a heat shock for activation (Russnak & Candido, 1985; Jones, Russnak, Kay, & Candido, 1986; Jones, Dixon, Graham, & Candido, 1989), but heat shock is known to affect life history traits, including fertility and life span (Lithgow, White, Hinerfeld, & Johnson, 1994; Lithgow, White, Melov, & Johnson, 1995). The cloning of genes that are expressed in an age-specific fashion may provide transcriptional promoters useful in aging studies (Fabian & Johnson, 1995). Fabian and Johnson identified mRNAs whose abundance decreased, increased, or remained constant with age by using a differential screening strategy. They identified nine mRNAs, the abundance of which declined with age. Three of these mRNAs encoded vitellogenin. In addition, two distinct cDNAs correspond to mRNAs that were shown to increase in abundance with age.

Two other methods for altering the function of specific genes may be useful to the nematode gerontologist. Expression of a candidate gene can be decreased by the production of antisense RNA (Fire, Albertson, Harrison, & Moerman, 1991), or expression can be abolished by insertional mutagenesis (Zwaal, Broeks, van Meurs, Groenen, & Plasterk, 1993). Although transposon tagging has been utilized for a number of years (Wood, 1988), a frozen bank of 5000 transposon-tagged mutant strains has been assembled (Zwaal, Broeks, van Meurs, Groenen, & Plasterk, 1993). This bank can be screened by the polymerase chain reaction (PCR) for an insertion in the desired gene. It is therefore relatively straightforward to establish genotype–phenotype relationships for genes of known sequence.

C. Age-Synchronous Cultures

Molecular and biochemical studies can require large amounts of biological material. Large quantities of mixed-stage *C. elegans* have been prepared by growth in liquid medium in shake flask cultures (Wood, 1988) and have been scaled up to 150 cultures in a 280-l stirred tank (Gbewonyo, Rohrer, Lister, Burgess, Cully, & Buckland, 1994). Methods have also been developed for the synchronous growth of large numbers of adult worms (Russell & Jacobson, 1984; Fabian & Johnson, 1994), which allow for the isolation of significant quantities of age-specific material. Synchrony is achieved initially by the isolation of eggs, either by allowing adult hermaphrodites to lay eggs for a limited period of time (3–24 hr) or by treatment of gravid adults with hypochlorite, which disintegrates the larval and adult carcasses, leaving intact only the resistant eggs. Age synchrony has also been obtained by velocity sedimentation (Sulston & Brenner, 1974) and by sieving through nylon membranes with specified pore sizes.

As adult hermaphrodites lay over 300 eggs in 5 days, maintenance of synchrony requires that the adults are routinely separated from the progeny. For large cultures this is not feasible, and methods to prevent

progeny production are required. This has been accomplished either by chemical sterilization with 5-fluoro- 2'-deoxyuracil (FUdR) (Hosono, 1978a; Mitchell, Stiles, Santelli, & Sanadi, 1979; Gandhi, Santelli, Mitchell, Stiles, & Sanadi, 1980; Zuckerman, 1980) or by the use of temperature-sensitive mutations blocking fertility. Although some fertility mutations may have an effect on life span (Van Voorhies, 1992), many such mutations do not (Johnson, 1984). Growth of strains mutant at the *fer-15*, *glp-4*, or *spe-9* loci at a restrictive temperature during development yields adults which produce very few or no progeny (Fabian & Johnson, 1994). Double mutant combinations, such as *fer-15* and *spe-9*, provide strains that produce no progeny at the restrictive temperature, allowing for the growth and maintenance of large numbers of age-synchronous adults to late ages (Fabian & Johnson, 1994). Thus, one can obtain age-synchronous protein and nucleic acid. Each adult worm contains about 0.4 μg of total protein (Johnson & Hirsh, 1979) and 10–30 ng of total RNA (Fabian, 1993). Dead worms can be removed from cultures by density gradient centrifugation, which also removes contaminating *E. coli* (Fabian & Johnson, 1994).

D. Life Span and Life Cycle

The mean life span of wild-type hermaphrodites range from 14 to 20 days at 20°C under monoxenic *ad libidum* feeding (Johnson & Hutchinson, 1993). The male life span is either significantly shorter or significantly longer, depending on the strain (Johnson & Hutchinson, 1993). Male life span is shorter for the N2 strain most commonly used in *C. elegans* research. An understanding of the *C. elegans* life cycle is necessary for critical reading of the aging literature (Wood & Johnson, 1994). Eggs laid on agar at 20°C will hatch into the first larval stage (L1) within 16 hr and proceed through three additional larval stages. During the first larval stage, a decision is made between two distinct developmental pathways. Under conditions of sufficient nutrition and low population density, the worms develop directly into adults. The hermaphrodite will begin to lay fertilized eggs 72 hr (3 days) after hatching. In conditions of overcrowding or poor nutrition, the L1 larva will molt into an alternative second stage larva (L2), which is called the L2d (Golden & Riddle, 1982, 1984a,b). An L2d will, if disadvantageous conditions continue, go on to form the dauer larva. The dauer is a non-reproducing, nonfeeding, long-lived larval stage (Riddle, 1988). Dauers live for at least 60 days and, under appropriate nutritional conditions, molt into a normal fourth larval stage worm and subsequently form reproducing adults that exhibit normal adult life span (Klass & Hirsh, 1976). The developmental switch is controlled in part by a pheromone produced by all life-cycle stages (Golden & Riddle, 1982, 1984a) in response to nutritional conditions and temperature. Genetic dissection of dauer larvae formation has revealed a complex signal transduction pathway with two parallel branches (Golden & Riddle, 1985; Albert & Riddle, 1988; Vowels & Thomas, 1992; Thomas, Birnby, & Vowels, 1993; Malone & Thomas, 1994; Gottlieb & Ruvkun, 1994), containing a member of the transforming growth factor–β-receptor superfamily (Estevez, Attisano, Wrana, Albert, Massaque, & Riddle, 1993) and also a serine/threonine kinase related to the *raf* proto-oncogene family (Georgi, Albert, & Riddle, 1990). This pathway has implications for nematode life span.

II. Demographics

Genetic effects on life span are best described by a detailed demographic analysis. Such models do not describe mechanistic processes, but may give clues about age-specific gene action or expression. Of particular interest to the physiologist or geneticist is the acceleration of mortality rate with age. Comparative analysis between genotypes can reveal a more complete picture of the action of an individual gene or the effects of multiple loci (Finch, 1990). Such an analysis of strains carrying a mutation of *age-1* revealed a change in the acceleration of age-specific mortality rates when mortality data were compared to the empirical Gompertz model (Johnson, 1990a). This was the first demonstration that the exponential increase in age-specific mortality rate could be influenced by a single gene. Interest has centered upon the applicability of the Gompertz model to large populations and diverse species. The exponential Gompertz component describes the acceleration of the age-specific mortality rate. Life tables compiled from large medfly and *Drosophila* populations demonstrated dramatic deviations from an exponential increase in mortality rate with age (Carey, 1991; Curtsinger, Fukui, Townsend, & Vaupel, 1992; Carey, Liedo, Orozco, & Vaupel, 1992; Vaupel & Carey, 1993; Fukui, Xiu, & Curtsinger, 1993). This may have been due to genetic heterogeneity within the population or due to some hitherto undetermined age-specific physiological change. A genetically heterogeneous population of *C. elegans* displayed a nonexponential increase in mortality rate with age (Brooks, Lithgow, & Johnson, 1994). By dividing this population into four quartiles on the basis of mean life span, the data showed a significantly improved fit to the exponential model. This is consistent with the notion that the nonexponential nature of the genetically heterogeneous population is due to the superposition of several exponential mortality rate increases. In contrast to the heterogeneous cohort, a large, genetically homogeneous cohort exhibited a generally exponential mortality rate increase (Brooks, Lithgow, & Johnson, 1994), which appears to be the product of two significantly different rates of mortality acceleration (Vaupel, Johnson, & Lithgow, 1994). One criticism of this study is that the mortality rates for the large population were derived by measuring the mortality rates of subpopulations. There is some inconsistency between the mortality rates observed and the number of animals remaining alive toward the end of the analysis (Vaupel, Johnson, & Lithgow, 1994). Even taking this into account, it is clear that genetically homogeneous populations of *C. elegans* do not display the dramatic inconsistencies with the Gompertz model that are displayed by *Drosophila* or the medfly.

Life tables have not yet been generated for large populations of mutant strains, such as *age-1*; a previous demographic analysis of *age-1* was limited to populations of under 200 worms (Johnson, 1990a). It may be that mutations that extend mean and maximum life spans display distinctive demographic characteristics. Life-span extension may be associated with either a decreased initial mortality rate, a decreased exponential Gompertz component, or a leveling off of mortality rates with increasing age. To date, all demographic alterations by genetic means in *C. elegans* result from changes in the exponential Gompertz component. Recombinant inbred strains with life spans that range from 10 to 31 days display different exponential Gompertz components and do not have significantly different initial mortality rates (Johnson, 1987). Johnson (1990a) also showed that mutation of *age-1* was clearly associated with a decrease in the exponential Gompertz component and that there was no significant change in the initial mortality rate. However, analysis of large populations may also reveal age-specific changes in the acceleration of mortality rate.

III. Genetics of *C. elegans* Life Span

Genetic analysis of invertebrate life span has provided some, if not most, of the evidence for the genetic determination of longevity (Finch, 1990; Rose, 1991). Significant estimates of the heritability of life span have been found in several studies (Johnson & Wood, 1982; Johnson, 1986; Brooks & Johnson, 1991; Ebert, Cherkasova, Dennis, *et al.*, 1993; Shook, Brooks, & Johnson, submitted). The genetics of life span is distinct from development and reproduction (Johnson, 1987; Friedman & Johnson, 1988a), and the mutation of single genes can dramatically affect mortality (Friedman & Johnson, 1988a,b; Johnson, 1990a; Van Voorhies, 1992; Kenyon, Chang, Gensch, Rudner, & Tabtiang, 1993). As *C. elegans* exhibits self-fertilizing, hermaphroditic reproduction, there is virtually no heterosis for life span (Johnson & Wood, 1982; Johnson & Hutchinson, 1993). This facilitates the isolation of recessive mutations, as homozygosity can be obtained without a depression in life span.

A. Mapping of QTLs Specifying Life Span

The life span of *C. elegans* is a quantitative trait, and in interstrain crosses it is determined by a number of quantitative trait loci (QTLs) (Johnson & Wood, 1982; Brooks & Johnson, 1991; Ebert, Cherkasova, Dennis, *et al.*, 1993; Shook, Brooks, & Johnson, submitted). Two studies have been undertaken to map the QTLs that specify this quantitative genetic variation. Both studies derive from Johnson and Wood (1982), who describes the effects on the F_2 life span of crosses between wild-type strains. When Bergerac–BO and Bristol–N2 were crossed, the F_1 progeny exhibited life spans similar to those of the parental strains. The F_2, however, had a 60% increase in variance for life span. RI lines, established by 19 rounds of self-fertilization, had reproducible mean life spans that ranged from 10 to 31 days (Johnson & Wood, 1982). The variance between RIs is polygenic (Brooks & Johnson, 1991), and these genes can be mapped by following the segregation of strain-specific, sequence-tagged sites (STSs). In a second study utilizing a cross between N2 and Bergerac, the variance in life span of a heterogeneous F_{12} population was 2.3 times that of the Bergerac parental strain and 1.9 times that of the N2 parental strain (Ebert, Cherkasova, Dennis, *et al.*, 1993).

The *C. elegans* transposable element, Tc1, which inserts at random genomic sites, creates STSs. The Bergerac haploid genome contains approximately 500 Tc1 transposable elements (Mori, Moerman, & Waterston, 1988), and the N2 haploid genome contains 31 elements (Liao, Rosenzweig, & Hirsh, 1983; Egilmez, Ebert, & Schmookler Reis, 1995). Williams Schrank, Huynh, Shownkeen, and Waterston (1992) sequenced chromosomal DNA adjacent to a number of Bergerac-specific Tc1 elements to design a set of PCR-amplifiable STSs in which one oligomer is Tc1-specific and thus will not be amplified by PCR unless that site contains a Tc1. Multiplex PCR reactions, in which a number of STSs are amplified simultaneously, allow for the scoring of a large number of physical markers in one PCR (Williams, Schrank, Huynh, Shownkeen, & Waterston, 1992). The correlation between an STS marker and mean life span suggests linkage to a gene influencing this phenotype.

The two studies use different strategies to map QTLs influencing longevity. Ebert *et al.* (1993) made the cross between Bergerac and N2 and then generated an F_{10-12} recombinant–inbred population by reproduction using male hermaphrodite crosses until the F_5 generation and then allowing self-fertilization until the F_{10}. These heterogeneous populations were then stored frozen in liquid nitrogen. These F_{10} populations were cultured in an age-synchronous fashion, and a number of individual animals were scored for 25 STSs at 5 days of age and the longest living 1–5% were scored for the same STSs. If an STS was linked to a gene specifying long life and the two parental alleles differed in their effect on longevity, then one allele should be present at a higher frequency in the last 5% of the population, compared with its frequency in 5-day-old worms. Ebert *et al.* (1993) identified STSs where allele frequency altered with age in two distinct environments: a cohort hand-transferred in Petri dishes maintained to 95% mortality and a much larger age-synchronous cohort maintained with FUdR from adulthood to 99% mortality. Four regions of the genome were shown to contain longevity-determining genes in both environments: one region is on chromosome II, one is on chromosome IV, and two are on the X chromosome. A fifth region, mapping to right-central chromosome V, was selected for only in the large-scale FUdR culture.

The second study (Shook, Brooks, & Johnson, submitted) follows the protocol developed previously for the generation of RIs (Johnson & Wood, 1982). The authors carried out a Bergerac–N2 cross, and then the hybrid F_1 progeny were identified by assessing fertility at 25°C (Bergerac is sterile at 25°C). Individual F_2 progeny were allowed to self-fertilize for an additional 20 generations. The resulting 81 recombinant–inbred strains were in excess of 99.99% homozygous. The mean life spans of the RIs ranged from 11 to 42 days. Fertility of the RIs was also measured. Individual animals from each RI were typed for each of 36 unique Tc1 STSs. The correlation of each STS with life span or fertility was derived. In this study, STSs linked to longevity were detected on chromosomes II, IV, and X.

Both studies have sought STSs that correlate with longevity, and both find such on chromosomes II, IV, and X. However, for chromosome II, Shook, Brooks, and Johnson (submitted) showed cosegregation of an N2-type allele with increased longevity, while Ebert *et al.* (1993) showed cosegregation of the Bergerac allele of the same marker with longevity. There is no obvious explanation for this inconsistency. Two genes that may influence longevity among the RIs, *age-1* and a gene for superoxide dismutase (*sod-1*), are present on this chromosome. It is not known whether these loci are polymorphic between N2 and Bergerac. Very significant increases in the resolution of these QTL maps are now required for progress toward the molecular identification of these gerontogenes and the physiological processes they specify.

The QTL mapping approach to identifying gerontogenes is limited in a number of ways. The most serious limitation is that only loci that differ between the parental genomes can be detected. Another limitation is that segregation analysis places a QTL within an interval on the genome, but does not provide a direct handle for gene cloning. Despite these deficiencies, high-resolution QTL mapping allows for the identification of genes specifying the considerable variation in life span in RI strains and may identify loci that cannot be identified by mutation.

B. Mutations and Life Span

The genetic basis of life-span determination in *C. elegans* is dramatically revealed by single gene mutations. The lack of heterosis for life span contributes to the power of this system for the isolation of mutations that extend life span (Johnson & Hutchinson, 1993).

Klass (1983) isolated the first long-lived strains, and Friedman and Johnson (1988a,b) used these strains to define the *age-1* locus. Mutation of *age-1* leads to a 70% increase in mean life span and a 110% increase in maximum life span (Friedman & Johnson, 1988a,b). The mutation was first associated with a fertility deficit, but subsequently this reduction in fertility was found to be associated with a linked mutation at the *fer-15* (fertility) locus (Johnson, Tedesco, & Lithgow, 1993). Life extension by mutation of *age-1* was unequivocally not due to lengthening the developmental or reproductive schedule or of a decrease in feeding rates (Friedman & Johnson, 1988a,b; Johnson & Lithgow,

1992). *age-1* shows increased resistance to oxidative stress (Larsen, 1993; Vanfleteren, 1993) and an increased thermotolerance (Lithgow, White, Hinerfeld, & Johnson, 1994; Lithgow, White, Mclov, & Johnson, submitted) and may show some residual effect on fertility (Lithgow, White, Hinerfeld, & Johnson, 1994). *age-1* is associated with two other phenotypes: a reduction in the rate of accumulation of mitochondrial DNA deletions (Melov, Lithgow, Fischer, Tedesco, & Johnson, 1995) and increased activity of the cytoplasmic Cu/Zn superoxide dismutase (SOD) and catalase (Larsen, 1993; Vanfleteren, 1993). SOD and catalase detoxify reactive oxygen species (ROS). It is tempting to suggest that the increased activity of these enzymes is responsible for the increased life span of *age-1*.

An interesting development has been the realization that genes that regulate alternative developmental processes can affect life span. Aging in *C. elegans* appears to have very little in common with development, in that there are no large changes in gene expression profiles (Johnson & McCaffrey, 1985; Fabian & Johnson, 1995). However, the signal transduction pathway controlling dauer formation does influence life span. Mutations of *daf-2* (*daf:* dauer formation) result in constitutive dauer formation at the restrictive temperature of 25°C. Kenyon *et al.* (1993) allowed *daf-2* mutants to pass through the critical period for dauer formation at the permissive temperature and then shifted young adults to the restrictive temperature. Such adult hermaphrodites display a mean life span some 100% greater than that of the wild type subjected to the same temperature regime. A second mutation, *daf-16*, which prevents the formation of dauer larvae upon starvation or overcrowding, suppresses both the dauer-forming and the age phenotype of *daf-2*. It is tempting to speculate that *daf-2* adults are expressing a subset of dauer-specific developmental genes, which extend life span; some part of dauer physiology is enabled in adults carrying this mutation.

Another gene is thought to interact with *daf-2* in determining the life span of adults. Larsen, Albert, and Riddle (submitted) have shown that animals mutant for both *daf-2* and *daf-12* have a nearly quadrupled life span, while *daf-12* alone slightly reduces life span. The *daf-12* gene encodes a transcription factor of the steroid/thyroid hormone receptor superfamily (Larsen, Albert, & Riddle, submitted). Larsen, Albert, and Riddle (1995) also demonstrated that *daf-23* doubles the life span and is suppressed by *daf-16*.

Dauer larvae are long-lived (Klass & Hirsh, 1976) and display a number of characteristics that may explain the link between *daf* mutations and life-span determination. In particular, dauers are resistant to oxidative stress, are thermotolerant (Anderson, 1978), and have high levels of the ROS-detoxifying SOD (Anderson, 1982; Larsen, 1993).

Perhaps the most surprising life extension mutation to emerge so far is *spe-26(hc138*ts), which affects the production of sperm (Van Voorhies, 1992). Although the relationship between longevity and fecundity has provoked widespread interest, there is little evidence of a direct correlation between these processes in *C. elegans.* The energetic cost of reproduction is thought to be an important determinant of mortality in many systems, and oocyte production is assumed to be costlier than sperm production (Partridge & Harvey, 1992). The *spe-26* mutation prevents normal primary spermatocytes from developing into spermatids. Male and hermaphrodite-mutant worms have an increased life span of 65% (Van Voorhies, 1992). The physiological basis of life-span extension in *spe-26* mutants is unknown, however.

Mutation of the *rad-8* gene also leads to a life-span extension contingent upon temperature. Hartman and co-workers isolated *rad-8* as a mutation conferring

sensitivity to UV radiation (Hartman & Herman, 1982). *rad-8* mutant strains were shown to be sensitive to methyl viologen and high oxygen concentrations. Life-span extension was observed at temperatures below that optimal for growth and reproduction (Ishii, Suzuki, Hartman, & Suzuki, 1994). At 16°C, under atmospheric partial pressure for oxygen, *rad-8* mutants exhibit an almost 50% longer mean life span than wild type. At 20 and 25°C there is no change in mean life span (Ishii, Suzuki, Hartman, & Suzuki, 1994).

IV. Testing Hypotheses

A. Testing Evolutionary Theories of Aging

Rose (1991) noted that the most satisfying method to test the evolutionary theory of aging is to undertake selection experiments in which the consequences on longevity can be observed. No such experiments have been published for the nematode. Nematode gerontologists seem preoccupied with mechanistic models of aging, and this is almost certainly a consequence of the existence of large effects of single gene mutations on life span. However, the nematode should be considered when testing evolutionary theory. We should look for consistency between our theoretical expectations of gerontogenes and the physiological alterations apparent in mutations that prolong life span; we may expect to observe phenotypes of mutations negatively covarying with life span.

The central principle of evolutionary theory, as developed by Medawar (1952), Hamilton (1966), and Charlesworth (1980), is that there is a decline in the force of natural selection with age (Rose, 1991). Thus, genes influencing longevity are not subject to natural selection as a consequence of their direct effect on longevity. Therefore, two classes of genes are expected. In the first class are genes that have a beneficial effect in early life and thus will be selected despite a detrimental effect in later life. These genes display antagonistic plciotropy (Williams, 1957). In thc sccond class are genes that have a detrimental effect in late life, but fail to be eliminated from the population because they show no detrimental effect early in life (Medawar, 1952). These are neutral genes and natural selection is blind to their presence.

The proximity of the *fer-15* fertility deficit to the *age-1* locus in the long-lived mutants isolated by Klass (1983) led Friedman and Johnson (1988a) and others (Rose, 1991) to propose that *age-1* is a clear example of a gene displaying antagonistic pleiotropy. When *age-1* was separated from the fertility deficit, the cost of the *age-1* mutation was not apparent (Johnson, Tedesco, & Lithgow, 1993). In fact, the enhanced stress response associated with *age-1* suggests that the mutation may be beneficial within certain environmental constraints (Lithgow, White, Hinerfeld, & Johnson, 1994; Lithgow, White, Melov, & Johnson, submitted). However, some strains that contain *age-1* and no other known mutations do exhibit slightly lower total fertility than wild-type strains (Lithgow, White, Hinerfeld, & Johnson, 1994).

The *spe-26* mutation appears to provide a straightforward example of antagonistic pleiotropy. At the restrictive temperature, *spe-26* worms produce no or very few progeny; thus, a "trade-off" is apparent between fertility and life span (Van Voorhies, 1992). Some commentators have been disturbed by the rather high cost of sperm production revealed by this mutation (Partridge & Harvey, 1992). There are two nonmutually exclusive interpretations of this result. First, the *spe-26* gene was selected for beneficial effects in early life, perhaps on fertility, and has a detrimental effect in late life. Second, a limited pool of resources is available, and prevention of sperm production results in more of the resources being available for increased longevity. We must now consider the fact that other mutations that are detrimental to fertility do not result in an altered life span (Johnson, 1984). In addition, fertility can be abolished by laser ablation of the gonad without alteration to life span (Kenyon, Chang, Gensch, Rudner, & Tabtiang, 1993), and the Age phenotype of *age-1* can be observed under conditions in which fertility is zero (Fabian & Johnson, 1994). Our first interpretation of the *spe-26* result is unaffected by these additional observations. However, the second interpretation, which envisions a partitioned pool of resources, is not consistent with a general failure of life span to covary with fertility. If abolition of sperm production alleviates an energy cost, then why do all mutations that depress sperm production not result in increased life span? Although the general principle of antagonistic pleiotropy holds true for *spe-26* and may hold true for *age-1*, the mechanisms by which life span is extended simply cannot be described in terms of the partitioning of limited energy stores between various life history traits, nor are the physiological mechanisms for such partitioning readily apparent.

daf-2 mutants provide another complex set of phenotypes to match with the evolutionary theory of aging. *daf-2* mutation results in the constitutive formation of dauer larvae, which is clearly a reproductive cost as the dauer larvae do not reproduce. Consequently, there is negative covariance of fertility with longevity. However, adult worms exhibit an extended life span and have near-normal fertility (Kenyon, Chang, Gensch, Rudner, & Tabtiang, 1993). Again, it is difficult to reconcile this result with a model in which resources saved in reproductive effort become available for longevity.

The QTL mapping of Shook, Brooks, and Johnson (submitted) is a direct attempt to map loci that affect life span and another life history trait, total fertility. The authors did not observe significant negative covariance for total fertility and life span. Perhaps the cloning of QTLs will provide more information on pleiotropic effects.

B. Damage to Mitochondrial DNA

An interesting correlate of the free radical theory of aging is the mitochondrial DNA damage theory of aging. Miquel and co-workers (1980) suggested that the mitochondrial genome is a major target of oxidative damage following from the generation of reactive oxygen species (ROS), resulting from byproducts of the electron transport chain. Mitochondrial DNA damage would lead to a deficit, presumably in energy (ATP) generation, which drives some senescent processes. This theory was strengthened by the observation of an increasing frequency of mitochondrial DNA deletions (dmtDNA) with age in humans (Corral-Debrinski, Horton, Lott, Shoffner, Flint-Beal, & Wallace, 1992; Cortopassi, Shibata, Soong, & Arnheim, 1992). Melov *et al.* (1994) have detected dmtDNA in aged *C. elegans*. PCR primers were chosen to yield a 4.3-kb band upon amplification. Deletions in this region appear as smaller amplicons. A number of smaller products were obtained, indicating that a number of distinct deletion events can occur. Sequence analysis of the break points shows that deletions occur at or immediately adjacent to direct repeats. Of eight deletion end points analyzed, six occur in or adjacent to tRNA genes. This implicates DNA secondary structure in deletion generation. In an extensive study of the frequency of deletion events, synchronous cohorts of some 900 individual animals in three distinct strains were assessed (Melov, Lithgow, Fischer, Tedesco, & Johnson, 1995). Both wild-type and *age-1* strains were analyzed daily over the life span. Wild-type strains showed an age-related increase in the occurrence of dmtDNAs, but the accumulation of dmtDNAs was retarded by the *age-1* mu-

tation. One interpretation of these results is that *age-1* strains are better able to cope with mitochondrial DNA damage from ROS. No *age-1*-associated increase in the activity of mitochondrial Mn SOD has been reported, and no other candidates for the attenuation of dmtDNA accumulation are obvious. The formal possibility exists that *age-1* encodes an activity directly involved in a mechanism that generates deletions.

C. Stress Response and Life Span

Harman's free radical theory of aging (Harman, 1956, 1992), and subsequent modifications, has prompted a number of important studies on *C. elegans* and other systems. This is a major mechanistic theory of aging with an increasing level of experimental support.

Response to oxidative stress is linked to life span in *Drosophila,* where a causative relationship between the expression of the oxidative-response enzymes, Cu/Zn SOD and catalase, and acceleration of mortality rates has been established (Orr & Sohal, 1994). The *age-1* mutation is associated with elevated levels of Cu/Zn SOD and catalase and resistance to the compounds paraquat and hydrogen peroxide, which increase oxidate stress (Larsen, 1993; Vanfleteren, 1993). Larsen (1993) demonstrated that hydrogen peroxide resistance and Cu/Zn SOD specific activities increase from mid to late life in *age-1* mutant strains. Catalase specific activity increases in both wild type and *age-1* until mid-life, at which point *age-1* strains continue to show an increase and wild type shows a decrease in specific activity. Vanfleteren (1993) showed that Cu/Zn SOD specific activity increased over the life spans of three age strains, while no increase in activity was observed in wild type. Vanfleteren's measurements of catalase are wholly consistent with Larsen's measurements. As elevation of these activities has been shown to increase life span in *Drosophila*, it is likely that these elevated activities contribute to the lower mortality rates in *age-1* strains. However, it is possible that these increased defenses against ROS are not directly related to the changes in life span. Vanfleteren reported that Age animals produce higher levels of the superoxide anion (O_2^-) than wild type in the third week of a cohort's life span. The rise in CU/Zn SOD and catalase activities may be an induced response to intrinsic O_2^- production.

Increased paraquat resistance of *age-1* strains has been observed at 10 (Vanfleteren, 1980) and 3 days of age (Melov, Jensen, & Johnson, unpublished data). Resistance to hydrogen peroxide was observed only in worms older than 15 days (Larsen, 1993). There is no information published on SOD or catalase enzyme activities in young *age-1* animals subjected to extrinsic oxidative stress.

Life-span extension by *age-1* may be a consequence of a more general enhancement in stress response. In addition to resistance to oxidative stress, Age strains are also resistant to thermal stress (Lithgow, White, Hinerfeld, & Johnson, 1994; Lithgow, White, Melov, & Johnson, 1995). Increased thermotolerance (Itt) was observed in a number of *age-1* strains and cosegragated with *age-1*. Mean survival for wild-type strains during thermal stress is 45% less than that for *age-1* mutant strains. This provides for a simple biological assay of genetically defined life span in young adult animals. *daf-2* mutants and *spe-26* mutants are also thermotolerant (Lithgow, White, Melov, & Johnson, 1995), suggesting that thermotolerance may be a characteristic of a number of long-lived mutants. Itt is associated with *age-1* throughout life span, but thermotolerance declines for both wild-type and *age-1* strains (Lithgow, White, Hinerfeld, & Johnson, 1994).

How would thermotolerance be linked to oxidative stress and the determination of life span? Distinct environmental in-

sults induce overlapping sets of stress response genes. For example, oxidative stress will elicit the transcription from the promoter of the *C. elegans* gene encoding heat shock protein 16 (hsp 16) (Candido, personal communication), and thermal stress can induce superoxide dismutase activity in mammalian tissue (Hass & Massaro, 1988). Therefore, tolerance to one stress can be acquired by exposure to another in some cases. *age-1* is both thermotolerant and resistant to oxidative stress, consistent with the wild-type *age-1* gene product being a negative regulator of genes specifying stress resistance. *age-1* may overexpress both radical-scavenging enzymes and heat shock proteins. No measurements of resistance to oxidative stress have been made for *daf-2* or *spe-26* mutant strains.

The effect of oxygen concentration on life span also provides supporting evidence for the detrimental effects of oxidative metabolism. With increasing partial pressures of O_2, mean and maximum life spans decrease, reflecting an increase in the Gompertz mortality rate (Honda & Matsuo, 1992). This effect is exaggerated in *mev-1* mutants. *mev-1* was isolated in a hunt for methyl viologen-sensitive mutants and was shown to exhibit half the Cu/Zn SOD activity of the wild type (Ishii, Takahashi, Tomita, *et al.*, 1990). One would predict that, under oxidative stress, the *mev-1* mutation would fair worse than the wild type, as was the case (Honda, Ishii, Suzuki, & Matsuo, 1993).

It is curious that *rad-8*, which prolongs life span at 16°C, is also hypersensitive to high oxygen partial pressures (Ishii, Suzuki, Hartman, & Suzuki, 1994). Although life span is not increased at normal temperatures, one would not expect a strain sensitive to oxidative stress to exhibit increased life span under any conditions. This observation is interesting in the light of a previous study, which failed to find any correlation between radiation sensitivity and life span in four recombinant–

inbred strains (Hartman, Simpson, Johnson, & Mitchell, 1988). Aside from *rad-8*, there is a general correlation between the ability of a strain to withstand oxidative or thermal stress and its age-specific mortality rate.

There is one more piece of evidence for a causal link between general stress response and life span. Life span can be enhanced in the nematode by transient exposure to a nonlethal stress. Significant extensions in mean life span have been obtained by exposure to ionizing radiation (Johnson & Hartman, 1988) and thermal stress (Lithgow, White, Melov, & Johnson, submitted). Mild thermal stress induces thermotolerance in worms (Lithgow, White, Melov, & Johnson, 1995). Induced thermotolerance has been studied in many systems, from bacteria to mammals, and is a consequence of the increased expression of heat shock proteins (Parsell & Lindquist, 1994). Cohorts of worms that have been induced by transient exposure to 30°C have elevated thermotolerance and modestly but significantly extended life spans (Lithgow, White, Melov, & Johnson, submitted). This suggests that the heat shock proteins, or other gene products induced by a mild thermal stress, influence mortality rate. Why would this be so? Many heat shock proteins exhibit chaperone activity that prevents the aggregation of malfolded protein and allows for the refolding of denatured protein or the targeting of denatured protein for degradation (Morimoto, Tissieres, & Georgopoulos, 1994). When we consider that conformationally altered (inactive) protein accumulates with age in the nematode (Zeelon, Gershon, & Gershon, 1973; Bolla & Brot, 1975; Sharma, Gupta, & Rothstein, 1976; Sharma & Rothstein, 1980), a possible explanation for life extension presents itself. ROS oxidize proteins, resulting in a conformational change. Since these proteins cannot function, mean life span is determined by the rate of accumulation of conformationally altered pro-

tein. This rate can be retarded either by neutralizing ROS or by refolding or removing damaged proteins. Induction of ROS-detoxifying enzymes and molecular chaperones, either by transient stress or by the *age-1, daf-2,* or *spe-26* mutations, slows the rate of accumulation of conformationally altered proteins, thus reducing mortality rates.

V. Summary and Outlook

Encouraging rumblings are emanating from the *C. elegans* aging laboratories. We are focusing on physiological mechanisms that may limit life span. This is almost wholly a consequence of studying the pleiotropic effects of single gene mutations that extend the life span. It is disappointing that clones are not available for these gerontogenes and that transgenic lines have not been constructed that display extended life span. The inability to regulate transgene expression across life span is a serious limitation that warrants attention. However, the sequencing of the genome will undoubtedly help cloning efforts, and additional mutations with significant positive effects on life span are appearing. Complete molecular and physiological analysis of these mutants should clarify the interpretation of associated phenotypes. It is interesting to note that only one of the age mutants currently being studied was isolated in a screen for life-span extension, *age-1*. This suggests that we may be able to isolate longevity mutants by selection for related phenotypes, such as stress resistance. However, it also illustrates the need to expand our current efforts to isolate age mutants by selecting for extended life span. This unstructured approach is not biased by our most cherished mechanistic theories.

A clear leader among mechanistic theories is the free radical theory and its correlates, such as the extent of stress response influencing life span and the mitochondrial theory of aging. Most of the literature discussed in this chapter is consistent with a causal role for ROS and the subsequent accumulation of conformationally altered macromolecules in limiting life span.

Having provided much of the experimental evidence for the genetic determination of life span, invertebrate systems are uniquely placed to quickly test specific mechanistic theories. Without a rapid determination of causality, it is difficult to justify research on the aging of *C. elegans*. Fortunately for those of us working with the worm, that goal is within reach.

Acknowledgments

I thank my colleagues for their helpful suggestions, particularly Simon Melov, Jacqui Brumfield, Tiffany M. White, Beth Bennett, Shin Murakami, David Shook, Tom E. Johnson, Pamela L. Larsen, and Robert J. Shmookler Reis. I am indebted to Pamela L. Larsen, Tom E. Johnson, and David Shook for openly discussing unpublished data.

References

Albert, P. S., & Riddle, D. L. (1988). Mutants of *Caenorhabditis elegans* that form dauer-like larvae. *Development Biology, 126,* 270–293.

Anderson, G. L. (1978). Responses of dauer larvae of *Caenorhabditis elegans* (Nematoda: Rhabditidae) to thermal stress and oxygen deprivation. *Canadian Journal of Zoology, 56,* 1786–1791.

Anderson, G. L. (1982). Superoxide dismutase activity in dauer larvae of *Caenorhabditis elegans* (Nematoda: Rhabditidae). *Canadian Journal of Zoology, 60,* 288–291.

Bolanowski, M. A., Russell, R. L., & Jacobson, L. A. (1981). Quantitative measures of aging in the nematode *Caenorhabditis elegans*. I. Population and longitudinal studies of two behavioral parameters. *Mechanims of Ageing and Development, 15,* 279–295.

Bolanowski, M. A., Jacobson, L. A., & Russell, R. L. (1983). Quantitative measures of aging in the nematode *Caenorhabditis elegans:* II. lysosomal hydrolases as markers of senes-cence. *Mechanisms of Ageing and Development, 21,* 295–319.

Bolla, R., & Brot, N. (1975). Age dependent changes in enzymes involved in macromolecular synthesis in *Turbatrix aceti*. *Archives of Biochemistry and Biophysics, 169,* 227–236.

Brenner, S. (1974). The genetics of *Caenorhabditis elegans*. *Genetics, 77,* 71–94.

Brenner, S. (1988). Foreword. In W. Wood (Ed.), *The Nematode Caenorhabditis elegans* (pp. ix–xiii). Cold Spring Harbor, NY: Cold Spring Harbor Laboratory Press.

Brooks, A., & Johnson, T. E. (1991). Genetic specification of life span and self-fertility in recombinant- inbred strains of *Caenorhabditis elegans*. *Heredity (Edinburgh), 67,* 19–28.

Brooks, A., Lithgow, G. J., & Johnson, T. E. (1994). Mortality rates in a genetically heterogeneous population of *Caenorhabditis elegans*. *Science, 263,* 668–671.

Broverman, S., MacMorris, M., & Blumenthal, T. (1993). Alteration of *Caenorhabditis elegans* gene expression by targeted transformation. *Proceedings of the National Academy of Sciences of the United States of America, 90,* 4359–4363.

Carey, J. R. (1991). Establishment of the Mediterranean fruit fly in California. *Science, 253,* 1369–1373.

Carey, J. R., Liedo, P., Orozco, D., & Vaupel, J. W. (1992). Slowing of mortality rates at older ages in large medfly cohorts. *Science, 258,* 457–461.

Charlesworth, B. (1980). *Evolution in Age-Structured Populations*. Cambridge: Cambridge University Press.

Corral-Debrinski, M., Horton, T., Lott, M. T., Shoffner, J. M., Flint-Beal, M., & Wallace, D. C. (1992). Mitochondrial DNA deletions in human brain: regional variability and increased with advanced age. *Nature Genetics, 2,* 324–329.

Cortopassi, G. A., Shibata, D., Soong, N. W., & Arnheim, N. (1992). A pattern of accumulation of a somatic deletion of mitochondrial DNA in aging human tissues. *Proceedings of the National Academy of Sciences of the United States of America, 89,* 7370–7374.

Coulson, A., Waterston, R., Kiff, J., Sulston, J., & Kohara, Y. (1988). Genome linking with yeast artificial chromosomes. *Nature, 335,* 184–186.

Coulson, A., Kozono, Y., Lutterbach, B., Shownkeen, R., Sulston, J., & Waterston, R. (1991). YACs and the *C. elegans* genome. *Bioessays, 13,* 413–417.

Croll, N. A., Smith, J. M., & Zuckerman, B. M. (1977). The aging process of the nematode *Caenorhabditis elegans* in bacterial and axenic culture. *Experimental Aging Research, 3,* 175–189.

Curtsinger, J. W., Fukui, H. H., Townsend, D. R., & Vaupel, J. W. (1992). Demography of genotypes: failure of the limited life-span paradigm in *Drosophila melanogaster*. *Science, 258,* 461–463.

Davis, B. O., Jr., Anderson, G. L., & Dusenbery, D. B. (1982). Total luminescence spectroscopy of fluorescence changes during aging in *Caenorhabditis elegans*. *Biochemistry, 21,* 4089–4095.

Duhon, S. A., & Johnson, T. E. (1995). Movement as an index of vitality: comparing wild-type and the *age-1* mutant of *Caenorhabditis elegans*. *Journal of Gerontology: Biological Sciences, 50,* B254–261.

Durbin, R., & Thierry-Mieg, J. (1991). acedb-A *C. elegans* Database, MRC Laboratory for Molecular Biology, Cambridge, UK, unpublished.

Ebert, R. H., Cherkasova, V. A., Dennis, R. A., Wu, J. H., Ruggles, S., Perrin, T. E., & Reis, R. J. S. (1993). Longevity-determining genes in *Caenorhabditis elegans:* chromosomal mapping of multiple noninteractive loci. *Genetics, 135,* 1003–1010.

Egilmez, N. K., & Shmookler Reis, R. J. (1994). Age-dependent somatic excision of transposable element Tc1 in *Caenorhabditis elegans*. *Mutation Research, 316,* 17–24.

Egilmez, N. K., Ebert, R. H., & Shmookler Reis, R. J. (1995). Strain evolution in *Caenorhabditis elegans:* Transposable elements as markers of interstrain evolutionary history. *Journal of Molecular Evolution, 40,* 372–381.

Emmons, S. W. (1988). The genome. In W. B. Wood (Ed.), *The Nematode Caenorhabditis Elegans* (pp. 47–79). Cold Spring Harbor, NY: Cold Spring Harbor Laboratory Press.

Estevez, M., Attisano, L., Wrana, J. L., Albert, P. S., Massague, J., & Riddle, D. L. (1993). The *daf-4* gene encodes a bone morphogenetic protein receptor controlling *C. elegans* dauer larva development. *Nature, 365,* 644–649.

Fabian, T. J. (1993). Analysis of transcript abundance during aging in the nematode *Caenorhabditis elegans*. University of Colorado. Ph.D. thesis.

Fabian, T. J., & Johnson, T. E. (1994). Production of age-synchronous mass cultures of *Caenorhabditis elegans*. *Journal of Gerontology: Biological Sciences, 49,* B145–B156.

Fabian, T. J., & Johnson, T. E. (1995). Identification of genes that are differentially expressed during aging in *Caenorhabditis elegans*. *Journal of Gerontology: Biological Sciences, 50,* 245–253.

Finch, C. E. (1990). *Longevity, Senescence and the Genome.* Chicago and London: University of Chicago Press.

Fire, A. (1986). Integrative transformation of *Caenorhabditis elegans*. *EMBO Journal, 5,* 2673–2680.

Fire, A., Kondo, K., & Waterston, R. (1990). Vectors for low copy transformation of *C. elegans*. *Nucleic Acids Research, 18,* 4269–4270.

Fire, A., Albertson, D., Harrison, S. W., & Moerman, D. G. (1991). Production of antisense RNA leads to effective and specific inhibition of gene expression in *C. elegans* muscle. *Development, 113,* 503–514.

Friedman, D. B., & Johnson, T. E. (1988a). A mutation in the *age-1* gene in *Caenorhabditis elegans* lengthens life and reduces hermaphrodite fertility. *Genetics, 118,* 75–86.

Friedman, D. B., & Johnson, T. E. (1988b). Three mutants that extend both mean and maximum life span of the nematode, *Caenorhabditis elegans*, define the *age-1* gene. *Journal of Gerontology: Biological Sciences, 43,* B102–9.

Fukui, H. H., Xiu, L., & Curtsinger, J. W. (1993). Slowing of age-specific mortality rates in *Drosophila melanogaster*. *Experimental Gerontology, 28,* 585–599.

Gandhi, S., Santelli, J., Mitchell, D. H., Stiles, J. W., & Sanadi, D. R. (1980). A simple method for maintaining large, aging populations of *Caenorhabditis elegans*. *Mechanisms of Ageing and Development, 12,* 137–150.

Gbewonyo, K., Rohrer, S. P., Lister, L., Burgess, B., Cully, D., & Buckland, B. (1994). Large scale cultivation of the free living nematode *Caenorhabditis elegans*. *Biotechnology, 12,* 51–54.

Georgi, L. L., Albert, P. S., & Riddle, D. L. (1990). daf-1, a *C. elegans* gene controlling dauer larva development, encodes a novel receptor protein kinase. *Cell, 61,* 635–645.

Golden, J. W., & Riddle, D. L. (1982). A pheromone influences larval development in the nematode *Caenorhabditis elegans*. *Science*, *218*, 578–580.

Golden, J. W., & Riddle, D. L. (1984a). A pheromone-induced developmental switch in *Caenorhabditis elegans:* Temperature-sensitive mutants reveal a wild-type temperature-dependent process. *Proceedings of the National Academy of Sciences of the United States of America*, *81*, 819–823.

Golden, J. W., & Riddle, D. L. (1984b). The *Caenorhabditis elegans* dauer larva: developmental effects of pheromone, food, and temperature. *Developmental Biology*, *102*, 368–378.

Golden, J. W., & Riddle, D. L. (1985). A gene affecting production of the *Caenorhabditis elegans* dauer-inducing pheromone. *Molecular and General Genetics*, *198*, 534–536.

Gottlieb, S., & Ruvkun, G. (1994). *daf-2, daf-16* and *daf-23:* Genetically interacting genes controlling dauer formation in *Caenorhabditis elegans*. *Genetics*, *137*, 107–120.

Hamilton, W. D. (1966). The moulding of senescence by natural selection. *Journal of Theoretical Biology*, *12*, 12–45.

Harman, D. (1956). Aging: a theory based on free radical and radiation chemistry. *Journal of Gerontology*, *11*, 298–300.

Harman, D. (1992). Free radical theory of aging. *Mutation Research*, *275*, 257–266.

Hartman, P. S., & Herman, R. K. (1982). Radiation-sensitive mutants of *Caenorhabditis elegans*. *Genetics*, *102*, 159–178.

Hartman, P. S., Simpson, V. J., Johnson, T. E., & Mitchell, D. (1988). Radiation sensitivity and DNA repair in *Caenorhabditis elegans* strains with different mean life spans. *Mutation Research*, *208*, 77–82.

Hass, M. A., & Massaro, D. (1988). Regulation of the synthesis of superoxide dismutase in rat lungs during oxidant and hyperthermic stresses. *Journal of Biological Chemistry*, *263*, 776–781.

Honda, S., & Matsuo, M. (1992). Lifespan shortening of the nematode *Caenorhabditis elegans* under higher concentrations of oxygen. *Mechanisms of Ageing and Development*, *63*, 235–246.

Honda, S., Ishii, N., Suzuki, K., & Matsuo, M. (1993). Oxygen-dependent perturbation of life span and aging rate in the nematode. *Journal of Gerontology: Biological Sciences*, *48*, B57–61.

Hosono, R. (1978a). Sterilization and growth inhibition of *Caenorhabditis elegans* by 5-fluorodeoxyuridine. *Experimental Gerontology*, *13*, 369–374.

Hosono, R. (1978b). Age dependent changes in the behavior of *Caenorhabditis elegans* on attraction to *Escherichia coli*. *Experimental Gerontology*, *13*, 31–36.

Hosono, R., Sato, Y., Aizawa, S. I., & Mitsui, Y. (1980). Age-dependent changes in mobility and separation of the nematode *Caenorhabditis elegans*. *Experimental Gerontology*, *15*, 285–289.

Ishii, N., Takahashi, K., Tomita, S., Keino, T., Honda, S., Yoshino, K., & Suzuki, K. A. (1990). Methyl viologen-sensitive mutant of the nematode *Caenorhabditis elegans*. *Mutation Research*, *237*, 165–171.

Ishii, N. Suzuki, N., Hartman, P. S., & Suzuki, K. (1994). The effects of temperature on the longevity of a radiation-sensitive mutant *rad-8* of the nematode *Caenorhabditis elegans*. *Journal of Gerontology: Biological Sciences*, *49*, B117–120.

Johnson, K., & Hirsh, D. (1979). Patterns of proteins synthesized during development of *Caenorhabditis elegans*. *Developmental Biology*, *70*, 241–248.

Johnson, T. E. (1984). Analysis of the biological basis of aging in the Nematode, with special emphasis on *Caenorhabditis elegans*. In D. H. Mitchell & T. E. Johnson (Eds.), *Invertebrate Models in Aging Research* (pp. 59–93). Boca Raton, FL: CRC Press Inc.

Johnson, T. E. (1986). Molecular and genetic analyses of a multivariate system specifying behavior and life span. *Behavioral Genetics*, *16*, 221–235.

Johnson, T. E. (1987). Aging can be genetically dissected into component processes using long-lived lines of *Caenorhabditis elegans*. *Proceedings of the National Academy of Sciences of the United States of America*, *84*, 3777–3781.

Johnson, T. E. (1988). Genetic specification of life span: processes, problems, and potentials. *Journal of Gerontology: Biological Sciences*, *43*, B87–92.

Johnson, T. E. (1990a). Increased life-span of *age-1* mutants in *Caenorhabditis elegans* and lower Gompertz rate of aging. *Science*, *249*, 908–912.

Johnson, T. E. (1990b). *Caenorhabditis elegans* offers the potential for molecular dissection of the aging process. In E. L. Schneider & J. W. Rowe (Eds)., *Handbook of the Biology of Aging* (pp. 45–59). New York: Academic Press.

Johnson, T. E. (1993). Genetic influences on aging in mammals and invertebrates. *Aging: Clinical and Experimental Research, 5*, 299–307.

Johnson, T. E., & Wood, W. B. (1982). Genetic analysis of life-span in *Caenorhabditis elegans. Proceedings of the National Academy of Sciences of the United States of America, 79*, 6603–6607.

Johnson, T. E., & McCaffrey, G. (1985). Programmed aging or error catastrophe? An examination by two-dimensional polyacrylamide gel electrophoresis. *Mechanisms of Ageing and Development, 30*, 285–297.

Johnson, T. E., & Hartman, P. S. (1988). Radiation effects on life span in *Caenorhabditis elegans. Journal of Gerontology: Biological Sciences, 43*, B137–41.

Johnson, T. E., & Lithgow, G. J. (1992). The search for the genetic basis of aging: the identification of gerontogenes in the nematode *Caenorhabditis elegans. Journal of the American Geriatrics Society, 40*, 936–945.

Johnson, T. E., & Hutchinson, E. W. (1993). Absence of strong heterosis for life span and other life history traits in *Caenorhabditis elegans. Genetics, 134*, 465–474.

Johnson, T. E., Conley, W. L., & Keller, M. L. (1988). Long-lived lines of *Caenorhabditis elegans* can be used to establish predictive biomarkers of aging. *Experimental Gerontology, 23*, 281–295.

Johnson, T. E., Tedesco, P. M., & Lithgow, G. J. (1993). Comparing mutants, selective breeding, and transgenics in the dissection of aging processes of *Caenorhabditis elegans. Genetica, 91*, 65–77.

Jones, D., Russnak, R. H., Kay, R. J., & Candido, E. P. (1986). Structure, expression, and evolution of a heat shock gene locus in *Caenorhabditis elegans* that is flanked by repetitive elements. *Journal of Biological Chemistry, 261*, 12006–12015.

Jones, D., Dixon, D. K., Graham, R. W., & Candido, E. P. (1989). Differential regulation of closely related members of the hsp16 gene family in *Caenorhabditis elegans. DNA, 8*, 481–490.

Kenyon, C., Chang, J., Gensch, E., Rudner, A., & Tabtiang, R. (1993). A *C. elegans* mutant that lives twice as long as wild type. *Nature, 366*, 461–464.

Kimble, J., Hodgkin, J., Smith, T., & Smith, J. (1982). Suppression of an amber mutation by microinjection of suppressor tRNA in *Caenorhabditis elegans. Nature, 299*, 456–458.

Klass, M. R. (1983). A method for the isolation of longevity mutants in the nematode *Caenorhabditis elegans* and initial results. *Mechanisms of Ageing and Development, 22*, 279–286.

Klass, M., & Hirsh, D. (1976). Non-ageing developmental variant of *Caenorhabditis elegans. Nature, 260*, 523–525.

Klass, M. R., & Johnson, T. E. (1985). *Caenorhabditis elegans. Interdisciplinary Topics in Gerontology, 21*, 164–187.

Klass, M., Nguyen, P. N., & Dechavigny, A. (1983). Age-correlated changes in the DNA template in the nematode *Caenorhabditis elegans. Mechanisms of Ageing and Development, 22*, 253–263.

Larsen, P. L. (1993). Aging and resistance to oxidative damage in *Caenorhabditis elegans. Proceedings of the National Academy of Sciences of the United States of America, 90*, 8905–8909.

Larsen, P. L., Albert, P. S., & Riddle, D. L. (1995). Genes that regulate development and longevity in *Caeorhabditis elegans. Genetics, 139*, 1567–1583.

Liao, L. W., Rosenzweig, B., & Hirsh, D. (1983). Analysis of a transposable element in *Caenorhabditis elegans. Proceedings of the National Academy of Sciences of the United States of America, 80*, 3585–3589.

Lithgow, G. J., White, T. M., Hinerfeld, D. A., & Johnson, T. E. (1994). Thermotolerance of a long-lived mutant of *Caenorhabditis elegans. Journal of Gerontology: Biological Sciences, 49*, B270–B276.

Lithgow, G. J., White, T. M., Melov, S., & Johnson, T. E. (1995). Thermotolerance and extended life span conferred by single-gene mutations and induced by thermal stress. *Proceedings of the National Academy of Sciences of the United States of America, 92*, 7540–7544.

Malone, E. A., & Thomas, J. H. (1994). A screen for nonconditional dauer-constitutive mutations in *Caenorhabditis elegans, Genetics, 136*, 879–886.

eval72 Gordon J. Lithgow

McCombie, W. R., Adams, M. D., Kelley, J. M., FitzGerald, M. G., Utterback, T. R., Khan, M., Dubnick, M., Kerlavage, A. R., Venter, J. C., & Fields, C. (1992). *Caenorhabditis elegans* expressed sequence tags identify gene families and potential disease gene homologues. *Nature Genetics, 1,* 124–131.

Medawar, P. B. (1952). *An Unsolved Problem of Biology.* London: H. K. Lewis.

Meheus, L., & Vanfleteren, J. R. (1986). Nuclease digestion of DNA and RNA in nuclei from young adult and senescent *Caenorhabditis elegans* (Nematoda). *Mechanisms of Ageing and Development, 34,* 23–34.

Meheus, L. A., Van Beeumen, J. J., Coomans, A. V., & Vanfleteren, J. R. (1987). Age-specific nuclear proteins in the nematode worm *Caenorhabditis elegans. Biochemical Journal, 245,* 257–261.

Mello, C. C., Kramer, J. M., Stinchcomb, D., & Ambros, V. (1991). Efficient gene transfer in *C. elegans:* extrachromosomal maintenance and integration of transforming sequences. *EMBO Journal, 10,* 3959–3970.

Melov, S., Hertz, G. Z., Stormo, G. D., & Johnson, T. E. (1994). Detection of deletions in the mitochondrial genome of *Caenorhabditis elegans. Nucleic Acids Research, 22,* 1075–1078.

Melov, S., Lithgow, G. J., Fisher, D. R., Tedesco, P. M., & Johnson, T. E. (1995). Increased frequency of deletions in the mitochondrial genome with age of *Caenorhabditis elegans. Nucleic Acids Research, 23,* 1419–1425.

Miquel, J., Economos, J., Fleming, J., & Johnson, J. E., Jr. (1980). Mitochondrial role in cell aging. *Experimental Gerontology, 15,* 575–591.

Mitchell, D. H., Stiles, J. W., Santelli, J., & Sanadi, D. R. (1979). Synchronous growth and aging of *Caenorhabditis elegans* in the presence of fluorodeoxyuridine. *Journal of Gerontology: Biological Sciences, 34,* 28–36.

Mori, I., Moerman, D. G., & Waterston, R. H. (1988). Analysis of a mutator activity necessary for germline transposition and excision of Tc1 transposable elements in *Caenorhabditis elegans. Genetics, 120,* 397–407.

Morimoto, R. I., Tissieres, A., & Georgopoulos, C. (1994). *The Biology of Heat Shock Proteins and Molecular Chaperones.* Cold Spring Harbor, NY: Cold Spring Harbor Laboratory Press.

Orr, W. C., & Sohal, R. S. (1994). Extension of life-span by overexpression of superoxide dismutase and catalase in *Drosophila melanogaster. Science, 263,* 1128–1130.

Parsell, D. A., & Lindquist, S. (1994). Heat shock proteins and stress tolerance. In R. I. Morimoto, A. Tissieres, & C. Georgopoulos (Eds.), *The Biology of Heat Shock Proteins and Molecular Chaperones* (pp. 457–494). Cold Spring Harbor, NY: Cold Spring Harbor Laboratory Press.

Patridge, L., & Harvey, P. H. (1992). What the sperm count costs. *Nature, 360,* 415.

Riddle, D. L. (1988). The dauer larva. In W. B. Wood (Ed.), *The Nematode Caenorhabditis elegans* (pp. 393–412). Cold Spring Harbor, NY: Cold Spring Harbor Laboratory Press.

Rose, M. R. (1991). *Evolutionary Biology of Aging.* New York: Oxford University Press, Inc.

Russell, R. L., & Jacobson, L. A. (1985). Some aspects of aging can be studied easily in nematodes. In *Handbook of the Biology of Aging.* New York: Van Nostrand Reinhold.

Russnak, R. H., & Candido, E. P. (1985). Locus encoding a family of small heat shock genes in *Caenorhabditis elegans:* two genes duplicated to form a 3.8-kilobase inverted repeat. *Molecular and Cellular Biology, 5,* 1268–1278.

Sarkis, G. J., Ashcom, J. D., Hawdon, J. M., & Jacobson, L. A. (1988). Decline in protease activities with age in the nematode *Caenorhabditis elegans. Mechanisms of Ageing and Development, 45,* 191–201.

Sharma, H. K., & Rothstein, M. (1980). Altered enolase in aged *Turbatrix aceti* results from conformational changes in the enzyme. *Proceedings of the National Academy of Sciences of the United States of America, 77,* 5865–5868.

Sharma, H. K., Gupta, S. K., & Rothstein, M. (1976). Age-related alteration of enolase in the free-living nematode. *Turbatrix aceti. Archives of Biochemistry and Biophysics, 174,* 324–332.

Spieth, J., MacMorris, M., Broverman, S., Greenspoon, S., & Blumenthal, T. (1988). Regulated expression of a vitellogenin fusion gene in transgenic nematodes. *Developmental Biology, 130,* 285–293.

Stinchcomb, D. T., Shaw, J. E., Carr, S. H., & Hirsh, D. (1985). Extrachromosomal DNA transformation of *Caenorhabditis elegans.*

Molecular and Cellular Biology, 5, 3484–3496.

Sulston, J. E., & Brenner, S. (1974). The DNA of *Caenorhabditis elegans. Genetics, 77,* 95–104.

Thomas, J. H., Birnby, D. A., & Vowels, J. J. (1993). Evidence for parallel processing of sensory information controlling dauer formation in *Caenorhabditis elegans. Genetics, 134,* 1105–1117.

Vanfleteren, J. R. (1980). Nematodes as nutritional models. In E. B. Zuckerman (Ed.), *Nematodes as Biological Models: Aging and Other Model Systems* (pp. 47–79). New York: Academic Press.

Vanfleteren, J. R. (1993). Oxidative stress and ageing in *Caenorhabditis elegans. Biochemistry Journal, 292,* 605–608.

Van Voorhies, W. A. (1992). Production of sperm reduces nematode lifespan. *Nature, 360,* 456–458.

Vaupel, J. W., & Carey, J. R. (1993). Compositional interpretations of medfly mortality. *Science, 260,* 1666–1667.

Vaupel, J. W., Johnson, T. E., & Lithgow, G. J. (1994). Rates of mortality in populations of *Caenorhabditis elegans. Science, 266,* 826.

Vowels, J. J., & Thomas, J. H. (1992). Genetic analysis of chemosensory control of dauer formation in *Caenorhabditis elegans. Genetics, 130,* 105–123.

Waterson, R., Martin, C., Craxton, M., Huynh, C., Coulson, A., Hillier, L., Durbin, R., Green, P., Shownkeen, R., Halloran, N., Metzstein, M., Hawkins, T., Wilson, R., Berks, M., Du, Z., Thomas, K., Thierry-Mieg, J., & Sulston, J. (1992). A survey of expressed genes in *Caenorhabditis elegans. Nature Genetics, 1,* 114–123.

Williams, B. D., Schrank, B., Huynh, C., Shownkeen, R., & Waterston, R. H. (1992). A genetic mapping system in *Caenorhabditis elegans* based on polymorphic sequence-tagged sites. *Genetics, 131,* 609–624.

Williams, G. C. (1957). Pleiotropy, natural selection, and the evolution of senescence. *Evolution, 11,* 398–411.

Wilson, R., Ainscough, R., Anderson, K., Baynes, C., Berks, M., Bonfield, J., Burton, J., Connell, M., Copsey, T., Cooper, J., Coulson, A., Craxton, M., Dear, S., Du, Z., Durbin, R., Favello, A., Fraser, A., Fulton, L., Gardner, A., Green, P., Hawkins, T., Hillier, L., Jier, M., Johnston, L., Jones, M., Kershaw, J., Kirsten, J., Laisster, N., Latreille, P., Lightning, J., Lloyd, C., Mortimore, B., O'Callaghan, M., Parsons, J., Percy, C., Rifken, L., Roopra, A., Saunders, D., Shownkeen, R., Sims, M., Smaldon, N., Smith, A., Smith, M., Sonnhammer, E., Staden, R., Sulston, J., Thierry-Mieg, J., Thomas, K., Vaudin, M., Vaughan, K., Waterston, R., Watson, A., Weinstock, L., Wilkinson-Sproat, J., & Wohldman, P. (1994). 2.2 Mb of contiguous nucleotide sequence from chromosome III of *C. elegans. Nature, 368,* 32–38.

Wood, W. B. (1988). Introduction to *C. elegans* biology. In W. B. Wood (Ed.), *The Nematode Caenorhabditis elegans* (pp. 1–16). Cold Spring Harbor, NY: Cold Spring Harbor Laboratory Press.

Wood, W. B., & Johnson, T. E. (1994). Stopping the clock. *Current Biology, 4,* 151–153.

Zeelon, P., Gershon, H., & Gershon, D. (1973). Inactive enzyme molecules in aging organisms. Nematode fructose-1, 6-diphosphate aldolase. *Biochemistry, 12,* 1743–1750.

Zuckerman, B. M. (1980). Achievement of age synchrony in *Caenorhabditis elegans* [letter]. *Journal of Gerontology: Biological Sciences, 35,* 282–283.

Zwaal, R. R., Broeks, A., van Meurs, J., Groenen, J. T., & Plasterk, R. H. (1993). Target-selected gene inactivation in *Caenorhabditis elegans* by using a frozen transposon insertion mutant bank. *Proceedings of the National Academy of Sciences of the United States of America, 90,* 7431–7435.

Five

Genetics of Aging in *Drosophila*

James E. Fleming and Michael R. Rose

I. Introduction

A. The Need for Genetic Studies

Unraveling of the genetics of aging constitutes a major area of investigation in contemporary experimental gerontology. At present, there is a dearth of information on the genes that play a major role in controlling the life spans of animals. As aptly noted by Finch (1990), "We cannot explain why age-related changes of mammals are generally so similar in their specific details and in the fraction of the lifespan in which they occur, despite thirtyfold differences in lifespan." Given these great differences between the life spans of different species, even when reared in similar environments, genetic differences must ultimately determine species life spans.

B. Good, Bad, and Ugly Genetics of Aging

Not all genetic effects on life span necessarily involve the mechanisms that determine normal life span. The genetic analysis of reduced life span has led to the identification of metabolic deficiencies

that can hasten death, such as acatalasemia in *Drosophila* mutants (Bewley & Mackay, 1990). Indeed, mutations of large effect generally shorten the life span of laboratory animals, particularly *Drosophila*. The analysis of mutant strains with short life spans is not likely to shed much light on the genetics of normal aging. Deterioration and death in such short-lived mutants may depend on the introduction of novel pathologies, rather than on an acceleration in the mechanisms of normal aging (Maynard Smith, 1966) (see examples given in II.A).

An alternative approach is to create stocks with genetically postponed aging. This has been achieved by means of mutagenesis and selection on recombinant inbreds in *Caenorhabditis elegans*, a nematode (Johnson & Wood, 1982), and genetic transformation in *Drosophila* (e.g., Reveillaud *et al.*, 1991; Orr & Sohal, 1994). It has also been achieved by selection on outbred *Drosophila* populations (Rose, 1991). The great advantage of the postponed-aging approach is that genetic interventions that prolong life and postpone the physiological symptoms of aging must, in some manner, affect the mechanisms that would

Handbook of the Biology of Aging, Fourth Edition
Copyright © 1996 Academic Press, Inc. All rights of reproduction in any form reserved.

otherwise give rise to aging of the organism at its normal time. Clearly, the identification of specific genes or sets of genes that can postpone aging in an experimental system such as *Drosophila* or *Caenorhabditis* would accelerate progress in the field of gerontology. In addition, genetic stocks such as *Drosophila melanogaster* with postponed aging have the potential to be model systems for biomedical research, in the sense that it is more convenient to use them to test basic technologies that could eventually be used to postpone aging in mammalian species. Thus, the postponement, rather than the acceleration, of aging is the experimental strategy of choice in the genetics of aging.

C. *Drosophila* as a Model System

The common laboratory fruit fly, *Drosophila melanogaster*, is an extremely well-known species from the standpoint of genetics, development, biochemistry, and phylogeny, which makes it an attractive model for any research program. Thus, it is not surprising that *Drosophila* provides an excellent system for the study of the genetics of aging (Rose *et al.*, 1992a). For example, if an investigator wishes to test one of the many hypotheses of aging, such as the somatic mutation theory, then an experimental test with an insect is as valid as a far more cumbersome test in a mammalian species (e.g., Fleming *et al.*, 1986). Given the short life span and small body size of *Drosophila* species, it is much easier to assay numerous flies for aging-related characteristics, including mean and maximum longevity. An example involves the use of *Drosophila* stocks by Curtsinger *et al.* (1992) to examine demographic models of aging. In addition, there are several important parallels between *Drosophila* and mammals that suggest analogous mechanisms in the control of aging for both groups of organisms. Both have diploid karyotypes, chromosomal sex determination, outbreeding, iteroparity, and abundant genetic polymorphism. Moreover, adult *Drosophila* show many of the age-dependent cellular, morphological, and biochemical changes also observed in mammals (Miquel *et al.*, 1981).

It is often argued that gerontological research on models such as *C. elegans* and *Drosophila* may not be directly relevant to understanding mammalian aging, since these models lack important physiological parallels with mammals. All animals, however, regardless of their level of organization, share common functional needs such as locomotion, sensory perception, feeding and digestion, water and ionic balance, excretion, respiration, and reproduction (Miquel *et al.*, 1981; Smith, 1968). Although there are clear differences between the internal organs of insects and mammals, they show similarities in cellular organization and function (Miquel *et al.*, 1981; Smith, 1968). For example, the muscular system and nervous system have different distributions of excitable cells, but the mechanisms of impulse conduction are identical. There are also similarities between the digestive systems and between the mammalian liver and the insect fat body.

Despite these similarities, there are several important differences between the physiological and cellular makeups of *Drosophila* and mammals. The transport of oxygen in insects is carried out by the use of tracheoles, whereas in mammals oxygen transport is accomplished by the circulatory system. In *Drosophila*, the circulatory system is involved only with the transport of nutrients (Miquel *et al.*, 1981). Thus, pigments such as hemoglobin, which function to transport oxygen in mammals, are not required in insects since oxygen is brought directly to the cells through the tracheoles. A collagen framework supports the organ architecture of insects, as in mammals; however, insects have no fibroblasts and collagen is not synthesized in the adult (Miquel *et al.*, 1981; Smith, 1968). In mammals, there are many cell types that can be categorized on the basis of their proliferative behavior (mammals have undifferentiated stem cells and several other dividing cell types), but in *Drosophila* all of the somatic cells are of the fixed postmitotic type (Bozuck, 1972).

It is pertinent that both insects and mammals show similar age-related, fine structural changes in their fixed postmitotic cells. These include nuclear inclusions, various cytoplasmic alterations, increased lipofuscin, decreased ribosome number, and significant alterations in the number and shape of mitochondria (Miquel *et al.*, 1980; Fleming *et al.*, 1982; Miquel & Fleming, 1986). Miquel has also noted some fundamental cellular differences between mammalian (C57BL/6J strain of mouse) and *Drosophila melanogaster* (Ore-R strain) aging. No alterations are apparent in the extracellular framework of senescent *Drosophila*. However, old mice experience significant changes in the integrity of their collagen matrix, especially around blood vessels where there is an increase in collagen (Miquel *et al.*, 1981). There is a conspicuous absence of significant structural changes in the replicating cells of old mice, whereas old *Drosophila* display dramatic changes in their somatic tissues (Miquel *et al.*, 1981). In their excellent comparative analysis, Miquel *et al.* conclude that the fine structural evidence suggests that mice and flies show very similar mechanisms of aging at the level of postmitotic cells (Miquel *et al.*, 1981).

While *Drosophila* is in no sense a miniature mammal, its aging nonetheless is broadly analogous to mammalian aging. In particular, as a genetic system it is much more analogous to a mammal than the rival yeast and nematode models, which are predominantly self-fertilizing, the many practical benefits of working with those systems notwithstanding.

II. Historical Background

A. Early Attempts To Unravel the Genetics of Aging in *Drosophila*

Attempts to unravel the genetics of aging in *Drosophila* date back to at least the early studies of Pearl and his colleagues (Pearl & Doering, 1923; Pearl *et al.*, 1923), in which heritable variations in life span were observed for inbred lines and genetic mutants. They demonstrated the inheritance of longevity by creating inbred lines in the laboratory that expressed abnormal morphological phenotypes (e.g., vestigial) that were associated with survivorship. The F_1 hybrids of these inbred lines had increased life spans. However, the mean life spans of these longer lived hybrids were similar to those of the parental outbred populations. Moreover, the F_2 generations showed longevities that were reduced to levels similar to those of the inbred lines. These results suggested that the reduced longevities observed in the inbred lines were the result of fixation of recessive deleterious alleles that affect longevity.

Genetic crossing of inbred lines continued in later years with the studies of Clarke and Maynard Smith (1955). They also demonstrated that F_1 hybrids from inbred lines of *Drosophila subobscura* had distinctively longer life spans, but were not morphologically distinct. The likely explanation of these results is that inbreeding leads to the fixation of genes with deleterious effects on survivorship (Crow, 1948; Wright, 1977). A similar effect was observed by Gowen in 1952 with the F_1 hybrids from a cross between various wild strains obtained from different regions of North America. Senescence in inbred lines of *Drosophila* is determined by how many and which deleterious alleles are fixed during inbreeding (Rose, 1984a). The use of such lines in studies of *Drosophila* aging is a matter of considerable debate. An understanding of the genetics of aging in inbred laboratory lines may not be relevant to what happens in outbred wild populations or may not even lead to an understanding of the genetics of aging of naturally inbred lines in the wild (Rose, 1991, pp. 35–6). This contrast was demonstrated experimentally by Rose (1984a), who showed that inbreeding *Drosophila* causes their genetic correlations between aging characters to reverse in sign. However, this is not an argument against the use of inbred lines in biology generally, nor even in aging research specifically (cf. Johnson & Wood, 1982).

Aging has been studied using mutant strains of *Drosophila* by a number of investigators over the years. In this approach, disruption of a specific gene is hypothesized to affect longevity in a mechanism-specific manner, so that a genetic analysis can be carried out. A number of mutants have been generated and described that affect the life span of *Drosophila*. In very early studies, Gowen (1931) carried out a study of diploid and triploid female *Drosophila melanogaster*. The results suggested that there is no influence of ploidy on life span. In related work outside of the genus *Drosophila*, Clark and Rubin (1961) carried out a very interesting study with haploid and diploid cohorts of the male wasp *Habrobracon serinopae*. They showed that there is no difference in the life spans of these two ploides under normal conditions, but that irradiation significantly reduced the life span of the haploid stocks relative to the diploid. Although the effect of gene dosage compensation on longevity in these species is not known nor is it known whether the critical tissues affecting longevity are polyploid, the results provide strong evidence against the importance of accumulation of somatic mutations with age in insects. Trout and Kaplan (1981) examined two neurological mutants, Hyperkinetic (Hk1) and Shaker (Sh3), and reported that they had reduced life spans of about 20% from control, with correspondingly

increased metabolic rates and physical activity. By using mosaic mutants of the Hk1 and Sh3 genes, they showed that expression of these genes in the ventral thorax tissue results in shorter life spans than mosaic controls. Although all of these mutants had reduced life spans, the technique might be employed in genetic transformation studies in which inserted genes have positive effects on life span.

Many of the mutant studies in insect aging have been reviewed extensively by Baker *et al.* (1985) and Mayer and Baker (1985) and discussed in an article by Arking and Dudas (1989). The reader is referred to these reports for more detail regarding the many mutations that have been examined in relation to the life span of *Drosophila*. Several are worthy of discussion here for their historical interest, as well as examples of mutations that do not lead to instances of accelerated senescence. The dunce gene, which affects the activity of cAMP phosphodiesterase II, results in decreased learning ability and shortened life span (Bellen & Kiger, 1987). This neurological mutation is also interesting in terms of the role of reproduction in regulating life span, since female mutants mate significantly more frequently than wild-type controls. Another neurological mutant, drop-dead (drd), is a short-lived mutant whose reduced life span is accompanied by neuron loss and rapid brain degeneration (Hotta & Benzer, 1972). It is not clear, however, whether the brain atrophy observed in the drop-dead mutant is similar to the atrophy of normal brain aging. Van Delden and Soliman (1988) have examined a well-characterized locus in *Drosophila*, the alcohol dehydrogenase (adh) allele. Alcohol dehydrogenase is required for the metabolism of ethanol in *Drosophila*, and the life spans of flies fed various concentrations of alcohol vary depending upon which allele is present. However, as noted by Arking and Dudas (1989), is this a gene that affects the aging process, or does it merely represent an example of a gene that "modulates the animals' ability to survive in particular environments?" Another mutation that shortens the life span of *Drosophila* is miniature (m), but, according to Flyg and Boman (1988), these flies are particularly susceptible to infection by the bacterium *Serratia maracescens* due to the increased vulnerability of the gut membrane to bacterial proteases. Of course, mutants like grandchildless, which increases life span substantially in *D. subobscura* (Maynard Smith, 1958), must mitigate normal aging processes. Such mutants are of considerable potential interest in aging research.

Several research groups have taken a somewhat different approach by examining the longevity of different strains or species of *Drosophila*. Fleming *et al.* (1987) compared the relationship between life span, oxygen consumption, and oxygen radical scavenging capacity of the Swedish C strain and the Samarkand strain of *Drosophila melanogaster*. The Swedish C strain (which is short-lived relative to the Samarkand strain) consumed oxygen at a significantly higher rate than the Samarkand strain and had a reduced ability to scavenge hydroxyl radicals (Fleming *et al.*, 1987). Spicer and Fleming (1991) examined seven different populations of *Drosophila melanogaster* with a worldwide geographic distribution using two-dimensional protein gel electrophoresis. The mean genetic similarity (F) found among the seven populations was 0.965, which was similar to previous studies showing low variation in population genetic surveys using two-dimensional electrophoresis. They noted that the historical relationships among these populations was somewhat congruent with the geographic distribution of the populations, but it was not exactly coincident. In addition, these authors found that there was no relationship between the life span of the seven populations and their two-dimensional protein pattern (unpublished data).

Unfortunately, such studies may be confounded by the usual problems associated with inbreeding depression, since the strains employed for many of these studies are highly inbred, and, as noted previously, comparisons of this nature may not necessarily reveal mechanistic differences that are related to normal aging processes. Outbred populations provide an alternative source of variants. For example, Templeton and co-workers have examined natural populations of *Drosophila mercatorum* in Hawaii for variations in fecundity and life span (Templeton *et al.*, 1987). They analyzed the naturally occurring polymorphism for abnormal abdomen (aa), which results in a phenotype that displays abnormalities in segmentation, color, and bristles and results in delaying the onset of eclosion. Moreover, the aa phenotype shows an increase in egg production, with a median life span that is 50% shorter but the same maximum life span (Templeton *et al.*, 1990).

B. Selection for Stocks with Postponed Aging

A fundamental misconception that many biologists, particularly cell biologists, have about aging is that it must be determined by cellular mechanisms and, thus, is best studied using the techniques of molecular and cell biology. This prejudice may arise from the phenomenon of the limited proliferative capacities of vertebrate somatic cells *in vitro* (Hayflick & Moorhead, 1961; Hayflick, 1965). However, the inference is certainly spurious; experimental strategies from organismal and evolutionary biology can be, and have been, brought to bear on aging with some success. The most dramatic illustration of this point is that evolutionary biologists have produced *Drosophila* stocks with substantially postponed aging, including increases in mean and maximum longevities.

An early experiment that gave negative results is of interest. Comfort (1953) reproduced an inbred *D. subobscura* stock at late ages for a number of generations, without producing any change in survival patterns. This experiment showed that breeding flies without genetic variations was not likely to produce stocks with different aging patterns.

Wattiaux (1968a,b) also reproduced *Drosophila pseudoobscura* and *D. subobscura* stocks at later ages and compared them to flies reproduced at early ages. Wattiaux appears to have been seeking evidence for some kind of Lamarckian effect, although his prose is too ambiguous in places to be certain. The effect of late reproduction was to increase the longevity of the later reproduced culture compared to the early-reproduced control. While the longevity increases were not extremely large, and the experiments were not properly replicated, this work indicated that it should be possible to breed *Drosophila* deliberately for postponed aging. Theoretically, this was predicted by Edney and Gill (1968) on the basis of the ideas of Medawar (1952): the force of natural selection on age-specific survival probability is expected to start to decline with the onset of reproduction. This has been shown mathematically in detail (Hamilton, 1966; Charlesworth, 1980): aging is shaped by evolutionary forces involving the timing of reproduction, not the specifics of any single biochemical mechanism (Rose, 1991). Therefore, if the timing of reproduction is changed, aging should evolve toward a different pattern. In particular, *Drosophila* stocks with genetic variability that are reproduced at later ages exclusively should evolve postponed aging.

Two laboratories working with *D. melanogaster* deliberately set out to produce stocks with postponed aging by using such late-reproduction cultures. Beginning in the mid-1970s, Rose and Charlesworth (1980, 1981a,b) studied an outbred population with respect to both quantitative genetics and response to selection. By 1979, they obtained a result like that of Wattiaux: an outbred line with modestly increased longevity compared to that of its control. In 1980, Rose (1984b) started a

replicated set of similar selection lines, in a follow-up experiment, which have since proven to have substantially increased mean and maximum longevities. The second laboratory was that of Luckinbill and Arking. Beginning in 1980, these workers also created a replicated set of late-reproduced and early-reproduced cultures. These lines too evolved postponed senescence like the lines of Rose (Luckinbill *et al.*, 1984; Luckinbill & Clare, 1985). While Wattiaux inadvertently anticipated the results of Rose, Luckinbill, and Arking, he had no cogent theoretical basis for his work. The later work was explicitly based on evolutionary theory and proceeded to postpone senescence directly. Therefore, it constitutes the key breakthrough.

Since the deliberate creation of stocks with postponed aging, other laboratories have created their own stocks of the same type (e.g., Partridge & Fowler, 1992) or used the extant stocks to study aging (e.g., Service, 1987, 1989). Further developments in the use of selection to postpone aging are discussed in Part III. Work on the biological analysis of the stocks resulting from selection is discussed in Part IV.

III. Current Approaches to Genetically Postponing Senescence

A. Transformation

1. P-Element Transformation

With the discovery of the p-transposable element in *Drosophila melanogaster* by Rubin and Spradling (1982), the method of germ line gene transfer in this organism has become relatively routine. A number of genes have been introduced and expressed in *Drosophila*, and several laboratories have now begun to exploit the p-element transformation technique in order to evaluate the role of specific genes in the aging process of *Drosophila*. For example, the gene for elongation factor 1 α (EF1-α)

was introduced into *Drosophila melanogaster* by Shepherd *et al.* (1989). These authors hypothesized that, since protein synthesis declines in *Drosophila* with age, attenuation of this decline might retard the rate of aging in flies. It had been shown previously by Webster and Webster (1983) that the decline in protein synthesis is correlated to a reduction in the synthesis of EF1-α (Shepherd *et al.*, 1989). EF1-α catalyzes a crucial step in protein synthesis, so it could be argued that transformants expressing an additional copy of this gene might show an augmentation of protein synthesis. EF1-α-transformed flies were shown to have significantly increased life spans (Shepherd *et al.*, 1989). However, Shikama *et al.* (1994) demonstrated that the transgenic lines generated by Shepherd *et al.* (1989) do not express more EF1-α mRNA or protein than control flies. The EF1-α transgene could be induced following a heat shock at 37°C, but no transgene product was detected at 29°C. Although these authors did replicate the finding that the EF1-α transgenics have a mean life span that is longer than that of control flies, it clearly is not the result of increased expression of EF1-α. It may be that the insertion of the EF1-α construct has induced a mutation that has a positive effect on life span. However, it is not likely that they have disrupted a gene analogous to *age-1* in *Caenorhabditis elegans*, as described by Friedman and Johnson (1988), since none of the EF1-α-transformed flies have life spans that exceed those of wild-type flies. Independently, Stearns and Kaiser (1993) carried out detailed genetic studies of the EF1-α transgenics, which suggested that genetic background and chromosomal position were more important factors affecting longevity in these lines than the expression of EF1-α.

2. Superoxide Dismutase and Catalase

Various laboratories have focused on a group of genes that are involved in protection against oxidative stress. The high concentration of oxygen in the atmosphere and the metabolic dependence of eukaryotes upon the respiratory utilization of oxygen confer upon these organisms the necessity of dealing with multiple toxic species of active oxygen (Phillips & Hilliker, 1990). Most organisms detoxify active oxygen through a complex system of defenses, which include enzymatic scavengers such as superoxide dismutase, catalase, and glutathione peroxidase, small-molecular-weight scavengers such as urate, ascorbate, vitamin E, and bilirubin, which convert active oxygen species to less reactive compounds, and other enzymatic mechanisms operating at the level of DNA repair (Gutteridge *et al.*, 1986; Saul *et al.*, 1987). The biological consequences of oxy radical damage originate from their destructive reaction with sensitive cellular macromolecules, including DNA, RNA, protein, lipid, and carbohydrate (Chow, 1988). Phillips and colleagues have been utilizing the genetic system of *Drosophila melanogaster* to investigate the biological consequences arising from directed genetic perturbation of specific components of oxygen defense metabolism (Phillips & Hilliker, 1990). For example, null mutation for Cu/Zn superoxide dismutase (CuZnSOD), one of two distinct superoxide dismutases found in higher animals, confers reduced adult life span, hypersensitivity to paraquat and $CuSO_4$, and male sterility (Phillips *et al.*, 1989). In contrast, moderate overexpression of native CuZnSOD generated by chromosomal duplications of the CuZnSOD gene (Staveley *et al.*, 1990) or by native CuZnSOD transgenes (Seto *et al.*, 1990) confers increased resistance to ionizing radiation, decreased resistance to paraquat toxicity, and marginal increase in adult life span.

Bewley and co-workers (1986, 1990) have examined catalase, another class of enzymatic scavengers of toxic oxygen metabolites. In their work, they used EMS mutagenesis to recover several hypo-morphic alleles of catalase, which were isolated and shown to be homozygous. Moreover, the flies were viable with cata-lase activities from 0 to 5%. The authors used these alleles to examine viability, fer-tility, and longevity in flies expressing var-ious levels of catalase (Bewley & Mackay, 1990). Although their data suggested that the mean and maximum life spans are di-rectly related to catalase activity at levels ranging from 0 to 50%, this has been ques-tioned by others (Orr *et al.*, 1992). Viability is affected at catalase levels below 3%, but above this level viability is near normal, suggesting that the expression of catalase at such a significantly reduced level appar-ently is not essential (Bewley & Mackay, 1990). However, as noted previously, the use of mutants that shorten the life spans of laboratory animals may not be partic-ularly useful for understanding the genet-ics of normal aging, since such animals of-ten have truncated life spans as a result of pathologies that are unrelated to normal aging (Rose *et al.*, 1992a).

Several laboratories have begun to in-vestigate the role of genes involved in oxy-gen metabolism and their effect on the aging process in *Drosophila* by using the p-element transformation technique (Seto *et al.*, 1990; Reveillaud *et al.*, 1991; Orr & Sohal, 1992). The oxyradical hypothesis has recruited a number of proponents over the last few years; however, most of the supporting evidence is still largely circum-stantial and indirect (Fleming *et al.*, 1982, 1992; Miquel & Fleming, 1986). So far, a modest amount of research has been car-ried out on the relationship between lon-gevity and antioxidant defenses. The first studies to report on the comparison of SOD to life span in *Drosophila* were car-ried out by Bartosz *et al.* (1979). These au-thors reported that a short-lived mutant of *Drosophila* was deficient in total SOD ac-tivity. However, Massie and co-workers have noted that SOD activity is not signifi-cantly different between wild strains of

Drosophila, whose life spans may differ by as much as 40% (Massie *et al.*, 1980). As discussed previously, Phillips *et al.* (1989) have reported that CuZn SOD null mu-tants in *Drosophila* are hypersensitive to paraquat and have reduced longevity. Un-doubtedly, SOD plays some role in regu-lating the life span of *Drosophila*. More-over, catalase, possibly in concert with SOD or other antioxidants, controls the level of toxic O_2 species in the cell, and that oxygen toxicity contributes to many aspects of cellular senescence. Until re-cently, a direct test of this concept, i.e., to up-regulate the intracellular levels of these enzymes and then determine the consequence on aging, was not possible. Such experiments can now be accom-plished with the use of transformation technologies that permit the introduction of new or additional genes into the genome of *Drosophila*.

In 1990, Seto *et al.* reported that the in-troduction of an extra gene for *Drosophila* CuZn SOD does not result in an increased life span. They argued that SOD trans-genics have the same life spans as control flies. Unfortunately, these authors did not provide a statistical analysis of their mor-tality data. Their results are interesting when compared to those of Reveillaud *et al.* (1991), who reported similar values for the life spans of their transgenic lines; however, they found that the moderate in-crease in mean life span observed in sev-eral SOD transgenic lines was statistically significant.

Reveillaud *et al.* (1991) have exploited p-element technology in order to examine, in more detail, the role of superoxide dis-mutase on the aging process in *Drosoph-ila*. Although catalase, glutathione per-oxidase, and vitamins C and E probably play major roles in intracellular free radi-cal detoxification, they initially focused their studies on CuZn superoxide dismu-tase (Reveillaud *et al.*, 1991). Transgenic strains of *Drosophila melanogaster* over-producing CuZn SOD were generated by microinjecting *Drosophila* embryos with p-elements containing bovine CuZn SOD cDNA under the control of the *Drosophila* actin 5C promoter (Klemenz *et al.*, 1987). The insertion of bovine CuZn SOD cDNA into the genome of *Drosophila* resulted in a mean increase of 32.5% in the level of total CuZn SOD activity in transformed adults compared to that in control flies. Twenty different strains of *Drosophila* expressing the bovine form of CuZn SOD were generated, and several of these stocks were examined for their resistance to oxidative stress and life span. Transgenic males are significantly more resistant to paraquat-induced killing than either the controls or the recipient lines. In these studies, it was reported that there was a slight, but statistically significant, increase in the mean life span of several strains (Reveillaud *et al.*, 1991).

Orr and Sohal (1992) have also used p-element transformation in *Drosophila* to examine the role of antioxidant genes in life span and resistance to oxidative stress. They initially introduced a genomic fragment containing the *Drosophila* catalase gene (Orr & Sohal, 1992). Levels of catalase expression in transgenics were increased by as much as 80%, but they reported that life span was not significantly different from controls. Moreover, resistance to hyperoxia and paraquat was not enhanced, although the catalase transgenics apparently were more resistant to hydrogen peroxide. These authors subsequently introduced a genomic fragment of the *Drosophila* CuZn SOD gene by using the same strategy (Orr & Sohal, 1993). Enhanced expression of SOD by 32–42% in their transgenic strains, again, did not result in significant protection from oxy radical damage induced by paraquat poisoning. Furthermore, this increased level of SOD did not result in significant effects on life span or resistance to exposure to hyperoxia. However, some transgenic lines showed a slight increase in mean life span, and these same strains were also more resistant to hyper-

oxia than their corresponding controls (Orr & Sohal, 1993). There were no changes in the maximum life span of flies overexpressing SOD, a finding noted previously by Reveillaud *et al.* (1991). These authors have found that transgenics overexpressing both CuZn SOD and catalase have a significant extension of life span (Orr & Sohal, 1994). These results underscore an important consideration in the use of transgenics for aging studies. The introduction of catalase or CuZn SOD alone had only moderate effects (and in some cases no effect) on the life spans of flies, whereas the simultaneous introduction of both genes presumably led to significant augmentation of both mean and maximum life spans. Increased levels of SOD, in the absence of a compensatory up-regulation of catalase, are thought to result in an accumulation of H_2O_2. This may give rise to cytotoxic effects such as that seen in Down's syndrome in which a 50% increase in cytoplasmic SOD has been associated with free radical-induced pathological changes (Elroy-Stein *et al.*, 1986; Krall *et al.*, 1988; Sinet *et al.*, 1979).

Reveillaud *et al.* (1994) introduced a synthetic bovine CuZnSOD transgene into a CuZnSOD–null mutant of *Drosophila*. The resulting transformants expressed bovine CuZnSOD exclusively to about 30% of normal *Drosophila* CuZnSOD levels. Expression of the *Drosophila*–bovine CuZnSOD transgene in the CuZnSOD–null mutant rescues male fertility and resistance to paraquat to apparently normal levels. However, adult life span was restored to only 30% of normal, and resistance to hyperoxia is 90% of that found in control flies. This striking differential restoration of pleiotropic phenotypes could be the result of a threshold of CuZnSOD expression necessary for normal male fertility and resistance to the toxicity of paraquat or hyperoxia, which is lower than the threshold required to sustain a normal adult life span. Alternatively, the differential rescue of fertility, resistance to active oxygen, and life span might indicate different cell-specific transcriptional requirements for these functions that are normally provided by the control elements of the native CuZnSOD gene, but which are only partly compensated for by the transcriptional control elements of the actin 5C promoter.

The observation that the *Drosophila*–bovine transgene does not completely restore adult life span may be related to the inability of the actin 5C promoter to restore CuZnSOD expression in those cells and tissues that are life-span-limiting in the CuZnSOD–null mutant. Although the whole body level of CuZnSOD in the transgenically rescued CuZnSOD–null mutant is elevated by 30%, the adult life span is restored to only 30% of normal. CuZnSOD–null heterozygotes that have 50% of normal CuZnSOD activity have a normal adult life span (Phillips *et al.*, 1989). Moreover, a mutant recovered from natural populations that has only 3% of normal whole body CuZnSOD activity has a life span nearly 70% of normal (Graf & Ayala, 1986).

B. Artificial Selection

There are two main selection techniques that are used to postpone aging in *Drosophila*. The first is the late-reproduction technique first tried by Comfort and Wattiaux, discussed earlier. It is well-established now that this technique will work, provided the experimenter begins with stocks having abundant genetic variations and employs appropriate larval densities (Clare & Luckinbill, 1985; Luckinbill & Clare, 1985; Service *et al.*, 1988). Some peculiar results of Lints and Hoste (1974, 1977), which had been the basis for various Lamarckian arguments against the evolutionary genetic analysis of aging, appear to have arisen from extremely low larval rearing densities (Clare & Luckinbill, 1985).

A second approach is to select on characters that are genetically correlated with postponed aging. Service *et al.* (1985) found that selectively postponed aging also gives rise to enhanced stress resistance, the stresses being starvation, desiccation, and exposure to 1.5% ambient ethanol. On the basis of this result, Rose *et al.* (1992b) selected for stress resistance characters by themselves. They found that longevity increased as stress resistance increased under selection: over about 20 generations in one experiment and about 45 generations in another. The significance of this experiment is that it shows that the longevity and aging phenotypes can be treated like other quantitative genetic characters, allowing both direct and indirect selection for postponed aging using characters that are genetically correlated with senescence.

There are a number of different *Drosophila* stocks that have been selected for postponed aging, directly or indirectly, in the United States and the United Kingdom. Additional stocks are readily created by selection, and such new stocks are now being developed. These stocks constitute excellent material for the biological analysis of aging at every level, from biochemistry to quantitative genetics, because they have undergone amelioration with respect to normal aging mechanisms. Such analyses are discussed in the next section.

IV. Levels of Analysis of Aging in *Drosophila*

A. Evolutionary Quantitative Genetics

Aging is a quantitative character in the same sense as body weight. Numerous loci affect it (Hutchinson & Rose, 1990), often of complicated or uncertain biochemical pathways. This may be contrasted with characters like catabolic enzyme activity or pigment synthesis, in which the pathways are relatively few and genetic dissection is relatively straightforward.

Aging is polygenic because it is both a "summative" character and it is related to fitness. Darwinian fitness is the sole focus of evolution, it is the reason for all of the transcribed, nonviroid, sequences in the genomes of metazoa, and, of course, it is the end result of many specific physiological mechanisms; thus, it is "summative." Although its evolutionary basis is very different, aging is similar in its organization, considered as a character subject to genetic analysis. It is the result of the evolutionary dereliction of natural selection at later adult ages in organisms without fissile reproduction (Rose, 1991). Thus, a fundamental starting point for research on aging in *Drosophila* must be its evolutionary quantitative genetics.

There is a surprisingly large number of studies of the evolutionary quantitative genetics of aging and related life history characters in *Drosophila* [see the survey in Rose (1991), Chapters 3 and 4]. Unfortunately, many of these studies founder because of two substantial artifacts: genotype-by-environment interaction (G × E) and inbreeding depression. Both of these artifacts arise from the necessity of studying *Drosophila* in laboratory cultures. If a population is sampled for live organisms in nature and that sample is then brought into the laboratory for culture, G × E will vitiate most evolutionary genetic interpretations. This arises because the laboratory constitutes a novel environment for the cultured sample, an environment, therefore, that the sample is not adapted to initially. The quantitative genetics of fitness-related characters, like aging, will not be in selective equilibrium. Not only will the quantitative genetic findings be uninterpretable under such conditions, but a culture that is not inbred will evolve rapidly to adapt to the laboratory. In effect, it will not even be possible to study such laboratory cultures as stable genetic entities, unless enough time is allowed for selective equilibrium

to be approximated. Hence, laboratory cultures of *Drosophila*, and indeed any other organism, require sufficient time for adaptation to the laboratory before they can be studied profitably.

Unfortunately, long-continued laboratory cultivation poses another problem: inbreeding depression. Most *Drosophila* cultures are maintained with dozens of flies. At such census numbers, effective population sizes (cf. Crow & Kimura, 1970) will be small enough that many deleterious recessive alleles will be fixed by genetic drift. This will give rise to reductions in fitness-related characters, like longevity. Upon crossing of these inbred lines, longevity shows marked hybrid vigor, as Clarke and Smith (1955) showed in *D. subobscura*. Thus, longevity is determined in such populations by accidents of fixation of deleterious alleles that are normally at low frequencies and do not normally determine longevity. One example of the artifacts that then arise for the quantitative genetics of aging is that such inbred lines are biased toward positive genetic correlations between aging and early fitness-related characters, as has been shown experimentally for *D. melanogaster* lines (Rose, 1984a).

This overview suggests a sorry prospect: the study of *Drosophila* aging requires laboratory cultivation, but such laboratory culture at first gives rise to G × E artifacts and later may produce inbreeding depression. What remedy is there for this situation? The solution that several laboratories (e.g., Rose, 1984b; Luckinbill *et al.*, 1984; Partridge & Fowler, 1992) have adopted is long-term selection on large laboratory cultures. While it appears that inbreeding artifacts have arisen in some of these cultures (Roper *et al.*, 1993), extensive hybridization tests reveal an absence of detectable inbreeding depression in other laboratories (e.g., Hutchinson & Rose, 1990). Such populations are then suitable material for further genetic research. The overall situation facing *Drosophila* aging genetics is one where the vast majority of stocks will not be suitable for most studies, but a few stocks nonetheless may be adequate to the task. From the quantitative genetic evidence, considerable caution is warranted, but not despair. In particular, quantitative genetic analysis of stocks with postponed aging strongly suggests that they can be valid systems for experimental investigation. However, some of these stocks may not be valid, and this can be ascertained by using these techniques. But virtually all other types of untransformed *Drosophila* stocks will not be useful material for the study of the genetics of aging.

It might also be noted that most of these strictures will apply to the genetic stocks of almost all other metazoa, including all mammals. Some species, such as *C. elegans*, do not suffer inbreeding depression because of their self-fertilization in nature (Johnson & Wood, 1982) and are free of the problems of inbreeding. However, all species will be subject to G × E effects upon initial culture in the laboratory. *Drosophila* with selectively postponed aging probably constitutes the best available "wild type" stocks, i.e., stocks that have not been mutated or transformed.

B. Organismal Physiology

The idea of studying the organismal physiology of aging in *Drosophila* is a reasonably old one. Aside from the historic studies of Pearl (1922) on the biology of aging in *Drosophila*, there have been numerous studies of the aggregate physiology of aging in *Drosophila* [see reviews in Lints and Soliman (1988)]. These developed, in part, out of Pearl's (1928) "rate of living" theory. Rate of living theories suppose that the organism has a fixed total amount of metabolism that it can undergo in a lifetime. If it undergoes this metabolism quickly, due to increased temperature, nutrition, or mating, then it is expected to die sooner. Conversely, decreased tempera-

ture, dietary restriction, and celibacy are expected to lead to postponed aging. Some of the oldest publications on aging in *Drosophila*, those on the effects of temperature on life span (Loeb & Northrop, 1916, 1917), illustrate the patterns expected from the rate of living theory.

This phenomenon has since been of sporadic interest to a variety of *Drosophila* workers. In particular, Maynard Smith (1963) sparked interest in this area by finding an example of the effect of temperature on *Drosophila* aging that apparently did not follow the rate of living pattern. Subsequent research (e.g., Lamb, 1968; Miquel *et al.*, 1976) did not manage to entirely sort out the puzzles raised by Maynard Smith (1963). One interpretation of the confusion about rate of living is that the modulation of aging by temperature is not merely the result of changing kinetic energy levels, but instead may reflect evolved adaptations for life span modulation based on the exploitation of varying thermodynamic conditions within an evolutionarily normal range of temperatures (Rose, 1991, pp. 112–114). Within the normal evolutionary range, the evolved facultative response of the organism to temperature variation may exhibit the trade-off pattern assumed by the rate of living theory. Beyond this range, this adaptation may break down, giving pathological variations in aging patterns that do not reflect a rate of living pattern. In effect, the rate of living may be shorthand for a complex underlying set of adaptations and maladaptations that are not, in fact, reducible to the mere tuning of a unified metabolic process.

An interesting focus of some *Drosophila* research has been physiological "biomarkers" of aging. Obviously, it would be desirable to have characteristics other than death that could be used to infer the degree to which a particular animal is "aged." Ganetzky and Flanagan (1978) attempted to study this question by comparing two different inbred stocks of *D.*

melanogaster, looking for biomarkers that matched the relative pattern of aging in these stocks. While enzymatic activities did not predict the pattern of aging, a measure of organismal function, negative geotaxis, did. Service *et al.* (1985, 1988), Service (1987), Rose *et al.* (1992b), and Graves *et al.* (1992) found strong correlations between stress resistance, caloric reserve substances (lipid and glycogen), and life span among *D. melanogaster* stocks selected for postponed senescence. Interestingly, while the mean level of starvation resistance partly predicts the mean life span of a stock, that same starvation resistance increases with female age. Thus, a good "biomarker" of population life span is a poor biomarker of the life expectancy of individual females. Luckinbill *et al.* (1984), Arking (1987), and Arking *et al.* (1991) also studied "biomarkers" in genetically based, long-lived strains of *Drosophila melanogaster.* They initially examined metabolic rate, phototactic and geotactic responses, female fecundity, and protein synthesis as potential biomarkers of physiological age in their long-lived stock (Arking & Wells, 1990). Their finding of a loss in phototactic behavior, which occurs significantly earlier in their normal-lived (R) strain than in their long-lived (L) strain, may be related to reports by Grigliatti (1987) that a decline in the physiological performance of the central nervous system is one of the early signs of aging in his short-lived mutant. Arking *et al.* (1991) reported that the increased longevity of their L strain is accompanied by an elevated resistance to paraquat, a herbicide that has been shown to generate the superoxide radical when metabolized *in vivo.* They have noted that a bioassay of paraquat resistance can be employed to determine the presence or absence of the long-lived phenotype in these stocks. Thus, paraquat resistance may turn out to be a "biomarker" of aging for their long-lived strain. But a major problem facing

work like that of Buck *et al.* (1993) is a lack of multiple, independent, selected lines. This renders the results suspect for general inferences because a single line may have undergone idiosyncratic differentiation.

Despite the paradoxes that await simple-minded "rate of living" or "biomarker" research, it is striking how strongly organismal physiology can be related to genetic differences in *Drosophila* life span. This may be contrasted with the relative failure of numerous attempts to connect molecular or cell biology phenotypes, like enzyme activity, to *Drosophila* aging. Insect physiology may have much more to contribute to this field than has been accepted to this point. In particular, *Drosophila* stock systems, which include flies with postponed aging, and their controls provide natural avenues for organismal physiology. One technique is to compare the physiological function of normal and long-lived flies, as in Service *et al.* (1985), Service (1987, 1989), and Graves *et al.* (1992). An additional possibility is to combine differentiated stocks with phenotypic manipulation, in order to test alternative hypotheses about physiological mechanisms underlying postponed aging. Experiments of this kind have been performed by Service (1989) using mating, Graves *et al.* (1992) using tethered flight, and Chippindale *et al.* (1993) using nutrition. Many of these experiments emulate aspects of earlier work in insect aging, but they have the additional strength that they can be connected to genetic research because they use differentiated stocks. All told, this work has strongly implicated energetic metabolism as a key determinant of aging patterns in *Drosophila.* Effectively, somatic sequestration of calories allows the postponement of aging, at the cost of reduced early reproduction. While the molecular genetic basis of this mechanism is not yet known, its discovery does constitute considerable achievement at the level of organismal physiology.

C. Molecular Biology and Biochemistry

From the foregoing discussion, it is apparent that the best stocks for discovering candidate loci controlling aging must be stocks that have been selected for postponed aging by one means or another. Of course, an entirely different strategy of great potential is that involving transformation, which is discussed in Section III. Here, discussion will be confined to the molecular analysis of stocks with postponed aging.

Fleming *et al.* (1993) analyzed postponed-aging stocks and their controls using high-resolution two-dimensional protein electrophoresis. 321 proteins were resolved and scored for their relative intensities from the five selected and the five control populations studied. Two proteins were found to be expressed only in the control lines, a highly significant result. Four additional proteins were statistically associated with selection, using a variety of statistical methods. It should be noted, however, that these statistical associations could arise from linkage disequilibrium between the alleles producing the differentiated protein and other, nearby, loci that have undergone allele frequency change as a result of selection. Thus, the differentiation of these proteins is a guide to either (i) the identity of the loci controlling aging or (ii) the location of the loci controlling aging. In either event, it would be of great interest to identify these loci using a molecular biological approach, which might proceed by determining the protein microsequence, generating oligonucleotide probes, cloning the gene, and then sequencing the gene. Definitive testing of alternatives (i) and (ii) could then proceed using transformation, as outlined in Section III. Finally, it would then be possible to test for the existence of homologous loci in other species, including mammals.

The appropriate molecular characterization of postponed aging in selected stocks of *Drosophila* is only beginning. Given the large amount of evolutionary genetic and physiological research that has been done on *Drosophila* with postponed aging, it would seem imperative now that the molecular and cell biology of the system be worked out in more detail. The vast molecular genetic database available for *Drosophila* should make this a very successful enterprise, given the creation of the appropriate selected stocks. The failure of previous efforts along these lines probably arose from the lack of appropriate lines with postponed aging.

V. Future Studies

A. From *Drosophila* to Other Species

Drosophila has historically been a jumping-off point for much biological research, in the sense of supplying the model that is then generalized to all or most other species, particularly eukaryotes and, among them, metazoa. Genetics, itself, was largely founded in this century by generalization from *Drosophila* experiments. Developmental genetics has been greatly enhanced by the extension of the homeo box model from *Drosophila* to other metazoa, especially vertebrates. The temptation is obvious: to unravel the genetics of aging in *Drosophila* and then generalize the *Drosophila* findings to most, or all, other metazoa.

This strategy is fraught with the most profound difficulties of evolutionary and genetic interpretation. A fundamental starting point for any debate on this topic is that aging is not a phenotype like eye pigment or segment number. Aging is not an adaptation. It may not even be a by-product of adaptation. It reflects, instead, a failure of adaptation at later ages, according to the formal analyses of theoretical population genetics (vid. Charlesworth,

1980; Rose, 1991). As such, all of the well-defined experimental analyses of fields like neurobiology and developmental genetics may come to naught when they are applied to aging, because their experimental strategies are based, implicitly or explicitly, on the hypothesis that the characteristics they study are adaptations. Therefore, the commonplace strategy of homologizing adaptations, such as the standard accounts of the evolution of the vertebrate heart (e.g., Romer, 1970), will fail when it is applied to aging.

This is not to say that there cannot be some large-scale generalization of mechanisms of aging, in principle. The point here is that any such generalization must find, as its warrant, a theoretical basis different from the extrapolation of adaptations. Some attempts have been made to develop such a new theoretical basis (e.g., Rose, 1991, Chapter 8; Rose & Finch, 1993). Among the key possibilities for generalization of aging mechanisms may be relationships between aging, reproduction, and hormones. If there is a cost to reproduction in terms of subsequent survival, in genetic terms antagonistic pleiotropy, then aging will be evolutionarily bound up with reproductive adaptations. As the key signaling mechanisms for reproduction, including hormones and their receptors, could be evolutionarily conserved among some taxa, these same signaling mechanisms could likewise give rise to phylogenetically general coordination of aging mechanisms. While it is not appropriate to elaborate on this theme here, the value of this example is that it illustrates how the generalization of mechanisms of aging, first unravelled in *Drosophila*, might be achieved. Vital to this generalization is the use of population genetic findings that have been almost entirely the product of that same *Drosophila* research. Whether at the mechanistic or evolutionary level, *Drosophila* will always be an indispensable system for aging research.

Acknowledgments

The authors are grateful to T. J. Nusbaum, Paige Ruchert, Lynn Noland, and Emile Zuckerkandl for their comments on the chapter. The research of J. E. Fleming was supported by The Glenn Foundation for Medical Research, by the Northwest Institute for Advanced Study, and by donations to the Institute of Molecular Medical Sciences. The research of M. R. Rose was supported by National Institute on Aging Grants US-PHS AG06346 and AG09970.

References

Arking, R. (1987). Successful selection for increased longevity in *Drosophila:* analysis of the survival data and presentation of a hypothesis on the genetic regulation of longevity. *Experimental Gerontology, 22,* 199–220.

Arking, R., & Dudas, S. P. (1989). Review of genetic investigations into the aging processes of *Drosophila. Journal of American Geriatrics Society, 37,* 757–773.

Arking, R., & Wells, R. A. (1990). Genetic alteration of normal aging processes is responsible for extended longevity in *Drosophila. Developmental Genetics, 11,* 141–148.

Arking, R., Buck, S., Berrios, A., Dwyer, S., & Baker, G. T., III (1991). Elevated paraquat resistance can be used as a bioassay for longevity in a genetically based long-lived strain of *Drosophila. Developmental Genetics, 12,* 362–370.

Baker, G. T., Jacobson, M., & Mokrynshi, G. (1985). Aging in *Drosophila.* In V. Cristofalo (Ed.), *Handbook of Cell Biology of Aging.* Boca Raton, FL: CRC Press.

Bartosz, G., Leyko, W., & Fried, R. (1979). Superoxide dismutase and life-span of *Drosophila melanogaster. Experientia, 35,* 1193–1194.

Bellen, H. J., & Kiger, J. A., Jr. (1987). Sexual hyperactivity and reduced longevity of *dunce* females of *Drosophila melanogaster. Genetics, 119,* 153–160.

Bewley, G. C., & Mackay, W. J. (1990). Development of a genetic model for acatalasemia: testing the oxygen free radical theory of aging. In D. E. Harrison (Ed.), *The Genetic Effects on Aging.* West Caldwell, NJ: Telford.

Bewley, G. C., Mackay, W. J., & Cook, J. L. (1986). Temporal variation for the expression of catalase in *Drosophila melanogaster:* Correlations between the rates of enzyme synthesis and levels of translatable catalase messenger RNA. *Genetics, 113,* 919–938.

Bozuck, A. N. (1972). DNA synthesis in the absence of somatic cell division associated with aging in *Drosophila subobscura. Experimental Gerontology, 7,* 147

Buck, S., Wells, R. A., Dudas, S. P., Baker, G. T., III, & Arking, R. (1993). Chromosomal localization and regulation of the longevity determinant genes in a selected strain of *Drosophila melanogaster. Heredity, 71,* 11–22.

Charlesworth, B. (1980). *Evolution in Age-Structured Populations.* Cambridge: Cambridge University Press.

Chippindale, A. K., Leroi, A. M., Kim, S. B., & Rose, M. R. (1993). Phenotypic plasticity and selection in *Drosophila* life-history evolution. I. Nutrition and the cost of reproduction. *Journal of Evolutionary Biology, 6,* 171–193.

Chow, C. K. (1988). *Cellular Antioxidant Defense Mechanisms* (Vols. I–III). Boca Raton, FL: CRC Press.

Clare, M. J., & Luckinbill, L. S. (1985). The effects of gene-environment interaction on the expression of longevity. *Heredity, 55,* 19–29.

Clark, A. M., & Rubin, M. A. (1961). The modification of X-irradiation of the life span of haploids and diploids of the wasp, *Habrobracon* sp. *Radiation Research, 15,* 244–253.

Clarke, J. M., & Smith, J. M. (1955). The genetics and cytology of *Drosophila subobscura.* XI. Hybrid vigor and longevity. *Journal of Genetics, 53,* 712–780.

Comfort, A. (1953). Absence of a lansing effect in *Drosophila subobscura. Nature, 172,* 83–84.

Crow, J. F. (1948). Alternative hypotheses of hybrid vigor. *Genetics, 33,* 477–487.

Crow, J. F., & Kimura, M. (1970). *An Introduction to Population Genetics Theory.* New York: Harper and Row.

Curtsinger, J. W., Fukui, H. H., Townsend, D. R., & Vaupel, J. W. (1992). Demography of genotypes: Failure of the limited life-span paradigm in *Drosophila melanogaster. Science, 358,* 461–463.

Edney, E. B., & Gill, R. W. (1968). Evolution of senescence and specific longevity. *Nature, 220,* 281–282.

Elroy-Stein, O., Bernstein, Y., & Groner, Y. (1986). Overproduction of human CuZn superoxide dismutase in transfected cells: extenuation of paraquat-mediated cytotoxicity and enhancement of lipid peroxidation. *European Molecular Biology Organization Journal, 5,* 615–622.

Finch, C. E. (1990). *Longevity, Senescence, and the Genome.* Chicago: The University of Chicago Press.

Fleming, J. E., Miquel, J., Cottrell, S. F., Yengoyan, L. S., & Economos, A. C. (1982). Is cell aging caused by respiration-dependent injury to the mitochondrial genome? *Gerontology, 28,* 44–53.

Fleming, J. E., Quattrocki, E., Latter, G., Miquel, J., Marcuson, Zuckerkandl, E., & Bensch, K. G. (1986). Age-dependent changes in proteins of *Drosophila melanogaster. Science, 231,* 1157–1159.

Fleming, J. E., Shibuya, R. B., & Bensch, K. G. (1987). Lifespan, oxygen consumption and hydroxyl radical scavenging capacity of two strains of *Drosophila melanogaster. Age, 10,* 86–89.

Fleming, J. E., Reveillaud, I., & Niedzwiecki, A. (1992). Role of oxidative stress in *Drosophila* aging. *Mutation Research, 275,* 267–279.

Fleming, J. E., Spicer, G. S., Garrison, R. C., & Rose, M. R. (1993). Two-dimensional protein electrophoretic analysis of postponed aging in *Drosophila. Genetica, 91,* 183–198.

Flyg, C., & Boman, H. G. (1988). *Drosophila* genes cut and minature are associated with the susceptibility to infection by *Serratia marcescens. Genetica, 52,* 51–56.

Friedman, D. B., & Johnson, T. E. (1988). A mutation in the age-1 gene in *Caenorhabditis elegans* lengthens life and reduces hermaphrodite fertility. *Genetics, 118,* 75–86.

Ganetzky, B., & Flanagan, J. R. (1978). On the relationship between senescence and age-related changes in two wild-type strains of *Drosophila melanogaster. Experimental Gerontology, 13,* 189–196.

Gowen, J. W. (1931). On chromosome balance as a factor in duration of life. *Journal of General Physiology, 14,* 447–461.

Gowen, J. W. (1952). Hybrid vigor in *Drosophila.*

In J. W. Gowen (Ed.), *Heterosis* (pp. 474–493). Ames, IA: Iowa State University Press.

Graf, J., & Ayala, F. J. (1986). Genetic variation for superoxide dismutase level in *Drosophila melanogaster*. *Biochemical Genetics, 24*, 153–168.

Graves, J. L., Toolson, E. C., Jeong, C., Vu, L. N., & Rose, M. R. (1992). Desiccation, flight, glycogen, and postponed senescence in *Drosophila melanogaster*. *Physiological Zoology, 65*, 268–286.

Grigliatti, T. A. (1987). Programmed cell death and aging in *Drosophila melanogaster*. In A. D. Woodhead & K. H. Thompson (Eds.), *Evolution of Longevity in Animals: A Comparative Approach* (pp. 193–207). New York: Plenum Press.

Gutteridge, J. M. C., Westermarck, T., & Halliwell, B. (1986). Oxygen radical damage in biological systems. In J. E. Johnson, Jr. (Ed.), *Free Radicals in Biology and Medicine* (pp. 99–140). New York: Alan R. Liss.

Hamilton, W. D. (1966). The moulding of senescence by natural selection. *Journal of Theoretical Biology, 12*, 12–45.

Hayflick, L. (1965). The limited *in vitro* lifetime of human diploid cell strains. *Experimental Cell Research, 37*, 614–636.

Hayflick, L., & Moorhead, P. S. (1961). The serial cultivation of human diploid cell strains. *Experimental Cell Research, 25*, 585–621.

Hotta, Y., & Benzer, S. (1972). Mapping of behaviour in *Drosophila* mosaics. *Nature, 240*, 527–535.

Hutchinson, E. W., & Rose, M. R. (1990). Quantitative genetic analysis of postponed aging in *Drosophila melanogaster*. In D. E. Harrison (Ed.), *Genetic Effects on Aging II* (pp. 66–87). Caldwell, NJ: Telford Press.

Johnson, T. E., & Wood, W. B. (1982). Genetic analysis of life-span in *Caenorhabditis elegans*. *Proceedings of the National Academy of Sciences of the United States of America, 79*, 6603–6607.

Klemenz, R., Weber, V., & Gehring, W. J. (1987). The white gene as a marker in a new P-element vector for gene transfer in *Drosophila*. *Nucleic Acids Research, 15*, 3947–3959.

Krall, J., Bagley, A. C., Mullenbach, G. T., Hallewell, R. A., & Lynch, R. E. (1988). Superoxide mediates the toxicity of paraquat for cultured mammalian cells. *Journal of Biological Chemistry, 263*, 1910–1914.

Lamb, M. J. (1968). Temperature and lifespan in *Drosophila*. *Nature, 220*, 808–809.

Lints, F. A., & Hoste, C. (1974). The lansing effect revisited. I. Life-span. *Experimental Gerontology, 9*, 51–69.

Lints, F. A., & Hoste, C. (1977). The lansing effect revisited. II. Cumulative and spontaneously reversible parental age effects on fecundity in *Drosophila melanogaster*. *Evolution, 31*, 387–404.

Lints, F. A., & Soliman, M. H. (1988). *Drosophila as a Model Organism for Aging Studies*. Glasgow: Blackie.

Loeb, J., & Northrop, J. H. (1916). Is there a temperature coefficient for the duration of life? *Proceedings of the National Academy of Sciences of the United States of America, 2*, 456–457.

Loeb, J., & Northrop, J. H. (1917). On the influence of food and temperature upon the duration of life. *Journal of Biological Chemistry, 32*, 103–121.

Luckinbill, L. S., & Clare, M. J. (1985). Selection for life span in *Drosophila melanogaster*. *Heredity, 55*, 9–18.

Luckinbill, L. S., Arking, R., Clare, M. J., Cirocco, W. C., & Buck, S. A. (1984). Selection for delayed senescence in *Drosophila melanogaster*. *Evolution, 38*, 996–1003.

Massie, H. R., Aiello, V. R., & Williams, T. R. (1980). Changes in superoxide dismutase activity and copper during development and ageing in the fruit fly *Drosophila melanogaster*. *Mechanisms of Ageing and Development, 12*, 279–286.

Mayer, P. J., & Baker, G. T., III (1985). Genetic aspects of *Drosophila* as a model system of eukaryotic aging. *International Review of Cytology, 95*, 61–102.

Maynard Smith, J. (1958). The effects of temperature and of egg-laying on the longevity of *Drosophila subobscura*. *Journal of Experimental Biology, 35*, 832–42.

Maynard Smith, J. (1963). Theories of aging. In P. L. Krohn (Ed.), *Topics in the Biology of Aging*. New York: Interscience.

Maynard Smith, J. (1966). Theories of aging. In P. L. Krohn (Ed.), *Topics in the Biology of Aging*. New York: Interscience.

Medawar, P. B. (1952). *An Unsolved Problem of Biology*. London: H. K. Lewis.

Miquel, J., & Fleming, J. E. (1986). Theoretical and experimental support for an "oxygen radical-mitochondrial injury" hypothesis of cell aging. In J. E. Johnson, R. Walford, D. Harman, & J. Miquel (Eds.), *Free Radicals, Aging, and Degenerative Diseases* (pp. 51–74). New York: Alan R. Liss, Inc.

Miquel, J., Lundgren, P. R., Bensch, K. G., & Atlan, H. (1976). Effects of temperature on the life span, vitality and fine structure of *Drosophila melanogaster. Mechanisms of Ageing and Development, 5,* 347–370.

Miquel, J., Economos, A. C., Fleming, J. E., & Johnson, J. E. (1980). Mitochondrial role in cell aging. *Experimental Gerontology, 15,* 575–591.

Miquel, J., Economos, A. C., & Bensch, K. G. (1981). Insect versus mammalian aging. *Aging and Cell Structure, 1,* 347–379.

Orr, W. C., & Sohal, R. S. (1992). The effects of catalase gene overexpression on life span and resistance to oxidative stress in transgenic *Drosophila melanogaster. Archives of Biochemistry and Biophysics, 297,* 35–41.

Orr, W. C., & Sohal, R. S. (1993). Effects of Cu-Zn superoxide dismutase overexpression on life span and resistance to oxidative stress in transgenic *Drosophila melanogaster. Archives of Biochemistry and Biophysics, 301,* 34–40.

Orr, W. C., & Sohal, R. S. (1994). Extension of life-span by overexpression of superoxide dismutase and catalase in *Drosophila melanogaster. Science, 263,* 1128–1130.

Orr, W. C., Arnold, L. A., & Sohal, R. S. (1992). Relationship between catalase activity, life span and some parameters associated with antioxidant defenses in *Drosophila melanogaster. Mechanisms of Ageing and Development, 63,* 287–296.

Partridge, L., & Fowler, K. (1992). Direct and correlated responses to selection on age at reproduction in *Drosophila melanogaster. Evolution, 46,* 76–91.

Pearl, R. (1922). *The Biology of Death, Being a Series of Lectures Delivered at the Lowell Institute in Boston in December 1920.* Philadelphia and London: J. B. Lippincott.

Pearl, R. (1928). *The Rate of Living.* New York: Alfred A. Knopf.

Pearl, R., & Doering, C. R. (1923). A comparison of mortality of certain lower organisms with that of man. *Science, 57,* 209.

Pearl, R., Parker, S. L., & Gonzalez, B. M. (1923). Experimental studies on the duration of life. 7. The Mendelian Inheritance of duration of life in crosses of wild type and quintuple stocks of *Drosophila melanogaster. American Naturalist, 57,* 153–192.

Phillips, J. P., & Hilliker, A. J. (1990). Genetic analysis of oxygen defense mechanisms in *Drosophila. Advances in Genetics, 28,* 43–71.

Phillips, J. P., Campbell, S. D., Michard, D., Charbonneau, M., & Hilliker, A. J. (1989). Null mutation of copper zinc superoxide dismutase in *Drosophila* confers hypersensitivity to paraquat and reduced longevity. *Proceedings of the National Academy of Sciences of the United States of America, 86,* 2761–2765.

Reveillaud, I., Niedzwiecki, A., Bensch, K. G., & Fleming, J. E. (1991). Expression of bovine superoxide dismutase in *Drosophila melanogaster* augments resistance to oxidative stress. *Molecular and Cellular Biology, 11,* 632–640.

Reveillaud, I., Phillips, J., Duyf, B., Hilliker, A., Kongpachith, A., & Fleming, J. E. (1994). Phenotypic rescue by a bovine transgene in a Cu/Zn superoxide dismutase-null mutant of *Drosophila melanogaster. Molecular and Cellular Biology, 14,* 1302–1307.

Romer, A. S. (1970). *The Vertebrate Body* (4th ed.). Philadelphia: W. B. Saunders.

Roper, C., Pignatelli, P., & Partridge, L. (1993). Evolutionary effects of selection on age at reproduction in larval and adult *Drosophila melanogaster. Evolution, 47,* 445–55.

Rose, M. R. (1984a). Genetic covariation in *Drosophila* life history: Untangling the data. *American Naturalist, 123,* 565–569.

Rose, M. R. (1984b). Laboratory evolution of postponed senescence in *Drosophila melanogaster. Evolution, 38,* 1004–1010.

Rose, M. R. (1991). *Evolutionary Biology of Aging.* New York: Oxford University Press.

Rose, M. R., & Charlesworth, B. (1980). A test of evolutionary theories of senescence. *Nature, 287,* 141–142.

Rose, M. R., & Charlesworth, B. (1981a). Genetics of life history in *Drosophila melanogaster.* I. Sib analysis of adult females. *Genetics, 97,* 173–186.

Rose, M. R., & Charlesworth, B. (1981b). Genetics of life history in *Drosophila melanogaster.*

II. Exploratory selection experiments. *Genetics, 97,* 187–196.

Rose, M. R., & Finch, C. E. (1993). The Janiform genetics of aging. *Genetica, 91,* 3–10.

Rose, M. R., Nusbaum, T. J., & Fleming, J. E. (1992a). *Drosophila* with postponed aging as a model for aging research. *Laboratory Animal Science, 42,* 114–118.

Rose, M. R., Vu, L. N., Park, S. U., & Graves, J. L. (1992b). Selection on stress resistance increases longevity in *Drosophila melanogaster. Experimental Gerontology, 27,* 241–250.

Rubin, G. M., & Spradling, A. C. (1982). Genetic transformation of *Drosophila* with transposable element vectors. *Science, 218,* 348.

Saul, R. L., Gee, P., & Ames, B. N. (1987). Free radicals, DNA damage, and ageing. In H. R. Warner *et al.* (Eds.), *Modern Biological Theories of Aging* (pp. 113–129). New York: Raven Press.

Service, P. M. (1987). Physiological mechanisms of increased stress resistance in *Drosophila melanogaster* selected for postponed senescence. *Physiological Zoology, 60,* 321–326.

Service, P. M. (1989). The effect of mating status on lifespan, egg laying, and starvation resistance in *Drosophila melanogaster* in relation to selection on longevity. *Journal of Insect Physiology, 35,* 447–452.

Service, P. M., Hutchinson, E. W., MacKinley, M. D., & Rose, M. R. (1985). Resistance to environmental stress in *Drosophila melanogaster* selected for postponed senescence. *Physiological Zoology, 58,* 380–389.

Service, P. M., Hutchinson, E. W., & Rose, M. R. (1988). Multiple genetic mechanisms for the evolution of senescence in *Drosophila melanogaster. Evolution, 42,* 708–716.

Seto, N. O. L., Hayashi, S., & Tener, G. M. (1990). Overexpression of Cu-Zn superoxide dismutase in *Drosophila* does not affect lifespan. *Proceedings of the National Academy of Sciences of the United States of America, 87,* 4270–4274.

Shepherd, J. C. W., Walldorf, V., Hug, P., & Gehring, W. J. (1989). Fruit flies with additional expression of the elongation factor EF-1 alpha live longer. *Proceedings of the National Academy of Sciences of the United States of America, 86,* 7520–7521.

Shikama, N., Ackermann, R., & Brack, C. (1994). Protein synthesis elongation factor EF-1 alpha expression and longevity in *Drosophila melanogaster. Proceedings of the National Academy of Sciences of the United States of America, 91,* 4199–4203.

Sinet, P. M., Lejeune, J., & Jerome, H. (1979). Trisomy 21 (Down's Syndrome) glutathione peroxidase, hexose monophosphate shunt and I.Q. *Life Sciences, 24,* 29–34.

Smith, D. S. (1968). *Insect Cells: Their Structure and Function.* Edinburgh: Oliver & Boyd.

Spicer, G. S., & Fleming, J. E. (1991). Genetic differentiation of *Drosophila melanogaster* populations as assessed by two-dimensional electrophoresis. *Biochemical Genetics, 29,* 389–401.

Staveley, B. E., Phillips, J. P., & Hilliker, A. J. (1990). Phenotypic consequences of copper/zinc superoxide dismutase overexpression in *Drosophila melanogaster. Genome, 33,* 867–872.

Stearns, S. C., & Kaiser, M. (1993). The effects of enhanced expression of EF-1 alpha on lifespan in *Drosophila melanogaster.* IV. A summary of three experiments. *Genetica, 91,* 167–182.

Templeton, A. R., Johnston, J. S., & Sing, C. F. (1987). The proximate and ultimate control of aging in *Drosophila* and humans. In A. D. Woodhead & K. H. Thompson (Eds.), *Evolution of Longevity in Animals: A Comparative Approach* (pp. 123–133). New York: Plenum.

Templeton, A. R., Hollocher, H., Lawler, S., & Johnston, J. S. (1990). The ecological genetics of abnormal abdomen in *Drosophila melanogaster.* In J. S. Barker & W. T. Starner (Eds.), *Ecological and Evolutionary Genetics of Drosophila.* San Diego: Academic Press.

Trout, W. E., & Kaplan, W. D. (1981). Mosaic mapping of foci associated with longevity in the neurological mutants Hk and Sh of *Drosophila melanogaster. Experimental Gerontology, 16,* 461–474.

Van Delden, W., & Soliman, M. H. (1988). Alcohol, Adh, and ageing. In F. A. Lints & M. H. Soliman (Eds.), *Drosophila as a Model Organism for Ageing Studies.* Glasgow: Blackie.

Wattiaux, J. M. (1968a). Cumulative parental effects in *Drosophila subobscura. Evolution, 22,* 406–421.

Wattiaux, J. M. (1968b). Parental age effects in *Drosophila pseudoobscura*. *Experimental Gerontology, 3*, 55–61.

Webster, G. C., & Webster, S. L. (1983). Decline in synthesis of elongation factor one (EF-1) precedes the decreased synthesis of total protein in aging *Drosophila melanogaster.*

Mechanisms of Ageing and Development, 22, 121–128.

Wright, S. (1977). *Evolution and the Genetics of Populations: A Treatise in Four Volumes* (Vol. 3, *Experimental Results and Evolutionary Deductions*). Chicago: University of Chicago Press.

Six
___

Genetic Control of Senescence and Aging in Plants

Larry D. Noodén and Juan J. Guiamét

"Why are we born only to suffer and die?"
"Because in the past, those who suffered and died outreproduced those who didn't."
GRAFFITI COLLECTED FROM A MEN'S LAVATORY IN THE UNIVERSITY OF MICHIGAN MUSEUM OF
ZOOLOGY BY RICHARD D. ALEXANDER, CA. 1976.

I. The Phenomena of Senescence and Aging

A. Introduction

1. What are Senescence and Aging in Plants?

One can argue with the specifics of the lament and response cited above, but they make the point that the degeneration of organisms with age may be selected for and may even reflect adaptive processes. Understanding why these processes occur or what role(s) they serve is helpful in determining what they are and how they are controlled by genes. Remarkably, in plants, genes, i.e., death genes, not only control localized death (apoptosis-like processes) but may directly cause the degeneration (monocarpic senescence) and death of the whole organism.

In plant biology, we are evolving a conceptual distinction between aging and senescence (Leopold, 1961; Noodén & Leopold, 1978; Noodén, 1988a). Both are degenerative in the sense of diminished function or vigor, and both have the potential to lead to death, either directly by cellular collapse or indirectly by increased vulnerability to external forces, e.g., environment, disease, predators. The primary distinction is that senescence is an active (internally programmed) developmental process and aging is a passive (non-programmed) process. While the factors that drive aging may be primarily external, internal factors may also be important. Since we do not know the primary biochemistry of these two processes well, they are more hypothetical than well-defined biochemical pathways.

Senescence and aging also differ from the sudden traumatic termination of life, which is sometimes called necrosis

Handbook of the Biology of Aging, Fourth Edition
Copyright © 1996 Academic Press, Inc. All rights of reproduction in any form reserved.

(Davies & Sigee, 1984; Noodén, 1988a). The term "functional senescence" is sometimes applied to the down-regulation of metabolism that does not lead to death. This is not senescence at all, but simply a negative feedback control of metabolism (Noodén & Guiamét, 1989; Sheen, 1990) or other metabolic declines (Noodén, 1988a).

Since this chapter is aimed primarily at nonplant specialists, it seems important to provide some general background on these phenomena in plants. In this background, reviews rather than primary sources will be cited.

2. Comparison of Plant and Animal Processes

The diverse views of aging and senescence in animals are well discussed by Arking (1991). At this time, it is difficult to reconcile all of the views of what aging and senescence are in animals, let alone to unify the plant and animal perspectives. Nonetheless, senescence in the animal context may be viewed as "age-related changes in an organism that adversely affect its vitality and function" (Finch, 1990). In particular, those changes occurring later in an animal's life, especially during the post-reproductive phase, seem more important (Arking, 1991). Although aging has often been used interchangeably with senescence in the animal literature, the term "aging" carries with it the implication of passive, time-dependent degeneration.

As the biochemistry of senescence and aging is unraveled, some similarities between animals and plants will probably appear. For example, it can be argued that cessation or curtailment of cell division sets the stage for senescence and aging processes to produce death by preventing the renewal of vital parts within plants (Noodén, 1980), and presumably this principle also applies in animals. Loss of telomeric DNA appears to play an important role in hampering mitosis in animal and yeast cells (Marx, 1994). Telomeric DNA is almost identical in higher animals and plants (Zakian, 1989), suggesting some commonality at this level. What is very clear in plants, but less clear in animals, is that active, rapid degeneration processes may be superimposed on this cessation of growth and regeneration. The rapid degeneration (monocarpic senescence) in whole plants resembles apoptosis in animals, except that the plant DNA does not seem to get fragmented (Section II.B). Plant monocarpic senescence does have a counterpart in those animals, such as certain species of salmon and some marsupial shrews, that die soon after their one and only reproductive episode (Finch, 1990).

B. Senescence—A Developmental Process

1. Biochemistry of the Senescence Syndrome

Ultimately, senescence results in the loss of homeostasis at the cell or organism level (Noodén, 1988a); however, the primary or causal reactions that drive senescence are not exactly clear. Because of these uncertainties, the term "senescence" is generally used to describe the broader senescence syndrome, which includes both causal and secondary reactions. In any case, this process is an active, orderly dismantling process.

The biochemistry of plant senescence will only be outlined here, but the details can be found elsewhere (Thimann, 1980; Lesham, Halevy, & Frenkel, 1986; Thomson, Nothnagel, & Huffaker, 1987; Noodén & Leopold, 1988; Borochov & Woodson, 1989; Brown, Paliyath, & Thompson, 1991; Matile, 1992; Feller & Fischer, 1994; Smart, 1994). The ultrastructural changes observed in senescing plant cells provide an informative outline of the process (Noodén & Leopold, 1978; Noodén, 1988a). The earliest changes are alterations of the photosynthetic membranes (thylakoids) and a decrease in the ribosomes and polysomes, both cytoplasmic and chloroplastic. Chlorophyll loss is related to thylakoid breakdown and is the most widely used measure of senescence in green tissues. Usually, the mitochondria, nuclei, and vacuolar membranes persist with little visible change until quite late. The plasma (cell) membranes appear to be the last to go, and this probably marks the collapse of homeostasis, i.e., death.

Although protein and RNA synthesis also decrease during senescence, some synthesis continues until quite late, and certain enzymes and mRNAs may increase (Section II.A.4). Senescence appears to require energy, which is probably why the integrity of the mitochondria is maintained until quite late (Noodén, 1988a). Indeed, activation or increase in key dismantling enzymes such as special proteases or lipases rather than a decrease in "housekeeping" or self-maintenance proteins may cause senescence (Section II.A).

2. Endogenous Control—Case Studies

Senescence may be triggered in the whole organism, in organs, in groups of cells, or even in individual cells, leaving neighboring cells alive and fully functional (Leopold, 1961; Noodén, 1988a). Often, but not always, the senescent organs are shed (Addicott, 1982). Some of the strongest evidence for endogenous control comes from correlative controls, which are the influences of an organ on other parts (Noodén, 1988a). Usually, the correlative controls are mediated by hormones.

The classic example of correlative control of senescence is the ability of roots to retard leaf senescence (Molisch, 1938) by producing the antisenescence hormone, cytokinin (Van Staden, Cook, & Noodén, 1988). Another conspicuous example is the senescence of peripheral flower parts following pollination (Mayak & Halevy, 1980; Gori, 1983), and this is often medi-

ated by the hormonal signal ethylene. Xylem cell differentiation, which ends in cell death and dissolution, is controlled by auxin coming from nearby leaves or from shoot apices (Roberts, Gahan, & Aloni, 1988).

Many plants, especially annuals and biennials, senesce and die as they produce seeds (monocarpic senescence) (Noodén, 1988a,b). Often, but not always, monocarpic senescence is controlled by the developing reproductive structures, particularly the seeds (Leopold, 1961; Noodén, 1988b). These and many other examples show that senescence is regulated by endogenous factors and therefore is programmed, i.e., genetically controlled.

C. Senescence as an Adaptive Process— Why It Pays To Die

1. Disposal of Unneeded Parts and Remodeling

Often, senescence serves to dispose of unneeded parts, such as tree leaves in autumn or flower petals following pollination. In fleshy and dry fruits, the peripheral parts senesce in final preparation for dispersal. The xylem cell protoplast is broken down to reduce resistance to sap flow (Roberts, Gahan, & Aloni, 1988). In some leaves, groups of cells senesce as a key part of morphogenesis (Noodén, 1988a), much like apoptosis in animals.

2. Reclamation and Reinvestment of Resources

Reclamation of the nutrient resources invested in the cells and organs of plants generally, but not always, proceeds along with senescence. Reclamation is particularly important in whole plant senescence, and the losses are most conspicuous in leaves, where the majority of the nitrogen is invested in the proteins of the photosynthetic apparatus (Lawlor, 1993). Usually during monocarpic senescence, nutrients (especially nitrogen in the form of amino acids) are released from the leaves and redistributed to the fruits, where they are used to make more or larger seeds (Molisch, 1938; Noodén, 1988b). Nonetheless, this breakdown may not be causal or central in the senescence process (Noodén, 1988b).

D. Aging—A Passive Process

1. Exogenous Control—Case Studies

The clearest illustration of aging in plants is the loss of viability (ability to germinate) in seeds over time, although similar processes occur in other tissues. Seeds may present a clearer view of aging processes because most of their repair metabolism is suspended. The rate of loss of viability in seeds is strongly influenced by environmental conditions (Priestley, 1986; McKersie, Senaratna, Walker, Kendall, & Hetherington, 1988; Roberts, 1988; Roos, 1988). However, the seeds of different species may differ greatly in their longevity.

The key to seed longevity may lie in the impermeability of the seed coats to oxygen and water, both of which decrease longevity. Since the seed coats and other self-protective mechanisms greatly influence seed aging, and these are under genetic control, seed aging is also under genetic control, albeit indirect.

2. Key Biochemical Lesions

Due to their economic importance, extensive studies have been made on the biochemical lesions that accumulate as seeds age. These lesions, reviewed in detail elsewhere (Anderson & Baker, 1983; Priestley, 1986; McKersie et al., 1988; Roberts, 1988), fall into three general groupings:

(a) decreased metabolism, especially respiration
(b) loss of membrane integrity
(c) damaged DNA

No doubt, reduced metabolism, especially respiration, and ATP synthesis hamper self-maintenance and repair, but the changes in the plasma membrane probably produce the collapse of homeostasis.

The lesions in DNA seem important and, from the viewpoint of this chapter, particularly relevant. Aged seeds produce more seedlings with developmental abnormalities and pigment deficiencies than young seeds (Nobbe, 1876; Priestley, 1986), and the progeny of aged seeds segregate more mutant phenotypes (Klekowski, 1988a,b). Interestingly, these mutations may not themselves cause loss of seed viability or at least not until the mutations reach a high frequency.

As the seed embryos age and lose their viability, the DNA becomes fragmented and the chromosomes may show breaks (Nilsson, 1931; Sax, 1962; Osborne, Sharon, & Ben-Ishai, 1980/81; Osborne & Cheah, 1982; Cherry & Skadsen, 1986; Priestley, 1986; Roberts, 1988; Roos, 1988). The frequency of cells with aberrant mitoses can be quite high, 80% or more, when the seed embryo cells start to divide during germination (Roberts, 1988). Figure 1 illustrates some of these aberrations. Significantly, the DNA fragments that form in aging seeds do not fall into discrete size classes ("laddering"), indicating that the fragmentation is random.

3. Causality and Recovery

Age-related lesions accumulate as a function of time, but the rate depends on the temperature and moisture content of the seeds (Priestley, 1986; Roos, 1986; Roberts, 1988; Hendry, 1993). Higher temperatures, moisture contents, and oxygen concentrations increase the rate of damage accumulation. Free radical scavengers offer some protection, suggesting that active oxygen species such as superoxide participate (Priestley, 1986; McKersie et al., 1988).

Highly reactive chemicals such as

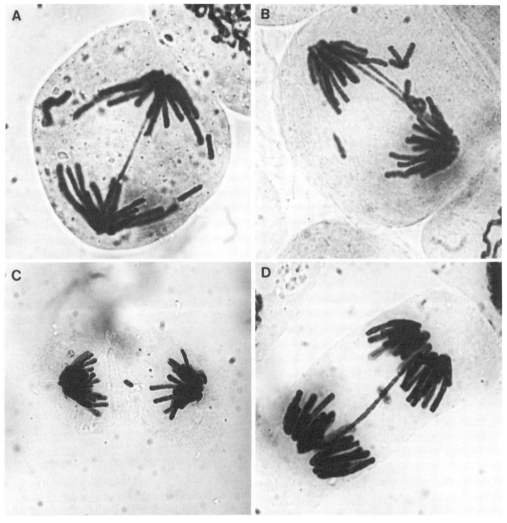

Figure 1. Chromosomal aberrations in anaphase cells from the embryonic root tip in broad bean (A, B) and onion (C, D) seeds during early germination. (A) shows a single bridge and several unequal fragments, (B) shows a double bridge and two pairs of unequal fragments plus other fragments, (C) shows a single fragment, and (D) shows a single bridge and fragment (from Roberts, 1988).

peroxides and superoxides can be generated as byproducts of normal cell metabolism (McKersie *et al.*, 1988; Vigo-Pelfrey, 1990; Halliwell & Aruoma, 1993; Lawlor, 1993; Yu, 1993), and these may also cause the lesions cited in Section I.D.2. Although these agents seem to blur the distinction between senescence and aging, in that they can be endogenous, it may be more appropriate to include them in the aging process because they usually seem to be generated as byproducts of normal metabolism. Sometimes, the endogenous production of these active agents is invoked as a driving force for senescence; however, they seem too indiscriminate to drive the orderly senescence process.

If aging-related degeneration has not progressed too far, seeds can recover remarkably (Table I; Abdulla & Roberts,

Table I

Chromosome Aberrations in *Allium cepa* Root
Tips at Successive Stages of Root Development[a]

Length of roots (mm)	Total cells analyzed	Percentage aberrations
2–5	450	10.4
7–9	58	6.6
10–12	138	5.8
25–30	190	2.1
80–100	116	1.7

[a]From Osborne (1983) after Nichols (1941).

1969; Murata, Tsuchiya, & Roos, 1984).
First, the various lesions may be repaired
through "unscheduled" DNA synthesis
(Osborne, 1983; Roberts, 1988). Second,
the defective cells may also be replaced
as cells with less damage out-multiply
those with more damage during seedling
growth. The same processes appear to take
place in tissues other than seeds; however,
because these other tissues are more active metabolically, they probably are better able to keep up with their repairs than
seeds are.

II. Senescence-Related Changes in Gene Expression

A. Evidence for Genetic Controls

Genetic control is implicit in the evidence
that senescence is an active process (Section I.B). More direct evidence comes from
four general lines of experimentation:

1. enucleation
2. selective inhibitors
3. mutations
4. changes in gene expression

1. Enucleation Studies

The chloroplasts in the nucleate *Elodea*
leaf protoplasts senesce, whereas those in
the enucleate protoplasts do not (Yoshida,
1961). Enucleation greatly prolongs the life
of the large, unicellular alga *Acetabularia*
(Hämmerling, 1953).

2. Use of Selective Inhibitors

Actinomycin D, a selective inhibitor of
DNA-dependent RNA synthesis, inhibits
senescence in leaves and petals (Noodén,
1988c). Thus, inhibitors indicate that nuclear gene expression is required for senescence.

Further insights can be obtained from
the two general classes of inhibitors of protein synthesis, i.e., those acting primarily
on cytoplasmic (eukaryotic) ribosomes,
such as cycloheximide, and those acting
mainly on chloroplast (prokaryotic) ribosomes, such as chloramphenicol. Generally, cycloheximide and similar inhibitors
retard senescence while chloramphenicol usually does not, which indicates
that senescence is driven mainly by nuclear genes and mRNAs translated in the
cytoplasm (Brady, 1988; Noodén, 1988c;
Matile, 1992). Nonetheless, chloramphenicol sometimes does inhibit senescence,
which suggests that genes and protein synthesis in the chloroplast may contribute to
the senescence process. The studies with
inhibitors also suggest that senescence is
not induced primarily by shutting genes
off, but instead by turning them on
(Noodén, 1988c).

3. Mutations Altering Senescence

A very wide range of mutations are known
to cause degeneration and premature
death. Most, if not all, of these interfere
with some essential process, i.e., auxin
hormone or chlorophyll production, and
most probably do not alter senescence directly.

Senescence-retarding mutations are easier to connect to senescence, and many
such mutants have been found (Table II;
Thomas & Smart, 1993). Without any
doubt, nonyellowing or stay-green types
are over-represented among the senescence-

Table II
Genetic Alterations of Senescence

Species	Genotype/inheritance	Phenotype	References
		A. Delay Whole Plant Death	
Cowpea	ND	Prolongs fruiting, residual green leaves after maturation of first set of fruits	Gwathmey, Hall, and Madore (1992)
Sorghum	ND	Increases green leaf retention, axillary bud growth (tillering); prolongs cytokinin production	Duncan, Bockholt, and Miller (1981); Ambler, Morgan, and Jordan (1992)
Soybean	Homozygosity for the recessive alleles at loci dt_1, dt_2, e_1, and e_2	Increases branching, slows decline in photosynthesis and nitrogen fixation	Phillips, Pierce, Edie, Foster, and Knowles (1984)
Pea	E Sn Hr	Delays apex senescence and ultimately plant death under short-day photoperiods	Proebsting, Davies, and Marx (1978); Kelly and Davies (1988)
		B. Inhibition of Chloroplast Breakdown	
Bean	Homozygosity for the recessive allele *ih* plus dominant *Gr*	Inhibits degradation of chloroplast membranes and thylakoid components (chlorophyll, light-harvesting complexes, cytochrome f)	Ronning, Bouwkamp, and Solomos (1991); Thomas and Smart (1993)
Corn	Nuclear, dominant	Inhibits chlorophyll and water loss	Ceppi, Sala, Gentinetta, Verderio, and Motto (1987)
Festuca pratensis	Sid^g (nuclear, recessive)	Inhibits degradation of thylakoid membranes, pigments, light-harvesting complexes, D1 protein, and cytochrome f	Thomas and Stoddart (1975); Thomas and Smart (1993)
Soybean	Homozygosity for the recessive alleles at loci d_1 and d_2 (nuclear)	Inhibits breakdown of chlorophyll and chlorophyll-binding proteins, rubisco, and soluble proteins	Guiamét, Schwartz, Pichersky, and Noodén (1991); Guiamét and Giannibelli (1994)
Soybean	G (nuclear, dominant)	Inhibits chlorophyll loss in seed coats	Bernard and Weiss (1973)
Soybean	*cytG* (cytoplasmic factor)	Inhibits degradation of chlorophyll, light-harvesting complex II and cytochrome f	Guiamét, Schwartz, Pichersky, and Noodén (1991); Guiamét, Pichersky, Green, and Noodén (1994)
Tomato	*gf* (nuclear, recessive)	Inhibits chlorophyll and thylakoid membrane breakdown	Grierson, Purton, Knapp, and Bathgate (1987)
		C. Abscission Mutants	
Soybean	*ab* (nuclear, recessive)	Delays leaf abscission, particularly under stress conditions	van Schaik and Probst (1958)
		D. Ethylene-Related Mutations	
Arabidopsis thaliana	*etr* (nuclear, dominant)	Decreases sensitivity to the plant hormone ethylene; delays leaf senescence	Bleecker, Estelle, Somerville, and Kende (1988)

Table II (*Continued*)

Species	Genotype/inheritance	Phenotype	References
Tomato	*Nr*	Reduces ethylene sensitivity; delays chlorophyll breakdown and flower senescence	Lanahan, Yen, Giovannoni, and Klee (1994)
Tomato	*rin*	Prevents climacteric rise in ethylene synthesis, slows degradation of chlorophyll and softening of cell walls	Grierson, Purton, Knapp, and Bathgate (1987)
Tomato	Transgenic line expressing EFE-antisense genes	Reduces synthesis of ethylene, delays senescence of leaves	Picton, Barton, Bouzayen, Hamilton, and Grierson (1993)
E. Cytokinin-Related Mutations			
Tobacco	Transgenic line expressing *tmr* under the control of a heat-shock promoter	Increases cytokinin levels and delays leaf senescence in transformed plants given a series of heat-shock treatments	Smart, Schofield, Bevan, and Dyer (1991)
Tobacco	Line transformed with *ipT* under the control of a SAVR promoter	Increases cytokinin levels and delays leaf senescence	Li, Hagen, and Guilfoyle (1992)
Sorghum, see part A			
F. Light-Signaling Mutations			
Arabidopsis thaliana	*det 2* (nuclear, recessive)	Delays chlorophyll loss; typical light phenotype in dark-grown plants	Chory, Nagpal, and Peto (1991)
Tobacco	Transgenic line expressing the photoreceptor phytochrome constitutively	Delays degradation of chlorophyll and protein; "light-exaggerated phenotype"	Cherry, Hershey, and Vierstra (1991)

retarding mutants, probably because they are very easy to identify and are not lethal. Genetic engineering has also produced "mutants" by changing specific processes that alter senescence.

During monocarpic senescence in soybean, the leaves and other parts normally turn yellow, followed by leaf shedding, and then the plant dies. The mutations $cytG$ and d_1d_2 prevent this yellowing (Guiamét, Teeri, & Noodén, 1990; Guiamét, Schwartz, Pichersky, & Noodén, 1991). $cytG$ exerts only a partial blockage of yellowing, selectively preserving only part of the chlorophyll antenna system, specifically the light-harvesting complex II, which is the major group of light-harvesting proteins (Lawlor, 1993). $cytG$ is of special interest because it shows a cytoplasmic inheritance pattern and presumably is coded in the chloroplast DNA (plastome). This indicates that the chloroplast may exert some control over its own dismantling.

By contrast, d_1d_2 exerts a wide array of antisenescence actions, apparently preserving overall photosynthetic capacity (Guiamét *et al.*, 1990, 1991; Guiamét & Giannibelli, 1994). Although d_1d_2 does not inhibit the decline in photosynthesis during seed maturation, the addition of G to form Gd_1d_2 does maintain photosynthesis possibly by maintaining the demand for photosynthate (Guiamét et al., 1990). Significantly, neither cytG nor Gd_1d_2 delays leaf abscission. Thus, disassembly of the photosynthetic apparatus and leaf abscission are parallel but separately regulated components of monocarpic senescence (Noodén, 1988b).

By far the most work has been done on the mutation Sid (senescence-induced degradation), which prevents leaf yellowing in meadow fescue grass, Festuca pratensis (Thomas & Stoddart, 1975; Thomas & Smart, 1993). F. pratensis is a perennial pasture grass, which forms bunches, sending up numerous shoots or ramets. Sid is a nuclear gene and can be designated Sid^g for stay-green (recessive) and Sid^Y for normal yellowing (Thomas & Smart, 1993). Sid^g prevents the normal yellowing of the leaves, but not the decline of photosynthesis and presumably not the death of the leaves. It may act by blocking a step in the breakdown of chlorophyll (Thomas, Bortlik, Rentsch, Schellenberg, & Matile, 1989; Thomas & Smart, 1993).

It is noteworthy that the stay-green phenotype can be produced by other means. In sorghum, sustaining the production of the senescence-inhibiting hormones, the cytokinins, by the roots seems to produce the nonsenescing phenotype (Ambler et al., 1992), but neither cytG nor Gd_1d_2 in soybean works this way (Kahanak, Okatan, Rupp, & Noodén, 1978).

Light is an important environmental cue for senescence (Noodén & Leopold, 1978; Biswal & Biswal, 1984), and it also controls the expression of a number of genes, including many of those coding for the photosynthetic apparatus (Quail, 1991; Thompson & White, 1991). Generally, light at low or moderate intensities delays senescence, or conversely, darkness promotes senescence. Some of the mutations that permanently (constitutively) turn on the light-stimulated signaling pathway also delay leaf senescence (Table II).

The gaseous hormone ethylene functions as a senescence-promoting signal in many tissues, particularly flowers and fruits, but the role of ethylene in leaf senescence has been less clear (Mayak & Halevy, 1980; Mattoo & Aharoni, 1988; Borochov & Woodson, 1989; Brady & Spiers, 1991; O'Neill et al., 1993). Antisense constructs for key enzymes in ethylene synthesis can inhibit ethylene production and delay ripening and senescence in tomato fruits (Table II). Some of these antisense genes aimed at fruits have also been found to inhibit flower and leaf senescence. In addition, a number of ethylene-insensitive mutants have been isolated, and these appear to inhibit senescence (Bleeker et al., 1988; Lanahan et al., 1994). Antisense genes for enzymes that cause softening in fruits also retard the softening and eventual senescence of tomato fruits (Oeller, Min-Wong, Taylor, & Pike, 1991).

The cytokinin hormone family plays an important role in preventing senescence or maintaining function in a variety of organs (Van Staden et al., 1988). Several groups have genetically engineered tobacco plants to produce higher levels of cytokinins, and these delay leaf senescence when the gene is expressed (Table II).

In summary, most of the stay-green mutations are recessive, which suggests that these mutations may knock out some enzyme or gene function that is required for senescence. Some of the stay-green genes such as d_1d_2 in soybean exert such broad pleiotropic antisenescence effects that one has to suspect that d_1 and d_2 are primary senescence-regulating or master genes. Genetic engineering has been employed to retard senescence through the alteration of some specific control function, i.e., hormone or light control. It is particularly promising that senescence-responsive promoters are starting to be identified (Ursin & Shewmaker, 1993).

4. Changes in Gene Expression

Ultimately, understanding senescence will require knowing which genes are turned on or off during senescence. Since senescence does not seem to be induced primarily by turning off RNA and protein synthesis (Section II.A.2), this section will emphasize up-regulated genes, mostly omitting down-regulated genes. Nonetheless, some down-regulation or turning off of functions is probably essential to the senescence process to prevent regeneration at the cell–subcell level, just as a curtailment of growth is required at a higher level to stop cell and organ replacement (Sections I.A and III.B).

Unfortunately, many of the studies on the biochemistry of senescence have used leaf tissues induced to senesce by excision and/or darkness. Although this type of senescence may not be fully representative of that that occurs in intact tissues (Noodén & Leopold, 1978), and it has been proposed that all such data be discarded (Woolhouse, 1987), these studies will probably reveal a lot about normal senescence (Noodén, 1988a); however, the discrepancies need to be recognized.

Both the amounts of RNA and protein and their syntheses decline during senescence and thereby affect the phenotypic expression of genes. The number of ribosomes, both cytoplasmic and chloroplastic, decreases early in senescence (Section I.B.1; Brady, 1988). Nonetheless, it is clear that RNA and protein synthesis continues during senescence, even quite late in senescence (Wollgiehn, 1967; Lamattina, Lezica, & Conde, 1985; Martin, Urteaga, & Sabater, 1986; Martin & Sabater, 1989; Bate, Strauss, & Thompson, 1990; Bate, Rothstein, & Thompson, 1991). Since RNA polymerase activities decrease during senescence, there seems to be a real decrease in RNA synthesis. It has been claimed that RNA polymerase activity completely disappears during early senescence in chloroplasts (Ness & Woolhouse,

1980), but this is incorrect, probably due to the failure to protect the RNA polymerase against proteolytic attack.

Individual proteins markedly differ in when and how rapidly they decline. It has been proposed that plastome-encoded proteins decrease ahead of nuclear-encoded proteins (Batt & Woolhouse, 1975; Ness & Woolhouse, 1980), but this clearly is not true (Gepstein, 1988). For example, the two subunits of the major CO_2-fixing enzyme ribulose bisphosphate carboxylase and the corresponding mRNAs drop together, even though one is encoded in the nucleus while the other is encoded in the plastome (Spiers & Brady, 1981). Similarly, plastome- and nucleus-encoded proteins in each complex, e.g., photosystems I and II, in the thylakoids decrease together (Gepstein, 1988; Lawlor, 1993; Guiamét, Pichersky, Green, & Noodén, 1994). Furthermore, the synthesis and the levels of some plastome-encoded mRNAs are maintained until quite late in senescence (Bate *et al.*, 1990, 1991; Droillard, Bate, Rothstein, & Thompson, 1992).

An implication of the genetic control of senescence (Sections II.A.1–3) is that changes in gene expression must accompany this syndrome, i.e., specific gene products should increase in abundance following the onset of senescence. Three general approaches have been used to analyze these changes (Table III).

First, analysis of the translation products of mRNAs isolated at various stages indicate that some mRNAs appear while others disappear during senescence.

Second, differential screening of cDNA libraries has identified several genes expressed preferentially in senescing petals and leaves.

Third, some progress has been made in identifying specific genes such as those producing ethylene or degradative enzymes whose expression increases during senescence, and some of these may even cause senescence.

In addition, several (usually unidentified)

Table III
Genes Up-Regulated in Senescing Tissues

Organ/type of senescence	Species	Observations	References
A. In vitro Translation of mRNAs			
Flower senescence	Carnation	Five translation products increase in senescing tissues	Woodson (1987)
Dark-induced (excised cotyledons)	Radish	Twenty-six translation products increase during senescence	Kawakami and Watanabe (1993)
Attached and detached leaves	*Festuca pratensis*	A small number of translation products appear *de novo* during senescence	Thomas, Ougham, and Davies (1992)
B. Isolation of cDNAs Corresponding to mRNAs That Increase in Senescing Tissues, but Whose Function Is Unknown			
Flower senescence	Carnation	Concentrations of two mRNAs increase in senescing petals	Lawton, Huang, Goldsbrough, and Woodson (1989)
Dark-induced, excised leaves	Barley	Concentrations of three mRNAs increase, but two of these are not detected in naturally senescing (attached) leaves	Becker and Apel (1993)
C. Expression of Ethylene Biosynthetic Genes			
Flower senescence	Petunia, carnation	Concentrations of mRNAs for ACC synthase and ACC oxidase increase	Woodson, Park, Drory, Larsen, and Wang (1992); Michael, Savin, Baudinette, Graham, Chandler, Lu, Caesar, Gautrais, Young, Nugent, Stevenson, O'Connor, Cobbett, and Cornish (1993)
Flower senescence	*Phalaenopsis* sp.	Concentrations of mRNAs for ACC synthase and ACC oxidase increase	Nadeau, Zhang, Nair, and O'Neill (1993); O'Neill, Nadeau, Zhang, Bui, and Halevy (1993)
D. Abscission-Related Genes			
Excised leaf explants	Bean	Cellulase mRNA increases in the abscission zone	Tucker, Matters, Koehler, Kemmerer, and Baird (1993)
E. Xylem Cell Differentiation			
Roots and cultured leaf mesophyll cells		Concentrations of several mRNAs increase and three are localized in the differentiating xylem cells	Demura and Fukuda (1994)
F. Proteases and Ribonucleases			
Leaf	*Arabidopsis thaliana*	Concentrations of an mRNA encoding a cysteine proteinase increase	Hensel, Grbic, Baumgarten, and Bleecker (1993)
Flower petals and leaves	*Arabidopsis thaliana*	Concentrations of an mRNA for ribonuclease (RNS2) increase	Taylor, Bariola, Del Cardayre, Raines, and Green (1993)
Leaf	*Arabidopsis thaliana*	Concentrations of six mRNAs including one encoding cysteine proteinase increases	Lohman, Gan, John, and Amasino (1994)

Table III (*Continued*)

Organ/type of senescence	Species	Observations	References
		G. Pathogenesis- or Stress-Related Proteins	
Dark-induced	Radish	Concentrations of a mRNA for a protein with high similarity to pathogenesis-related proteins increase; repressed by cytokinins	Azumi and Watanabe (1991)
Progressive	Soybean	Concentrations of an mRNA that also accumulates in response to stress increase; similar to pathogenesis-related proteins	Crowell, John, Russell, and Amasino (1992)

proteins have been shown to appear or disappear during senescence.

Finally, there is probably some shared biochemistry between senescence and environmental stress responses in plants (Noodén, 1988a; Van Staden *et al.*, 1988; Ohashi & Ohshima, 1992; Scholes, 1992; Smart, 1994). Similarly, the expression of genes coding for "pathogenesis-related proteins" increases during senescence in some species (Azumi & Watanabe, 1991; Crowell, John, Russell, & Amasino, 1992). Ethylene may be responsible for inducing some of these proteins/genes common to both pathogenesis and senescence (Eyal & Fluhr, 1991).

Some of the genes whose expression is up-regulated during senescence clearly are not causal, but secondary or they accommodate senescence (Sections I.B and I.C). For example, enzymes of the glyoxylic acid cycle increase in order to convert the breakdown products of the released fatty acids to sugars, which can be transported and utilized elsewhere (Gut & Matile, 1988; DeBellis, Tsugeki, & Nishimura, 1991; Graham, Leaver, & Smith, 1992). Likewise, the breakdown of proteins releases large quantities of amino acids, which can themselves be toxic, and they need to be converted to less toxic and more readily transported forms, e.g., glutamine and asparagine (Kamachi, Yamaya, Hayakawa, Mae, & Ojima, 1992; Vicentini & Matile, 1993). Several other metabolic functions increase. Some, e.g., glutathione S-transferases, may help to protect against the damaging effects of lipid hydroperoxides formed (Meyer, Goldsbrough, & Woodson, 1991), and metallothionein-like proteins may protect against some of the metal ions released during senescence (Buchanan-Wollaston, 1994).

Because degradation of proteins, nucleic acids, and membranes may be an integral part of senescence, much effort has been focused on degradative enzymes, especially the proteases, as causal factors (see Noodén & Leopold, 1978; Brady, 1988; Peoples & Dalling, 1988; Feller & Fischer 1994). Certainly, there are cases where protease activity rises during senescence, but there are also some noncorrelations and even negative correlations. Some of the studies that focus on a single enzyme or its mRNA offer the beginning of a clearer picture of the biochemistry of senescence (Table III). While these degradative enzymes no doubt are important components of the broader senescence syndrome, they do not necessarily cause senescence.

In addition, several hormones (i.e., ethylene, jasmonates, and cytokinins) are known to regulate senescence and also to alter gene expression, i.e., mRNA levels (Mattoo & Suttle, 1991; Abeles, Morgan, & Saltveit, 1992; Pech, Latché, & Balagué, 1992; Crowell & Amasino, 1994). In some cases, the hormones have been shown to increase or decrease particular mRNAs as they induce or retard senescence. This linkage between the hormones and gene expression does provide stronger evidence, but again not definitive proof, of a connection between those genes and senescence.

5. Antagonistic Pleiotropy

The concept of antagonistic pleiotropy has been so significant in the thinking about animal aging (Alexander, 1987; Kirkwood & Rose, 1991; Finch, 1990; Finch & Johnson, 1990; Rose, 1991) that it warrants some discussion here. Basically, the antagonistic pleiotropy theory holds that certain genes that are highly beneficial at younger stages are detrimental later, causing degeneration. A central feature of this theory is that these genes could not be selected against because their detrimental effects are expressed post-reproductively. Otherwise, the detrimental genes would rapidly be selected for a more favorable expression pattern. In the case of monocarpic plants (Section III.A), senescence takes place during the reproductive phase. In fact, there is little or no post-reproductive life, so that a mechanism of this type cannot explain monocarpic senescence or any other programmed degeneration.

A specific case in point for plants may be the hydrolytic enzymes such as proteases, which mobilize the nutrients stored in seeds enabling the early development of the seedling. Later, when a new generation of seeds is forming, extensive breakdown and mobilization of resources occur in different structures, the assimilatory organs, of the parent plant (Section I.C). These changes may indeed increase the vulnerability of the parent plant to external forces, but many of these plants seemed to be programmed to die even under the best

conditions (Noodén, 1988b). Furthermore, these changes are not post-reproductive. In addition, the breakdown of seed storage depots and parent plant assimilatory organs probably involves different enzymes or isoenzymes controlled by quite different genetic regulatory elements. They probably also occur in different subcellular compartments. For example, those in the germinating seeds occur in vacuole-like vesicles (Laidman, 1982), and those in the assimilatory organs (Section I.B) seem to be outside the vacuole. Thus, it is difficult to apply the antagonistic pleiotropy explanation for genetic control of senescence when one gets down to actual biochemical mechanisms.

B. Genetic Integrity in Senescing Tissues

In contrast to aging seeds (Section I.D), senescing plant cells seem to maintain their genetic integrity until quite late. The evidence comes from three lines of observations:

First, the ultrastructure of the nucleus generally does not change until very late in senescence in most tissues (Brady, 1988; Noodén, 1988a). However, the nucleus does degenerate early in xylem cell differentiation (Lai & Srivastava, 1976), which suggests that xylogenesis may be different from other patterns of senescence.

Second, total DNA generally stays about the same in senescing leaves or decreases only slightly (Noodén & Leopold, 1978; Brady, 1988). Some of the repeated DNA sequences may be eliminated preferentially (Chang, Miksche, & Dhillon, 1985), but at least the redundant DNAs that code for rRNA do not drop preferentially (Keegan & Timmis, 1981). Some of the DNA lost could be chloroplast DNA (Wollgiehn, 1967; Brady, 1988; Gepstein, 1988; Sodmergen, Tano, & Kuroiwa, 1991).

As senescence progresses in mustard cotyledons, the size distribution profile of DNA extracted does not change (Osborne & Cheah, 1982). Restriction fragment polymorphism analyses employing two gene probes also indicate that the structural integrity of the DNA is maintained in senescing cucumber cotyledons (Abeles & Dunn, 1990). Thus, DNA does not seem to fragment during senescence.

Third, and last, the genetic capacity of the senescing tissues seems to be maintained until quite late. Plant cells do not lose their genetic capacity (totipotency) when they differentiate (Noodén & Thompson, 1985), but it is not clear how late in senescence this applies. Moreover, the issue is complicated by the fact that some species do not regenerate well (Thomas, 1994). Nonetheless, leaves and green cotyledons (Brady, 1988; Noodén, 1988a) can regenerate even after all visible chlorophyll or 85% of the protein has been lost. These demonstrate that the essential coding capacities of the DNA, including that of the chloroplasts, remain intact until late. The apparent stability of the plant DNA in senescing tissues contrasts with apoptosis in animal cells where the DNA is markedly fragmented (Martin, Green, & Cotter, 1994).

III. Longevity in Plants

A. Major Patterns

Plant longevities fall into several fairly discrete categories relative to the annual seasonal cycle. Basically, these are annuals (longevity equal or less than 1 year), biennials (longevity of more than 1 year but less than 2 years), and perennials (longevity of more than 2 years). Plants can also be classified on the basis of the number of reproductive episodes that an individual undergoes before it dies. Monocarpy (semelpary) refers to a single reproductive episode followed by death, whereas polycarpy (iteropary) designates more than one reproductive output (Molisch, 1938; Noodén, 1980). Annuals and biennials are generally monocarpic, while perennials tend to be polycarpic (Noodén, 1988a,b; Begon, Harper, & Townsend, 1990).

B. Clonal Growth—What Does Clonal Longevity Mean?

Usually, monocarpic plants show a well-defined end point. For polycarpic plants, especially for clonal plants, it is sometimes difficult to decide what constitutes an individual organism (Klekowski, 1988a,b; Noodén, 1988b), and therefore it is difficult to determine when the individual has died. The concepts of genet and ramet are useful here. The genet is the product of a single zygote, no matter what size or however subdivided (White, 1979; Klekowski, 1988b). The ramet is a single shoot complex, and individual ramets may have their own roots. In clonal organisms, a genet may contain many ramets, each existing separately from other ramets. For example, quaking aspen clones can become quite large with many ramets spreading over 81 hectares, and these clones apparently live for a very long time, probably more than 10,000 years (Kemperman & Barnes, 1976; Noodén, 1988b). However, the ramets, which are more like individual trees, do not live long.

In this way, the clonal genet escapes the determinate growth that limits most genets (Section VI.A). These ramets certainly are separate individuals independent from the rest of the genet, just as identical human twins (clones) are separate organisms (Noodén, 1988b). Nonetheless, clones also degenerate and die (Sax, 1962; Noodén, 1988b; Van Groenendael & De Kroon, 1990), possibly due to genetic load (Section VI.B), but sometimes due to low-grade virus infections or changing environments.

C. Evolution of Annuals from Perennials

In general, annuals and biennials appear to be derived from perennials (Stebbins,

1974; Fox, 1990). Annuality, together with monocarpic senescence, has evolved repeatedly and independently in many different groups (Noodén, 1980, 1988a).

Why would annuals (monocarpy) evolve from perennials (polycarpy) or vice versa? Basically, annuals tend to evolve where adult or established plant survival is low relative to the juveniles or seedlings (Law *et al.*, 1977; Rathke & Lacey, 1985; Fox, 1990; Begon *et al.*, 1990; Garnier, 1992; Young & Peacock, 1992). In other words, annuals are favored where small, short-lived plants reproduce more successfully than larger, longer lived plants. Environments that favor annuality tend to have highly variable (unpredictable) climates or very high predation, for example, deserts, alpine habitats, and areas disturbed by human activity. In contrast, stable woodland habitats favor perennials (Begon *et al.*, 1990). Interestingly, many crop plants have been selected for annuality (monocarpy) and synchronous maturation (Hancock, 1992; Harlan, 1992). It is less clear why monocarpy should evolve among perennials, but some good ideas have been ventured (Janzen, 1976; Schaffer & Schaffer, 1977; Lacey, 1986).

Annual (monocarpic) individuals reproduce rapidly with large numbers of offspring and little investment in the parent generation (r patterns; Begon *et al.*, 1990). Perennial (polycarpic) individuals reproduce less rapidly, produce fewer offspring at a time, invest more in the parental generation, i.e., perenniating structures, and tend to be larger (K patterns). Thus, it is clear that longevity is usually (always?) tied to reproductive needs.

D. Longevity Is a Species Characteristic

Obviously, longevity is a characteristic of the species in the sense of annuality, bienniality, and perenniality; however, polycarpic perennials also have characteristic longevities (Noodén, 1988b). While polycarpic perennials do not undergo a well-defined, distinctive senescence phase as seen in most monocarpic plants, older individuals tend to be less vigorous (Sax, 1962; Noodén, 1988b; Meier-Dinkel & Kleinschmit, 1990). The exact causes of this decline in perennials are not clear (Section III.B). Nonetheless, genetic factors seem to determine their longevity, even if it is mainly by enhancing their resistance to environmental stress, disease, or predation.

IV. How Plants Protect Their Genetic Heritage—A Special Body Design

A. Modular Construction vs Embryonic Regions

Plants, especially the higher or vascular plants, have some special body design and developmental features that mainly serve environmental adaptive purposes, but also help the organism to combat aging processes. Overall, plants are open systems with potential for unlimited growth, tissue renewal, and immortality primarily due to the localized regions of cell divisions, the meristems (Fig. 2). As long as the production of new cells continues, this genetic population of cells, the genet, can live on indefinitely. However, this unlimited growth potential often gets truncated, i.e., determinate growth, in organs and even in meristems (Noodén, 1980, 1988b). Some plants, such as clonal species, are able to escape determinacy, and they propagate themselves asexually, producing new individuals indefinitely (Begon *et al.*, 1990; Van Groenendael & De Kroon, 1990).

B. Somatic Selection in a Cell Metapopulation

Plants do not maintain separate somatic and germ lines as animals do (Watkinson

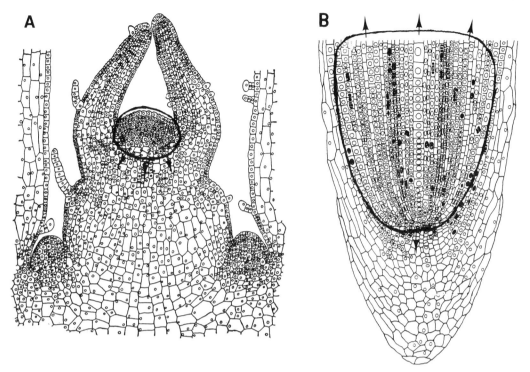

Figure 2. Root (A) and shoot (B) apical meristems showing the tissues derived from them. The apical meristems are encircled, and the arrows indicate the direction of cell production. Also, note the lineages (files) of cells arising from the apical meristem. Cell division may continue even after these files of cells have progressed out of the apical meristem.

& White, 1985; Lyndon, 1990). Even though the cells in the meristematic zones (Fig. 2) produce orderly files of cells, they still form a metapopulation (White, 1979) with some resemblance to a chemostat (Klekowski, 1988a,b).

Both macro- and micromutations accumulate with age in the somatic cells, even within the meristems themselves (Crumpacker, 1967; Klekowski, 1988a,b; Klekowski & Godfrey, 1989); however, most are not immediately life-threatening (Klekowski, 1988a,b). Of particular interest, long-lived plants acrue a greater mutational load than short-lived ones (Klekowski & Godfrey, 1989). Likewise, the abortion rates for ovules tend to be much higher in perennials (50%) than in annuals (15%) (Wiens, 1984). In spite of all this somatic mutation, species and even specific cultivars *can retain* their phenotypes over a very long time (Sax, 1962; Noodén & Thompson, 1985; Noodén, 1988b).

Although there is some competition among cells and elimination of mutant phenotypes in the somatic cell population, this selection process is complex. Sometimes mutant cells (e.g., chloroplast-deficient) have an advantage over normal cells (Klekowski, Kazarinova-Fukshansky, & Mohr, 1985). While diploidy buffers the mutations within a plant, a small haploid gametophytic phase precedes gamete formation, providing an opportunity to filter out some mutant (defective) genes (Klekowski, 1988b). This filtration may be a reason why passage through the sexual process rejuvenates polycarpic plants (Noodén, 1988b).

C. Disposable Soma as a Factor in Senescence

The disposable soma theory holds that it may be advantageous to make only a minimal investment in the construction or maintenance of an organism or just an organ (Kirkwood & Rose, 1991). It is difficult to make an accurate assessment of this idea; however, it is true that different plants and their parts have distinctive longevities (Molisch, 1938; Noodén, 1988b), and it may be particularly applicable in short-lived species such as *Arabidopsis* (Hensel *et al.*, 1993).

While it is true that defective genes do accumulate in somatic tissues (Section IV.B), it is less clear how much influence they actually exert on those tissues (Klekowski, 1988a,b). Plants have very effective mechanisms for disposing of body parts, especially leaves, once they become defective, and the resources invested in these parts may be transferred for reuse elsewhere, so that the loss is minimized. Indeed, senescence may dispose of organs before the mutational load becomes a problem (Klekowski, 1988a,b). Nonetheless, such accumulations of lesions may contribute to the decline of perennial plants (Section III.D).

V. Prospective Benefits

A. Agricultural Spinoffs

Two general areas of agriculture have benefited from studies of senescence. The first is postharvest physiology. Following harvest, or perhaps even before harvest, vegetables, fruits, and flowers undergo senescence and this may result in diminished quality and ultimately spoilage (Kays, 1991). Genetic engineering has been employed to block ethylene production and responses, e.g., synthesis of key enzymes such as polygalacturonase, which play a major role in fruit ripening and related processes, have yielded practical results (Section II.A.3). Plants genetically engineered to produce greater levels of cytokinin also show promise.

Second, field crop production sometimes seems to be limited by senescence (Noodén 1988b). For example, most field crops are monocarpic, senescing during their reproductive phase, and retardation of this senescence could increase yields (Guiamét *et al.*, 1990). Stay-green varieties of corn (maize) with retarded senescence have already been utilized successfully (Arnold & Josephson, 1975; Section II.A.3). It probably will also be beneficial to retard the senescence of the lower leaves of forage and hay crops such as alfalfa and pasture grasses, but little has been done in this direction.

B. Biomedical Implications

The large amount of biochemical literature on aging in plants provides some data that should be applicable to aging in active human cells, but the seed data should be particularly useful in understanding the changes in human tissues and reproductive cells during long-term storage in an inactive state.

Because the senescence programs are clearly defined in plants, an understanding of how these programs function in plants in terms of development, adaptive value, and their specific biochemistry should help to identify ways of probing for similar phenomena in humans.

Acknowledgments

Supported in part by a Rockefeller Foundation Biotechnology Career Fellowship to J.J.G. Juan J. Guiamét is a researcher at C.I.C., Pcia de Buenos Aires, Argentina. We thank Sarah Noodén for her help in editing this manuscript.

Note added in proof. Since this review was submitted, many important findings have been reported and it seems important to relate a few of them here, not only to update this review but also to show the dynamism of this field. First, nuclear degeneration with DNA fragmentation akin to that often seen in apoptosis of animal cells has been reported to occur during xylem formation (Section I.B.2) and in the hypersensitive response, a rapid collapse of cells as part of a defense against pathogens (Mittler *et al.*, *Plant Cell*, 7, 29, 1995; Mittler and Lam, *Plant Physiology*, 108, 489, 1995). The old observation (Phillips and Hawkins, *Journal of Experimental Botany*, 36, 119, 1985) that 3-aminobenzamide, an inhibitor of ADP-ribosyl transferase and apoptosis, also inhibits xylogenesis now becomes more significant. These observations show some similarity between animals and plants, indicating an early evolutionary origin for apoptosis (Section I.A.2 and Vaux *et al.*, *Cell*, 76, 777, 1994). Second, one of the stay-green mutations (Section II.A.3) appears to alter one of the enzymes in chlorophyll breakdown leading to an accumulation of chlorophyll and/or partial breakdown products which in turn stabilize chlorophyll-binding proteins and some other proteins in the photosynthetic membranes (Vicenti *et al.*, *New Phytologist*, 129, 247, 1995). Third, ethylene is a major senescence signal in plants (Section III.A.3), and evidence now indicates that it induces DNA-binding proteins (Ohme-Takagi and Shinshi, *Plant Cell*, 7, 173, 1995) and activates protein kinases (Chang, Kwok, Bleecker, and Myerowitz, *Science*, 262, 539, 1993). In addition, a host of genes have been shown to be up-regulated (increased mRNA) during senescence, but most are very abundant mRNAs and probably play ancillary roles (see Section II.A.4) as opposed to causing senescence. Perhaps the most interesting feature of these genes is the number which are also up-regulated in disease and environmental stress responses.

References

Abdulla, F. M., & Roberts, E. H. (1969). The effects of temperature and moisture on the induction of genetic changes in seeds of barley, broad beans and peas during storage. *Annals of Botany*, 33, 153–167.

Abeles, F. B., & Dunn, L. J. (1990). Restriction fragment length polymorphism analyses of DNA from senescing cotyledon tissue. *Plant Science*, 72, 13–17.

Abeles, F. B., Morgan, P. W., & Saltveit, M. E., Jr. (1992). *Ethylene in Plant Biology* (2nd ed.). San Diego: Academic Press, Inc.

Addicott, F. T. (1982). *Abscission.* Berkeley, CA: University of California Press.

Alexander, R. D. (1987). *The Biology of Moral Systems.* Hawthorne, NY: Aldine De Gruyter.

Ambler, J. R., Morgan, P. W., & Jordan, W. R. (1992). Amounts of zeatin and zeatin riboside in xylem sap of senescent and nonsenescent sorghum. *Crop Science*, 32, 411–419.

Anderson, J. D. (1973). Metabolic changes associated with senescence. *Seed Science Technology*, 1, 401–416.

Anderson, J. D., & Baker, J. E. (1983). Deterioration of seeds during aging. *Phytopathology*, 73, 321–325.

Arking, R. (1991). *Biology of Aging.* Englewood Cliffs, NJ: Prentice Hall.

Arnold, J. M., & Josephson, L. M. (1975). Inheritance of stalk quality characteristics in maize senescent stalks, crushing strength and rind thickness. *Crop Science*, 15, 338–340.

Azumi, Y., & Watanabe, A. (1991). Evidence for a senescence-associated gene induced by darkness. *Plant Physiology*, 95, 577–583.

Barber, J., & Andersson, B. (1992). Too much of a good thing: Light can be bad for photosynthesis. *Trends in Biochemical Sciences*, 17, 61–66.

Bate, N. J., Strauss, N. A., & Thompson, J. E. (1990). Expression of chloroplast photosynthesis genes during leaf senescence. *Physiologia Plantarum*, 80, 217–225.

Bate, N. J., Rothstein, S. J., & Thompson, J. E. (1991). Expression of nuclear and chloroplast photosynthesis-specific genes during leaf senescence. *Journal of Experimental Botany*, 42, 801–811.

Batt, T., & Woolhouse, H. W. (1975). Changing activities during senescence and sites of synthesis of photosynthetic enzymes in leaves of the Labiate *Perilla frutescens* (L). *Journal of Experimental Botany, 26,* 569–579.

Becker, W., & Apel, W. (1993). Differences in gene expression between natural and artificially induced leaf senescence. *Planta, 189,* 74–79.

Begon, M., Harper, J. L., & Townsend, C. R. (1990). *Ecology* (2nd ed.). Oxford, UK: Blackwell Scientific Publications Ltd.

Bernard, R. L., & Weiss, M. G. (1973). Qualitative Genetics. In B. E. Caldwell (Ed.), *Soybeans: Improvement, Production and Uses.* Madison, WI: American Society of Agronomy.

Biswal, U. C., & Biswal, B. (1984). Photocontrol of leaf senescence. *Photochemistry and Photobiology, 39,* 875–879.

Bleeker, A. B., Estelle, M. A., Somerville, C., & Kende, H. (1988). Insensitivity to ethylene conferred by a dominant mutation in *Arabidopsis thaliana. Science, 241,* 1086–1089.

Borochov, A., & Woodson, W. (1989). Physiology and biochemistry of flower petal senescence. *Horticultural Reviews, 11,* 2–43.

Brady, C. J. (1988). Nucleic acid and protein synthesis. In L. D. Noodén & A. C. Leopold (Eds.), *Senescence and Aging in Plants* (pp. 147–179). San Diego: Academic Press.

Brady, C. J., & Spiers, J. (1991). Ethylene in fruit ontogeny and abscission. In A. K. Mattoo & J. C. Suttle (Eds.), *The Plant Hormone Ethylene* (pp. 235–258). Boca Raton, FL: CRC Press.

Brown, J. H., Paliyath, G., & Thompson, J. E. (1991). Physiological mechanisms of plant senescence. In R. G. S. Bidwell (Ed.), *Plant Physiology. A Treatise. Vol. X: Growth and Development* (pp. 227–275). San Diego: Academic Press.

Buchanan-Wollaston, V. (1994). Isolation of cDNA clones for genes that are expressed during leaf senescence in *Brassica napus.* Identification of a gene encoding a senescence-specific metallothionein-like protein. *Plant Physiology, 105,* 839–846.

Ceppi, D., Sala, M., Gentinetta, E., Verderio, A., & Motto, M. (1987). Genotype-dependent leaf senescence in maize. *Plant Physiology, 85,* 720–725.

Chang, D. Y., Miksche, J. P., & Dhillon, S. S. (1985). DNA changes involving repeated sequences in senescing soybean (*Glycine max*) cotyledon nuclei. *Physiologia Plantarum, 64,* 409–417.

Cherry, J. H., & Skadsen, R. W. (1986). Nucleic acid and protein metabolism during seed deterioration. In M. B. McDonald, Jr. and C. J. Nelson (Eds.), *Physiology of Seed Deterioration* (pp. 65–87). Madison, WI: Crop Science Society of America.

Cherry, J. R., Hershey, H. P., & Vierstra, R. D. (1991). Characterization of tobacco expressing functional oat phytochrome. *Plant Physiology, 96,* 775–785.

Chory, J., Nagpal, P., & Peto, C. A. (1991). Phenotypic and genetic analysis of *det2,* a new mutant that affects light-regulated seedling development in *Arabidopsis. Plant Cell, 3,* 445–459.

Crowell, D. N., & Amasino, R. M. (1994). Cytokinins and plant gene regulation. In D. W. Mok & M. C. Mok (Eds.), *Cytokinins, Chemistry, Activity and Function* (pp. 233–242). Boca Raton, FL: CRC Press.

Crowell, D. N., John, M. E., Russell, D., & Amasino, R. M. (1992). Characterization of a stress-induced, developmentally regulated gene family from soybean. *Plant Molecular Biology, 18,* 459–466.

Crumpacker, D. W. (1967). Genetic loads in maize (*Zea mays* L.) and other cross-fertilized plants and animals. *Evolutionary Biology, 1,* 306–424.

Davies, I., & Sigee, D. C. (1984). Cell ageing and cell death: perspectives. In I. Davies & D. C. Sigee, (Eds.), *Cell Ageing and Cell Death* (pp. 347–350). Cambridge, UK: Cambridge University Press.

DeBellis, L., Tsugeki, R., & Nishimura, M. (1991). Glyoxylate cycle enzymes in peroxisomes isolated from petals of pumpkin (*Cucurbita* sp.) during senescence. *Plant Cell Physiology, 32,* 1227–1235.

Demura, R., & Fukuda, H. (1994). Novel vascular cell-specific genes whose expression is regulated temporally and spatially during vascular system development. *Plant Cell, 6,* 967–981.

Droillard, M. J., Bate, N. J., Rothstein, S. J., & Thompson, J. E. (1992). Active translation of the D-1 protein of photosystem II in senescing leaves. *Plant Physiology, 99,* 589–594.

Duncan, R. R., Bockholt, A. J., & Miller, F. R. (1981). Descriptive comparison of senescent and nonsenescent sorghum genotypes. *Agronomy Journal, 73,* 849–853.

Eyal, Y., & Fluhr, R. (1991). Cellular and molecular biology of pathogenesis related proteins. In B. J. Miflin (Ed.), Oxford Surveys of Plant Molecular and Cell Biology (Vol. 7, pp. 223–254). Oxford UK: Oxford University Press.

Feller, U., & Fischer, A. (1994). Nitrogen metabolism in senescing leaves. *Critical Reviews in Plant Sciences, 13,* 241–273.

Finch, C. E. (1990). *Longevity, Senescence and the Genome.* Chicago: University of Chicago Press.

Finch, C. E., & Johnson, T. E. (Eds.) (1990). *Molecular Biology of Aging.* New York: Wiley-Liss.

Fox, G. A. (1990). Perenniation and the persistence of annual life histories. *American Naturalist, 135,* 829–840.

Garnier, E. (1992). Growth analysis of congeneric annual and perennial grass species. *Journal of Ecology, 80,* 665–675.

Gepstein, S. (1988). Photosynthesis. In L. D. Noodén & A. C. Leopold (Eds.), *Senescence and Aging in Plants* (pp. 85–109). San Diego: Academic Press.

Gori, D. F. (1983). Post-pollination phenomena and adaptive floral changes. In C. E. Jones & R. J. Little (Eds.), *Handbook of Experimental Pollination Biology* (pp. 31–45). New York: Van Nostrand Reinhold Co., Inc.

Graham, I. A., Leaver, C. J., & Smith, S. M. (1992). Induction of malate synthase gene expression in senescent and detached organs of cucumber. *Plant Cell, 4,* 349–357.

Grierson, D., Purton, M. E., Knapp, J. E., & Bathgate, B. (1987). Tomato ripening mutants. In H. Thomas & D. Grierson (Eds.), *Developmental Mutants in Higher Plants* (pp. 73–94). Cambridge, UK: Cambridge University Press.

Guiamét, J. J., & Giannibelli, M. C. (1994). Inhibition of the degradation of chloroplast membranes during senescence in nuclear "stay green" mutants of soybean. *Physiologia Plantarum, 91,* 395–402.

Guiamét, J. J., Teeri, J. A., & Noodén, L. D. (1990). Effects of nuclear and cytoplasmic genes altering chlorophyll loss on gas exchange during monocarpic senescence in soybean. *Plant Cell Physiology, 31,* 1123–1130.

Guiamét, J. J., Schwartz, E., Pichersky, E., & Noodén, L. D. (1991). Characterization of cytoplasmic and nuclear mutations affecting chlorophyll and chlorophyll-binding proteins during senescence in soybean. *Plant Physiology, 96,* 227–231.

Guiamét, J. J., Pichersky, E., Green, B. R., & Noodén, L. D. (1994). Disassembly of the thylakoids during monocarpic senescence in the soybean and alterations by the stay green gene cytG. *Plant Physiology, 105,* 247.

Gut, H., & Matile, P. (1988). Apparent induction of key enzymes of the glyoxylic acid cycle in senescent barley leaves. *Planta, 176,* 548–550.

Gwathmey, C. O., Hall, A. E., & Madore, M. A. (1992). Adaptive attributes of cowpea genotypes with delayed monocarpic leaf senescence. *Crop Science, 32,* 765–772.

Halliwell, B., & Aruoma, O. I. (1993). *DNA and Free Radicals.* New York: Ellis Horwood.

Hämmerling, J. (1953). Nucleocytoplasmic relationships in the development of *Acetabularia. International Reviews of Cytology, 2,* 475–498.

Hancock, J. F. (1992). *Plant Evolution and the Origin of Crop Species.* Englewood Cliffs, NJ: Prentice Hall.

Harlan, J. R. (1992). *Crops and Man* (2nd ed.). Madison, WI: American Society of Agronomy, CSSA.

Hendry, G. A. F. (1993). Oxygen, free radical processes and seed longevity. *Seed Science Research, 3,* 141–153.

Hensel, L. L., Grbic, V., Baumgarten, D. A., & Bleecker, A. B. (1993). Development and age-related processes that influence the longevity and senescence of photosynthetic tissues in *Arabidopsis. Plant Cell, 5,* 553–564.

Johnson, T. E. (1988). Genetic specification of life span: Processes, problems and potentials. *Journal of Gerontology, 43,* 1387–1392.

Kahanak, G. M., Okatan, Y., Rupp, D. C., & Noodén, L. D. (1978). Hormonal and genetic alteration of monocarpic senescence in soybeans. *Plant Physiology, 61* (Suppl.), 26.

Kamachi, D., Yamaya, T., Hayakawa, R., Mae, T., & Ojima, K. (1992). Changes in cytosolic glutamine synthetase polypeptide and its mRNA in a leaf blade of rice plants during natural senescence. *Plant Physiology, 98,* 1323–1329.

Kar, M., Streb, P., Hertwig, B., & Feierabend, J. (1993). Sensitivity to photodamage increases during senescence in excised leaves. *Journal of Plant Physiology, 141,* 538–544.

Kawakami, N., & Watanabe, A. (1993). Translatable mRNAs for chloroplast-targeted proteins in detached radish cotyledons during senescence in darkness. *Plant Cell Physiology, 34,* 697–704.

Kays, S. J. (1991). *Postharvest Physiology of Perishable Plant Products.* New York: Van Nostrand Reinhold.

Keegan, L. P., & Timmis, J. N. (1981). Ribosomal RNA gene redundancy and aging in radish (*Raphanus sativus*) cotyledons. *Journal of Life Sciences, 2,* 171–180.

Kelly, M. O., & Davies, P. J. (1988). The control of whole plant senescence. *Critical Reviews in Plant Science, 7,* 139–173.

Kemperman, J. A., & Barnes, B. V. (1976). Clone size in American aspens. *Canadian Journal of Botany, 54,* 2603–2607.

Kirkwood, T. B., & Rose, M. R. (1991). Evolution of senescence: Late survival sacrificed for reproduction. *Philosophical Transactions of the Royal Society, London, 332,* 15–24.

Klekowski, E. J., Jr. (1988a). *Mutation, Developmental Selection, and Plant Evolution.* Irvington, NY: Columbia University Press.

Klekowski, E. J., Jr. (1988b). Mechanisms that maintain the genetic integrity of plants. In W. Greuter & B. Zimmer (Eds.), *Proceedings XIV International Botany Congress* (pp. 137–152). Germany: Koeltz, Königstein Taunus.

Klekowski, E. J., Jr., & Godfrey, P. J. (1989). Ageing and mutation in plants. *Nature, 340,* 389–391.

Klekowski, E. J., Jr., Kazarinova-Fukshansky, N., & Mohr, H. (1985). Shoot apical meristems and mutation: Stratified meristems and angiosperm evolution. *American Journal of Botany, 72,* 1788–1800.

Lacey, E. P. (1986). Onset of reproduction in plants: size- versus age-dependency. *Trends in Ecology and Evolution, 1,* 72–76.

Lai, V., & Srivastava, L. M. (1976). Nuclear changes during differentiation of xylem vessel elements. *Cytobiologie, 12,* 220–243.

Laidman, D. L. (1982). Control mechanisms in the mobilisation of stored nutrients in germinating cereals. In A. A. Khan (Ed.), *The Physiology and Biochemistry of Seed Development, Dormancy and Germination* (pp. 371–405). Amsterdam: Elsevier Biomedical Press.

Lamattina, L., Lezica, R. P., & Conde, R. D. (1985). Protein metabolism in senescing wheat leaves. Determination of synthesis and degradation rates and their effects on protein loss. *Plant Physiology, 77,* 587–590.

Lanahan, M. B., Yen, H.-C., Giovannoni, J. J., & Klee, H. J. (1994). The *never ripe* mutation blocks ethylene perception in tomato. *Plant Cell, 6,* 521–530.

Law, R., Bradshaw, A. D., & Putwain, P. D. (1977). Life history variation in *Poa annua. Evolution, 31,* 233–246.

Lawlor, D. W. (1993). *Photosynthesis: Molecular, Physiological and Environmental Processes* (2nd ed.). Marlow, England: Longman.

Lawton, K. A., Huang, B., Goldsbrough, P. B., & Woodson, W. R. (1989). Molecular cloning and characterization of senescence-related genes from carnation flower petals. *Plant Physiology, 90,* 690–696.

Leopold, A. C. (1961). Senescence in plant development. *Science, 134,* 1727–1732.

Lesham, Y. Y., Halevy, A. H., & Frenkel, C. (1986). *Processes and Control of Plant Senescence.* Amsterdam: Elsevier.

Li, Y., Hagen, G., & Guilfoyle, T. J. (1992). Altered morphology in transgenic tobacco plants that overproduce cytokinins in specific tissues and organs. *Developmental Biology, 153,* 386–395.

Lohman, K. N., Gan, S., John, M. C., & Amasino, R. M. (1994). Molecular analysis of natural leaf senescence in *Arabidopsis thaliana. Physiologia Plantarum, 92,* 322–328.

Lyndon, R. F. (1990). *Plant Development. The Cellular Basis.* London: Unwin Hyman Ltd.

Martin, M., & Sabater, B. (1989). Translational control of chloroplast protein synthesis during senescence of barley leaves. *Physiologia Plantarum, 75,* 374–381.

Martin, M., Urteaga, B., & Sabater, B. (1986). Chloroplast protein synthesis during barley leaf growth and senescence: Effect of leaf excision. *Journal of Experimental Botany, 37,* 230–237.

Martin, S. J., Green, D. R., & Cotter, T. G. (1994). Dicing with death: dissecting the components of the apoptosis machinery. *Trends in Biochemical Science, 19,* 26–30.

Marx, J. (1994). Chromosome ends catch fire. *Science, 265,* 1656–1658.

Matile, P. (1992). Leaf senescence. In N. Baker & H. Thomas (Eds.), *Crop Photosynthesis: Spatial and Temporal Determinants* (pp. 413–440). Amsterdam: Elsevier.

Mattoo, A. K., & Aharoni, N. (1988). Ethylene and plant senescence. In L. D. Noodén &

A. C. Leopold (Eds.), *Senescence and Aging in Plants* (pp. 241–280). San Diego: Academic Press.

Mattoo, A. K., & Suttle, J. C. (Eds.) (1991). *The Plant Hormone Ethylene.* Boca Raton, FL: CRC Press.

Mayak, S., & Halevy, A. H. (1980). Flower senescence. In K. V. Thimann (Ed.), *Senescence in Plants* (pp. 131–156). Boca Raton, FL: CRC Press.

McKersie, B. D., Senaratna, T., Walker, M. A., Kendall, E. J., & Hetherington, P. R. (1988). Deterioration of membranes during aging in plants: Evidence for free radical mediation. In L. D. Noodén & A. C. Leopold (Eds.), *Senescence and Aging in Plants* (pp. 441–464). San Diego: Academic Press, Inc.

Meier-Dinkel, A., & Kleinschmit, J. (1990). Aging in tree species: Present knowledge. In R. Rodríguez, R. Sánchez Tamés, & D. J. Durzan (Eds.), *Plant Aging: Basic and Applied Approaches* (pp. 51–63). New York: Plenum Press.

Meyer, R. C., Jr., Goldsbrough, P. B., & Woodson, W. R. (1991). An ethylene-responsive flower senescence-related gene from carnation encodes a protein homologous to glutathuione *S*-transferases. *Plant Molecular Biology, 17,* 277–281.

Michael, M. Z., Savin, K. W., Baudinette, S. C., Graham, M. W., Chandler, S. F., Lu, C.-Y., Caesar, C., Gautrais, I., Young, R., Nugent, G. D., Stevenson, K. R., O'Connor, E. L.-J., Cobbett, C. S., & Cornish, E. C. (1993). Cloning of ethylene biosynthetic genes involved in petal senescence of carnation and petunia, and their antisense expression in transgenic plants. In J. C. Pech, A. Latché, & C. Balagué (Eds.), *Cellular and Molecular Aspects of the Plant Hormone Ethylene* (pp. 298–303). Dordrecht, The Netherlands: Kluwer Academic Publishers.

Molisch, H. (1938). *The Longevity of Plants* (translated by H. Fulling). Lancaster, PA: Science Press.

Murata, M., Tsuchiya, T., & Roos, E. E. (1984). Chromosome damage induced by artificial seed aging in barley. *Theoretical and Applied Genetics, 67,* 161–170.

Nadeau, J. A., Zhang, X. S., Nair, H., & O'Neill, S. D. (1993). Temporal and spatial regulation if 1-aminocyclopropane 1-carboxylate oxidase in pollination-induced senescence of orchid flowers. *Plant Physiology, 103,* 31–39.

Ness, P. J., & Woolhouse, H. W. (1980). RNA synthesis in *Phaseolus* chloroplasts II. Ribonucleic acid synthesis in chloroplasts from developing and senescing leaves. *Journal of Experimental Botany, 31,* 235–245.

Nichols, C. (1941). Spontaneous chromosome aberrations in *Allium. Genetics, 26,* 89–100.

Nilsson, N. H. (1931). Sind die induzierten Mutanten nur selektive Erscheinungen. *Hereditas, 15,* 320–328.

Nobbe, F. (1876). *Handbuch der Samenkunde.* Berlin: Hempel and Parey.

Noodén, L. D. (1980). Senescence in the whole plant. In K. V. Thimann (Ed.), *Senescence in Plants* (pp. 219–258). Boca Raton, FL: CRC Press, Inc.

Noodén, L. D. (1988a). The phenomena of senescence and aging. In L. D. Noodén & A. C. Leopold (Eds.), *Senescence and Aging in Plants* (pp. 1–50). San Diego: Academic Press.

Noodén, L. D. (1988b). Whole plant senescence. In L. D. Noodén & A. C. Leopold (Eds.), *Senescence and Aging in Plants* (pp. 391–439). San Diego: Academic Press.

Noodén, L. D. (1988c). Postlude and prospects. In L. D. Noodén & A. C. Leopold (Eds.), *Senescence and Aging in Plants* (pp. 499–517). San Diego: Academic Press.

Noodén, L. D., & Guiamét, J. J. (1989). Regulation of assimilation and senescence by the fruit in monocarpic plants. *Physiologia Plantarum, 77,* 267–274.

Noodén, L. D., & Leopold, A. C. (1978). Phytohormones and the endogenous regulation of senescence and abscission. In D. S. Letham, P. B. Goodwin, & T. J. Higgins (Eds.), *Phytohormones and Related Compounds— A Comprehensive Treatise* (Vol. II, pp. 329–369). Amsterdam: Elsevier/North-Holland Biomedical Press.

Noodén, L. D., & Leopold, A. C. (Eds.) (1988). *Senescence and Aging in Plants.* San Diego: Academic Press.

Noodén, L. D., & Thompson, J. W. (1985). Aging and senescence in plants. In C. E. Finch & E. L. Schneider (Eds.), *Handbook of the Biology of Aging* (2nd ed., pp. 105–127). New York: Van Nostrand Reinhold.

Oeller, P. W., Min-Wong, L., Taylor, L. P., & Pike, D. A. (1991). Reversible inhibition of tomato fruit senescence by antisense RNA. *Science, 254,* 437–439.

Ohashi, Y., & Ohshima, M. (1992). Stress-induced expression of genes for pathogenesis-related proteins in plants. *Plant Cell Physiology*, 33, 819–826.

O'Neill, S. D., Nadeau, J. A., Zhang, X. S., Bui, A. Q., & Halevy, A. H. (1993). Interorgan regulation of ethylene biosynthetic genes by pollination. *Plant Cell*, 5, 419–432.

Osborne, D. J. (1983). DNA integrity in plant embryos and the importance of DNA repair. In M. M. Burger & R. Weber (Eds.), *Embryonic Development* (pp. 577–592). New York: Liss.

Osborne, D. J., & Cheah, K. S. E. (1982). Hormones and foliar senescence. In M. B. Jackson, B. Grout, & I. A. Mackenzie (Eds.), *Growth Regulators in Plant Senescence* (Monograph No. 8). Wantage, England: British Plant Growth Regulator Group.

Osborne, D. J., Sharon, R., & Ben-Ishai, R. (1980/81). Studies on DNA integrity and DNA repair in germinating embryos of rye (*Secale cereale*). *Israel Journal of Botany*, 29, 259–272.

Pech, J. C., Latché, A., & Balagué, C. (Eds.) (1992). *Cellular and Molecular Aspects of the Plant Hormone Ethylene*. Dordrecht, The Netherlands: Kluwer Academic Publishers.

Peoples, M. B., & Dalling, M. J. (1988). The interplay between proteolysis and amino acid metabolism during senescence and nitrogen reallocation. In L. D. Noodén & A. C. Leopold (Eds.), *Senescence and Aging in Plants* (pp. 181–217). San Diego: Academic Press.

Phillips, D. A., Pierce, R. O., Edie, S. A., Foster, K. W., & Knowles, P. F. (1984). Delayed leaf senescence in soybean. *Crop Science*, 24, 518–522.

Picton, S., Barton, S., Bouzayen, M., Hamilton, A., & Grierson, D. (1993). Altered fruit ripening and leaf senescence in tomatoes expressing and antisense ethylene-forming transgene. *Plant Journal*, 3, 469–481.

Priestley, D. A. (1986). *Seed Aging*. Ithaca, NY: Comstock Publ. Assocs.

Proebsting, W. M., Davies, P. J., & Marx, G. A. (1978). Photoperiod-induced changes in gibberellin metabolism in relation to apical growth and senescence in genetic lines of peas (*Pisum sativum* L.). *Planta*, 141, 231–238.

Quail, P. H. (1991). Phytochrome: A light activated molecular switch that regulates gene expression. *Annual Review of Genetics*, 25, 389–409.

Rathke, B., & Lacey, E. P. (1985). Phenological patterns of terrestrial plants. *Annual Review of Ecology and Systematics*, 16, 179–214.

Roberts, E. H. (1988). Seed aging: The genome and its expression. In L. D. Noodén & A. C. Leopold (Eds.), *Senescence and Aging in Plants* (pp. 465–498). San Diego: Academic Press, Inc.

Roberts, L. W., Gahan, P. B., & Aloni, R. (1988). *Vascular Differentiation and Plant Growth Regulators*. Berlin: Springer-Verlag.

Ronning, C. M., Bouwkamp, J. C., & Solomos, T. (1991). Observations on the senescence of a mutant nonyellowing genotype *Phaseolus vulgaris* L. *Journal of Experimental Botany*, 42, 235–241.

Roos, E. E. (1988). Precepts of successful seed storage. In M. B. McDonald, Jr., & C. J. Nelson (Eds.), *Physiology of Seed Deterioration* (pp. 1–25). Madison, WI: Crop Science Society of America.

Rose, M. R. (1991). *Evolutionary Biology of Aging*. New York: Oxford University Press.

Sax, K. (1962). Aspects of aging in plants. *Annual Review of Plant Physiology*, 13, 489–506.

Scholes, J. D. (1992). Photosynthesis: Cellular and tissue aspects in diseased leaves. In *Pests and Pathogens, Plant Responses to Foliar Attack* (pp. 85–106). Oxford, UK: BIOS Scientific Publishers, Ltd.

Sheen, J. (1990). Metabolic repression of transcription in higher plants. *Plant Cell*, 2, 1027–1038.

Smart, C. M. (1994). Gene expression during leaf senescence. *New Phytologist*, 126, 419–448.

Smart, C. M., Schofield, S. R., Bevan, M. W., & Dyer, T. A. (1991). Delayed leaf senescence in tobacco plants transformed with *TMR*, a gene for cytokinin production in *Agrobacterium*. *Plant Cell*, 3, 647–656.

Sodmergen, S. K., Tano, S., & Kuroiwa, T. (1991). Degradation of chloroplast DNA in second leaves of rice (*Oryza sativa*) before leaf yellowing. *Protoplasma*, 160, 89–98.

Spiers, J., & Brady, C. J. (1981). A coordinated decline in the synthesis of subunits of ribulose bisphosphate carboxylase in ageing wheat leaves. II. Abundance of messenger RNA. *Australian Journal of Plant Physiology*, 8, 608–618.

Stebbins, G. L. (1974). *Flowering Plants. Evolution above the Species Level*. Cambridge, MA: Harvard University Press.

Taylor, L. B., Bariola, P. A., Del Cardayre, S. B., Raines, R. T., & Green, P. J. (1993). RNS2: A senescence-associated RNase of *Arabidopsis* that diverged from the S-RNases before speciation. *Proceedings of the National Academy of Sciences of the United States of America, 90*, 5118–5122.

Thimann, K. V. (Ed.) (1980). *Senescence in Plants*. Boca Raton, FL: CRC Press, Inc.

Thomas, H. (1994). Aging in the plant and animal kingdoms—the role of cell death. *Reviews in Clinical Gerontology, 4*, 5–20.

Thomas, H., & Smart, C. M. (1993). Crops that stay green. *Annals of Applied Biology, 123*, 193–219.

Thomas, H., & Stoddart, J. L. (1975). Separation of chlorophyll degradation from other senescence processes in leaves of a mutant genotype of meadow fescue (*Festuca pratensis* L.). *Plant Physiology, 56*, 438–441.

Thomas, H., Bortlik, K., Rentsch, D., Schellenberg, M., & Matile, P. (1989). Catabolism of chlorophyll *in vivo:* significance of polar chlorophyll catabolites in a non-yellowing senescence mutant of *Festuca pratensis. New Phytologist, 111*, 3–8.

Thomas, H., Ougham, H. J., & Davies, T. G. E. (1992). Leaf senescence in a non-yellowing mutant of *Festuca pratensis.* Transcripts and translation products. *Journal of Plant Physiology, 139*, 403–412.

Thompson, W. R., & White, M. J. (1991). Physiological and molecular studies of light-regulated nuclear genes in higher plants. *Annual Review of Plant Physiology and Plant Molecular Biology, 42*, 423–466.

Thomson, W. W., Nothnagel, E. A., & Huffaker, R. C. (Eds.) (1987). *Plant Senescence: Its Biochemistry and Physiology*. Rockville, MD: American Society of Plant Physiologists.

Tucker, M. L., Matters, G. L., Koehler, S. M., Kemmerer, E. C., & Baird, S. L. (1993). Hormonal and tissue-specific regulation of cellulase gene expression in abscission. In J. C. Pech, A. Latché, & C. Balagué (Eds.), *Cellular and Molecular Aspects of the Plant Hormone Ethylene* (pp. 265–271). Dordrecht, The Netherlands: Kluwer Academic Publishers.

Ursin, V. M., & Shewmaker, C. K. (1993). Demonstration of a senescence component in the regulation of the mannopine synthase promoter. *Plant Physiology, 102*, 33–36.

Van Groenendael, J., & De Kroon, H. (1990). *Clonal Growth in Plants: Regulation and Function*. The Hague, The Netherlands: SPB Academic Publishing.

van Schaik, P. H., & Probst, A. H. (1958). The inheritance of influorescence type, peduncle length, flowers per node, and percent flower shedding in soybeans. *Agronomy Journal, 50*, 99–102.

Van Staden, J., Cook, E. L., & Noodén, L. D. (1988). Cytokinins and senescence. In L. D. Noodén & A. C. Leopold (Eds.), *Senescence and Aging in Plants* (pp. 281–328). San Diego, Academic Press.

Vicentini, F., & Matile, P. (1993). Gerontosomes, a multifunctional type of peroxisome in senescent leaves. *Journal of Plant Physiology, 142*, 50–56.

Vigo-Pelfrey, V. (1990). *Membrane Lipid Oxidation* (Vols. I–III). Boca Raton, FL: CRC Press.

Watkinson, A. R., & White, J. (1985). Some life-history consequences of modular construction in plants. *Philosophical Transactions of the Royal Society, London, Series B, 313*, 31–51.

White, J. (1979). The plant as a metapopulation. *American Reviews of Ecology and Systematics, 10*, 109–145.

Wiens, D. (1984). Ovule survivorship, life history, breeding systems and reproductive success in plants. *Oecologia, 64*, 47–53.

Wollgiehn, R. (1967). Nucleic acid and protein metabolism of excised leaves. *Symposia of the Society for Experimental Biology, 21*, 231–246.

Woodson, W. R. (1987). Changes in protein and mRNA populations during the senescence of carnation petals. *Physiologia Plantarum, 71*, 495–502.

Woodson, W. R., Park, K. Y., Drory, A., Larsen, P. B., & Wang, H. (1992). Expression of ethylene biosynthetic pathway transcripts in senescing carnation flowers. *Plant Physiology, 99*, 526–532.

Woolhouse, H. W. (1987). Regulation of senescence in the chloroplast. In W. W. Thomson, E. A. Nothnagel, & R. C. Huffaker (Eds.), *Plant Senescence: Its Biochemistry and*

Physiology (pp. 132–145). Rockville, MD: American Society of Plant Physiologists.

Yoshida, Y. (1961). Nuclear control of chloroplast activity in *Elodea* leaf cells. *Protoplasma, 54,* 476–492.

Young, T. P., & Peacock, M. M. (1992). Giant senecios and alpine vegetation of Mount Kenya. *Journal of Ecology, 80,* 141–148.

Yu, B. P. (Ed.) (1993). *Free Radicals in Aging.* Boca Raton, FL: CRC Press.

Zakian, V. A. (1989). Structure and function of telomeres. *Annual Review of Genetics, 23,* 579–604.

Part Three

Molecular and Cellular Biology

Edited by Nikki J. Holbrook

Seven

Control of Replicative Senescence

Judith Campisi, Goberdhan Dimri, and Eiji Hara

I. Introduction

Most, if not all, eukaryotic cells divide only a limited number of times. This property, termed the finite replicative life span of cells, restricts cell division by a process known as replicative or cellular senescence. Replicative senescence entails a stable, irreversible arrest of cell proliferation and selective changes in differentiated cell functions. Several lines of evidence suggest that senescent cells accumulate with age *in vivo*, where they may contribute to age-related pathology. In addition, there is substantial evidence that replicative senescence constitutes a powerful, albeit imperfect, tumor suppressive mechanism.

Replicative senescence appears to be controlled by multiple, dominant-acting genes. Cells escape senescence due to a loss of gene function or genetic loci, some of which have been mapped to specific human chromosomes. In addition, oncogenes encoded by certain DNA tumor viruses can lead to cell immortalization by inactivating cellular tumor suppressor proteins. In either case, immortalization is a multistep process and a rare occurrence, particularly in human cells.

What determines replicative life span? And what prevents cell division and alters differentiation once replicative capacity is exhausted? Cell division may be limited by progressive telomere shortening. Once the replicative limit is reached, dominant growth inhibitors appear to institute and maintain the growth arrest. Presenescent and senescent cells express many genes in common, but some genes whose activities are needed for cell cycle progression are repressed. This repression may be the immediate cause of the failure of senescent cells to proliferate. The ultimate cause most likely resides in the expression of dominant repressors. Whether and how these repressors participate in the change in differentiation are not yet known. We may well need to understand both the growth arrest and the altered differentiation that occur during replicative senescence in order to understand its role in organismic aging.

II. Replicative Senescence—What Is It?

A. Cell Division Potential Is Limited

Normal eukaryotic cells do not divide indefinitely. This property, termed the finite

Handbook of the Biology of Aging, Fourth Edition
Copyright © 1996 Academic Press, Inc. All rights of reproduction in any form reserved.

replicative life span of cells, limits cell division by a process known as cellular or replicative senescence. The finite replicative life span of cells was first described over 30 years ago in cultures of human fibroblasts (Hayflick & Moorhead, 1961; Hayflick, 1965). Since then, many cell types from many animal species have been shown to have a limited division potential [reviewed in Stanulis-Praeger (1987); Cristofalo & Pignolo, 1993]. Replicative senescence may be a very primitive process because it occurs in some simple single-celled organisms such as *Saccharomyces cerevisiae* (Jazwinski, 1990).

Replicative senescence is generally studied in culture. In culture, cells can be stimulated to proliferate (used here interchangeably with growth) in a controlled fashion for the many doublings that are needed for most or all cells in a population to senesce. By contrast, cell proliferation is not easily manipulated or controlled *in vivo*. Despite the difficulties of *in vivo* studies, the proliferative potential of some tissues and cell types has been studied in intact animals (Krohn, 1962, 1966; Daniel *et al.*, 1968; Daniel, 1972). Results from these studies, together with the evidence discussed in Section II.A, strongly suggest that replicative senescence is not an artifact of cell culture.

Replicative senescence depends on the number of cell divisions—not time. Thus, the maintenance of proliferative cells such as fibroblasts under nongrowing conditions for long periods of time does not reduce their replicative potential (Hayflick, 1965; Dell'Orco *et al.*, 1973; Goldstein & Singal, 1974). Likewise, the cell cycle time, or interval between divisions, does not affect the number of divisions through which cells can proceed. On the other hand, replicative potential depends very much on the cell type and the species and age of the donor (see Section II.A.1; Stanulis-Praeger, 1987; Cristofalo & Pignolo, 1993).

Only two, perhaps three, types of cells may fail to senesce, that is, may have an indefinite or immortal replicative life span. Certainly the germ line is capable of unlimited replication. In addition, many tumors contain cells that are immortal. Finally, some primitive somatic stem cells may divide indefinitely, but this has yet to be proven. Replicative senescence is exceedingly stringent in human cells. In sharp contrast to many rodent cells, human cells rarely—if ever—spontaneously fail to senesce (Ponten, 1976; Sager, 1984; McCormick & Maher, 1988; Shay & Wright, 1989).

B. The Senescent Phenotype

Senescent cells, that is, cells that have reached the end of their replicative life span, remain viable and metabolically active for long periods of time (Matsumura *et al.*, 1979; Pignolo *et al.*, 1994). Thus, replicative senescence is not programmed cell death or apoptosis. In fact, senescent cells may be substantially more resistant to apoptotic death than presenescent cells (Wang *et al.*, 1994). Although some cells may die during passage in culture (Pignolo *et al.*, 1994), it is well-established that, with increasing cell division, the fraction of senescent cells in a proliferating population rises more or less exponentially (Smith & Hayflick, 1974; Smith & Whitney, 1980). Eventually, the population consists entirely of senescent cells.

Senescent cells continue to metabolize RNA and protein, respond to environmental signals, and retain many presenescent characteristics. Presenescent and senescent cells express numerous genes in common, and several genes remain inducible by external stimuli throughout the replicative life span (Hornsby *et al.*, 1986; Rittling *et al.*, 1986; Seshadri & Campisi, 1990; Choi *et al.*, 1995). Two features distinguish senescent cells from their presenescent counterparts. First, senescent cells are incapable of proliferation (Section I.B.1). Second, senescent cells show selected changes in differentiated functions (Section I.B.2).

1. Irreversible Arrest of Cell Division

The universal characteristic of replicative senescence is a stable, essentially irreversible loss of cell proliferative capacity. At the end of their replicative life span, normal eukaryotic cells arrest their growth with a G1 DNA content. Once this growth arrest occurs, physiological mitogens cannot induce senescent cells to enter the S phase of the cell cycle [reviewed in Goldstein (1990); McCormick & Campisi, 1991; Shay & Wright, 1991; Cristofalo & Pignolo, 1993].

The failure of senescent cells to initiate DNA replication is not due to a *general* breakdown in growth factor signal transduction. This has been most clearly established in human fibroblast cultures, in which the replicative senescence and mitogen responsiveness of many genes have been well-characterized (Goldstein, 1990). Many genes, including at least three proto-oncogenes (c-jun, c-myc, and c-ras-Ha), remain fully mitogen-inducible in senescent human fibroblasts (Rittling *et al.*, 1986; Chang & Chen, 1988; Seshadri & Campisi, 1990; Phillips *et al.*, 1992).

A small number of mitogen-inducible, growth-regulatory genes remain repressed in senescent cells (Section IV.B.2). The mechanisms responsible for these repressions are not known. They could entail *selective* blocks to mitogen signaling pathways. Indeed, this may be the case for senescent melanocytes. Mitogen-stimulated tyrosine phosphorylation and nuclear translocation of ERK-2 (extracellular signal-regulated kinase-2; MAPK, mitogen-activated protein kinase-2) fail to occur once adult human melanocytes undergo replicative senescence (Medrano *et al.*, 1994). Interestingly, senescent human fibroblasts also fail to phosphorylate ERK-2 in response to mitogens, although ERK-1 is constitutively phosphorylated in

these cells (Afshari *et al.*, 1993). Alternatively, and/or in addition, the selective repression of growth-regulatory genes may be a consequence of the senescence-specific expression of dominant, upstream growth inhibitors (Sections IV.B.2 and IV.B.3).

2. Altered Differentiated Function

In addition to an arrest of cell proliferation, replicative senescence entails selected changes in differentiation. The altered differentiation of senescent cells is frequently overlooked. Unlike growth arrest, the cell functions that change upon senescence largely depend on the cell type. In fact, replicative senescence and terminal differentiation may be analogous processes (Bayreuther *et al.*, 1988; Seshadri & Campisi, 1990; Peacocke & Campisi, 1991). Certainly, by the criteria of stable irreversible growth arrest and a change in function, senescent cells resemble terminally differentiated cells. In contrast to terminal differentiation, however, replicative senescence occurs as a consequence of completing a finite number of cell divisions.

Several general phenotypic changes are associated with replicative senescence in most, if not all, cell types. These include increased cell size, increased lysosome biogenesis, and decreased rates of protein synthesis and degradation [reviewed in Stanulis-Praeger (1987)]. In addition, the expression or regulation of genes that participate in cell type-specific functions is altered. Tables I–III include examples of such alterations in senescent human fibroblasts. In other types of cells, different functions may change as the cells senesce. For example, in senescent human endothelial cells, there is a marked increase in the expression of interleukin-1α and the cell-specific adhesion molecule I-CAM (Maier *et al.*, 1990, 1993). Likewise, there is an increase in the retinoic acid receptor β isoform in senescent human mammary

Table I
Some Genes That Are Repressed or Underexpressed in Senescent Human Fibroblasts

Gene/protein	Description/function	Expression	References
cdk2	Cyclin-dependent protein kinase-2	G1	Afshari *et al.* (1993)
cycA	Cyclin A, activator of cdk kinase	Late G1	Stein *et al.* (1991); Afshari *et al.* (1993)
cycB, cdc2	Active cdc2 kinase components	G2/M	Stein *et al.* (1991)
DHFR	Dihydrofolate reductase	Late G1/S	Pang and Chen (1993, 1994)
E2F1	Component of E2F transcription factor	Mid–late G1	Dimri *et al.* (1994)
EPC1	Serine protease inhibitor	G0	Pignolo *et al.* (1993)
c-fos	Component of AP-1 transcription factor	Early G0/G1	Seshadri and Campisi (1990)
gas1, gas6	Growth arrest-specific genes	G0	Cowled *et al.* (1994)
his2a,2b,3,4	Replication-dependent histones	Late G1/S	Zambetti *et al.* (1987); Seshadri and Campisi (1990)
hsp70, 90	Heat shock proteins 70 and 90	Stress-inducible late G1/S	Liu *et al.* (1989); Choi *et al.* (1990); Luce and Cristofalo (1992)
Id1, Id2	Inhibitors of bHLH transcription factors	Early and mid-G1	Hara *et al.* (1994)
IGF1	Insulin-like growth factor-1	G1	Ferber *et al.* (1993)
IL-6	Interleukin-6 multifunctional cytokine	G1	Goodman and Stein (1994)
L7	Large ribosomal subunit protein	Constitutive	Seshadri *et al.* (1993)
mig-5	Tissue inhibitor of metalloproteinase	G0/G1	Wick *et al.* (1994)
PCNA	Proliferating cell nuclear antigen/ DNA polymerase δ function	Late G1/S	Chang *et al.* (1991)
polα	DNA polymerase α	Late G1/S	Pendergrass *et al.* (1991)
RNR	Ribonucleotide reductase	Late G1/S	Pang and Chen (1993, 1994)
TIMP-1	Tissue inhibitor of metalloproteinase	G0	West *et al.* (1989); Millis *et al.* (1992)
TK	Thymidine kinase	Late G1/S	Pang and Chen (1993, 1994)
TS	Thymidylate synthetase	Late G1/S	Pang and Chen (1993, 1994)

epithelial cells (Swisshelm *et al.*, 1994), and an induction of cornifin in senescent human mammary epithelial cells and keratinocytes (Saunders *et al.*, 1994). Virtually nothing is known about how the altered differentiation associated with replicative senescence is regulated. The altered phenotype of senescent cells may be the result of an altered complement of transcription factors expressed by these cells (Dimri & Campisi, 1994a). However, very little is known about the functional repercussions of the transcriptional changes that occur as a consequence of cell senescence.

The altered differentiation associated with senescence can have rather profound consequences for cell—and, at least in principle, tissue—function. For example, over their replicative life span, adrenocortical epithelial cells progressively lose the ability to induce 17α-hydroxylase, a key enzyme in cortisol biosynthesis (Hornsby *et al.*, 1987; Cheng *et al.*, 1989). Other steroidogenic enzymes are not affected in this way. Thus, replicative senescence alters the spectrum of steroids produced by adrenocortical cells. Similarly, presenescent dermal fibroblasts express low levels of collagenase and stromelysin (proteases that degrade extracellular matrix proteins) and high levels of TIMP 1 and 3 (the pro-

Table II
Some Genes That Are Overexpressed by Senescent Human Fibroblasts

Gene/protein	Description/function	References
Cathepsin B	Protease	DiPaolo et al. (1992)
Collagen, α1, 2 (I)	Extracellular matrix component	Murano et al. (1991)
Collagenase	Protease; extracellular matrix remodeling	West et al. (1989); Millis et al. (1992)
Cyclins E and D	Regulatory components of cdks	Dulic et al. (1993)
EF1α	Protein synthesis elongation factor	Giordano et al. (1989)
Fibronectin	Extracellular matrix component	Porter et al. (1990); Murano et al. (1991)
IGFBP-3	Insulin-like growth factor binding protein	Murano et al. (1991)
IL-1	Interleukin-1α and -1β cytokines	Kumar et al. (1992)
p21 (sdi1)	Cyclin-dependent kinase inhibitor	Noda et al. (1994)
SAG	Senescence-associated gene, function unknown	Wistrom and Villeponteau (1992)
Statin	Nuclear protein, associates with pRb	Wang (1985)
Stromelysin	Protease; extracellular matrix remodeling	Millis et al. (1992)
WS3-10	Calcium binding protein	Liu et al. (1994a)

tease inhibitors tissue inhibitor of metalloproteinases 1 and 3). Upon senescence, collagenase and stromelysin expression rises and TIMP expression falls (West et al., 1989; Millis et al., 1992; Wick et al., 1994). Thus, senescence entails a switch in the phenotype of dermal fibroblasts from matrix-producing to matrix-degrading.

As discussed in the following, replicative senescence may suppress tumorigenesis and contribute to aging. Most likely, the growth arrest associated with senescence is the most important feature vis-à-vis its role in tumor suppression. By contrast, the altered differentiation associated with senescence may be most important for its role in aging.

III. Replicative Senescence— Significance

There are two ideas regarding the physiological significance of replicative senescence.

Table III
Some Gene-Specific Posttranslational Modifications in Senescent Fibroblasts

Gene/protein	Description/function	Modification	References
cdk	Cyclin-dependent protein kinase; G1 progression	Inhibition of activity; p21 association	Dulic et al. (1993)
Fibronectin	Extracellular matrix component	Novel antigenic determinant	Porter et al. (1990)
Mortalin	hsp70-related	Intracellular localization	Wadhwa et al. (1993)
pRb	Tumor suppressor, growth inhibitor	Lack of phosphorylation	Stein et al. (1990)
Prohibitin	Growth inhibitor	Loss of low-MW form; phosphorylation?	Liu et al. (1994b)
Terminin	Lysosomal?/unknown	Proteolysis to smaller peptide	Wang and Tomaszewski (1991)

One holds that replicative senescence is a tumor suppressive mechanism; the other holds that senescent cells accumulate with age and contribute to age-related dysfunction. The evidence for these ideas is discussed here. At first glance, they may seem unrelated or even at odds with each other. However, evolutionary theories of aging suggest that some traits that were selected to maintain health during the period of reproductive fitness may have unselected and deleterious post-reproductive effects (see Finch, 1990; Rose, 1991). Thus, at least in higher eukaryotes, replicative senescence may contribute to the relative freedom from neoplasia that is seen early in life. Later in life, replicative senescence may be deleterious because dysfunctional senescent cells accumulate. From the rise in cancer incidence with age, it also appears that replicative senescence fails increasingly with age. At least among mammals, there is a very close relationship between the rate of aging and rate at which cancers arise. In fact, it has been proposed that these processes may derive from a shared mechanism(s) (Miller, 1991). One possibility is that the finite replicative life span of cells links the rate of aging with that of tumor incidence.

A. Replicative Senescence and Aging

1. Correlative Evidence

The idea that replicative senescence is related to organismic aging derives from four lines of correlative evidence.

First, cells cultured from old donors tend to senesce after fewer population doublings (PD) than cells from young donors (Martin et al., 1970; Le Guilly et al., 1973; Rheinwald & Green, 1975; Schneider & Mitsui, 1976; Bierman, 1978; Bruce et al., 1986). There is considerable scatter in the data, particularly among humans, although this may be due to genetic and life history differences. Nonetheless, human fetal fibroblasts generally senesce after 60–80 PD, fibroblasts from young to middle-aged adults may do so after 20–40 PD, and cells from old adults may senesce after 10–20 PD. These findings suggest that the replicative life span of cells in renewable tissues may be progressively exhausted during the chronological life span of organisms.

Second, cells from short-lived species tend to senesce after fewer PD than comparable cells from long-lived species (Goldstein, 1974; Hayflick, 1977; Rohme, 1981). Thus, mouse fetal fibroblasts senesce after 10–15 PD, whereas fibroblasts from the Galapagos tortoise proliferate for >100 PD. Overall, cells from organisms with intermediate life spans generally senesce at an intermediate PD. These results suggest that the genes that control the chronological life span of organisms may overlap, at least in part, with genes that control the replicative life span of cells.

Third, cells from humans with hereditary premature aging syndromes senesce much more rapidly than cells from age-matched controls (Goldstein, 1978; Martin, 1978; Salk et al., 1985; Brown, 1990). This has been best studied in cells from donors with the Werner syndrome, a segmental adult-onset, premature aging syndrome (Goldstein, 1978; Martin, 1978) that is caused by a recessive mutation on chromosome 8 (Goto et al., 1992). Cells from young adults with Werner syndrome generally senesce within 10–20 PD, well ahead of cells from age-matched controls. These findings further support the idea that organismic life span and replicative life span are related and may be controlled by overlapping genes.

Finally, the regulation of at least some genes is altered similarly by senescence in culture and aging in vivo. For example, the c-fos protooncogene becomes refractory to induction by mitogens in human fibroblasts that have undergone senescence in culture (Seshadri & Campisi, 1990). c-fos also becomes refractory to induction by a pressure overload to the heart (Takahashi *et al.*, 1992) or an electroconvulsive shock to the brain (D'Costa *et al.*, 1991) in aged rats or mice. Likewise, the induction of heat shock protein 70 (hsp70) by stress is attenuated by replicative senescence in cultured human fibroblasts (Liu *et al.*, 1989) and by chronological age in rats (Fargnoli *et al.*, 1990; Heydari *et al.*, 1993). In addition, telomeres have been shown to shorten progressively with PD in culture and with age *in vivo* (Section IV.A).

2. A Biomarker for Replicative Senescence in Culture and *in Vivo*

The idea that senescent cells accumulate with age has lacked direct evidence. However, we found a marker for senescent human cells that may provide the first *in situ* evidence that senescent cells accumulate in aged tissue. Several human cell types expressed an unusual β-galactosidase (β-gal) upon senescence in culture (Dimri *et al.*, 1995). This activity, which we term senescence-associated or SA-β-gal, was detectable in individual cells by histochemical

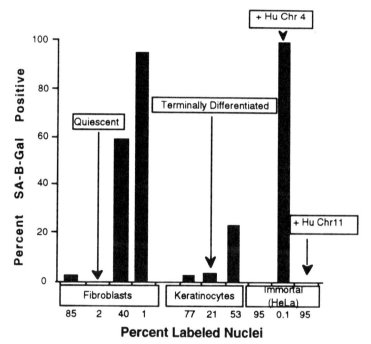

Figure 1. Expression of SA-β-gal in cultured cells. Human neonatal foreskin fibroblasts and epidermal keratinocytes were passaged in culture, and proliferative capacity was assessed by the incorporation of radiolabeled thymidine in 48–72 h, detectable by autoradiography (percent labeled nuclei, %LN). Early passage presenescent cells (%LN = 85) were made quiescent by serum deprivation for 3 days. Keratinocytes were induced to terminally differentiate by the addition of 2 mM calcium chloride to the medium for 4 days. HeLa cells were fused to microcells containing normal human chromosome 4 or 11. The cells were fixed in 1% formaldehyde for 5 min and then stained for β-galactosidase using X-gal as a substrate, using the standard protocol except that the staining solution was buffered at pH 6.0 with citrate/phosphate buffer. The cells were viewed by light microscopy 12–16 hr later.

staining at pH 6 using the artificial substrate X-gal. SA-β-gal differed in pH optimum from the lysosomal β-gal (pH 4) and the bacterial β-gal (pH 7.5) commonly used as a reporter gene.

In culture, SA-β-gal was expressed by senescent human fibroblasts and keratinocytes (Fig. 1), as well as senescent endothelial and mammary epithelial cells. It was not expressed by quiescent fibroblasts or terminally differentiated keratinocytes (Fig. 1). It also was not expressed by immortal human cells, including HeLa. However, HeLa cells expressed SA-β-gal after the introduction of a normal human chromosome 4, which induces senescence in these cells (Ning et al., 1991a), but not with chromosome 11, which does not (Figure 1). Thus, SA-β-gal expression was linked to senescence, but not quiescence or terminal differentiation.

The origin and function of SA-β-gal are not known. Nonetheless, it provided a means by which to distinguish senes-cent cells from quiescent or terminally differentiated cells in tissue. In collaboration with Monica Peacocke (Columbia-Presbyterian Hospital), we surveyed frozen sections of skin samples from young and old donors for SA-β-gal activity. SA-β-gal positive cells ranged from undetectable (0) to multiple clusters in multiple fields (+3) (Fig. 2). The positive cells were fibroblasts (in the dermis) and basal keratinocytes (in the epidermis) (Peacocke & Scott, unpublished). Both clearly were more abundant in skin from older donors (Fig. 2).

These findings support the ideas that replicative senescence occurs during organismic aging and that senescent cells accumulate in aged tissue. Whether this accumulation contributes to age-associated pathology has yet to be determined. Nonetheless, it is possible that the age-associated decline in regenerative capacity and function may at least partly derive from the accumulation of senescent cells, which cannot proliferate, are resistant to

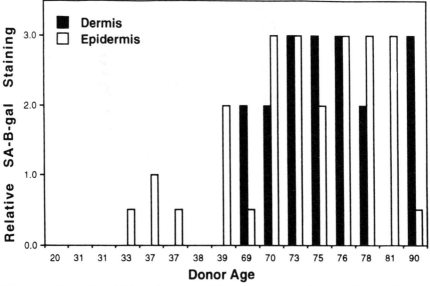

Figure 2. Expression of SA-β-gal positive cells *in vivo.* Human skin samples were frozen, mounted, and sectioned, and the sections were mounted onto glass slides. The sections were stained for β-galactosidase as described earlier, counterstained with eosin, and assessed blind for relative (scale = 0–3) β-galactosidase staining in the dermis and epidermis.

apoptotic death, and have an altered differentiated phenotype.

B. Replicative Senescence and Tumor Suppression

The idea that replicative senescence constitutes a tumor suppressive mechanism derives from several lines of evidence.

First, many, if not most, tumors contain cells that have bypassed the limit imposed by replicative senescence (Ponten, 1976; Newbold et al., 1982; Sager, 1991). That is, tumors very often contain immortal cells or cells that have an extended replicative life span. This is not to say that immortality is required for tumorigenesis (although it may be for metastasis). Rather, there appears to be a strong selection for cells with an increased proliferative potential in the development of neoplasia. Immortality, or even an extended replicative life span, greatly increases the susceptibility to malignant progression because it permits the extensive cell division that is necessary to acquire successive mutations.

Second, certain oncogenes act at least in part by immortalizing or extending the replicative life span of cells (Ruley, 1983; Weinberg, 1985; Galloway & McDougall, 1989; Hinds et al., 1989; Sugden, 1989; Shay & Wright, 1991). These include mutated or deregulated cellular genes (e.g., p53 or c-myc, which readily immortalize rodent cells), as well as the oncogenes of certain viruses that are implicated in the etiology of some human cancers (e.g., Epstein–Barr or human papilloma viruses). Thus, mutations that lead to tumorigenesis, or the strategies of oncogenic viruses, may and do involve mechanisms that permit cells to escape replicative senescence.

Finally, among the genes that are essential for establishing and/or maintaining replicative senescence are two well-recognized tumor suppressor genes: the p53 gene and the retinoblastoma susceptibility gene (Rb) (Hara et al., 1991; Shay & Wright, 1991; Dimri & Campisi, 1994b). The evidence for the involvement of p53 and Rb in replicative senescence is discussed in Section III.B.1. For the moment, suffice to say that the activities of p53 and Rb are together perhaps the most commonly lost functions in human cancers (Bookstein & Lee, 1991; Hollstein et al., 1991; Weinberg, 1991), and these activities are necessary for replicative senescence.

IV. Genetic Control of Replicative Senescence

Replicative senescence is genetically controlled. Earlier ideas that cellular senescence results from random accumulated damage or errors in translation or transcription are not supported by consistent data [reviewed in Stanulis-Praeger (1987)], although some of these ideas cannot be unequivocally ruled out. By contrast, the idea that replicative senescence is controlled by specific genetic loci is now well-substantiated. This is not to say that extrinsic factors do not influence the course of replicative senescence. For example, the PD at which a cell culture completely senesces depends on the oxygen tension at which it is grown (low oxygen tension extends replicative life span) (Packer & Feuhr, 1977; Balin et al., 1977; Chen et al., 1995). This finding suggests that oxidative damage may influence the replicative life span. Likewise, an as yet unconfirmed report suggests that inhibition of protein glycation by the dipeptide carnosine retards the senescence of human fibroblasts (McFarland & Holliday, 1994). Thus, as is the case for the growth and senescence of organisms, replicative senescence in cells is very likely governed by genetic programs that are influenced by nongenetic and environmental factors.

A. Somatic Cell Genetics

1. Dominance

The growth arrest associated with replicative senescence and the finite replicative life span of cells are clearly dominant traits in somatic cell fusion experiments [see, for example, Norwood et al. (1974); Muggleton-Harris & Hayflick, 1976; Bunn & Tarrant, 1980; Muggleton-Harris & De-Simone, 1980; Stein et al., 1982, 1985; Pereira-Smith & Smith, 1983]. The most conclusive of these studies has relied almost entirely on human cells because of their extreme resistance to spontaneous immortalization.

When proliferating presenescent cells are fused to senescent cells, they fail to initiate DNA replication in response to mitogens. Moreover, when most immortal tumor cells are fused to senescent cells, DNA replication is inhibited. Thus, the growth-stimulatory genes expressed by proliferating cells, as well as the cellular oncogenes expressed by tumor cells, do not overcome the growth arrest associated with senescence. Rather, the growth of normal and tumor cells is suppressed, presumably by genes expressed by senescent cells. This suggests that senescent cells do not fail to proliferate due to a deficiency in positive growth signals or defects in critical cellular components. Rather, senescent cells must express one or more factors that act in a trans-dominant fashion to inhibit progression into the S phase of the cell cycle.

Similarly, when proliferating presenescent cells are fused to immortal tumor cells, the hybrid cells acquire a finite replicative capacity. Immortal cells often emerge from these hybrid cell populations, and this frequently correlates with a loss of normal chromosomes. These findings suggest that normal cells express dominant genes that limit replicative life span and that such genes are lost or inactivated in immortal cells. This idea is strengthened by the finding that different immortal cell lines often (but not always, as discussed in the following) produce hybrids that have a limited cell division potential (Pereira-Smith & Smith, 1983). Thus, a finite replicative life span is a dominant trait, whereas immortality is a recessive trait.

The relationship between the genes that limit replicative life span and those that induce the growth arrest of senescent cells is not known. Given that the final senescent state requires multiple steps and that replicative life span is controlled by multiple genetic loci (both discussed in the following), it is possible that limited division potential and the senescent state are directed by independent, albeit interacting, pathways.

2. Complementation Groups

Most immortal cell lines, when fused to each other, form hybrid cells that senesce. However, some immortal cell pairs form hybrids that are immortal, even though each member of that pair, upon fusion to a third cell line, produces hybrids that senesce. This suggests that immortality can result from the inactivation of more than one gene. Thus, immortal cells with legions in different genes can complement one another, producing hybrids with a finite replicative life span; immortal cells with lesions in the same gene cannot complement, and the hybrids remain immortal. Fusions between many different immortal human cells have revealed four distinct complementation groups for immortality (designated A, B, C, and D) (Pereira-Smith & Smith, 1988). Three of these have been assigned to specific human chromosomes (discussed in the following). The suggestion that the complementation shown by immortal cells is in fact delayed toxicity of the drugs used to select the hybrids (Ryan et al., 1994) is difficult to reconcile with the stable viability of the senescent hybrids, the complementation of some but not all immortal cell pairs, and the fact that specific chromosomes complement cells assigned to specific complementation groups. Taken together, the data strongly suggest that the finite replicative life span of cells is controlled by multiple, dominant genetic loci.

One particularly interesting result has emerged from the complementation group studies: cells of diverse tissue origins may belong to the same complementation group. This suggests that the genes that control replicative senescence do not act in a cell type- or tissue-specific manner.

3. Human Chromosomes

The human chromosomes that have been reported to induce a finite replicative life span and senescence when introduced into specific immortal cell lines include 1, 4, 6, 7, 11, 18, and X (see Table IV for references). Of particular importance is that the abilities of chromosomes 1, 4, and 7 to limit replicative potential are restricted to cells assigned to complementation groups C, B, and D, respectively (Table IV) (Hensler et al., 1994; Ning et al., 1991a; Ogata et al., 1993). Thus, the chromosomes on which three of the four complementation group genes reside are known,

although the genes of interest have yet to be identified.

At present, the number of human chromosomes reported to induce senescence exceeds the number of complementation groups. Moreover, some immortal cells can be assigned to more than one complementation group (Duncan et al., 1993; Berry et al., 1994). It is possible that some immortal cells have lost more than one senescence-regulatory gene (and, thus, may assign to more than one complementation group) and that some chromosomes may arrest cell division by mechanisms that are independent of the growth arrest associated with senescence [see, for example, Loh et al. (1992); Koi et al., 1993; Barbanti-Brodano & Croce, 1994; Ning et al., 1991b). Until the senescence-inducing genes are identified and studied, the basis for the complementation of immortal cells, and mechanisms by which normal genetic loci induce immortal cells to senesce, will remain speculative.

B. Viral Genes That Overcome Replicative Senescence

The finding that multiple dominant genes control replicative senescence predicts

Table IV
Chromosomes That Induce a Finite Division Potential in Immortal Cells

Chromosome	Complementation group	References
Human 1	C	Sugawara et al. (1990); Yamada et al. (1990); Hensler et al. (1994)
Human 4	B	Ning et al. (1991a)
Human 6	Unassigned	Barbanti-Brodano and Croce (1994); Sandhru et al. (1994); Gualandi et al. (1994)
Human 7	D	Ogata et al. (1993)
Human 11	Unassigned	Kano and Little (1989); Loh et al. (1992); Koi et al. (1993); see Ning et al. (1991b)
Human 18	Unassigned	Sake et al. (personal communication)
Human/hamster X	Unassigned (Epigenetic?)	Klein et al. (1991); Wang et al. (1992)

that it should not be possible to immortalize normal cells or reactivate the growth of senescent cells by providing them with growth-stimulatory cellular genes, including cellular oncogenes. Indeed, from the somatic cell fusion experiments and the data discussed in Section IV.B, this appears to be the case. However, the oncogenes of certain DNA tumor viruses are capable of extending the replicative life span of human cells and reactivating DNA synthesis in senescent cells. The best studied of these is the large T-antigen of SV40 virus (Fanning, 1992). T-antigen is the only single gene that can stimulate senescent human fibroblasts to synthesize DNA (Ide et al., 1984; Gorman & Cristofalo, 1985; Shay & Wright, 1991). Two genes encoded by certain other viruses can provide the equivalent of these activities of T-antigen. These include the E1a and E1b genes of adenoviruses (Boulanger & Blair, 1991) and E6 and E7 genes of papilloma viruses (Galloway & McDougall, 1989).

1. Immortalization

When introduced into presenescent cells, T-antigen (or E1a + E1b or E6 + E7) will extend the replicative life spans of cells and immortalize them. However, the efficiency of immortalization is species-dependent. Immortalization is fairly efficient in rodent cells (Ponten, 1976; Newbold et al., 1982; Ruley, 1983; Shay & Wright, 1991). In human cells, by contrast, these viral genes are capable only of reliably extending the replicative life span (Girardi et al., 1965; Ide et al., 1984; Neufeld et al., 1987; Shay & Wright, 1989; Hawley-Nelson et al., 1989; Munger et al., 1989; Boulanger & Blair, 1991; Shay & Wright, 1991). This life span extension amounts to about 20 PD for human fetal fibroblasts (Ide et al., 1984; Shay & Wright, 1989; Hara et al., 1991), but can be as great as >60 PD for some cell types (Rinehart et al., 1991; Ryan et al., 1992).

At the end of their replicative life span,

T-antigen-expressing cells do not undergo normal senescence. Rather, they enter a state termed crisis, in which cell growth is approximately balanced by cell death. Human cell cultures may spend weeks or months in crisis, after which rare immortal cells may emerge.

T-antigen immortalizes only about 3 in 10^{-7} human fetal lung fibroblasts (Shay & Wright, 1989). This frequency suggests that immortality requires at least one mutational event in addition to T-antigen. In one study, T-antigen immortalized human adult mammary epithelial cells more readily (about 1 in 10^{-5}) than fetal lung fibroblasts (Shay et al., 1993a). The T-antigen-expressing fibroblasts became largely pseudotetraploid as they approached crisis, whereas the T-antigen-expressing epithelial cells maintained a sizable pseudodiploid population (Shay et al., 1993a). One possibility is that if one allele of a dominant senescence-inducing gene spontaneously mutates, the genomic instability induced by T-antigen may favor its conversion to homozygosity. Thus, fewer non-dysjunction events may have been needed to immortalize the epithelial cells (Shay et al., 1993a). The basis for the ploidy difference between the fibroblasts and epithelial cells in this study is not known, but may explain why some epithelial cells, but not fibroblasts, are immortalized by E6 or E7 alone (Band et al., 1991; Halbert et al., 1991; Shay et al., 1993b; Reznikoff et al., 1994). An intrinsic difference in genomic stability between fibroblasts and epithelial cells may contribute to the fact that most adult cancers are epithelial in origin.

The preceding findings suggest that a finite replicative life span entails at least two (mortality) mechanisms, termed M1 and M2 (Wright et al., 1989; Shay & Wright, 1991). T-antigen appears to inactivate one mechanism (M1), but both must be inactivated before human cells can escape senescence and become immortal. The relation between M1 and M2 and the growth arrest of senescent cells is discussed here and in Section IV.B.1.

2. Reactivation of DNA Synthesis in Senescent Cells

In addition to extending replicative life span by inactivating M1, T-antigen stimulates limited cell cycle progression in cells that have already reached senescence (Tsuji *et al.*, 1983; Ide *et al.*, 1983; Gorman & Cristofalo, 1985; Lumpkin *et al.*, 1986; Dimri *et al.*, 1994). T-antigen induces senescent cells to progress through and complete DNA replication, but does not induce senescent cells to undergo mitosis (Ide *et al.*, 1983; Gorman & Cristofalo, 1985). Moreover, human fibroblasts immortalized by a conditional T-antigen reversibly arrest growth in G1 when T-antigen is conditionally inactivated (Radna *et al.*, 1989; Wright *et al.*, 1989). Thus, the growth arrest associated with replicative senescence appears to entail two blocks to cell cycle progression. One block is T-antigen (or E1a + E1b or E6 + E7) sensitive, and it prevents cells from entering the S phase. A second, T-antigen-insensitive block prevents cells from undergoing mitosis (Fig. 3).

3. Inactivation of p53 and Rb Tumor Suppressor Genes

T-antigen and the combinations E1a + E1b or E6 + E7 have two functions in common: they bind and/or inactivate the p53 and pRb tumor suppressor proteins (Galloway & McDougall, 1989; Boulanger & Blair, 1991; Fanning, 1992). T-antigen binds and inactivates both p53 and pRb, as well as the pRb-related proteins p107 and p130. E1a and E7, on the other hand, bind only pRb and its related proteins. By contrast, E1b binds and E6 inactivates p53 only.

Both p53 and pRb must be inactivated in order to maximally extend the replicative life span of presenescent cells and to reactivate DNA synthesis in senescent cells. This conclusion derives from several lines of evidence. First, Rb and p53 antisense oligomers, which inhibited pRb and p53 expression, extended the replicative life span of human fibroblasts to the same extent as T-antigen (Hara *et al.*, 1991). Antisense Rb alone extended life span about half as well as T-antigen, whereas antisense p53 alone was without effect. Similarly, E6 and E7 were both required for maximal life span extension of human

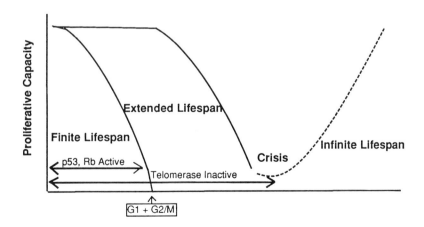

Number of Population Doublings

Figure 3. Steps required to escape replicative senescence. See text for explanation.

fibroblasts; alone, each extended to a lesser extent than the two together (White *et al.*, 1994). Second, human fibroblasts immortalized by a conditional T-antigen arrested growth when T-antigen was inactivated; growth was rescued by E6 and E7 together, but not by either alone (Shay *et al.*, 1991). Third, T-antigen mutants that are defective in either pRb (Sakamoto *et al.*, 1993) or p53 binding failed to reactivate DNA synthesis in senescent human fibroblasts (Dimri & Campisi, 1994b; Hara *et al.*, submitted).

Taken together, these findings suggest that at least two tumor suppressor genes, p53 and Rb, are responsible for the T-antigen-sensitive step that establishes and maintains the growth arrest of senescent cells. Inactivation of both Rb and p53 is necessary in order for cells to overcome this first block to unlimited cell proliferation.

V. Molecular Control of Replicative Senescence

The molecular bases for replicative senescence are just beginning to be unraveled. Insights into three critical questions have emerged. What is the "counting" mechanism responsible for a finite replicative capacity? What is the immediate cause for the failure of senescent cells to initiate DNA synthesis? What is the nature of the dominant repressors expressed by senescent cells?

A. Counting Mechanisms: The Telomere Hypothesis

An intriguing question regarding replicative senescence is how do cells sense the number of divisions through which they have gone? This number can be substantial—more than 60–80 for human fetal fibroblasts (Section II.A.1). Moreover, for a given cell population, the PD at which senescence occurs is reproducible.

At present, the telomere hypothesis is perhaps the most viable explanation for a cell division "counting" mechanism (Levy *et al.*, 1992).

Telomeres, the termini of linear chromosomes, consist of a highly repetitive sequence (TTAGGG in humans and other vertebrates) that forms a distinct three-dimensional structure. Because DNA polymerase requires a labile primer to initiate unidirectional $5' \rightarrow 3'$ DNA replication, each round of DNA replication leaves some $3'$ bases within the telomere unreplicated. Germ cells express telomerase, a unique DNA polymerase that adds telomeric repeats to chromosome ends *de novo*. However, most somatic cells do not appear to express this enzyme. This is particularly true of cells from adult human tissue (Harley & Villeponteau, 1995).

The telomere hypothesis predicts that telomeres should progressively shorten throughout the replicative life span (Harley *et al.*, 1990; Allsopp *et al.*, 1992; Levy *et al.*, 1992). Indeed, mean telomere length decreases by about 50 bp per doubling for human fibroblasts in culture. Moreover, mean telomere length decreases by about 15 bp per year in cells from different aged donors. Because homologous chromosomes segregate randomly during mitosis, there may be considerable variability in telomere length from chromosome to chromosome and from cell to cell. Nonetheless, these findings support the idea that cells sense replicative age by the degree of telomere shortening, both in culture and *in vivo*.

Telomere length stabilizes, and sometimes increases, in immortal cells. This very likely is due to the expression of telomerase (Counter *et al.*, 1992, 1994; Kim *et al.*, 1994). As noted earlier, most normal somatic cells do not express this enzyme. However, most immortal cells are telomerase-positive. Thus, induction of telomerase activity may be required for the unlimited cell division potential of immortal cells. By contrast, telomerase is not necessary for the extension of replicative life span. Human cells expressing T-antigen, or E1a and E1b, remained devoid of telomerase activity throughout the resulting extension of life span. However, immortal variants arising from these cultures did express the activity (Counter *et al.*, 1992). Thus, the T-antigen-insensitive, or M2, mechanism that ensures a finite replicative life span may entail, at least in part, repression of telomerase activity.

The telomerase hypothesis is based on correlations, albeit strong ones. It is not yet possible to critically test it in higher eukaryotic cells (for example, by preventing or accelerating telomere shortening). However, yeasts express telomerase (and in this regard resemble immortal cells), and telomeres and telomerase can be manipulated by genetic means. In yeast, loss of a single telomere arrests cell growth, but only transiently (Sandell & Zakian, 1993). Senescent mammalian cells, by contrast, are irreversibly growth-arrested. Moreover, inactivation of yeast telomerase by mutation leads to cell death (Lundblad & Szostak, 1989), whereas senescent mammalian cells remain viable. There may, of course, be fundamental differences between yeast and mammalian cells in the mechanisms by which a short telomere signals growth arrest. The cloning of the RNA component of human telomerase (Feng *et al.*, 1995) should greatly facilitate the cloning of other human telomerase components and critical testing of the telomere hypothesis in higher eukaryotic cells.

The mechanism by which short telomeres arrest cell proliferation is not known. In yeast, a DNA damage-response pathway mediates the growth arrest caused by telomere loss (Sandell & Zakian, 1993). It is possible, therefore, that replicative senescence is a DNA damage response to a shortened telomere (Levy *et al.*, 1992). Counter to this argument, the senescent state is remarkably stable (Section I.B), whereas most damage-arrested states are not. In addition, p53 protein and

DNA binding activity, which increases markedly in the mammalian DNA damage response, is not elevated in senescent cells (Afshari, *et al.*, 1993; Oshima *et al.*, 1995; Hara *et al.*, submitted). Another view (Wright & Shay, 1992) suggests that telomeric chromatin creates a field that affects genes located near telomeres and that this field, and consequently gene expression, changes as telomeres shorten. This hypothesis is consistent with the genetics discussed in Section III, if it invokes a growth-inhibitory gene that is repressed by a long telomere and activated upon shortening. Finally, it is possible that, as telomeres shorten, a constitutively expressed telomere binding protein may accumulate and repress transcription, as do the RAP1 or RIF1 proteins in yeast (Lustig *et al.*, 1990; Hardy *et al.*, 1992), or may induce a dominant inhibitor.

B. Growth Arrest Mechanisms

The mechanisms responsible for establishing and maintaining the growth arrest of senescent cells are exceedingly stringent, particularly in human cells. Several growth-related genes have been identified whose expression or regulation is altered in senescent cells (Tables I–III), principally cultured human fibroblasts. Although there is little doubt that the growth arrest associated with replicative senescence is controlled by multiple mechanisms, it is unlikely that each of the changes in gene expression is independently controlled. The difficulty at present is sorting out how these changes in gene expression are related to each other, and how they relate to the dominance of the growth arrest, the inability to enter S phase and mitosis, and the functions of p53 and pRb.

1. Multiple Steps Establish and Maintain Replicative Senescence

The growth arrest induced by replicative senescence and escape from senescence or immortalization are both multistep processes (Sections III.B and IV.A). These steps are summarized here and in Fig. 3.

Senescent cells arrest growth with a G1 DNA content. T-antigen, by inactivating p53 and pRb, will stimulate senescent cells to initiate and complete S phase. T-antigen cannot, however, stimulate mitosis. Thus, T-antigen-stimulated senescent cells arrest growth with a G2 DNA content. These findings suggest that senescent cells fail to proliferate due to at least two blocks to cell cycle progression. We refer to these as the G1 and G2/M cell cycle blocks. Together, these blocks may constitute the M1 mortality mechanism (or the first block to immortality) described by Shay and Wright (1991).

Prior to senescence, T-antigen bypasses not only the G1 cell cycle block but the G2/M block as well. Hence, presenescent cells expressing T-antigen overcome the entire M1 mechanism and proliferate beyond their normal replicative life span. The basis for the disparate effects of T-antigen in senescent vs presenescent cells is not known. One possibility is that the G2/M cell cycle block is imposed only after the G1 block is instituted. Thus, the G1 and G2/M cell cycle blocks may not be independently initiated (see Section IV.B.2). Once initiated, however, they may act independently.

At the end of their replicative life span, T-antigen-expressing cells enter an unstable state termed crisis. Some cells in crisis may arrest growth because the normal senescence mechanisms prevail, others may continue to proliferate, and yet others may experience both stimulatory and inhibitory signals and die. Eventually, most cells in crisis either senesce or die. Thus, T-antigen alone (and, hence, abrogation of only M1) is not sufficient for replicative immortality.

Immortal cells may arise from human cell cultures in crisis at a very low frequency. These immortal cells very likely have acquired a mutation that bypasses a second immortality block or the M2 mechanism (Shay & Wright, 1991). The appearance of immortal cells correlates strongly with the induction of telomerase activity. Thus, the M2 mechanism may entail the repression of either a component(s) of telomerase or a telomerase inducer.

2. Immediate Causes

We now have at least a superficial understanding of some of the immediate causes for the failure of senescent cells, principally senescent human fibroblasts, to proliferate. Several positive growth regulators are now known to be repressed or refractory to induction by mitogens. Table I lists some of the genes that senescent human fibroblasts fail to express or underexpress. In addition, some growth-inhibitory genes are overexpressed or are constitutively active in senescent cells (Tables II and III). The idea that senescent cells arrest growth at the G1/S boundary [see, for example, Stanulis-Praeger (1987)] is not a very tenable concept, given the diversity of changes in gene expression that occurs in senescent cells (Tables I–III).

a. Repression of Early Response Genes Early response genes are induced within an hour or so of mitogen stimulation, and their induction is independent of prior gene expression. Many early response genes are induced more or less normally in senescent human fibroblasts (Rittling et al., 1986; Chang & Chen, 1988; Seshadri & Campisi, 1990; Phillips et al., 1992). However, two early response genes, whose expression appears to be essential for fibroblasts to initiate DNA synthesis, fail to respond to mitogens. These are the c-fos protooncogene (Seshadri & Campisi, 1990), which encodes a component of the AP1 transcription factor (Cohen & Curran, 1989), and the Id1 and Id2 genes (Hara et al., 1994), which encode negative regulators of basic helix–loop–helix (bHLH) transcription factors (Benezra *et al.*, 1990; Sun *et al.*, 1991). Because both c-fos and Id are needed for entry into S phase, the repression of either gene can explain why senescent cells fail to proliferate.

The mechanism(s) responsible for the repression of Id1 and Id2 is unknown. c-fos, on the other hand, may remain repressed in senescent cells because the serum response factor (SRF) fails to bind the serum response element (SRE) in the c-fos promoter. SRF is hyperphosphorylated in senescent cells, and this may prevent its binding to the SRE and, thus, prevent mitogen-inducible c-fos expression (Atadia *et al.*, 1994). Although mitogen-dependent c-fos induction is lost in senescent cells, c-fos remains inducible by DNA-damaging agents (Choi *et al.*, 1995). It is not known whether or how the repression of c-fos and Id is related, nor is it known how the repression of these early response genes relates to the repression of G1/S genes (discussed in the following).

b. Repression of G1/S Genes   Several genes that are normally induced in late G1 or at the G1/S boundary are not expressed by senescent cells (see Table I). The replication-dependent histone genes are not expressed (Seshadri & Campisi, 1990; Zambetti *et al.*, 1987). In addition, senescent cells do not express genes encoding a variety of enzymes needed for DNA replication, including thymidine kinase (TK), thymidylate synthetase, and dihydrofolate reductase (DHFR) (Pang & Chen, 1993, 1994).

The mechanism responsible for the repression of at least some of the G1/S genes is now known: senescent human fibroblasts are markedly deficient in the activity of E2F (Dimri *et al.*, 1994). E2F is a heterodimeric transcription factor that is essential for the induction of many G1/S genes (Nevins, 1992; Farnham *et al.*, 1993). The deficiency in E2F activity, in turn, is very likely due to the repression of E2F1, the cell cycle-regulated component

of E2F. E2F1 mRNA is normally induced about 4 hr before S phase. This induction is thought to be rate-limiting for the expression of DHFR and other G1/S genes (Slansky *et al.*, 1993; Sala *et al.*, 1994) and fails to occur in senescent cells (Dimri *et al.*, 1994). The mechanism responsible for the repression of E2F1 is not yet known.

c. Repression of Selected Cyclins and Cyclin-Dependent Protein Kinases   Senescent cells also fail to express several cyclins and cyclin-dependent protein kinases (cdks), whose activities regulate progression through the G1 and G2 phases of the cell cycle (Ohtsubo & Roberts, 1993; Pines, 1993; Sherr, 1993). Senescent human fibroblasts underexpress cdk2 mRNA (Afshari *et al.*, 1993); cyclins A and B, and cdc2 (the first cdk identified) mRNA (Stein *et al.*, 1991). In addition, senescent cells are deficient in cyclin E- and D-dependent cdk activities (Dulic *et al.*, 1993).

The repression of cyclin A and cdc2 may be another downstream consequence of the repression of E2F1, because both cyclin A and cdc2 require E2F activity for their expression (Yamamoto *et al.*, 1994; Dalton, 1991). In addition, because cyclin B and cdc2 are important for regulating progression through G2 (Nishimoto *et al.*, 1992; Pines, 1993), the repression of cyclin B and cdc2 may be among the immediate causes of the G2/M block in senescent cells. If so, the repression of E2F1 and deficiency in E2F activity may be the link that connects the G1 block to the G2/M block in senescent cells.

d. Over- or Constitutive Expression of Growth Inhibitors   Senescent cells overexpress or constitutively express at least three growth inhibitors.

First, senescent cells overexpress p21, which very likely also constitutes an immediate cause for their failure to proliferate. p21 was independently cloned as an overexpressed gene in senescent human fibroblasts (Noda *et al.*, 1994), a p53-inducible gene (El-Deiry *et al.*, 1993), and a cdk-interacting protein (Gu *et al.*, 1993; Harper *et al.*, 1993; Xiong *et al.*, 1993). p21 inhibits the kinase activity of a variety of cyclin–cdk complexes. It is a particularly potent inhibitor of the G1 cyclin–cdk2 complexes. Thus, the senescence-associated deficiency in cyclin E- and D-dependent kinase activity (Dulic *et al.*, 1993) is very likely due to the overexpression of p21.

The inhibition of cyclin-dependent kinases, in turn, very likely causes the constitutive underphosphorylation of pRb in senescent cells (Stein *et al.*, 1990). pRb is growth-suppressive in its underphosphorylated form; mitogens induce pRb phosphorylation, which relieves its growth-inhibitory activity (Hamel *et al.*, 1992). pRb remains underphosphorylated in mitogen-stimulated senescent cells (Stein *et al.*, 1990). Thus, pRb remains a constitutive growth suppressor and may well constitute an immediate cause for the failure to proliferate. Because pRb is an important substrate of cdk's (Hamel *et al.*, 1992; Ohtsubo & Roberts, 1993; Pines, 1993; Sherr, 1993), one immediate cause for the G1 block of senescent cells (pRb underphosphorylation) can be traced to the overexpression of p21. The mechanism responsible for p21 overexpression is not yet known. Another growth-inhibitory protein, prohibitin, has also been reported to lack posttranslational modification, presumably phosphorylation, in senescent human fibroblasts (Liu *et al.*, 1994b). In contrast to pRb, the biological function of this modification is not known, nor is it known whether prohibitin is a substrate for cdk, much less an indirect target of p21.

Finally, p53 remains constitutively active in senescent human fibroblasts (Hara *et al.*, submitted). As discussed earlier (Section IV.A), p53 protein and DNA binding activities are similar in quiescent and senescent cells. When quiescent cells are stimulated by mitogens, p53 binding activity declines sharply as the cells enter the S phase. This decline in p53 activity is undoubtedly due to the induction, in late G1, of mdm2. mdm2 encodes a protein that binds and inactivates p53 (Momand *et al.*, 1992) and participates in an auto-regulatory feedback loop to control p53 function (Wu *et al.*, 1993). mdm2 is not induced by mitogens in senescent cells (Hara *et al.*, submitted).

In summary, the immediate causes for the failure of senescent cells to initiate DNA replication appear to be the repression of a few key positive growth regulators and the overexpression of a key growth inhibitor. Minimally, these include the repression of three transcriptional regulators (c-fos, Id, and E2F) and the overexpression of a cdk inhibitor (p21). Together, these changes in gene expression may account for many of the other changes in senescence-associated changes in gene expression. In addition, the p53 and pRb tumor suppressors are rendered constitutive growth inhibitors in senescent cells. This is very likely due to the repression of mdm2 and the overexpression of p21, respectively. In principle, each of these senescence-associated changes can account for the failure of senescent cells to enter the S phase of the cell cycle.

3. Prime Causes

The dominance of the growth arrest associated with replicative senescence dictates that the failure to proliferate ultimately cannot be explained by deficiencies in gene expression. Indeed, we have been unable to reactivate DNA synthesis in senescent human fibroblasts by providing them with expression vectors encoding c-fos, Id-1, Id-2, mdm2, or E2F1, alone or in combination (unpublished). This suggests that senescent cells express one or more genes that override the stimulatory effects of c-fos, Id, mdm2, and E2F1. This idea is, of course, consistent with the results of the somatic cell fusion studies.

Thus far, p21 overexpression is the only senescence-associated change in gene expression that has the potential to act in a dominant fashion. Given what is known about how p21 inhibits cell proliferation (Section IV.B.2), it is very likely that p21 plays a causal role in the growth arrest associated with senescence. However, because p21 antisense vectors may not stimulate senescent human fibroblasts to progress normally through the S phase (J. Smith, personal communication), it is also likely that additional mechanisms may cooperate with p21 to suppress the growth of senescent cells.

p21 overexpression may be a direct consequence of a senescence-inducing signal (for example, a shortened telomere), or it may be due to an as yet unidentified upstream regulator. One possible candidate for a dominant inhibitor is a bHLH transcription factor that is normally inactivated by Id proteins. We have found that an Id-1 expression vector complements an Rb-binding defective T-antigen for the ability to reactivate DNA synthesis in senescent human fibroblasts [Hara *et al.*, in press; reviewed in Dimri and Campisi (1994b)]. This suggests that senescent cells may express one or more growth-inhibitory bHLH proteins that cooperate with pRb. In addition, we identified a senescence-associated DNA binding activity (SNF, senescence factor) that has transcription silencer activity (Dimri & Campisi, 1994b). We do not yet know whether this activity mediates the repression of c-fos, Id, or E2F1 or the overexpression of p21 or whether it acts on an entirely different set of genes.

In summary, in contrast to the immediate causes, the prime causes for the growth arrest associated with replicative senescence are largely unknown. Although there are now several candidates for dominant-acting growth repressors (p21, a bHLH protein, SNF, and prohibitin), with the exception of p21, very little is known about how they act, and virtually nothing is known about how the expression of these genes relates to the primary senescence-inducing signal(s).

VI. Implications for Aging

As discussed in Section II.A, there is now substantial correlative evidence, and some direct evidence, that replicative senescence occurs *in vivo* and that senescent cells accumulate in tissues with age. Does the accumulation of senescent cells cause or contribute to the functional decrements and/or pathologies that occur during aging? Unfortunately, at this time, there is only conjecture and no direct evidence that this is the case. However, the ability to detect, much less manipulate, senescent cells *in vivo* is at a very embryonic stage. There is little doubt that the idea that replicative senescence is a causal factor in aging will be subjected to increasingly more critical testing in the next few years. This said, let us speculate on how the accumulation of senescent cells might contribute to aging.

The key features of senescent cells are their inability to proliferate, altered differentiated functions (Section I.B), and resistance to apoptotic death (Wang *et al.*, 1994). The failure to proliferate clearly would retard the ability of tissues that accumulate senescent cells to regenerate or repair. Indeed, wound healing is generally slower in the elderly. However, substantial numbers of proliferative cells can often be recovered from even very old tissues, and wounds do heal even in very old mammals. Moreover, the results of the SA-β-gal staining discussed in Section II.A.2 suggest that senescent cells may comprise only a few percent of the cells in old skin. Thus, the proliferative failure of senescent cells may not have a major impact on tissue function, although it certainly might compromise the organism by retarding tissue repair.

By contrast, the altered differentiation of senescent cells might have a substantial impact on tissue function and integrity. The examples of an altered profile of steroids produced by senescent adreno-cortical cells and increased collagenase produced by senescent dermal fibroblasts are discussed in Section I.B.2. Senescent cells may also overexpress or underexpress inflammatory or host-defense cytokines, such as interleukin-1 (Kumar *et al.*, 1992) and interleukin-6 (Goodman & Stein, 1994). These types of senescence-associated changes would certainly be expected to affect neighboring (nonsenescent) cells or even other tissues. Moreover, the fraction of senescent cells needed to have adverse local or systemic effects need not be large.

Finally, the relative resistance of senescent cells to apoptosis, or programmed cell death, may explain why senescent cells accumulate *in vivo*. Thus, senescent cells are much less responsive to the mechanisms by which cells with abnormal phenotypes are cleared from tissues. In addition, senescent cells, and some tissues in old animals, fail to mount an adequate heat shock or stress response (discussed in Section II.A.1), and thus damaged senescent cells may accumulate in tissues after a local or systemic stress.

What is needed now is a better understanding of the phenotype of senescent cells *in vivo* and reagents to modulate this phenotype *in vivo*.

VII. Unanswered Questions/Future Directions

At present, we have only a scaffold of molecular understanding regarding the control of replicative senescence. Many gaps remain in our knowledge of how this process is controlled and its physiological consequences for the organism.

We have very little information as to whether and how senescent cells contribute to the functional decrements that are the hallmarks of organismic aging. In this regard, the SA-β-gal marker for senescent cells should facilitate the ability to identify senescent cells at sites of age-dependent pathology. This biomarker may also help identify or develop compounds that can re-

verse some features of the senescent phenotype, without the dangerous side effect of inducing immortalization, and help identify the genes responsible for the immortality complementation groups.

The identification and cloning of the immortality complementation group genes, and other genes that may limit the proliferative capacity of normal cells, is another important and as yet unfulfilled goal. In light of the rapid advances that are being made in genomics, it may well be reached in the not too distant future. There is every likelihood that new genes will be identified in this search and that these genes may provide new insights into both tumor suppression and aging.

There are also many gaps in our understanding of the mechanism(s) responsible for the inability of senescent cells to initiate DNA replication and mitosis. Despite the realization that pRb and p53 have critical roles in the block to entry into the S phase, and the tentative identification of candidate dominant growth repressors, we know almost nothing about how the tumor suppressor proteins act in senescent cells, much less interact with putative senescence-specific repressors. Moreover, the mechanism(s) responsible for the block to mitosis is virtually unknown. We also do not yet understand the relationship between the block to entry into the S phase and mitosis and the M1 and M2 mechanisms that are bypassed during immortalization. Finally, we have virtually no knowledge of how the mechanisms responsible for growth arrest associated with senescence relate to those responsible for the altered differentiation of senescent cells.

References

Afshari, C. A., Vojta, P. J., Annab, L. A., Futreal, P. A., Willard, T. B., & Barrett, J. C. (1993). Investigations of the role of G1/S cell cycle mediators in cellular senescence. *Experimental Cell Research, 209,* 231–237.

Allsopp, R. C., Vaziri, H., Patterson, C., Goldstein, S., Younglai, E. V., Futcher, A. B., Greider, C. W., & Harley, C. B. (1992). Telomere length predicts replicative capacity of human fibroblasts. *Proceedings of the National Academy of Sciences of the United States of America, 89,* 10114–10118.

Atadja, P. W., Stringer, K. F., & Riabowol, K. T. (1994). Loss of serum response element binding activity and hyperphosphorylation of serum response factor during cellular aging. *Molecular and Cellular Biology, 14,* 4991–4999.

Balin, A. K., Goodman, D. B. P., Rasmussen, H., & Cristofalo, V. J. (1977). The effect of oxygen and vitamin E on the lifespan of human diploid cells in vitro. *Journal of Cell Biology, 74,* 58–67.

Band, V., DeCaprio, J. A., Delmolino, L., Kulesa, V., & Sager, R. (1991). Loss of p53 protein in human papillomavirus type 16 E6-immortalized human mammary epithelial cells. *Journal of Virology, 65,* 6671–6676.

Barbanti-Brodano, D., & Croce, C. M. (1994). Suppression of tumorigenicity of breast cancer cells by microcell-mediated chromosome transfer: Studies on chromosomes 6 and 11. *Cancer Research, 54,* 1331–1336.

Bayreuther, K., Rodemann, H. P., Hommer, R., Dittman, K., Albiez, M., & Francz, P. I. (1988). Human skin fibroblasts in vitro differentiate along a terminal cell lineage. *Proceedings of the National Academy of Sciences of the United States of America, 85,* 5112–5116.

Benezra, R., Davis, R. L., Lockshon, D., Turner, D. L., & Weintraub, H. (1990). The protein Id: A negative regulator of helix-loop-helix DNA binding proteins. *Cell, 61,* 49–59.

Berry, I. J., Burns, J. E., & Parkinson, E. K. (1994). Assignment of two human epidermal squamous cell carcinoma cell lines to more than one complementation group for the immortal phenotype. *Molecular Carcinogenesis, 9,* 134–142.

Bierman, E. L. (1978). The effect of donor age on the in vitro lifespan of cultured human arterial smooth-muscle cells. *In Vitro, 14,* 951–955.

Bookstein, R., & Lee, W. H. (1991). Molecular genetics of the retinoblastoma tumor suppressor gene. *Critical Reviews in Oncology, 2,* 211–227.

Boulanger, P. A., & Blair, G. E. (1991). Expression and interactions of human adenovirus oncoproteins. *Biochemistry Journal, 275,* 281–299.

Brown, W. T. (1990). Genetic diseases of premature aging as models of senescence. *Annual Review of Gerontology and Geriatrics, 10,* 23–42.

Bruce, S. A., Deamond, S. F., & T'so, P. O. P. (1986). In vitro senescence of Syrian hamster mesenchymal cells of fetal to aged adult origin. Inverse relationship between *in vivo* donor age and *in vitro* proliferative capacity. *Mechanisms in Ageing and Development, 34,* 151–173.

Bunn, C. L., & Tarrant, G. M. (1980). Limited lifespan in somatic cell hybrids and cybrids. *Experimental Cell Research, 127,* 385–396.

Chang, Z. F., & Chen, K. Y. (1988). Regulation of ornithine decarboxylase and other cell-cycle dependent genes during senescence of IMR90 human fibroblasts. *Journal of Biological Chemistry, 263,* 11431–11435.

Chang, C. D., Phillips, P. D., Lipson, K. E., Cristofalo, V., & Baserga, R. (1991). Senescent human fibroblasts have a posttranscriptional block in the expression of proliferating cell nuclear antigen gene. *Journal of Biological Chemistry, 266,* 8663–8666.

Chen, Q., Fischer, A., Reagan, J. D., Yan, L. J., & Ames, B. N. (1995). Oxidative DNA damage and senescence of human diploid fibroblast cells. *Proceedings of the National Academy of Sciences of the United States of America,* in press.

Cheng, C. Y., Ryan, R. F., Vo, T. P., & Hornsby, P. J. (1989). Cellular senescence involves stochastic processes causing loss of expression of differentiated functions: SV40 as a means for dissociating effects of senescence on growth and on differentiated function gene expression. *Experimental Cell Research, 180,* 49–62.

Choi, H. S., Lin, Z., Li, B., & Liu, A. Y. C. (1990). Age-dependent decrease in the heat-inducible, DNA sequence-specific DNA binding activity in human diploid fibroblasts. *Journal of Biological Chemistry, 265,* 1–7.

Choi, A. M. K., Pignolo, R. J., ap Rhys, C. M. I., Cristofalo, V. J., & Holbrook, N. J. (1995). Alterations in the molecular response to DNA damage during cellular aging of cultured fibroblasts: Reduced AP1 activation and collagenase gene expression. *Journal of Cellular Physiology,* in press.

Cohen, D. R., & Curran, T. (1989). The structure and function of the fos protooncogene. *Critical Reviews in Oncogenesis, 1,* 65–88.

Counter, C. M., Avillon, A. A., LeFeuvre, C. E., Stewart, N. G., Greider, C. W., Harley, C. B., & Bacchetti, S. (1992). Telomere shortening associated with chromosome instability is arrested in immortal cells which express telomerase activity. *EMBO Journal, 11,* 1921–1929.

Counter, C. M., Hirte, H. W., Bacchetti, S., & Harley, C. B. (1994). Telomerase activity in human ovarian carcinoma. *Proceedings of the National Academy of Sciences of the United States of America, 91,* 2900–2904.

Cowled, P. A., Ciccarelli, C., Coccia, E., Philipson, L., & Sorrentino, V. (1994). Expression of growth arrest specific (gas) genes in senescent murine cells. *Experimental Cell Research, 211,* 197–202.

Cristofalo, V. J., & Pignolo, R. J. (1993). Replicative senescence of human fibroblast-like cells in culture. *Physiological Reviews, 73,* 617–638.

Dalton, S. (1991). Cell cycle regulation on the human cdc2 gene. *EMBO Journal, 11,* 1979–1984.

Daniel, C. W. (1972). Aging of cells during serial propagation *in vivo. Advanced Gerontological Research, 4,* 167–199.

Daniel, C. W., De Orne, K. B., Young, J. T., Blair, P. B., & Faulkin, L. J., Jr. (1968). The *in vivo* life span of normal and preneoplastic mouse mammary glands: A serial transplantation study. *Proceedings of the National Academy of Sciences of the United States of America, 61,* 53–60.

D'Costa, A., Breese, C. R., Boyd, R. L., Booze, R. M., & Sonntag, W. E. (1991). Attenuation of fos-like immunoreactivity induced by a single electroconvulsive shock in brains of aged mice. *Mice Research, 567,* 204–211.

Dell'Orco, R. T., Mertens, J. G., & Kruse, P. F. (1973). Doubling potential, calendar time and senescence of human diploid cells in culture. *Experimental Cell Research, 77,* 356–360.

Dimri, G. P., & Campisi, J. (1994a). Altered profile of transcription factor binding activities in senescent human fibroblasts. *Experimental Cell Research, 212,* 132–140.

Dimri, G. P., & Campisi, J. (1994b). Molecular and cell biology of replicative senescence. *Cold Spring Harbor Symposia on Quantitative Biology: Molecular Genetics of Cancer, 54,* 67–73.

Dimri, G. P., Hara, E., & Campisi, J. (1994). Regulation of two E2F related genes in presenescent and senescent human fibroblasts. *Journal of Biological Chemistry, 269,* 16180–16186.

Dimri, G. P., Lee, X., Basile, G., Acosta, M., Scott, G., Roskelley, C., Medrano, E. E., Linskens, M., Rubelj, I., Pereira-Smith, O., Peacocke, M., & Campisi, J. (1995). A bio-marker that identifies senescent human cells in culture and in aging skin *in vivo. Proceedings of the National Academy of Sciences of the United States of America, 92,* 9363–9367.

DiPaolo, B. R., Pignolo, R. J., & Cristofalo, V. J. (1992). Overexpression of the two chain form of cathepsin B in senescent WI38 cells. *Experimental Cell Research, 201,* 500–505.

Dulic, V., Drullinger, L. F., Lees, E., Reed, S. I., & Stein, G. H. (1993). Altered regulation of G1 cyclins in senescent human diploid fibroblasts: Accumulation of inactive cyclin E-cdk and cyclin D-cdk complexes. *Proceedings of the National Academy of Sciences of the United States of America, 90,* 11038–11043.

Duncan, E. L., Whitaker, N. J., Moy, E. L., & Reddel, R. R. (1993). Assignment of SV40-immortalized cells to more than one complementation group for immortalization. *Experimental Cell Research, 205,* 337–344.

El-Deiry, W. S., Tokino, T., Velculescu, V. E., Levy, D. B., Parsons, R., Trent, J. M., Lin, D., Mercer, W. E., Kinzler, K. W., & Vogelstein, B. (1993). WAF1, a potential mediator of p53 tumor suppression. *Cell, 75,* 817–825.

Fanning, E. (1992). Structure and function of simian virus 40 large tumor antigen. *Annual Review of Biochemistry, 61,* 55–85.

Fargnoli, J., Kunisada, T., Fornace, A. J., Schneider, E. L., & Holbrook, N. J. (1990). Decreased expression of heat shock protein 70 mRNA and protein after heat treatment in cells of aged rats. *Proceedings of the National Academy of Sciences of the United States of America, 87,* 846–850.

Farnham, P. J., Slansky, J. E., & Kollmar, R. (1993). The role of E2F in the mammalian cell cycle. *Biochimica et Biophysica Acta, 1155,* 125–131.

Feng, J., Funk, W. D., Wang, S. S., Weinrich, S. L., Avilion, A. A., Chiu, C. P., Adams, R. P., Chang, E., Allsopp, R. C., Yu, J., Harley, C. B., & Villeponteau, B. (1995). The RNA component of human telomerase. *Science, 269,* 1236–1241.

Ferber, A., Chang, C., Sell, C., Ptasznik, A., Cristofalo, V. J., Hubbard, K., Ozer, H. L., Adam, M., Robert, C. T., Jr., Le Roith, D., Dumenil, G., & Baserga, R. (1993). Failure of senescent human fibroblasts to express the insulin like growth factor-1 gene. *Journal of Biological Chemistry, 268,* 17883–17888.

Finch, C. E. (1990). *Longevity, Senescence, and the Genome.* Chicago: University of Chicago Press.

Galloway, D. A., & McDougall, J. K. (1989). Human papillomaviruses and carcinomas. *Advances in Virus Research, 37,* 125–171.

Giordano, T., Kleinseck, D., & Foster, D. N. (1989). Increase in abundance of a transcript hybridizing to elongation factor α during cellular senescence and quiescence. *Experimental Gerontology, 24,* 501–513.

Girardi, A. J., Fensen, F. C., & Koprowski, H. (1965). SV40-induced transformation of human diploid cells: Crisis and recovery. *Journal of Cellular Comparative Physiology, 65,* 69–84.

Goldstein, S. (1974). Aging in vitro: Growth of cultured cells from the Galapagos tortoise. *Experimental Cell Research, 83,* 297–302.

Goldstein, S. (1978). Human genetic disorders that feature premature onset and accelerated progression of biological aging. In E. L. Schneider (Ed.), *The Genetics of Aging* (pp. 171–224). New York: Plenum Press.

Goldstein, S. (1990). Replicative senescence: The human fibroblast comes of age. *Science, 249,* 1129–1133.

Goldstein, S., & Singal, D. P. (1974). Senescence of cultured human fibroblasts: Mitotic versus metabolic time. *Experimental Cell Research, 88,* 359–364.

Goodman, L., & Stein, G. H. (1994). Basal and induced amounts of interleukin-6 mRNA decline progressively with age in human fibroblasts. *Journal of Biological Chemistry, 269,* 19250–19255.

Gorman, S. D., & Cristofalo, V. J. (1985). Reinitiation of cellular DNA synthesis in BrdU-selected nondividing senescent WI38 cells by simian virus 40 infection. *Journal of Cellular Physiology, 125,* 122–126.

Goto, M., Rubenstein, M., Wever, J., Wood, K., & Drayna, D. (1992). Genetic linkage of Werners syndrome to five markers on chromosome 8. *Nature, 355,* 735–738.

Gu, Y., Turek, C. W., & Morgan, D. O. (1993). Inhibition of cdk2 activity in vivo by an associated 20 K regulatory subunit. *Nature, 366,* 707–710.

Gualandi, F., Morelli, C., Pavan, J. V., Rimessi, P., Sensi, A., Bonfatti, A., Gruppioni, R., Possati, L., Stanbridge, E. J., & Barbanti-Brodano, G. (1994). Induction of senescence and control of tumorigenicity in BK virus transformed mouse cells by human chromosome 6. *Genes, Chromosomes and Cancer, 10,* 77–84.

Halbert, C. L., Demers, G. W., & Galloway, D. A. (1991). The E7 gene of human papillomavirus type 16 is sufficient for immortalization of human epithelial cells. *Journal of Virology, 65,* 473–478.

Hamel, P. A., Gallie, B. L., & Phillips, R. A. (1992). The retinoblastoma protein and cell cycle regulation. *Trends in Genetics, 8,* 180–185.

Hara, E., Tsuri, H., Shinozaki, S., & Oda, K. (1991). Cooperative effect of antisense-Rb and antisense-p53 oligomers on the extension of lifespan in human diploid fibroblasts, TIG-1. *Biochemical and Biophysical Research Communication, 179,* 528–534.

Hara, E., Yamaguchi, T., Nojima, H., Ide, T., Campisi, J., Okayama, H., & Oda, K. (1994). Id related genes encoding helix loop helix proteins are required for G1 progression and are repressed in senescent human fibroblasts. *Journal of Biological Chemistry, 269,* 2139–2145.

Hara, E., Uzman, J. A., Dimri, G. P., Nehliu, J. O., Testori, A., & Campisi, J. (in press). The helix–loop–helix protein Id-1 and a retinoblastoma protein binding mutant of SV-40 T antigen synergize to reactivate DNA synthesis in senescent human fibroblasts. *Developmental Genetics.*

Hardy, C. F. J., Sussel, L., & Shore, D. (1992). A RAP1-interacting protein involved in transcriptional silencing and telomere length regulation. *Genes and Development, 6,* 801–814.

Harley, C. B., Futcher, A. B., & Greider, C. W. (1990). Telomeres shorten during ageing of human fibroblasts. *Nature, 345,* 458–460.

Harley, C. B., & Villeponteau, B. (1995). Telomeres and telomerase in aging and cancer. *Current Opinion in Genetics & Development, 5,* 249–255.

Harper, J. W., Adami, G. R., Wei, N., Keyomarsi, K., & Elledge, S. J. (1993). The p21-cdk-interacting protein Cip1 is a potent inhibitor of G1 cyclin-dependent kinases. *Cell, 75,* 805–816.

Hawley-Nelson, P., Vousden, K. H., Hubbert, N. L., Lowy, D. R., & Schiller, J. T. (1989). HPV16 E6 and E7 proteins cooperate to immortalize human foreskin keratinocytes. *EMBO Journal, 8,* 3905–3910.

Hayflick, L. (1965). The limited *in vitro* lifetime of human diploid cell strains. *Experimental Cell Research, 37,* 614–636.

Hayflick, L. (1977). The cellular basis for biological aging. In C. E. Finch & L. Hayflick (Eds.), *Handbook of the Biology of Aging* (pp. 159–186). New York: Van Nostrand Reinhold Co.

Hayflick, L., & Moorhead, P. S. (1961). The serial cultivation of human diploid cell strains. *Experimental Cell Research, 25,* 585–621.

Hensler, P., Annab, L. A., Barrett, J. C., & Pereira-Smith, O. M. (1994). A gene involved in control of human cellular senescence on human chromosome 1q. *Molecular and Cell Biology, 14,* 2292–2297.

Heydari, A. R., Wu, B., Takahashi, R., Strong, R., & Richardson, A. (1993). Expression of heat shock protein 70 is altered by age and diet at the level of transcription. *Molecular and Cellular Biology, 13,* 2909–2918.

Hinds, P., Finlay, C., & Levine, A. J. (1989). Mutation is required to activate the p53 gene for cooperation with the ras oncogene and transformation. *Journal of Virology, 63,* 739–746.

Hollstein, M., Sidransky, D., Vogelstein, B., & Harris, C. C. (1991). p53 mutation in human cancer. *Science, 253,* 49–53.

Hornsby, P. J., Aldern, K. A., & Harris, S. E. (1986). Clonal variation in response to adrenocorticotropin in cultured bovine adrenocortical cells: Relationship to senescence. *Journal of Cellular Physiology, 129,* 395–402.

Hornsby, P. J., Hancock, J. P., Vo, T. P., Nason, L. M., Ryan, R. F., & McAllister, J. M. (1987). Loss of expression of a differentiated function gene, steroid 17α-hydroxylase, as adrenocortical cells senesce in culture. *Proceedings of the National Academy of Sciences of the United States of America, 84,* 1580–1584.

Ide, T., Tsuji, Y., Ishibashi, S., & Mitsui, Y. (1983). Reinitiation of host DNA synthesis in senescent human diploid cells by infection with simian virus 40. *Experimental Cell Research, 143,* 343–349.

Ide, T., Tsuji, Nakashima, T., & Ishibashi, S. (1984). Progress of aging in human diploid cells transformed with a tsA mutant of simian virus 40. *Experimental Cell Research, 150,* 321–328.

Jazwinski, S. M. (1990). Aging and senescence in the budding yeast *Saccharomyces cerevisiae. Molecular Microbiology, 4,* 337–344.

Kano, Y., & Little, J. B. (1989). Efficient immortalization by SV40 T DNA of skin fibroblasts from patients with Wilm's tumor association with chromosome 11p. *Molecular Carcinogenesis, 2,* 314–321.

Kim, N. W., Platyszek, M., Prowse, K. R., Harley, C. B., West, M. D., Ho, P. L. C., Coviello, G. M., Wright, W. E., Weinrich, S. L., & Shay, J. W. (1994). Specific association of human telomerase activity with immortal cells and cancer. *Science, 266,* 2011–2015.

Klein, C. B., Conway, K., Wang, X. W., Bhamra, L., Cohen, M. D., Annab, L., Barrett, J. C., & Costa, M. (1991). Senescence of Nickel-transformed cells by an Y chromosome: Possible epigenetic control. *Science, 251,* 796–799.

Koi, M., Johnson, L. A., Kalikin, L. M., Little, P. F. R., Nakamura, Y., & Feinberg, A. P. (1993). Tumor cell growth arrest caused by subchromosomal transferable DNA fragments from chromosome 11. *Science, 260,* 361–364.

Krohn, P. L. (1962). Review lectures on senescence. II. Heterochronic transplantation in the study of aging. *Proceedings of the Royal Society of London, 157,* 128–147.

Krohn, P. L. (1966). Transplantation and aging. In P. L. Krohn (Ed.), *Topics of the Biology of Aging* (pp. 125–138). New York: John Wiley.

Kumar, S., Millis, A. J., & Baglioni, C. (1992). Expression of interleukin 1-inducible genes and production of interleukin 1 by aging human fibroblasts. *Proceedings of the National Academy of Sciences of the United States of America, 89,* 4683–4687.

Le Guilly, Y., Simon, M., Lenoir, P., & Bourel, M. (1973). Long-term culture of human adult liver cells: Morphological changes related to *in vitro* senescence and effect of donor's age on growth potential. *Gerontologia, 19,* 303–313.

Levy, M. Z., Allsopp, R. C., Futcher, A. B., Greider, C. W., & Harley, C. B. (1992). Telomere end-replication problem and cell aging. *Journal of Molecular Biology, 225,* 951–960.

Liu, A. Y., Lin, Z., Choi, H. S., Sorhage, F., & Boshan, L. (1989). Attenuated induction of heat shock gene expression in aging diploid fibroblasts. *Journal of Biological Chemistry, 264,* 12037–12045.

Liu, S., Thweat, R., Lumpkin, C. K., & Gold-stein, S. (1994a). Suppression of calcium de-pendent membrane currents in human fi-broblasts by replicative senescence and forced expression of a genes encoding a puta-tive calcium binding protein. *Proceedings of the National Academy of Sciences of the United States of America, 91,* 2186–2190.

Liu, X. T., Stewart, C. A., King, R. L., Danner, D. A., Dell'Orco, R. T., & McClung, J. K. (1994b). Prohibitin expression during cellu-lar senescence of human diploid fibroblasts. *Biochemical and Biophysical Research Com-munications, 201,* 409–414.

Loh, W. E., Scrable, H. J., Livanos, E., Arboleda, M. J., Cavenee, W. K., Oshimura, M., & Weiss-man, B. (1992). Human chromosome 11 con-tains two different growth suppressor genes for embryonal rhabdomyosarcoma. *Proceedings of the National Academy of Sciences of the United States of America, 89,* 1755–1759.

Luce, M. C., & Cristofalo, V. J. (1992). Reduc-tion in heat shock gene expression correlates with increased thermosensitivity in senes-cent human fibroblasts. *Experimental Cell Research, 202,* 9–16.

Lumpkin, C. K., Knepper, J. E., Butel, J. S., Smith, J. R., & Pereira-Smith, O. M. (1986). Mitogenic effects of the protooncogene and oncogenc forms of c-H-ras DNA in human diploid fibroblasts. *Molecular and Cellular Biology, 6,* 2990–2993.

Lundblad, V., & Szostak, J. W. (1989). A mutant with a defect in telomere elongation leads to senescence in yeast. *Cell, 57,* 633–643.

Lustig, A. J., Kurtz, S., & Shore, D. (1990). In-volvement of the silencer and UAS binding protein RAP1 in regulation of telomere length. *Science, 250,* 549–553.

Maier, J. A. M., Voulalas, P., Roeder, D., & Ma-ciag, T. (1990). Extension of the life-span of human endothelial cells by an interleukin-1a antisense oligomer. *Science, 249,* 1570–1574.

Maier, J. A. M., Statuto, M., & Ragnoti, G. (1993). Senescence stimulates U037-endothelial cell interactions. *Experimental Cell Research, 208,* 270–274.

Martin, G. M. (1978). Genetic syndromes in man with potential relevance to the pathol-ogy of aging. In D. Bergsma & D. E. Harrison (Eds.), *Genetic Effects on Aging, Birth De-fects: Original Article Series* (pp. 5–39). New York: Alan Liss.

Martin, G. M., Sprague, C. A., & Epstein, C. J. (1970). Replicative life-span of cultivated hu-man cells. Effect of donor's age, tissue and geno-type. *Laboratory Investigation, 23,* 86–92.

Matsumura, T., Zerrudo, Z., & Hayflick L. (1979). Senescent human diploid cells in cul-tures: survival, DNA synthesis and morphol-ogy. *Journal of Gerontology, 34,* 328–334.

McCormick, J. J., & Maher, V. M. (1988). To-wards an understanding of the malignant transformation of diploid human fibroblasts. *Mutation Research, 199,* 273–291.

McCormick, A., & Campisi, J. (1991). Cellular aging and senescence. *Current Opinion in Cell Biology, 3,* 230–234.

McFarland, G. A., & Holliday, R. (1994). Retar-dation of the senescence of cultured human diploid fibroblasts by carnosine. *Experimen-tal Cell Research, 212,* 167–175.

Medrano, E. E., Yang, F., Boissy, R., Farooqui, J., Shah, V., Matsumoto, K., Norlund, J. J., & Park, H. Y. (1994). Terminal differentiation and senescence in the human melanocyte: Repression of tyrosine-phosphorylation of the extracellular signal-regulated kinase 2 se-lectively defines the two phenotypes. *Mo-lecular Biology of the Cell, 5,* 497–509.

Miller, R. A. (1991). Gerontology as oncology: Research on aging as a key to the understand-ing of cancer. *Cancer, 68,* 2496–2501.

Millis, A. J., Hoyle, M., McCue, H. M., & Mar-tini, H. (1992). Differential expression of met-alloproteinase and tissue inhibitor of metal-loproteinase genes in aged human fibroblasts. *Experimental Cell Research, 201,* 373–379.

Momand, J., Zambetti, G. P., Olson, D. C., George, D., & Levine, A. J. (1992). The mdm2 oncogene product forms a complex with p53 protein and inhibits p53-mediated transac-tivation. *Cell, 64,* 1237–1245.

Muggleton-Harris, A. L., & Hayflick, L. (1976). Cellular aging studied by the reconstruction of replicating cells from nuclei and cyto-plasms isolated from normal human diploid cells. *Experimental Cell Research, 103,* 321–330.

Muggleton-Harris, A. L., & DeSimone, D. W. (1980). Replicative potentials of fusion prod-ucts between WI38 and SV40-transformed WI38 cells and their components. *Somatic Cell Generation, 6,* 689–698.

Munger, K., Phelps, W. C., Bubb, V., Howley, P. M., & Schlegel, R. (1989). The E6 and E7 genes of human papillomavirus type 16 together are necessary and sufficient for transformation of primary human keratinocytes. *Journal of Virology, 63*, 4417–4421.

Murano, S., Thweatt, R., Shmookler-Reis, R. J., Jones, R. A., Moerman, E. J., & Goldstein, S. (1991). Diverse gene sequences are overexpressed in Werner syndrome fibroblasts undergoing premature replicative senescence. *Molecular and Cellular Biology, 11*, 3905–3914.

Neufeld, D. S., Ripley, S., Henderson, A., & Ozer, H. L. (1987). Immortalization of human fibroblasts transformed by origin-defective simian virus 40. *Molecular and Cellular Biology, 7*, 2794–2802.

Nevins, J. (1992). E2F: A link between the Rb tumor suppressor protein and viral oncoproteins. *Science, 258*, 1300–1303.

Newbold, R. F., Overell, R. W., & Connell, J. R. (1982). Induction of immortality is an early event in malignant transformation of mammalian cells by carcinogens. *Nature, 299*, 633–635.

Ning, Y., Weber, J. L., Killary, A. M., Ledbetter, D. H., Smith, J. R., & Pereira-Smith, O. M. (1991a). Genetic analysis of indefinite division in human cells: Evidence for a senescence-related gene(s) on human chromosome 4. *Proceedings of the National Academy of Sciences of the United States of America, 88*, 5635–5639.

Ning, Y., Shay, J. W., Lovell, M., Taylor, L., Ledbetter, D. H., & Pereira-Smith, O. M. (1991b). Tumor suppression by chromosome 11 is not due to cellular senescence. *Experimental Cell Research, 192*, 220–226.

Nishimoto, T., Uzawa, S., & Schlegel, R. (1992). Mitotic checkpoints. *Current Opinion in Cell Biology, 4*, 174–179.

Noda, A., Ning, Y., Venable, S. F., Pereira-Smith, O. M., & Smith, J. R. (1994). Cloning of senescent cell derived inhibitors of DNA synthesis using an expression screen. *Experimental Cell Research, 211*, 90–98.

Norwood, T. H., Pendergrass, W. R., Sprague, C. A., & Martin, G. M. (1974). Dominance of the senescent phenotype in heterokaryons between replicative and post-replicative human fibroblast-like cells. *Proceedings of the National Academy of Sciences of the United States of America, 71*, 2231–2235.

Ogata, T., Ayusawa, D., Namba, M., Takahashi, E., Oshimura, M., & Oishi, M. (1993).

Chromosome 7 suppresses indefinite division of nontumorigenic immortalized human fibroblast cell lines KMST-6 and SUSM-1. *Molecular and Cellular Biology, 13*, 6036–6043.

Ohtsubo, M., & Roberts, J. M. (1993). Cyclin-dependent regulation of G1 in mammalian fibroblasts. *Science, 259*, 1908–1912.

Oshima, J., Campisi, J., Tannock, C. A., Sybert, V. P., & Martin, G. M. (1995). Regulation of c-fos in senescing Werner syndrome fibroblasts differs from that observed in senescing fibroblasts from normal donors. *Journal of Cellular Physiology*, in press.

Packer, L., & Feuhr, K. (1977). Low oxygen concentration extends the lifespan of cultured human diploid cells. *Nature, 267*, 423–425.

Pang, J. H., & Chen, K. Y. (1993). A specific CCAAT binding protein CBP/tk may be involved in the regulation of thymidine kinase gene expression in human IMR-90 diploid fibroblasts during senescence. *Journal of Biological Chemistry, 268*, 2909–2916.

Pang, J. H., & Chen, K. Y. (1994). Global change of gene expression at late G1/S boundary may occur in human IMR-90 diploid fibroblasts during senescence. *Journal of Cell Physiology, 160*, 531–536.

Peacocke, M., & Campisi, J. (1991). Cellular senescence: A reflection of normal growth control, differentiation or aging? *Journal of Cell Biochemistry, 45*, 147–155.

Pendergrass, W. R., Angello, J. C., Kirschner, M. D., & Norwood, T. H. (1991). The relationship between the rate of entry into S phase, concentration of DNA polymerase alpha and cell volume in human diploid fibroblast like monokaryon cells. *Experimental Cell Research, 192*, 418–425.

Pereira-Smith, O. M., & Smith, J. R. (1983). Evidence for the recessive nature of cellular immortality. *Science, 221*, 964–967.

Pereira-Smith, O. M., & Smith, J. R. (1988). Genetic analysis of indefinite division in human cells: Identification of four complementation groups. *Proceedings of the National Academy of Sciences of the United States of America, 85*, 6042–6046.

Phillips, P. D., Pignolo, R. J., Nishikura, K., & Cristofalo, V. J. (1992). Renewed DNA synthesis in senescent WI38 cells by expression of an inducible chimeric c-fos construct. *Journal of Cell Physiology, 151*, 206–212.

Pignolo, R. J., Cristofalo, V. J., & Rotenberg,

M. O. (1993). Senescent WI-38 cells fail to express EPC-1, a gene induced in young cells upon entry into the G0 state. *Journal of Biological Chemistry, 268,* 8949–8957.

Pignolo, R. J., Rotenberg, M. O., & Cristofalo, V. J. (1994). Alterations in contact and density-dependent arrest state in senescent WI-38 cells. *In Vitro Cell & Developmental Biology, 30A,* 471–476.

Pines, J. (1993). Cyclins and their associated cyclin-dependent protein kinases in the human cell cycle. *Biochemical Society Transactions, 21,* 921–925.

Ponten, J. (1976). The relationship between in vitro transformation and tumor formation in vivo. *Biochimica et Biophysica Acta, 458,* 397–422.

Porter, M. B., Pereira-Smith, O. M., & Smith, J. R. (1990). Novel monoclonal antibodies identify antigenic determinants unique to cellular senescence. *Journal of Cellular Physiology, 142,* 425–433.

Radna, R. L., Caton, Y., Jha, K. K., Kaplan, P., Li, G., Traganos, F., & Ozer, H. L. (1989). Growth of immortal simian virus 40 ts-A transformed human fibroblasts is temperature dependent. *Molecular and Cell Biology, 9,* 3093–3096.

Reznikoff, C. A., Belair, C., Savelieva, E., Zhai, Y., Pfeifer, K., Yeager, T., Thompson, K. J., De Vries, S., Bindley, C., Newton, M. A., Kekhon, G., & Waldman, F. (1994). Long-term genome stability and minimal genotypic and phenotypic alterations in HPV16 E7-, but not E6-, immortalized human uroepithelial cells. *Genes and Development, 8,* 2227–2240.

Rheinwald, J. R., & Green, H. (1975). Serial cultivation of strains of human epidermal keratinocytes: The formation of keratinizing colonies from single cells. *Cell, 6,* 331–344.

Rinehart, C. A., Haskill, J. S., Morris, J. S., Butler, T. D., & Kaufman, D. G. (1991). Extended life span of human endometrial stromal cells transfected with cloned origin-defective temperature sensitive simian virus 40. *Journal of Virology, 65,* 1458–1465.

Rittling, S. R., Brooks, K. M., Cristofalo, V. J., & Baserga, R. (1986). Expression of cell cycle dependent genes in young and senescent WI38 fibroblasts. *Proceedings of the National Academy of Sciences of the United States of America, 83,* 3316–3320.

Rohme, D. (1981). Evidence for a relationship between longevity of mammalian species and lifespans of normal fibroblasts *in vitro* and erythrocytes *in vivo*. *Proceedings of the National Academy of Sciences of the United States of America, 78,* 5009–5013.

Rose, M. R. (1991). *The Evolutionary Biology of Aging.* Oxford: Oxford University Press.

Ruley, H. E. (1983). Adenovirus early region 1A enables viral and cellular transforming genes to transform primary cells in culture. *Nature, 304,* 602–606.

Ryan, Q. C., Goonewardene, I. M., & Murasko, D. M. (1992). Extension of lifespan of human T lymphocytes by transfection with SV40 large T antigen. *Experimental Cell Research, 199,* 387–391.

Ryan, P. A., Maher, V. M., & McCormick, J. J. (1994). Failure of infinite life span human cells from different immortality complementation groups to yield finite life span hybrids. *Journal of Cellular Physiology, 159,* 151–160.

Sager, R. (1984). Resistance of human cells to oncogenic transformation. *Cancer Cells, 2,* 487–493.

Sager, R. (1991). Senescence as a mode of tumor suppression. *Environmental Health Perspectives, 93,* 59–62.

Sakamoto, K., Howard, T., Ogryzko, V., Xu, N. Z., Corsico, C. C., Jones, D. H., & Howard, B. (1993). Relative mitogenic activities of wild-type and retinoblastoma binding defective SV40 T antigens in serum deprived and senescent human fibroblasts. *Oncogene, 8,* 1887–1893.

Sala, A., Nicolaides, N. C., Engelhard, A., Bellon, T., Lawe, D. C., Arnold, A., Grana, X., Giordano, A., & Calabretta, B. (1994). Correlation between E2F1 requirement in S phase and E2F1 transactivation of cell cycle related genes in human cells. *Cancer Research, 54,* 1402–1406.

Salk, D., Bryant, E., Hoehn, H., Johnston, P., & Martin, G. M. (1985). Growth characteristics of Werner syndrome cells in vitro. *Advances in Experimental Medicine and Biology, 190,* 305–311.

Sandell, L. L., & Zakian, V. A. (1993). Loss of a yeast telomere: Arrest, recovery and chromosome loss. *Cell, 75,* 729–739.

Sandhu, A. K., Hubbard, K., Kaur, G. P., Jha, K. K., Ozer, H. L., & Athwal, R. S. (1994). Senescence of immortal human fibroblasts by introduction of normal human chromosome 6. *Proceedings of the National Academy of Sciences of the United States of America, 91*, 5498–5502.

Saunders, N. A., Smith, R. J., & Jetten, A. M. (1994). Regulation of proliferation-specific and differentiation-specific genes during senescence of human epidermal keratinocytes and mammary epithelial cells. *Biochemical and Biophysical Research Communication, 197*, 46–54.

Schneider, E. L., & Mitsui, Y. (1976). The relationship between *in vitro* cellular aging and *in vivo* human aging. *Proceedings of the National Academy of Sciences of the United States of America, 73*, 3584–3588.

Seshadri, T., & Campisi, J. (1990). c-fos repression and an altered genetic program in senescent human fibroblasts. *Science, 247*, 205–209.

Seshadri, T., Uzman, J. A., Oshima, J., & Campisi, J. (1993). Identification of a transcript that is downregulated in senescent human fibroblasts. *Journal of Biological Chemistry, 268*, 18474–18480.

Shay, J. W., & Wright, W. E. (1989). Quantitation of the frequency of immortalization of normal human diploid fibroblasts by SV40 large T antigen. *Experimental Cell Research, 184*, 109–118.

Shay, J. W., & Wright, W. R. (1991). Defining the molecular mechanisms of human cell immortalization. *Biochimica et Biophysica Acta, 1071*, 1–7.

Shay, J. W., Pereira-Smith, O. M., & Wright, W. E. (1991). A role for both Rb and p53 in the regulation of human cellular senescence. *Experimental Cell Research, 196*, 33–39.

Shay, J. W., Van Der Haegen, B. A., Ying, Y., & Wright, W. E. (1993a). The frequency of immortalization of human fibroblasts and mammary epithelial cells transfected with SV40 large T antigen. *Experimental Cell Research, 209*, 45–52.

Shay, J. W., Wright, W. E., Brasiskyte, D., & Van Der Haegen, B. A. (1993b). E6 of human papillomavirus type 16 can overcome the M1 stage of immortalization in human mammary epithelial cells but not in human fibroblasts. *Oncogene, 8*, 1407–1413.

Sherr, C. J. (1993). Mammalian G1 cyclins. *Cell, 73*, 1059–1065.

Slansky, J. E., Li, Y., Kaelin, W. G., & Farnham, P. J. (1993). A protein synthesis-dependent increase in E2F1 mRNA correlates with growth regulation of the dihydrofolate reductase promoter. *Molecular and Cellular Biology, 13*, 1610–1618.

Smith, J. R., & Hayflick, L. (1974). Variation in the lifespan of clones derived from human diploid strains. *Journal of Cell Biology, 62*, 48–53.

Smith, J. R., & Whitney, R. G. (1980). Intraclonal variation in proliferative potential of human diploid fibroblasts: Stochastic mechanism for cellular aging. *Science, 207*, 82–84.

Stanulis-Praeger, B. (1987). Cellular senescence revisited: A review. *Mechanisms of Ageing and Development, 38*, 1–48.

Stein, G. H., Yanishevsky, R. M., Gordon, L., & Beeson, M. (1982). Carcinogen-transformed human cells are inhibited from entry into S phase by fusion to senescent cells but cells transformed by DNA tumor viruses overcome the inhibition. *Proceedings of the National Academy of Sciences of the United States of America, 79*, 5287–5291.

Stein, G. H., Namba, M., & Corsaro, C. M. (1985). Relationship of finite proliferative lifespan, senescence, and quiescence in human cells. *Journal of Cellular Physiology, 122*, 343–349.

Stein, G. H., Beeson, M., & Gordon, L. (1990). Failure to phosphorylate the retinoblastoma gene product in senescent human fibroblasts. *Science, 249*, 666–669.

Stein, G. H., Drullinger, L. F., Robetorye, R. S., Pereira-Smith, O. M., & Smith, J. R. (1991). Senescent cells fail to express cdc2, cycA and cycB in response to mitogen stimulation. *Proceedings of the National Academy of Sciences of the United States of America, 88*, 11012–11016.

Sugawara, O., Oshimura, M., Koi, M., Annab, L. A., & Barrett, J. C. (1990). Induction of cellular senescence in immortalized cells by human chromosome 1. *Science, 247*, 707–710.

Sugden, B. (1989). An intricate route to immortality. *Cell, 57*, 5–7.

Sun, X. H., Copeland, N. G., Jenkins, N. A., & Baltimore, D. (1991). Id proteins Id1 and Id2 selectively inhibit DNA binding by one class of helix-loop-helix proteins. *Molecular and Cellular Biology, 13*, 7874–7880.

Swisshelm, K., Ryan, K., Lee, X., Tsou, H., Peacocke, M., & Sager, R. (1994). Downregulation of retinoic acid receptor β in mammary carcinoma cell lines and its up-regulation in senescing normal mammary epithelial cells. *Cell Growth and Differentiation, 5,* 133–141.

Takahashi, T., Schunkert, H., Isoyama, S., Wei, J. Y., Nadal-Ginard, B., Grossman, W., & Izumo, S. (1992). Age-related differences in the expression of protooncogene and contractile protein genes in response to pressure overload in the rat myocardium. *Journal of Clinical Investigation, 89,* 939–946.

Tsuji, Y., Ide, T., & Ishibani, S. (1983). Correlation between the presence of T antigen and the reinitiation of host DNA synthesis in senescent human diploid fibroblasts after SV40 infection. *Experimental Cell Research, 144,* 165–169.

Wadhwa, R., Kaul, S. C., Sugimoto, Y., & Mitsui, Y. (1993). Induction of cellular senescence by transfection of cytosolic mortalin cDNA in NIH3T3 cells. *Journal of Biological Chemistry, 268,* 22239–22242.

Wang, E. (1985). A 57 kDa protein uniquely present in nonproliferating and senescent human fibroblasts. *Journal of Cell Biology, 100,* 545–551.

Wang, E., & Tomaszewski, G. (1991). The granular presence of terminin is the marker to distinguish between senescent and quiescent states. *Journal of Cellular Physiology, 147,* 514–522.

Wang, X. W., Lin, X., Klein, C. B., Bhamra, R. K., Lee, Y. W., & Costa, M. (1992). A conserved region in human and Chinese hamster X chromosomes can induce cellular senescence of nickel-transformed Chinese hamster cell lines. *Carcinogenesis, 13,* 555–561.

Wang, E., Lee, M. J., & Pandey, S. (1994). Control of fibroblast senescence and activation of programmed cell death. *Journal of Cell Biochemistry, 54,* 432–439.

Weinberg, R. A. (1985). The action of oncogenes in the cytoplasm and nucleus. *Science, 230,* 770–774.

Weinberg, R. A. (1991). Tumor suppressor genes. *Science, 254,* 1138–1146.

West, M. D., Pereira-Smith, O. M., & Smith, J. R. (1989). Replicative senescence of human skin fibroblasts correlates with a loss of regulation and overexpression of collagenase activity. *Experimental Cell Research, 184,* 138–147.

White, A. E., Livanos, E. M., & Tlsty, T. D. (1994). Differential disruption of genomic integrity and cell cycle regulation in normal human fibroblasts by the HPV oncoproteins. *Genes and Development, 8,* 666–677.

Wick, M., Burger, C., Brusselbach, S., Lucibello, F. C., & Muller, R. (1994). A novel member of human tissue inhibitor of metalloproteinases (TIMP) gene family is regulated during G1 progression, mitogenic stimulation, differentiation and senescence. *Journal of Biological Chemistry, 269,* 18953–18960.

Wistrom, C., & Villeponteau, B. (1992). Cloning and expression of SAG, a novel marker of cellular senescence. *Experimental Cell Research, 199,* 355–362.

Wright, W. E., & Shay, J. W. (1992). Telomere position effects and the regulation of cellular senescence. *Trends in Genetics, 8,* 193–197.

Wright, W. E., Pereira-Smith, O. M., & Shay, J. W. (1989). Reversible cellular senescence: Implications for immortalization of normal human diploid fibroblasts. *Molecular and Cell Biology, 9,* 3088–3092.

Wu, X., Bayle, J. H., Olson, D., & Levine, A. J. (1993). p53–mdm2 autoregulatory feedback loop. *Genes and Development, 7,* 1126–1132.

Xiong, Y., Hannon, G., Zhang, H., Casso, D., & Beach, D. (1993). p21 is a universal inhibitor of cyclin kinases. *Nature, 366,* 701–704.

Yamada, H., Wake, N., Fujumoto, S., Barrett, J. C., & Oshimura, M. (1990). Multiple chromosomes carrying tumor suppressor activity for a uterine endometrial carcinoma cell line identified by microcell-mediated chromosome transfer. *Oncogene, 5,* 1141–1147.

Yamamoto, M., Yoshida, M., Ono, K., Fujita, T., Ohtani-Fujita, N., Sakai, T., & Nikaido, T. (1994). Effect of tumor suppressors on cell cycle-regulatory genes: RB suppresses p34/cdc2 expression and normal p53 suppresses cyclin A expression. *Experimental Cell Research, 210,* 94–101.

Zambetti, G., Dell'Orco, R., Stein, G., & Stein, J. (1987). Histone gene expression remains coupled to DNA synthesis during in vitro cellular senescence. *Experimental Cell Research, 172,* 397–403.

Eight

Mechanisms of Altered Gene Expression with Aging

John Papaconstantinou, Peter D. Reisner, Li Liu, and David T. Kuninger

I. Introduction

Aging affects the constitutive levels of gene expression, as well as their regulation by various hormonal and growth factors. These changes have been detected by studies of rates of transcription and changes in mRNA and protein pool levels, indicating that transcription, mRNA processing, mRNA stability, or protein turnover may be the underlying processes affected by aging. The effect of aging on many of these regulatory processes has been reviewed in detail (Van Remmen *et al.*, 1994). Alteration of any of these regulatory processes, e.g., transcription, could account for the establishment of new steady-state levels of mRNA and protein pool levels. In fact, some trans-acting factors exhibit positive while others exhibit negative regulatory effects, thus pointing to the importance of their activity in aged tissues. Since the activity of many trans-acting factors is regulated by mediators, such as cytokines and hormones, any age-associated changes in their homeostatic levels could affect the activity of trans-acting factors and the expression of their target genes. Thus, to understand the mechanisms of altered gene

expression, it is essential to understand the processes by which the signals initiated by mediators are transmitted to the trans-acting factors. In this chapter, we discuss the age-associated changes in trans-acting factors that regulate families of stress response genes. This small group of trans-acting factors is regulated by cytokines, growth factors, and hormones, and an attempt is made to link the role of mediators and signal pathways to the activity of these regulatory proteins and to the age-associated changes in expression and regulation of their target genes.

II. Regulation of Eukaryotic Gene Expression

Regulation of eukaryotic and prokaryotic gene expression involves processes that mediate both gene activation and repression. In multicellular organisms, where different cell types carry out specific physiological functions, the basis for this tissue specificity and diversity lies in differential gene expression, i.e., the activation of some genes and repression of others. Furthermore, each tissue exhibits the ability

Handbook of the Biology of Aging, Fourth Edition
Copyright © 1996 Academic Press, Inc. All rights of reproduction in any form reserved.

to respond to specific hormones, growth factors, etc. by differential gene regulation.

Gene expression can be regulated at several stages in the pathway from DNA to RNA to protein. Transcriptional control, which involves the transfer of genetic information from DNA to RNA, involves specific interactions of transcription regulatory proteins (trans-acting factors) with specific regulatory DNA sequences (cis-acting sequences) in the promoter and enhancer regions of the gene. The cis-acting DNA sequences are usually at the 5' end of the coding region, although in some cases these regulatory protein-binding sites are found within the introns of the coding region. These cis-acting sequences are usually ~20 nucleotides or less in length and serve as recognition sites for the binding of specific trans-acting factors that serve to activate and/or repress gene expression. An important feature of the cis-acting sequences is the palindromic arrangement of their nucleotides, which is the basis for their recognition by the trans-acting regulatory proteins.

The ability of trans-acting factors to interact with cis-acting DNA sequences involves specific structural characteristics of these proteins. These are the ability to (a) dimerize, (b) recognize DNA-binding sites, and (c) interact with other proteins to effect transcriptional regulation. Dimerization of most trans-acting factors is critical to their ability to bind to their specific promoter-binding sites. The formation of a dimer brings together two DNA-binding domains that are able to recognize the palindromic DNA-binding site sequences. This establishes the DNA–protein interaction between the regulatory protein and its specific DNA-binding site. The transcription activation domain is a part of the protein that interacts with other proteins (including components of the RNA-polymerase) to form either an activation or a repression complex.

III. Molecular Responses to Stress in Eukaryotic Organisms

Eukaryotic organisms possess natural defense mechanisms triggered by rapid environmental changes, such as injuries due to inflammation, infection, oxidative stress, heavy metals, hyperthermia, and radiation. Exposure of cells and tissues to these cell-damaging conditions evokes a cascade of genetically programmed events that involves the activation of families of stress response genes. Interestingly, these families of genes are regulated by a relatively small number of trans-acting factors, e.g., the NFκB/rel family, the bZIP families of proteins, which include AP-1 (fos, jun) and the C/EBPs, the heat shock factors (HSF), and the glucocorticoid receptor (GR). This suggests that stimuli such as bacterial lipopolysaccharide (LPS), oxidative radicals, phorbol esters (TPA), heavy metals, hyperthermia, and UV can elicit a cascade of stress response gene activities, whose functions are to protect against further injury and to initiate the processes of tissue regeneration. Although the types of genes induced are dependent upon the nature of the stress, there is significant overlap in the genes that respond to the same factors so that a particular stress stimulus, such as those listed earlier, can elicit a cascade of genetic events within each family of genes. The expression of many of these genes is either activated or attenuated in aging. This is due, in part, to age-associated changes in the activity of specific trans-acting factors that regulate their transcription. The functions of these key regulatory proteins are sensitive to changes in levels of both intrinsic (biological mediators) and extrinsic (pollutants) factors.

Furthermore, since many of the responses to stress are mediated by factors such as cytokines, growth factors, hormones, etc., the activation of most stress response genes must be initiated via ligand–receptor complexes linked to complex signal transduction pathways. Biological mediators of the stress response, such as cytokines, H_2O_2, oxygen radicals, and extrinsic environmental factors such as pollutants, act as second messengers that target the cytoplasmic signaling molecules, thereby regulating the activity of trans-acting proteins that regulate stress response genes. These factors are also the mediators whose homeostatic levels are altered by aging and, therefore, may play a critical role in the development of changes in gene expression characteristic of aging. A model has been presented that correlates the mechanisms by which the intrinsic and extrinsic factors may play a role in the development of age-specific biochemical characteristics (Papaconstantinou, 1994). In this chapter, attempts are made to argue that trans-acting factors are targets of components of the same signal transduction and redox pathways and that these signaling processes may be affected by aging, thus establishing the age-associated changes in gene expression. Emphasis is placed on the effect of aging on NFκB, AP-1 (fos, jun), and heat shock factors, although other trans-acting factors such as C/EBPs and GR are also essential for stress response and are affected by aging.

Because of the complexity of the question of how aging may affect gene expression, we have summarized in Table I the results of studies on how aging affects trans-acting factors. This summary indicates that the effect of aging on trans-acting factors is not widespread and that tissues and organs appear to develop specific characteristics of aging with respect to gene regulation, i.e., some exhibit an increased level of activity of transactivators, while others exhibit a decrease in these regulatory proteins. This would explain tissue and organ-specific differences in age-associated gene activities and emphasize the fact that organs and tissues

may exhibit differential susceptibility to aging.

IV. Families of Stress Response Genes Whose Expressions Are Altered by Aging

Acute-phase reactants (APR), metallothioneins (MT), heat shock proteins (HSP), and extracellular matrix (ECM) proteins are the products of families of genes induced by various physical, chemical, and biological stress stimuli (Koj, 1985; Nover, 1984; Oh *et al.*, 1978). The responses of many of these genes are altered in aging and senescent cells due to age-associated properties, such as changes in DNA-binding activity of their trans-acting factors, or protein–protein interactions that inhibit trans-acting factor activity (Baeuerle & Baltimore, 1988b; Carter *et al.*, 1991; Choi *et al.*, 1990; Fargnoli *et al.*, 1990; Heydari *et al.*, 1993; Liu, *et al.*, 1989; Post *et al.*, 1991; Fawcett *et al.*, 1994). The expression and regulation of APR genes, α_1-acid glycoprotein (Carter *et al.*, 1991; Post *et al.*, 1991), T-kininogen (Sierra *et al.*, 1989), angiotensinogen, the MT genes (Yiangou & Papaconstantinou, in preparation), and the heat shock protein genes (Blake *et al.*, 1990, 1991a,b; Fargnoli *et al.*, 1990; Heydari *et al.*, 1993; Liu *et al.*, 1989) are affected by aging, and this altered gene expression (either over- or underexpression) appears to correlate with changes in the activity of their trans-acting factors, i.e., C/EBP, NFκB, AP-1, and HSF. Cytokines and products of oxidative metabolism, as well as environmental stress factors, target intermediates of the signal transduction–redox pathways that regulate the modification and activation of these trans-acting factors (Fig. 1). Through this mechanism, intrinsic factors (biological mediators) and extrinsic factors (pollutants) can activate the same cascade of stress response genes by targeting common components of the signal transduction–

Table I
Transcription Factors and Aging[a]

Transcription Factor	Assay	Effect of aging and/or conclusions	Ages studied	Species/tissue	Reference
AP-1 (binding activity)	Band shift after PTZ injection (CTAGTGAT-GAGTCAGCCGG-ATC)	No change (both young and aged tissue show robust stimulation upon PTZ injection; however, aged show more pronounced stimulation)	4 vs 24 months	Rat (Wistar)/hippocampus	Kaminska and Kaczmarek (1993)
	Band shift (CGCTTGATGAGT-CAGCCGGAA)	Decrease in senescent fibroblasts as compared to presenescent dividing fibroblasts	Presenescent quiescent and/or dividing fibroblasts vs senescent fibroblasts	Human/WI38 fetal lung fibroblasts	Dimri and Campisi (1994)
	Band shift (CGCTT-GATGAGTCAGCC-GGAA)	No change	4 vs 30 months	Rat (Wistar males)/brain	Ammendola et al. (1992)
	Band shift after serum stimulation (TCGAC-GGTATCGATAAG-CTATGACTCATCC-GGGGATC)	Overall decrease of 10–20-fold of basal and induced binding; qualitative difference indicates a possible Jun–Jun:DNA complex in senescent fibroblasts	In vitro young (30–45 MPD) fibroblasts vs senescent (75–80 MPD) fibroblasts	Human/diploid fibroblasts (Hs68)	Riabowol et al. (1992)
	Band shift following PHA stimulation (22-mer Stratagene Kit)	"Strong" decrease in DS subjects and "slight" decrease in NCL-afflicted subjects as compared to stimulated control subjects	Healthy individuals vs "prematurely aged" DS and NCL patients	Human/PHA-stimulated pbl's	Sikora et al. (1993)
	Band shift after serum stimulation, immunostaining, 2-D protein electrophoresis (TCGACGGTATCG-ATAAGCTATGACT-CATCCGGGGATC)	10-fold decrease in binding activity; qualitative change in DNA:protein complex; may favor Jun–Jun complex in senescent cells; decrease in fos protein by immunostaining; decrease in fos protein isoforms in senescent cells	Young (42 MPD) fibroblasts vs presenescent aged fibroblasts (77 MPD)	Human/diploid fibroblasts (Hs68)	Riabowol et al. (1992) (PNAS)
	Band shift after Con A stimulation (AP-1 Stratagene)	Decrease in basal and Con A-stimulated DNA-binding activity	3 vs 20 months	Mouse (Swiss albinol)/from cultured lymphocytes	Sikora et al. (1992)

(continued)

Table I (*Continued*)

Transcription Factor	Assay	Effect of aging and/or conclusions	Ages studied	Species/tissue	Reference
c-fos	mRNA after Con A stimulation (RT-PCR)	Decrease, no message detected in aged mice even after stimulation, whereas young mice demonstrated a "dramatic elevation" after stimulation	3 vs 20 months	Mouse (Swiss albino)/from cultured lymphocytes	Sikora *et al.* (1992)
	mRNA after PHA activation	No change	32.3 ± 1.6 vs 74.4 ± 3.5 years	Human/PHA-stimulated pbl's	Song *et al.* (1992)
	mRNA after hemodynamic stress	Decrease (stimulation was "significantly reduced" in the 18-month rat)	9 vs 18 months	Rat (Fisher 344, male)/heart (left ventricle)	Takahashi *et al.* (1992)
	mRNA, immunoprecipitation after serum stimulation	Decrease (up to 95% reduction in mRNA) (aged fibroblasts "fail to synthesize fos at levels similar to young")	Young fibroblasts (35–40 MPD) vs *in vitro*-aged fibroblasts (75–80 MPD)	Human/fibroblasts	Riabowol *et al.* (1992)
	Immunocytochemical staining after ECS	Decreased stimulation of 58–62% in aged brain as compared to young	6 month vs 13 vs 28 months	Mouse (B6C3)/brain	D'Costa *et al.* (1991)
	mRNA	"Significant elevation" seen in all aged animals	6–7 vs 24 months	Rat (Wistar, male and female)/liver	Fujita and Maruyama (1991)
	Immunofluorescent cell staining, and reporter gene expression	Microinjection of c-Ha-Ras into senescent fibroblasts increased c-fos expression and AP-1-binding activity; however, senescence was not reversed	Senescent human fibroblasts (47–55 pd's)	Human/senescent fibroblasts/IMR-90	Rose *et al.* (1992)
c-jun	mRNA after Con A stimulation (RTPCR)	Increased basal level in aged mice; additionally, aged mice showed a diminished response to stimulation	3 vs 20 months	Mouse (Swiss albino)/from cultured lymphocytes	Sikora *et al.* (1992)
	mRNA	No change between 4 and 24 months; however, there was a 55% decrease between 4 and 12 months	4 vs 12 vs 24 months	Mouse (male B10.R11, C57BL10 and B10.BR/liver)	Mote *et al.* (1991)

	Method	Result	Age comparison	Species/tissue	Reference
	mRNA after PHA activation	Reduced "significantly" ($p < 0.01$) in aged subjects	32.3 ± 1.6 vs 74.4 ± 3.5 years	Human/PHA-stimulated pbl's	Song et al. (1992)
	mRNA	No change	4 vs 16 vs 30 months	Mouse (female C3B10RFI/liver)	Spindler et al. (1991)
	mRNA after anti-CD2 activation	No change	32.3 ± 1.6 vs 74.4 ± 3.5 years	Human/purified T-cells (anti-CD2 activated)	Song et al. (1992)
	mRNA after hemodynamic stress	Decrease (stimulation was "significantly reduced" in the 18-month rat)	9 vs 18 months	Rat (male Fisher 344)/heart (left ventricle)	Takahashi et al. (1992)
	mRNA and immunoprecipitation after serum stimulation	No change	Young fibroblasts (35–40 MPD) vs in vitro-aged fibroblasts (75–80 MPD)	Human/diploid fibroblasts (Hs68)	Riabowol et al. (1992)
	mRNA	Increase of 7-fold	6–7 vs 24–25 months	Rat (Wistar/Slc male and female)/liver	Fujita and Maruyama (1991)
jun-B	mRNA after anti-CD2 or PHA activation	No change	32.3 ± 1.6 vs 74.4 ± 3.5 years	Human/purified T-cells (anti-CD2 activated)	Song et al. (1992)
AP-2	Band shift (AP-2 Stratagene Kit)	No change	3 vs 20 months	Mouse (Swiss albino)/from cultured lymphocytes	Sikora et al. (1992)
AP-3	Band shift (AP-3 Stratagene Kit)	No change	3 vs 20 months	Mouse (Swiss albino)/from cultured lymphocytes	Sikora et al. (1992)
C/EBP	Band shift (TTTTCCATCTTACTCAACATCCTCC)	No quantitative "decrease" reported	3 vs 26 months	Rat (Fisher 344)/liver	Supakar et al. (1993)
C/EBPα	mRNA	No change	4 vs 16 vs 30 months	Mouse (female C3B10RFI/liver)	Spindler et al. (1991)
	mRNA	No change	4 vs 24 months	Mouse (B10.R11, C57BL10 and B10.BR)/liver	Mote et al. (1991)

(continued)

Table I (*Continued*)

Transcription Factor	Assay	Effect of aging and/or conclusions	Ages studied	Species/tissue	Reference
Sp1	Band shift (ATTCGATC-GGGGCGGGGCG-AGC)	No change	Presenescent quiescent and/or dividing fibroblasts vs senescent fibroblasts	Human/WI38 fetal lung fibroblasts	Dimri and Campisi (1994)
	mRNA	No change	4 vs 16 vs 30 months	Mouse (female C3B10RFl)/liver	Spindler *et al.* (1991)
	Western blot/band shifts/DNAse protection (ATCGGGGC-GGGGCGGGGC-GGGGCGGGGC)	Protein levels show no change; binding activity is decreased 60-fold; DNAse protection is decreased	4 vs 30 months	Rat (Wistar, males)/brain	Ammendola *et al.* (1992)
	mRNA	No change	4 vs 24 months	Mouse (male B10.R11, c57BL10 and B10.BR)/liver	Mote *et al.* (1991)
	Band shift after serum stimulation (ATC-GGGGCGGGGATC-GGGGCGGGGATC-GGGGCGGGGATC)	No change	Young fibroblasts (22 MPD) vs *in vitro*-aged fibroblasts (49 MPD)	Human/IMR-90 diploid fibroblasts	Pang and Chen (1993)
GREBP	Band shift (TCGACTG-TACAGGATGTTC-TAGCTACT)	No change	Senescent fibroblasts vs presenescent quiescent and/or dividing fibroblasts	Human/WI38 fetal lung fibroblasts	Dimri and Campisi (1994)
CREBP	Band shift (AGAGATTGCC-TGACGTCAGAGAG-CTAG)	Decrease by 8-fold in senescent cells	Presenescent quiescent and/or dividing fibroblasts vs senescent fibroblasts	Human/WI38 fetal lung fibroblasts	Dimri and Campisi (1994)
	Band shift after PTZ injection (GATTGGCT-GACGTCAGAG-AGCT)	No change (basal activity);no change (after PTZ injection)	4 vs 24 months	Rat (Wistar)/hippocampus	Kaminska and Kacz-marek (1993)

TFIID (one specific complex)	Band shift (GCAGAG-CATATAAGGTGA-GGTAGGA)	Increase of 4-fold in senescent cells vs quiescent presenescent cells.	Presenescent quiescent and/or dividing fibroblasts vs senescent fibroblasts	Human/WI38 fetal lung fibroblasts	Dimri and Campisi (1994)
TFIID (two specific complexes)	Band shift (GCAGAG-CATATAAGGTGA-GGTAGGA)	No change	Presenescent quiescent and/or dividing fibroblasts vs senescent fibroblasts	Human/WI38 fetal lung fibroblasts	Dimri and Campisi (1994)
NFκB	Band shift (AGTTGA-GGGGACTTTCCC-AGGC)	No change	Presenescent quiescent and/or dividing fibroblasts vs senescent fibroblasts	Human/WI38 fetal lung fibroblasts	Dimri and Campisi (1994)
Myc	mRNA after serum stimulation	Reduced stimulation of expression in senescent cells at 0, 4, and 16 hr after serum stimulation	Senescent fibroblasts vs young fibroblasts	Human/WI38 fetal lung fibroblasts	Rittling et al. (1986)
Oct B	Band shift (TGTCGAATGC-AAATCACTAGAA)	Increase of 1.6–2.0-fold in senescent cells	Presenescent quiescent and/or dividing fibroblasts vs senescent fibroblasts	Human/WI38 fetal lung fibroblasts	Dimri and Campisi et al. (1994)
ADF	Band shift (TAGGCTT-GTCTGTTAAAAAA)	Decrease (binding activity is "markedly reduced" in aged rats)	3 vs 26 months	Rat (Fisher 344)/liver	Supakar et al. (1993)
AF	Band shift (TCGCTCC-AAGTTAAAGCTT-CTGCTT)	Decrease (binding activity is "markedly reduced" in aged rats)	3 vs 26 months	Rat (Fisher 344)/liver	Supakar et al. (1993)
AR	mRNA using RTPCR	Decrease of 100-fold	100 vs 600 days	Rat (Fisher 344)/liver	Supakar et al. (1993)
	mRNA (RNAse protection)	Decrease in aged to "nearly undetectable" level	75–85 vs 750 days	Rat/liver	Song et al. (1991)
HSTF	Band shift after heat shock (CTAGAAGC-TTCTAGAAGCTT-CTAG)	Decrease in heat shock-stimulated binding activity of 1.7-fold in aged rats	4–7 vs 22–28 months	Rats (Fisher 344)/isolated hepatocytes (heat shock treated)	Heydari et al. (1993)

(continued)

Table I (*Continued*)

Transcription Factor	Assay	Effect of aging and/or conclusions	Ages studied	Species/tissue	Reference
	Band shift following heat shock (GCCTCGAA-TGTTCGGCGAAG-TTTCG)	Decrease; longer times and higher temperatures required to elicit response in aged fibroblasts	*In vitro*-aged fibroblasts; 15 vs 40 doublings	Human/diploid lung fibroblasts/IMR-90	Liu *et al.* (1991)
	Band shift, Scatchard analysis, Southwestern after H S (GCCTC-GAATGTTCGGCGAAA-GTTTCG)	Decrease of 2.5-fold in binding activity, no change in affinity by Scatchard analysis, Southwestern reveals a slight decrease in an 83-kDa factor in high pd fibroblasts	22 vs 35 vs 45 pdl's	Human/IMR-90 fibroblasts	Choi *et al.* (1990)
CBP/TK	Band shift after serum stimulation (AGGT-CAGCGGCCGGG-CGCTGATTGGCCC)	Decrease (prominent complex formed only in young fibroblasts)	Young fibroblasts (22 MPD) vs *in vitro*-aged fibroblasts (49 MPD)	Human/IMR-90 diploid fibroblasts	Pang and Chen (1993)
eIF-2	Western blot/activity assays/mRNA	Decreased protein level; decreased activity; mRNA unchanged, suggesting translational deficiency	1 vs 10 months	Rat (Sprague–Dawley)/liver and brain	Kimball *et al.* (1992)
GR	mRNA	increase of 17–37% in 16 and 30 months (observed in females only)	4 vs 16 vs 30 months	Mouse (female C3B10RFl)/liver	Spindler *et al.* (1991)
	mRNA	No change	4 vs 24 months	Mouse (B10.R11, c57BL10 and B10.BR)/liver	Mote *et al.* (1991)

Factor	Detection method	Change	Age comparison	Species/tissue	Reference
EF-SII	mRNA	No change	4 vs 16 vs 30 months	Mouse (female C3B10RF1)/liver	Spindler et al. (1991)
	mRNA	No change	4 vs 24 months	Mouse (B10.R11, c57BL10 and B10.BR)/liver	Mote et al. (1991)
DBP	mRNA, Western blot, band shift (TGGTA-TGATTTTGTAAT-GGGGTGGTA)	Increase of 20-fold in adult mRNA and protein, increase of 3.5-fold binding activity in band shift	1 month vs adult	Rat/brain, liver, spleen, testis	Mueller et al. (1990)
HNF-1	mRNA	No "significant" change	6–7 vs 24 months	Rat (Wistar, male and female)/liver	Fujita and Maruyama (1991)
NF-1/CTF	Band shift (TTATTTT-GGATTGAAGCCAA-TATGATAA)	No change	4 vs 30 months	Rat (Wistar, male)/brain	Ammendola et al. (1992)
CTF	Band shift (CCTTTGG-CATGCCAATATG)	Decrease by 30-fold in senescent cells	Presenescent quiescent and/or dividing fibroblasts vs senescent fibroblasts	Human/WI38 fetal lung fibroblasts	Dimri and Campisi (1994)

[a] List of abbreviations: AR, androgen receptor; ADF, age-dependent factor, binds to AR promoter sequence, ubiquitous; AF, associated factor with ADF, tissue specific; CBP/tk, CCAAT binding protein for thymidine kinase gene; C/EBP, CCAAT and enhancer binding protein; Con A, concanavalin A; CREBP, cAMP response element binding protein; CTF, CAAT binding transcription factor (synonymous with NF-1); DBP, D-binding protein; DS, Down's syndrome; ECS, electroconvulsive shock; EF-SII, RNA polymerase elongation factor; eIF-2, eukaryotic initiation factor; GREBP, glucocorticoid response element binding protein; HS, heat shock; HSTF, heat shock transcription factor; MPD, mean population doublings; NCL, neuronal ceroid lypofuscinosis; NF-1, nuclear factor 1; NFκB, nuclear factor κ B; OctB, octamer binding protein; PBL, peripheral blood lymphocytes; pdl's, population doublings; PHA, phytohemagglutinin; PTZ, pentylenetetrazole; Sp1, promoter-specific transcription factor; TFIID, transcription factor II D.

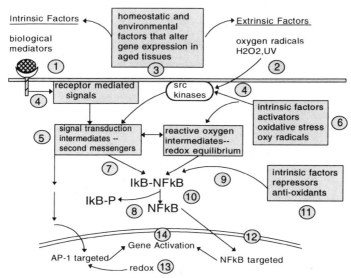

Figure 1. Model outlining the general interactions of the signal transduction–redox pathways that regulate trans-acting factors of the stress response genes. (1) Biological mediators (intrinsic factors) such as cytokines activate stress response genes via a receptor–ligand complex that transmits signals to the cytoplasm. The early response signals may be transmitted from the membrane to signal transduction second messengers. A prooxidant state is induced by intrinsic factors, thus affecting the redox equilibrium. (2) Extrinsic factors such as oxygen radicals and UV radiation exert their effects upon the early response cytoplasmic intermediate, i.e., src kinases. (3) Homeostatic and environmental changes of intrinsic and/or extrinsic factors could result in altered gene expression and regulation in aged tissues. (4) Membrane-bound src kinases (P-tyrosine kinases) are the earliest cytoplasmic factors activated by extrinsic factors (UV, H_2O_2, etc.) and biological mediators (cytokines). (5) Signal transduction intermediates conduct a cascade of modifications (phosphorylation, dephosphorylation) that lead to gene regulation. An age-associated change in these modifications could be the basis for increased (or decreased) gene activity seen in aged tissues. (6) Oxidative metabolism is a source of oxy radicals that can act as second messengers to stimulate signal transduction intermediates (src kinases, etc.) and affect the redox equilibrium by stimulation of antioxidants such as TRX and GSH levels. An age-associated increase in oxidative metabolism would affect the redox equilibrium in the direction of activation of stress response genes; prolonged exposure to similar extrinsic factors would enhance this age-associated steady-state level of the redox equilibrium. (7–8) Activation of NFκB requires its release from IκB. This is initiated by cytokines via the signal pathway that phosphorylates IκB, thus mediating the release and activation of NFκB. This activation is also mediated by oxidative stress, suggesting that these factors may initiate this process through src kinases. (4) NFκB is a trans-acting factor activated by intrinsic and extrinsic factors and is, therefore, an important target in aged tissues. (9–10) NFκB is sequestered in the cytoplasm in the oxidized state and must be reduced to function as a transactivator. Steps 9–10 link the redox equilibrium to the reduction of NFκB as a step in its activation and its ability to activate stress response genes. Antioxidant processes prevent oxidative stress and may be looked upon as intrinsic factors that repress the response to oxidative stress. The redox equilibrium in this case is shifted so that antioxidant intermediates such as TRX, GSH, etc. are not stimulated. This explains the activation *in vivo* of NFκB by oxidative processes and its inhibition by reducing agents. The *in vivo* response is dependent upon a change in the redox state of the cell, so that peroxide treatment would activate and reducing agents inhibit levels of intermediates such as TRX, which are important for maintenance of the redox equilibrium. (12) Nuclear translocation is mediated by a specific carrier protein. (13) NFκB activation and its ability to transactivate stress response genes involve extracellular intrinsic or extrinsic signals; phosphorylation, dephosphorylation, and redox represent modifications of the proteins that carry the signals through the cytoplasm. This cascade of events demonstrates how NFκB can respond to intrinsic and extrinsic factors via common pathway intermediates. Thus, NFκB can respond to these factors. Any age-associated effect on this cascade of events from the external signals to gene activation will affect the expression and regulation of stress response.

redox pathways. Age-associated changes in the homeostatic levels of intrinsic mediators as well as of extrinsic factors can accelerate the development of age-associated characteristics of gene regulation.

The mechanisms of regulation of the NFκB–IκB, AP-1, and HSF complexes are presented as representative models of how these pathways may affect the activity of these transactivators and their target genes in aging tissues.

V. NFκB Family of Transcription Factors

NFκB is a multisubunit transcription factor (Sen & Baltimore, 1986a) that plays a critical role in the cascade of regulations involved in the rapid activation of genes during the inflammatory, immune, and acute-phase responses (Baeuerle & Baltimore, 1991; Blank et al., 1991; Grilli et al., 1993; Schreck et al., 1991). Although NFκB was originally described as a heterodimer composed of a p50 and a p65 subunit (Baeuerle & Baltimore, 1989; Ghosh & Baltimore, 1990), there are five different proteins known to participate in dimer formation (Nabel & Verma, 1993). Thus, the NFκB/Rel family consists of p50, p52, p65 (rel A), c-rel, and rel B (I-rel) and is related to the c-rel oncogene and to the Drosophila morphogene dorsal (Ballard et al., 1992; Ghosh et al., 1990; Kieran et al., 1990; Nolan et al., 1991; Ruben et al., 1991, 1992; Ryseck et al., 1992; Schmid et al., 1991).

NFκB has been characterized best in pre-B-, B-, and T-lymphocytes and macrophages (Baeuerle & Henkel, 1994). Most of the NFκB-targeted genes fall into four classes: genes encoding (a) immunomodulatory cytokines (TNF-α, IL-6, and GM-CSF), (b) immunoregulatory cell surface receptors (MHC class I antigens; nonpolymorphic subunits of MHC genes; IL-2 cytokine receptors), (c) acute-phase proteins (serum amyloid A; angiotensinogen),

and (d) the human immunodeficiency virus (HIV-1), cytomegalovirus (Sambucetti et al., 1989), and SV40 (Baeuerle, 1991). NFκB is of relevance to aging because of its key role in the regulation of stress response genes. Studies indicate that aging affects the activity of members of the NFκB/Rel family (Liu et al., in preparation). NFκB DNA-binding activity, for example, is significantly increased in liver nuclear extracts of aged mice, in the absence of a challenging stress factor. Furthermore, mRNA levels of the angiotensinogen gene, an NFκB-regulated gene, are superinduced by LPS in aged mouse liver (Yiangou & Papaconstantinou, in preparation). Thus, the age-associated increase in this transcription factor may be the basis for this overexpression of a stress response gene. The increased NFκB binding activity in unstimulated aged liver nuclei also suggests that the constitutive level of activity of other stress response genes could be affected.

A. Regulation, Structure, and Function

In most cells, NFκB is sequestered in a cytoplasmic non-DNA-binding form (Baeuerle & Baltimore, 1988a,b) that is composed of three subunits: p50, which contains DNA-binding, dimerization, and nuclear translocation (NLS) domains (Ghosh et al., 1990; Kieran et al., 1990); p65, which shares in the DNA-binding and dimerization activity and contains a transcription activation domain (Baeuerle & Baltimore, 1989; Ruben et al., 1991); and an inhibitory subunit, IκB, which binds to p65 (Baeuerle & Baltimore, 1988b) (Fig. 2). The fact that NFκB is sequestered in the cytoplasm explains the observation that NFκB-binding activity occurs rapidly and in the absence of protein synthesis (Sen & Baltimore, 1986b; Hohmann et al., 1991).

The p50 subunit of NFκB is processed from the amino-terminal end of a 105-kDa precursor (p105). The resultant p50 then associates with p65, thus linking the p50–

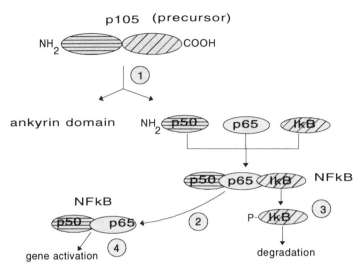

Figure 2. Model of the NFκB–IκB cytoplasmic complex and the sites that may affect the function of this trans-acting factor that are relevant to aging. (1) Activators such as oxy radicals and viruses may accelerate the activity of p105 protease and the processing of p105 to p50 subunit. (2) Various intrinsic and extrinsic factors mediate the activation of NFκB by phosphorylation of IκB and dephosphorylation of p65. The latter modification leads to transactivation. (3) NFκB is released when IκB is phosphorylated. At this step NFκB is in the oxidative state and may be reduced in the cytoplasm prior to its translocation. Reduction of p50 increases NFκB activity. (4) NFκB is translocated to the nucleus, where it activates a cascade of stress response genes.

p65 heterodimer with IκB in the cytoplasm (Blank *et al.*, 1992; Ghosh *et al.*, 1990; Kieran *et al.*, 1990) (Fig. 2). Another functionally important domain of p50 is the nuclear localization sequence (NLS), which consists of 4–5 basic amino acids (Gilmore, 1991; Blank *et al.*, 1991; Beg *et al.*, 1992). Specific proteins that mediate nuclear translocation bind to this domain. The transactivator function of NFκB is mediated by p65, which contains the transcription activation domain and is responsible for the strong transactivation mediated by the p50–p65 heterodimer (Schmitz & Baeuerle, 1991; Ruben *et al.*, 1992).

IκB is responsible for the cytoplasmic localization of the NFκB complex (Baeuerle & Baltimore, 1988b). The IκB family of proteins is composed of five members, all of which contain an ankyrin repeat motif, which inhibits DNA binding and nuclear

translocation of NFκB (Nabel & Verma, 1993; Kerr *et al.*, 1991; Wulczyn *et al.*, 1992; Zabel & Baeuerle, 1990; Blank *et al.*, 1991; Ghosh *et al.*, 1990; Hatada *et al.*, 1992; Kieran *et al.*, 1990). These functions are attributed to a protective action of the C-terminal ankyrin-containing domain, achieved by protein folding over the DNA-binding and NLS domains (Henke *et al.*, 1992). It is the signal transduction-mediated phosphorylation of IκB that releases the p50–p65 heterodimer from the complex and that triggers NFκB activation and its translocation to the nucleus. Thus, each of the components of the cytoplasmic NFκB–IκB complex, i.e., their synthesis, processing, activation, and translocation, are potential cytoplasmic targets for age-associated alteration in the functions of this regulatory complex.

Both the p50 and p65 subunits of NFκB

are regulated by redox modification (Hayashi, et al., 1993; Matthews et al., 1992; Mosialos et al., 1991). Studies have shown that reduced Cys^{62} is the crucial redox site needed for high-affinity binding of p50 to DNA and suggest that both intrinsic and extrinsic factors significantly affect NFκB DNA-binding and transactivation functions via the redox state of this protein. The redox state of aged tissues may, therefore, be an important factor in the age-associated activity of NFκB and the genes it targets. Phosphorylation of p50 is also believed to play a role in regulating transcriptional activity of the p50–p65 complex (Mosialos et al., 1991).

B. Intrinsic and Extrinsic Stress Factors Act as Second Messengers for Activation of NFκB

Many different intrinsic and extrinsic agents can induce NFκB DNA-binding activity (Baeuerle, 1991; Baeuerle & Baltimore, 1988a, 1991; Lenardo & Baltimore, 1989; Lenardo et al., 1989; Schmitz et al., 1991). These include viruses (HIV-1, cytomegalovirus, or dsRNA), bacterial lipopolysaccharide (LPS), protein synthesis inhibitors, cytokines, (TNF-α, TNF-β, and IL-1), T-cell mitogens (phorbol esters, lectins), calcium ionophores, antibodies against T-cell receptors, agents provoking oxidative stress (Schreck et al., 1992; Schutze-Osthoff et al., 1992), and reducing agents such as dithiothreitol (DTT) and thioredoxin (TRX). Although it is not fully known how such diverse agents can induce the signal transduction–redox pathways that activate the NFκB pathway, it is certain that p50, p65, and IκB are targets of these pathways (Ghosh & Baltimore, 1990; Schmitz & Baeuerle, 1991; Blank et al., 1991; Bours et al., 1990; Logeat et al., 1991; Lux et al., 1990; Meyer et al., 1991; Nolan et al., 1991; Schmitz et al., 1991).

NFκB is activated by phorbol ester (PMA) via protein kinase C (PKC). Phosphorylation of IκB through PKC releases the inhibitor, thereby activating NFκB (Ghosh & Baltimore, 1990; Shirakawa & Meijel, 1989; Hatada et al., 1992; Lux et al., 1990; Ten et al., 1992). Studies suggest that the pathway involves PMA→PKC→Ras p21→Raf-1→IκB-NFκB (Finco & Baldwin, 1993; Li & Sedivy, 1993). However, activation of NFκB by TNF-α appears to be independent of PKC (Meichle et al., 1990). Although TNF-α induces a rapid and transient activation of PKC (Schutze et al., 1990), depletion of the kinase by prolonged PMA treatment and the use of the PKC inhibitor, staurosporine, do not affect NFκB activation by TNF-α (Feuillard et al., 1991). In fact, studies have shown that the signaling pathway for TNFα is mediated via the sphingomyelin pathway. In summary, this pathway involves the activation of NFκB via the production of ceramide and the activation of PKCζ, which is not sensitive to PMA treatment (Kolesnick & Golde, 1994; Diaz-Meco et al., 1994; Dominguez et al., 1993; Lozano et al., 1994; Machleidt et al., 1994; Schutze et al., 1992). This also explains the failure of PMA to inhibit the TNF-α pathway of activation of NFκB. Alternatively, induction by IL-1 acts via an increase in cAMP levels and PKA phosphorylation of IκB (Shirakawa & Meijel, 1989), whereas another study suggests that the diacylglycerol phosphate activation of PKC is also a pathway of NFκB activation (Rosoff et al., 1988). There is now evidence that the IL-1-mediated activation of NFκB can proceed via the sphingomyelin pathway (Kolesnick & Golde, 1994), linking PKCζ and/or Raf-1, and via the Ras p21 pathway to Raf-1. This demonstrates how intrinsic (TNF-α and IL-1) and extrinsic (PMA) factors activate NFκB via phosphorylation, presumably via different components of the signal transduction pathway. Thus, the signals initiated by intrinsic and extrinsic factors converge to common sites, i.e., PKCζ and Ras-1, to mediate the activation of NFκB via the phosphorylation of IκB (Dominguez et al., 1993).

Studies have shown that the IκBα- complexes are direct targets for Raf-1-mediated phosphorylation (Li & Sedivy, 1993; Beg et al., 1993; Beg & Baldwin, 1993). This phosphorylation prevents the binding of IκBα to p50–p65 and *rel* (Ghosh & Baltimore, 1990; Shirakawa & Meijel, 1989; Kerr et al., 1991, 1992), suggesting that phosphorylation regulates the complex formation *in vivo*. The present mechanism invokes that stimulation by factors such as LPS results in the release and rapid loss, by degradation, of phosphorylated IκBα and the release of the NFκB complex and its transport to the nucleus followed by DNA binding and gene activation (Brown et al., 1993; Sun et al., 1993; Rice & Ernst, 1993).

C. Models of the *in Vivo* Control of NFκB

There are two key features of IκBα regulation of NFκB in the constitutive, unstimulated cell (Rice & Ernst, 1993). The synthesis of new IκBα is very rapid, so that most liberated dimers are efficiently captured and retained in the cytoplasm. Thus, IκBα complexes themselves are unstable, with frequent dissociation and/or degradation of the IκBα (Beg & Baldwin, 1993; Rice & Ernst, 1993; Beg et al., 1993; Shirakawa & Meijel, 1989; Machleidt et al., 1994). The release by phosphorylation and rapid degradation of IκBα make up another important regulatory pathway that may determine the level of NFκB activity in aged cells. LPS is one of several agents that induces the loss of IκBα from p65 and *c-rel*-containing complexes. Dissociation of the complexes correlates with the appearance of *NFκB (rel)* family members in the nucleus (Beg & Baldwin 1993; Beg et al., 1993; Brown et al., 1993; Cordle et al., 1993; Sun et al., 1993) and with the rapid rise in DNA-binding activity. In aging liver cells, both the constitutive and LPS-induced levels of NFκB are significantly increased in the nucleus, suggesting that a

regulatory process for sequestering NFκB in the cytoplasm may be altered during aging (Liu et al., in preparation). These studies also show that the IκBα pool level is not altered in aged liver, suggesting there is no change in the turnover of the inhibitor. However, both IκBα and Raf-1 are hyperphosphorylated in aged liver. This age-associated increase in the activity of these intermediates of the signal transduction pathway could explain the increased binding activity of NFκB in nuclei of aged liver.

VI. Leucine Zipper (bZIP) Families of Transcription Factors

The leucine zipper motif was discovered as a conserved sequence pattern in several transcription factors, including the C/EBPs, Jun, Fos, Myc, and the HSFs (Johnson & McKnight 1989; Kerppola & Curran 1991; Landschulz et al., 1988). These transcription factors are characterized by three distinct domains: the leucine zipper region, which consists of a heptad repeat of leucines within a sequence of about 30 amino acids that form an α-helix. Dimerization occurs via the "zippering" of two such helices, mediated by interactions between leucine residues along the hydrophobic face of each helix. The leucine zipper domain is usually located at the carboxy-terminal portion of the protein. There are some exceptions, the most obvious being that of the heat shock factors (HSFs), which have multiple leucine zipper domains, one of which is at the carboxy terminus. The basic region, which contains the DNA-binding domain, contains about 30 amino acid residues and is high in arginines and lysines. The basic regions are immediately amino-terminal to the leucine zipper domain. Studies have shown that the basic regions form the DNA contact surface, and mutations of these regions block DNA binding but not dimerization. The transcription activation domain, which is amino-terminal to the basic region, is the most divergent region of these proteins and is involved in the protein–protein interactions that activate or repress gene expression.

A. Structure of AP-1–Fos–Jun Trans-Acting Factors

The AP-1 cis-acting DNA-binding site was first identified in the enhancer regions of SV40, human metallothionein II$_A$ (hMII$_A$), and several phorbol ester responsive genes (Angel et al., 1987, 1988; Lee et al., 1987). Members of the Fos and Jun family belong to the bZIP family of trans-acting factors and bind to the AP-1 DNA sequence. These proteins consist of distinct DNA-binding, dimerization, and transcriptional activation domains, which are required for the formation of functional hetero- and homodimers (Kouzarides & Ziff, 1988; Turner & Tjian, 1989; Gentz et al., 1989; O'Shea et al., 1989). Although the DNA-binding domains are contributed by both Fos and Jun, Fos does not bind to the hMTII$_A$ AP-1 site, and Jun homodimers bind with relatively low affinity. However, Fos enhances the binding of the Fos–Jun heterodimer primarily by stabilizing the protein–DNA interaction (Rauscher et al., 1988). Since the leucine zipper and basic region motifs of c-fos and c-jun are highly conserved, multiple protein complexes can form between members of this family. Homodimeric Jun–Jun and heterodimeric Fos–Jun complexes interact with the same DNA motif; both proteins make direct contact to the DNA. The members of the bZIP families and their heterodimerizing abilities are discussed by Lamb and McKnight (1991).

B. Signal Transduction and AP-1

The AP-1 (Fos–Jun dimers) proteins are members of a super family of trans-acting factors induced by biological mediators, such as polypeptide hormones, growth factors, cytokines, and neurotransmitters (intrinsic factors), and by extrinsic factors such as ultraviolet irradiation (UV-C), DNA-damaging agents (Devary et al., 1991; Stein et al., 1989), and phorbol esters (TPA) (12-O-tetradecanoylphorbol 13-acetate) (Fig. 3). The signaling pathways that transmit an external stimulus to AP-1 occur via membrane-associated tyrosine kinases or phospholipid turnover, the latter giving rise to PKC activity. In addition, the transforming oncogenes, v-Src, Ha-Ras, and v-Raf, act as intermediates in the signal pathway that transmit information from the cell surface tyrosine kinases to the AP-1 in the nucleus. Oxidative stress due to physical (UV-C) and chemical factors (phorbol esters, alkylating agents) also activates a signaling pathway that is initiated with the stimulation of membrane associated tyrosine kinases (Devary et al., 1992). Thus, in pathways initiated by either intrinsic or extrinsic factors, tyrosine-specific protein kinases act rapidly at the initial stages of signaling; this leads to increased Ras activity, which appears to play a central role in activation of downstream serine/threonine-specific protein kinases such as Raf-1 and the mitogen-activated protein kinases (MAP kinases), which include extracellular signal-regulated kinases (ERK) and jun kinases (JNK).

C. Posttranslational Modification of c-fos and c-jun

Posttranslational modifications by phosphorylation and reduction are basic reactions that determine the level of activity of these transcription factors. Exposure to UV-C results in a dramatic increase in the phosphorylation of c-jun on two serine residues, Ser[63] and Ser[73], which are located in the transactivation domain. Phosphorylation of these sites enhances the ability of c-jun to activate the transcription of AP-1 target genes (Binetruy et al., 1991; Rauscher et al., 1988; Smeal et al., 1991, 1992). Phosphorylation of Ser[63] and Ser[73]

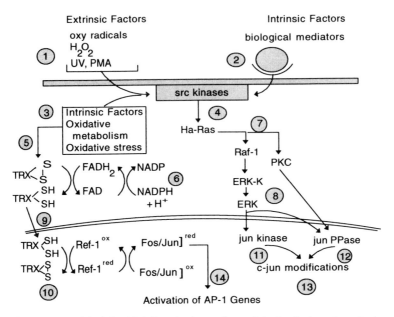

Figure 3. Model of the AP-1 (Fos–Jun) complex and the intrinsic and extrinsic factors that affect its activity as a transactivator of stress response genes. The earliest response to (1) extrinsic and (2) intrinsic factors involves the activation of src kinases. (3) Intrinsic factors produced by oxidative metabolism may act as second messengers to activate src kinases. (4) Src kinases lead to the activation of Raf-1 and subsequent signal transduction intermediates. These lead to the phosphorylation of the activation domain via jun kinase (11), which stimulates its transactivator function, and the dephosphorylation of its DNA-binding domain (12), which stimulates its binding activity. (13) The overall effect of these modifications is the activation of c-jun. (5) Intrinsic and (1) extrinsic factors stimulate the level of antioxidants such as TRX, which is a reducing factor for the nuclear protein Ref-1. (9–10) TRX reduces Ref-1, which then reacts to reduce essential cysteines in c-fos and c-jun. (14) These modifications result in AP-1 activation.

is also stimulated by *v-src* and requires the function of Ras (Smeal *et al.*, 1992), thus suggesting the cascade of processes that leads to AP-1 (*c-jun*) activation (Fig. 3). These observations suggest that phosphorylation potentiates transactivation by affecting the conformation of the activation domains by mediating protein–protein interactions and thereby interaction with a target that is part of the transcription machinery.

Ha-Ras has been shown to activate two protein kinases, Raf-1 and MEK (MAPK or ERK kinase) kinase (MEKK). These are intermediates in the pathway leading to *c-jun* response to mitogen, cytokines, and UV irradiation. Both Ha-Ras and Raf-1 operate downstream of cell surface-associated tyrosine kinases (Karin, 1992; Karin & Smeal, 1992; Cantley *et al.*, 1991); Raf-1 directly contributes to ERK activation, but not to JNK activation, whereas MEKK activates JNK (Minden *et al.*, 1994). These studies demonstrate the existence of two distinct Ras-dependent MAPK cascades, one initiated by Raf-1 leading to ERKI activation and the other initiated by MEKK leading to JNK activation. The pathway leading to the stimulation of AP-1 by mitogens (intrinsic) and UV (extrinsic) factors is shown in Fig. 3.

Studies have shown that c-Jun N-terminal kinases (JNK) phosphorylate the amino-terminal sites of c-Jun (Hibi *et al.*, 1993; Derijard *et al.*, 1994). It has also been reported that ERK kinases phosphorylate one of the carboxy-terminal inhibitory sites, which results in inhibition of c-Jun.

The carboxy-terminal phosphorylation of c-Jun occurs at Thr^{231}, Ser^{243}, and Ser^{249}. These amino acids are localized in the DNA-binding domain. Thr^{231} and Ser^{243} are phosphorylated by CKII, whereas Ser^{249} is phosphorylated (*in vitro*) by ERK (MAP) kinases. *In vitro* phosphorylation of Thr^{231} and Ser^{249} by CKII inhibits the DNA-binding activity of c-Jun. These studies suggest that the role of phosphatases is to increase DNA-binding activity by relieving the inhibitory effect of phosphorylation by CKII. Presumably the dephosphorylation increases c-Jun binding to the TRE of the *c-jun* promoter, leading to increased *c-jun* expression. Thus, although phosphorylation of the DNA-binding domain inhibits binding activity, phosphorylation of the activation domain stimulates transactivation. This suggests that the activity of c-Jun can be either up- or down-regulated, depending on the protein site phosphorylated (Devary *et al.*, 1992). Since aging affects AP-1 activity, these modification sites are potential targets for age-associated processes that affect AP-1 gene activity.

Activation of Src family tyrosine kinases is the earliest signal of the UV-signaling cascade, followed by activation of Ha-Ras and Raf. It is proposed that the UV response is initiated at the cell surface membrane rather than within the nucleus (Cantley *et al.*, 1991). Thus, AP-1 represents a major nuclear transcription factor that transmits the activity of signal transduction–redox pathways to stress response genes in response to intrinsic and extrinsic factors. These signaling pathways affect AP-1 activity at the transcriptional and posttranscriptional levels. The constitutive levels of *c-fos* and *c-jun* gene transcription are very low in most non-stimulated cells and are induced in response to extracellular stimuli. Thus, the age-associated rise in rat hepatocyte constitutive levels of both *c-fos* and *c-jun* in the absence of stress factors is an indication of chronic stress or constant stimulation of these genes (Fujita & Maruyama, 1991). Furthermore, the constitutive levels of *c-fos* gene expression and AP-1-binding activity in the brain are an indication of the development of age-associated tissue-specific effects on the AP-1 family of transcription factors (Kitrabi *et al.*, 1993). Further indications of an age-associated tissue-specific alteration of AP-1-binding activity is suggested by observations that AP-1 is more strongly induced in the hippocampus of aged rats treated with the proconvulsant pentylenetetrazole (Kaminska & Kaczmarek, 1993). This correlates well with the occurrence, in various tissues, of an alteration of constitutive and regulatory patterns of AP-1-targeted genes.

VII. Oxidative Stress and the Signal Transduction Pathway

Oxidative stress caused by UV or alkylating agents activates signal transduction pathways and stress response genes. The fact that *N*-acetyl-L-cysteine (NAC), a precursor to glutathione (GSH) (Meister, 1991), attenuates c-Src activation and induction of *c-jun* by UV-C suggests that oxidative stress may be an activator of this signaling cascade. The importance of redox equilibrium is suggested by the observation that oxidative stress caused by either oxidizing or alkylating agents activates certain tyrosine kinases (Karin & Smeal, 1992; Bauskin *et al.*, 1991; Garcia-Morales *et al.*, 1990) and inhibits tyrosine phosphatases (Garcia-Morales *et al.*, 1990; Heffetz & Zick, 1989), possibly through the oxidation or alkylation of a highly reactive essential cysteine residue at their catalytic centers (Hunter & Karin, 1992).

Since the phosphorylation of Tyr[416] of c-Src is believed to augment its activity (Hunter & Karin, 1992), and the dephosphorylation of this site attenuates its activity, the ability of the redox state to regulate these processes would be a direct linkage between the redox equilibrium, signal transduction pathway, intrinsic factors, and extrinsic factors in the activation of stress response genes.

Perturbation of the cellular redox equilibrium appears to affect the activity of several tyrosine kinases and phosphatases. Activation of Src kinases is the earliest detectable response to UV irradiation leading to the activation of nuclear transcription factors. This provides a good explanation for the induction of NFκB activity by UV and other DNA-damaging agents (Stein *et al.*, 1989). Both AP-1 and NFκB are, therefore, induced by oxidative stress and blocked by free radical scavengers, suggesting a common intermediate(s) along the signaling–redox pathways. In addition, other agents that cause oxidative stress, such as UV-A (Cerutti, 1985; Cerutti & Trump, 1991) and arsenite (Devary *et al.*, 1991), are also effective inducers of nuclear transcription factors associated with the activation of stress response genes.

A. Identification of Intermediates of the Redox Pathway

The H_2O_2-mediated activation of NFκB in Jurkat cells suggests that extrinsic oxidative radicals can link into the signal transduction–redox pathway. An intrinsic increase in oxidative metabolism and homeostatic levels of products of oxidative metabolism, which occur in aging, could alter the overall regulation of NFκB–IκB in the cytoplasm. This is supported by observations that treatment of cells with oxidizing agents causes a homeostatic response involving increased synthesis and activity of antioxidants and reducing enzymes such as thioredoxin (TRX) and GSH (Holmgren, 1984, 1985, 1989; Meister &

Anderson, 1983). Interestingly, TRX cannot reduce NFκB(p50) when it is complexed to IκB, whereas reduction occurs when the p50–p65 complex is released (Hayashi *et al.*, 1993). Thus, it appears that the sequence of events leading to NFκB activation involves signal transduction, which phosphorylates IκB and releases NFκB, followed by reduction of p50 (Cys[62]) and translocation to the nucleus. TRX appears, therefore, to play a direct role in regulating the DNA-binding activity of NFκB.

Redox factor-1 (Ref-1) has been shown to stimulate the DNA-binding activity of several transcription factors *in vitro* (Xanthoudakis & Curran, 1992; Xanthoudakis *et al.*, 1992). These include Fos, Jun, AP-1, NFκB, Myb, and CREB (Xanthoudakis *et al.*, 1992). The redox activity of Ref-1 is mediated through a conserved cysteine basic amino acid motif (KCR) that is present in all of the Fos- and Jun-related proteins identified to date. Similar cysteine residues have been detected in the DNA-binding domains of p65–NFκB (KICR) and Myb (KQCR) (Toledano & Leonard, 1991). However, the efficiency of Ref-1-mediated reduction of NFκB was low in comparison to TRX, suggesting that Ref-1 is not the primary *in vivo* redox factor for NFκB. Furthermore, TRX mediates the reduction of NFκB in the cytoplasm, whereas Ref-1 mediates the reduction of Fos–Jun in the nucleus. Thus, the redox pathways involving TRX- and Ref-1-mediated reduction of transcription factors may be compartmentalized. Interestingly, Ref-1 activity is significantly increased by TRX *in vitro*, indicating that the reduction of Fos–Jun involves the following redox pathway: TRX→Ref-1→Fos/Jun (Fig. 3). Furthermore, since Ref-1 is a nuclear protein it is possible that the TRX→Ref-1 interaction occurs in the cytoplasm, and since Ref-1 has nuclear translocation sequences (Xanthoudakis & Curran, 1992; Xanthoudakis *et al.*, 1992), it may be rapidly translocated to the nucleus upon reduction. Alternatively, TRX may function as a redox factor in the nucleus as well as the cytoplasm. The actual mechanism remains to be worked out.

Current data strongly suggest that redox processes are involved in NFκB signal transduction. *In vivo*, active oxygen has been implicated as a common intermediate in the cytoplasmic activation of NFκB by phorbol esters, TNF-α, and H_2O_2 (Schreck *et al.*, 1991; Staal *et al.*, 1990). Indeed, the treatment of cells with phorbol esters, which induce NFκB and AP-1 activity, generates a prooxidant state (Cerutti, 1985). Although redox-mediated regulation may affect many transcription factors, it appears that there may be differences in their mechanisms of action. A crucial difference between NFκB–p50 and Fos–Jun is that TRX directly stimulates the DNA-binding activity of NFκB and that a free SH group at Cys^{62} (p50) is required for DNA binding (Hayashi *et al.*, 1993; Matthews *et al.*, 1992). In the case of Fos–Jun, TRX does not act directly, but manifests its effect via Ref-1 (Xanthoudakis *et al.*, 1992). Furthermore, it is proposed that the oxidized cysteine in Fos and Jun may be in the form of a reversible sulfonic acid derivative (Abate *et al.*, 1990) and that the reaction with Ref-1 would involve the reduction of a sulfur–oxygen bond.

VIII. Heat Shock Proteins

Hyperthermia results in the induction of synthesis of a family of heat shock proteins (HSP), which are essential for the survival of cells and tissues exposed to this tissue-damaging factor (Lindquist, 1986; Morimoto *et al.*, 1990). All organisms from archaebacteria to plants and animals express HSPs, although the number varies from organism to organism and between cell types within an organism (Lindquist, 1986). At least four groups of genes make up the HSP70 family; of these, HSP70 is expressed at very low levels by nonstressed cells and is the most strongly induced by hyperthermia. It is the most highly conserved protein known throughout the evolution of prokaryotes and eukaryotes (Lindquist, 1986) and plays a critical role in protecting cells and tissues against hyperthermic damage (Johnston & Kucey, 1988; Angelidis *et al.*, 1991; Li *et al.*, 1991; Riabowol *et al.*, 1988). The other members of this family include HSC70, which is expressed constitutively and is only slightly induced by heat, GRP78, which is induced by glucose starvation but not by hyperthermia, and GRP75, which is localized within the mitochondria (Mizzen *et al.*, 1989).

HSPs present constitutively, as well as those induced in response to stress, appear to serve vital cell functions, e.g., they act as chaperones to assist in the assembly, disassembly, and transport of other intracellular proteins (Welch, 1993; Craig *et al.*, 1994; Gething & Sambrook, 1992). As chaperones, the HSPs facilitate the removal as well as the replacement of damaged proteins. Induction of the HSPs in response to stress factors is, therefore, related to an increased requirement for such chaperone functions. It appears, therefore, that the regulation of HSP expression serves beneficial effects during stress, e.g., the state of thermotolerance or resistance to other stress factors (Riabowol *et al.*, 1988; Johnston & Kucey, 1988; Li *et al.*, 1991; Angelidis *et al.*, 1991). It has been demonstrated by a number of investigators that mammalian aging is associated with an age-associated alteration in the ability of cells to express HSP in response to thermal stress (Holbrook & Richardson, 1995).

A. Heat Shock Response by Senescent Cells in Culture

The regulation of HSP70 expression is an excellent example of a cellular mechanism that evolved as a protective response to hyperthermia and other types of stress. Inhibition of HSP70 activity, by microinjection of monoclonal antibody (Riabowol et al., 1988), or inhibition of HSP70 transcription renders fibroblasts thermosensitive (Johnston & Kucey, 1988), whereas transfection of cells with expression vectors that constitutively expressed HSP70 confers thermotolerance (Angelidis et al., 1991; Li et al., 1991). A major characteristic of senescent organisms is their reduced ability to respond to hyperthermic stress, and changes in HSP70 expression and/or function may be an important survival factor in aging (Shock et al., 1984). This view is supported by the fact that, in response to heat and other stressors, HSP70 expression has been shown to decline in senescent human diploid fibroblasts, and this is associated with a decrease in the ability of cells to withstand hyperthermic stress (Liu et al., 1989, 1991; Luce & Cristofalo, 1992).

The induction of HSP70 expression also occurs after heat stress in primary cultures of rat lung and skin fibroblasts and in primary hepatocytes. The age-related impairment of HSP70 expression persists in these primary cultures, suggesting that the age-associated inhibition of HSP70 is stable in cultured cells (Fargnoli et al., 1990; Heydari et al., 1993).

B. Heat Shock Response in Aging Tissues *in Vivo*

A large number of cell types and tissues show an age-associated decline in HSP70 expression in response to heat shock. This includes skin fibroblasts (Fargnoli et al., 1990), hepatocytes (Heydari et al., 1993), splenocytes (Pahlavani et al., 1995), and mononuclear cells (Deguchi et al., 1988). Heat-induced HSP70 expression has also been measured in whole lung tissue heat-stressed *in vitro* (Fargnoli et al., 1990) and in the brain hippocampus of intact animals subjected to heat stress (Pardue et al., 1992), where it has also been shown to de-

cline with age. In addition, induction of HSP70 synthesis by mitogens decreases with age in lymphocytes isolated from young and elderly human subjects (Faassen et al., 1989).

Studies have shown that restraint or immobilization stress can induce the expression of HSP70 mRNA selectively in rodent adrenal cortex and vascular smooth muscle cells of the thoracic and abdominal aorta and vena cava (Blake et al., 1991a; Udelsman et al., 1993; Fawcett, et al., 1994). Unlike most stress paradigms used to elicit the heat shock response, restraint is not associated with overt injury to cells or tissues. Viewed more as a behavioral stress, this model has been used to induce physiological stress response syndromes by the activation of the hypothalamic–pituitary–adrenal (HPA) and sympathetic neuroendocrine axes (Pare & Galvin, 1986). The adrenal and vascular responses have been well-characterized, and it has been shown that both are dependent upon hormonal responses (Blake et al., 1991a; Udelsman et al., 1993). The adrenal response is localized in the cortical region and is dependent on adrenocorticotropic hormone, while the vascular response is localized in the smooth muscle cell layer of the vessel and is mediated by α_1-adrenergic receptors. Both of these tissue responses are reduced in aged rats, suggesting that the host defenses are attenuated with aging. This could contribute to the reduced stress tolerance seen in elderly people and aged animals.

C. Trans-Acting Factors of hsp Genes— Heat Shock Factors (HSFs)

The heat shock response occurs within minutes and involves transcriptional activation mediated by heat shock transcription factors (HSFs), which bind to the promoter elements (HSE) of heat shock-responsive genes (Morimoto, 1993; Bienz & Pelham, 1986; Xiao & Lis, 1988; Abravaya et al., 1991; Amin et al., 1988;

Perisic *et al.*, 1989; Xiao *et al.*, 1991). The following model (Fig. 4) has been proposed for the mechanism of activation of HSP gene induction via regulation of HSF (Morimoto, 1993): (1) HSF is maintained in a monomeric, non-DNA-binding form in both the cytoplasm and nucleus of un-stressed cells. The inability to bind to DNA is achieved by interaction of HSF with HSP70, which stabilizes a specific non-DNA-binding conformation of HSF (Zimarino & Wu, 1987; Kingston *et al.*, 1987; Mosser *et al.*, 1988). (2) In response to heat shock, HSF assembles into a trimer and is translocated to the nucleus, where it binds to the heat shock DNA-binding site (HSE) in the promoter regions of heat shock response genes (Morimoto, 1993; Sorger & Nelson, 1989; Abravaya *et al.*, 1991, 1992; Kingston *et al.*, 1987; Mosser *et al.*, 1990; Sarge *et al.*, 1993; Westwood *et al.*, 1991; Zimarino, *et al.*, 1990). This activation process is associated with the removal of the inhibitor of HSF-binding activity. (3) Activation of DNA-binding activity occurs when HSF is released and assembles into trimers. Activation of HSF DNA-binding activity leads to the induction of transcription of the HSP70 gene and the accumulation of HSP70. (4) At this time the HSF is phosphorylated. (5) The heat transcriptional response attenuates upon return to physiological temperature. (6) Attenuation of the response is accompanied by conversion of the active trimeric HSF to the non-DNA-binding monomer and a return to the normal subcellular distribution (5 and 6). According to the proposed model, the newly synthesized HSP70 associates with HSF, mediating its conversion back to a monomeric form and thereby turning off or reducing HSP70

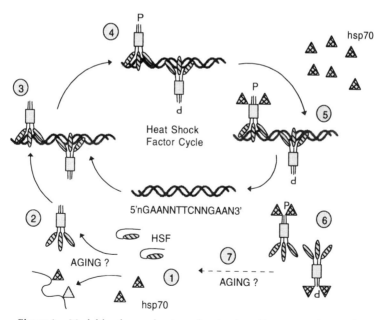

Figure 4. Model for the mechanism of activation of hsp gene induction by HSF. The steps of HSF-mediated activation of the HSP70 gene are depicted in the text. Current data suggest that the age-associated attenuation of HSP70 activation is due to the failure of activation of HSF and may occur at steps (1) and/or (7). The model is according to that proposed by Morimoto (1993).

gene transcription. Importantly, while the general model is well-supported by experimental data, the role of HSP70 in inhibiting the DNA-binding activity and in converting it back to a monomeric state is subject to much debate (see Holbrook & Richardson, 1995).

At least two HSFs are present in mammalian cells, HSF1 and HSF2 (Clos *et al.*, 1990; Rabindran *et al.*, 1991, 1993; Schutze *et al.*, 1991). Both HSF genes are present as single copies and share the following structural features: a DNA-binding domain at the N-terminus, an adjacent cluster of hydrophobic amino acids organized into heptad repeats (leucine zippers 1, 2, and 3), and a distally located heptad repeat near the C-terminus (leucine zipper 4). HSFs 1 and 2 are simultaneously expressed in most cells, and the DNA-binding activity of each is negatively regulated (Nakai & Morimoto, 1993). There are regions of extensive homology within the DNA-binding and dimerization domains. Most of the homology is located in the amino-terminal DNA-binding domain and in the arrays of hydrophobic amino acid heptad repeats, which comprise the oligomerization domains in the NH_2-terminal half (leucine zippers 1–3) and the carboxy terminus (leucine zipper 4) of the proteins (Clos *et al.*, 1990; Rabindran *et al.*, 1991; Schutze *et al.*, 1991). The highly conserved carboxy-terminal leucine zipper 4 motif is speculated to be involved in the formation of the inactive state of HSF under non-shock conditions, as deletion of this region results in constitutive DNA-binding activity (Rabindran *et al.*, 1991; Nakai & Morimoto, 1993; Rabindran *et al.*, 1993).

D. Regulation of HSF Activity in Response to Heat Shock

Analyses of heat-shocked NIH-3T3 cells indicate that levels of HSF1 and HSF2 mRNAs are not altered by heat shock and that there is no change in their transcription. Gel shift analyses have shown that HSF1 binds to HSE only after heat shock, whereas HSF2 exhibits binding in unstressed constitutive conditions at 0 or 37°C, but not at 43°C (Sarge *et al.*, 1991). Thus, HSF1 and HSF2 show DNA-binding activity that is differentially altered by heat treatment. These changes in DNA-binding activity occur in the absence of changes in transcription, mRNA and protein pools, or protein degradation. Although in most cells the primary level of heat shock gene regulation occurs via transcriptional activation involving the interaction of HSF1 with the heat shock promoter element (HSE), the transcription of the HSF genes themselves is not activated (Bienz & Pelham, 1986; Xiao & Lis, 1988; Kingston *et al.*, 1987; Mosser *et al.*, 1990; Perisic *et al.*, 1989; Sarge *et al.*, 1993; Westwood *et al.*, 1991; Xiao *et al.*, 1991; Zimarino *et al.*, 1990). HSF1 is the mediator of stress-induced heat shock gene transcription and displays heat-induced DNA-binding activity, oligomerization, and nuclear translocation in the absence of new protein synthesis (Sarge *et al.*, 1993).

E. Regulation of HSF Activity during Aging

Induction of HSP70 expression by heat shock, sodium arsenite, or the amino acid analogue canavanine is significantly lower in late-passage or senescent diploid fibroblasts (Liu *et al.*, 1989, 1991; Luce & Cristofalo, 1992). In all cases this decrease is attributed to a reduction in the transcription of HSP70 (Liu *et al.*, 1989) and correlates well with the loss of heat shock factor (HSF) binding activity, which activates the HSP70 gene (Liu *et al.*, 1991; Choi *et al.*, 1990). Similarly, the age-related decline in *in vitro* heat-induced HSP70 expression in freshly isolated hepatocytes likewise is associated with a reduction in the DNA-binding activity of HSF (Heydari *et al.*, 1993). Finally, examination of relative HSF-binding activity in adrenal extracts of old and young rats showed that the total HSE-binding activity was significantly lower in old rats both in control (absence) and under conditions of restraint stress. The binding activity in extracts of control old rats was only 40% of that seen in extracts of young rats. Importantly, however, Western analyses showed that there are no significant differences in HSF1 protein pool levels or in protein size in control or restraint groups.

It has been proposed that the decreased DNA-binding activity of HSF1 in senescent diploid fibroblasts may be due to the presence of an inhibitor of DNA-binding activity in the aged cells (Choi *et al.*, 1990). However, no evidence for such an inhibitor was found in studies with either aged adrenal extracts or hepatocytes (Holbrook & Richardson, 1995).

F. Intrinsic and Extrinsic Factors That Activate HSFs—Second Messengers

In addition to heat shock, agents such as heavy metals, oxidative and restraint stresses, and amino acid analogues induce HSF-binding activity and HSP70 gene transcription (Mosser *et al.*, 1988). Mouse 3T3 cells treated with either cadmium sulfate or the proline analogue azetidine at 37°C result in maximal levels of HSF-binding activity (Sarge *et al.*, 1993). The HSF DNA-binding activity induced by cadmium sulfate or L-azetidine-2-carboxylic acid, like that induced by heat, is composed primarily of HSF1. Cadmium sulfate treatment also results in HSF1 phosphorylation (Sarge *et al.*, 1993), whereas treatment with azetidine is identical to that of untreated cells, i.e., it is not accompanied by an increase in phosphorylation (Jakobsen & Pelham, 1991; Sorger & Pelham, 1988). HSF2, on the other hand, is not activated by any of these treatments, but rather is activated by hemin-induced differentiation of erythroleukemia cells and abundantly expressed during mouse spermatogenesis (Morimoto *et al.*, 1992; Sarge *et al.*, 1993; Sistonen *et al.*, 1992).

Thus, differences between the roles of HSF1 and HSF2 lie in their differential response to stress factors. No studies have yet been conducted on the activity of HSF2 during aging.

IX. Importance of Understanding How Aging Affects Response to Stress

There have been several reports of age-dependent alterations of thermoregulation in humans, as well as experimental animals (Finch & Landfield, 1979; Wollner & Spalding, 1978). Hyperthermia is an increasingly recognized clinical disorder in older individuals exposed to high temperatures (Hoffman-Goetz & Keir, 1984), and there is a strong correlation between age and mortality from hyperthermia in human subjects. The number of deaths associated with high environmental temperature increases progressively with age, e.g., deaths increase by 10-fold between 80 and 90 years of age (Oeschli & Buechley, 1970). Aged rats fed a calorie-restricted (CR) diet are more thermoresistant than *ad libitum*-aged rats. This is supported by the observation that 75% of rats fed a CR diet survived a period of hyperthermia in which only 16% of the *ad libitum* old rats survived. Thus, the old CR-fed rats showed a greater ability to survive hyperthermic conditions than old rats (Heydari *et al.*, 1993). Interestingly, hepatocytes of aged CR-fed rats also show little decline in HSF DNA-binding activity of HSP70 expression compared to non-CR rats (Heydari *et al.*, 1993). These findings suggest that CR may delay or prevent the age-related decline in the host defense.

X. Importance of Understanding Biological Processes of Aging

It is clear that the transcriptional factor activities are tightly linked to the signal transduction and/or redox pathways. Each of these processes regulates binding activities of trans-acting factors that activate cascades of stress response genes. This is very relevant to aging because there are a variety of inducing agents, intrinsic and extrinsic, ranging from cytokines to intermediates of oxidative metabolism, that regulate these transactivators. Thus, modifications such as phosphorylation, dephosphorylation, redox, or protein–protein interactions appear to play a crucial role in the regulation of transcription factors, and aging affects these processes. Thus, age-associated increases (NFκB and AP-1) or decreases (HSFs) in binding activity occur in the absence of an obvious stimulus or stress factor. Furthermore, these changes are stable and establish a new spectrum of gene regulations characteristic of aged tissues. Since the mechanisms of activation, translocation, and regulation of these trans-acting factors are well-known, experiments to determine how aging mediates their increased or decreased activity in aged animals are indeed feasible. The arguments presented in this chapter suggest that this mechanism may involve the intermediates of signal transduction–redox pathways, which are sensitive to the mediators whose homeostatic levels are altered in aging. They are also sensitive to the external environmental factors that accelerate the development of aging characteristics. The fact that the development of age-associated autoimmune diseases, such as rheumatoid arthritis, and the activation of viruses such as influenza and HIV-I may be associated with overproduction (and/or overexposure) of oxygen free radicals and H_2O_2 supports this concept. A series of major questions arises from these arguments: (a) How and why are the homeostatic changes in aging initiated and stabilized? (b) Do age-associated changes in response to stress result in the decline in tissue function? (c) Can aged cells and tissues be induced to properly regulate their response to stress? (d) Are constitu-

tive levels of intrinsic factors (mediators) that elicit the response to stress increased to the extent that the aged tissues are in a state of chronic stress? (e) Is the combination of age-associated changes in mediator homeostasis and environmental pollutants a basis for the altered regulation of stress response genes?

References

Abate, C. L., Patel, L., Rauscher, F. J., III, & Curran, T. (1990). Redox regulation of fos and jun DNA-binding activity in vitro. *Science, 249,* 1157–1161.

Abravaya, K., Phillips, B., & Morimoto, R. I. (1991). Heat shock-induced interactions of heat shock transcription factor and the human hsp 70 promoter examined by in vivo footprinting. *Molecular and Cellular Biology, 11,* 586–592.

Abravaya, K., Myers, M. P., Murphy, S. P., & Morimoto, R. I. (1992). The heat shock protein hsp 70 interacts with HSF, the transcription factor that regulates heat shock gene expression. *Genes and Development, 6,* 1153–1164.

Amin, J., Ananthan, J., & Voellmy, R. (1988). Key features of heat shock regulatory elements. *Molecular and Cellular Biology, 8,* 3761–3769.

Ammendola, R., Mesuraca, M., Russo, T., & Cimino, F. (1992). Sp1 DNA binding efficiency is highly reduced in nuclear extracts from aged rat tissues. *Journal of Biological Chemistry, 267,* 17944–17948.

Angel, P., Imagaura, M., Chiu, R., Stein, B., Imbra, R. J., Rahmsdorf, H., Jonat, C., Herrlick, P., & Karin, M. (1987). Phorbol ester-inducible genes contain a common cis element recognized by a TPA modulated trans-acting factor. *Cell, 49,* 729–739.

Angel, P., Hattori, K., Smeal, T., & Karin, M. (1988). The jun proto-oncogene is positively autoregulated by its product, Jun/AP1. *Cell, 55,* 875–885.

Angelidis, C. E., Lazaridis, I., & Pagoulatos, G. N. (1991). Constitutive expression of heat shock protein 70 in mammalian cells confers thermoresistance. *European Journal of Biochemistry, 199,* 35–39.

Baeuerle, P. A. (1991). The inducible transcription activator NF kappa B: regulation by distinct protein subunits. *Biochimica et Biophysisca Acta, 1072,* 63–80.

Baeuerle, P. A., & Baltimore, D. (1988a). Activation of DNA-binding activity in the apparently cytoplasmic precursor of the NF kappa B transcription factor. *Cell, 53,* 211–217.

Baeuerle, P. A., & Baltimore, D. (1988b). I kappa B: a specific inhibitor of the nuclear factor kappa B transcription factor. *Science, 242,* 540–546.

Baeuerle, P. A., & Baltimore, D. (1989). A 65-kappa D subunit of active NF Kappa B is required for inhibition of NF Kappa B by I kappa B. *Genes and Development, 3,* 1689–1698.

Baeuerle, P. A., & Baltimore, D. (1991). Molecular aspects of cellular regulation. In P. Cohen & J. G. Faulkes (Eds.), *The Hormonal Control of Gene Transcription* (Vol. 6, pp. 409–432). Amsterdam: Elsevier, North Holland Biomedical Press.

Baeuerle, P. A., & Henkel, T. (1994). Function and activation of NF-kB in the immune system. *Annual Review in Immunology, 12,* 141–179.

Ballard, D. W., Dixon, E. P., Peffer, N. J., Bogerd, H., Doerre, S., Stein, B., & Greene, W. C. (1992). The 65-kDa subunit of human NF-kappa B functions as a potent transcriptional activator and a target for v-Rel-mediated repression. *Proceedings of the National Academy of Sciences of the United States of America, 89,* 1875–1879.

Bauskin, A. R., Alkalay, I., & Ben-Neriak, Y. (1991). Redox regulation of a protein tyrosine kinase in the endoplasmic reticulum. *Cell, 66,* 685–696.

Beg, A. A., & Baldwin, A. S., Jr. (1993). The IκB proteins: multifunctional regulators of Rel/NF-κB transcription factors. *Genes and Development, 7,* 2964–2970.

Beg, A. A., Ruben, S. M., Scheinman, F. I., Haskill, S., Rosen, C. A., & Baldwin, A. S., Jr. (1992). I kappa B interacts with the nuclear localization sequences of the subunits of NF-kappa B: a mechanism for cytoplasmic retention. *Genes and Development, 6,* 1899–1913.

Beg, A. A., Finco, T. S., Nantermet, P. V., & Baldwin, A. S., Jr. (1993). TNF and IL-1 lead to phosphorylation and loss of I kappa B alpha: a mechanism for NF kappa B activation. *Molecular and Cellular Biology, 13,* 3301–3310.

Bienz, M., & Pelham, H. R. B. (1986). Heat shock regulatory elements function as an inducible enhancer in the *Xenopus* hsp 70 gene and when linked to a heterologous promotor. *Cell, 45,* 753–760.

Binetruy, B., Smeal, T., & Karin, M. (1991). Ha-Ras augments c-jun activity and stimulated phosphorylation of its activation domain. *Nature, 351,* 122–127.

Blake, M. J., Gershon, J., Fargnoli, J., & Holbrook, N. J. (1990). Discordant expression of heat shock protein mRNAs in tissues of heat-stressed rats. *Journal of Biological Chemistry, 265,* 15275–15279.

Blake, M. J., Udelsman, R., Feulner, G. J., Norton, D. D., & Holbrook, N. J. (1991a). Stress-Induced heat shock protein 70 expression in adrenal cortex: An adrenocorticotropic hormone-sensitive, age-dependent response. *Proceedings of the National Academy of Sciences of the United States of America, 88,* 9873–9877.

Blake, M. J., Fargnoli, J., Gershon, D., & Holbrook, N. J. (1991b). Concomitant decline in heat induced hyperthermia and HSP 70 mRNA expression in aged rats. *American Journal of Physiology, 260,* R663–R667.

Blank, V., Kourilsky, P., & Israel, A. (1991). Cytoplasmic retention, DNA binding and processing of the NF kappa B p50 precursor are controlled by a small region in its c-terminus. EMBO *Journal, 10,* 4159–4167.

Blank, V., Kourilsky, P., & Israel, A. (1992). NF-kappa B and related proteins: Rel/dorsal homologies meet ankyrin-like repeats. *Trends in Biochemical Science, 17,* 135–140.

Bours, V., Villalobos, J., Burd, P. R., Kelly, K., & Siebenlist, U. (1990). Cloning of a mitogen-inducible gene encoding a kappa B DNA-binding protein with homology to the rel oncogene and to cell-cycle motifs. *Nature, 348,* 76–78.

Brown, K., Pank, S., Kanno, T., Franzoso, G., & Siebenlist, U. (1993). Mutual regulation of the transcriptional activator NF-kappa B and its inhibitor, I kappa B-alpha. *Proceedings of the National Academy of Sciences of the United States of America, 90,* 2532–2536.

Cantley, L., Auger, K. A., Carpenter, C., Duckworth, B., Graziani, A., Kaperley, R., & Soltoff, S. (1991). Oncogenes and signal transduction. *Cell, 64,* 281–302.

Carter, K. C., Post, D. G., & Papaconstantinou,

J. (1991). Differential expression of the mouse alpha 1-acid glycoprotein genes (AGP-1 and AGP-2) during inflammation and aging. *Biochimicaet Biophysica Acta, 1089,* 197–205.

Cerutti, P. A. (1985). Prooxidant states and tumor promotion. *Science, 227,* 375–381.

Cerutti, P. A., & Trump, B. F. (1991). Inflammation and oxidative stress in carcinogenesis. *Cancer Cells, 3,* 1–7.

Choi, H.-S., Lin, Z., Li, B., & Liu, A. Y.-C. (1990). Age-dependent decrease in the heat-inducible DNA sequence-specific binding activity in human diploid. *Journal of Biological Chemistry, 265,* 18005–18011.

Clos, J., Westwood, J. T., Becker, P. B., Wilson, S., Lambert, K., & Wu, C. (1990). Molecular cloning and expression of a hexameric *Drosophila* heat shock factor subject to negative regulation. *Cell, 63,* 1085–1097.

Cordle, S. R., Donald, R., Read, M. A., & Hawiger, J. (1993). Lipopolysaccharide induces phosphorylation of MADS and activation of c-Rel and related NF-kappa B proteins in human monocytic THP-1 cells. *Journal of Biological Chemistry, 268,* 11803–11810.

Craig, E. A., Weissman, J. S., & Harwich, A. L. (1994). Heat shock proteins and molecular chaperones: mediators of protein confirmation and turnover in the cell. *Cell, 78,* 365–372.

D'Costa, A. D., Breese, C. R., Boyd, R. L., Booze, R. M., & Sonntag, E. (1991). Attenuation of fos-like immunoreactivity induced by a single electroconvulsive shock in brains of aging mice. *Brain Research, 567,* 204–211.

Deguchi, Y., Negoro, S., Kishimoto, S. (1988). Age-related changes of heat shock protein gene transcription in human peripheral blood mononuclear cells. *Biochemical and Biophysical Research Communications, 157,* 580–584.

Derijard, B., Hibi, M., Wu, I. H., Barrett, T., Su, B., Deng, T., Karin, M., & Davis, R. J. (1994). JNK1: a protein kinase stimulated by UV light and Ha-Ras that binds and phosphorylates the c-jun activation domain. *Cell, 76,* 1025–1037.

Devary, Y., Gottlieb, R., Lau, L. F., & Karin, M. (1991). Rapid and preferential activation of the c-jun gene during the mammalian UV response. *Molecular and Cellular Biology, 11,* 2804–2811.

Devary, Y., Gottlieb, R. A., Smeal, T., & Karin, M. (1992). The mammalian ultraviolet response is triggered by activation of Src tyrosine kinases. *Cell, 71,* 1081–1091.

Diaz-Meco, M. T., Dominguez, I., Sanz, L., Dent, P., Lozano, J., Municio, M. M., Berra, E., Hay, R. T., Sturgill, T. W., & Moscat, J. (1994). ζPKC induces phosphorylation and inactivation of IκB-α *in vitro. EMBO Journal 13,* 2842–2848.

Dimri, G. P., & Campisi, J. (1994). Altered profile of transcription factor-binding activities in senescent human fibroblasts. *Experimental Cell Research, 212,* 132–140.

Dominguez, I., Sanz, L., Arenzana-Seisdedos, F., Diaz-Meco, M. T., Virelizier, J.-L., & Moscat, J. (1993). Inhibition of protein kinase C ζ subspecies blocks the activation of an NF-κB-like activity in *Xenopus laevis* oocytes. *Molecular and Cellular Biology, 13,* 1290–1295.

Faassen, A. E., O'Leary, J. J., Rodysill, K. J., Bergh, N., & Hallgren, H. M. (1989). Diminished heat-shock protein synthesis following mitogen stimulation of lymphocytes from aged donors. *Experimental Cell Research, 183,* 326–334.

Fargnoli, J., Kunisada, T., Fornace, A. J., Jr., Schneider, E. L., & Holbrook, N. J. (1990). Decreased expression of heat shock protein 70 mRNA and protein after heat shock in cells of aged rats. *Proceedings of the National Academy of Sciences of the United States of America, 87,* 846–850.

Fawcett, T. W., Sylvester, S. L., Sarge, K. D., Morimoto, R. I., & Holbrook, N. J. (1994). Effects of neurohormonal stress and aging on the activation of mammalian heat shock factor 1. *Journal of Biological Chemistry, 269,* 32272–32278.

Feuillard, J., Gouy, H., Bismuth, G., Lee, L. M., Debre, P., & Korner, M. (1991). NF kappa B activation by tumor necrosis factor alpha in the Jurkat T cell line is independent of protein kinase A, protein kinase C, and Ca(2+)-regulated kinases. *Cytokine, 3,* 257–265.

Finch, C. E., & Landfield, P. W. (1979). In C. E. Finch & E. L. Schneider (Eds.), *Handbook of the Biology of Aging* (pp. 567–594). New York: Van Nostrand Reinhold.

Finco, T. S., & Baldwin, A. S., Jr. (1993). κB site-dependent induction of gene expression by diverse inducers of nuclear factor kappa B requires Raf-1. *Journal of Biological Chemistry, 268,* 176/6–17679.

Fujita, T., & Maruyama, N. (1991). Elevated levels of c-jun and c-fos transcripts in the aged rat liver. *Biochemical and Biophysical Research Communications, 178*, 1485–1491.

Garcia-Morales, P., Minami, Y., Luong, E., Kausner, R. D., & Samelson, L. E. (1990). Tyrosine phosphorylation in T cells is regulated by phosphatase activity: studies with phenylarsine oxide. *Proceedings of the National Academy of Sciences of the United States of America, 87*, 9225–9259.

Gentz, R., Raucher, F. J., III, Abate, C., & Curran, T. (1989). Parallel association of Fos and Jun leucine zippers juxtaposes DNA binding domains. *Science, 243*, 1695–1699.

Gething, M. J., & Sambrook, J. (1992). Protein folding in the cell. *Nature, 355*, 33–34.

Ghosh, S., & Baltimore, D. (1990). Activation in vitro of nuclear factor kappa B by phosphorylation of its inhibitor I kappa B. *Nature, 344*, 678–682.

Ghosh, S., Giffor, A. M., Riviere, L. R., Tempst, P., Nolan, G. P., & Baltimore, D. (1990). Cloning of the p50 DNA binding subunit of NF-Kappa B: homology to rel and dorsal. *Cell, 62*, 1019–1029.

Gilmore, T. D. (1991). Malignant transformation by mutant Rel proteins. *Trends in Genetics, 7*, 318–322.

Grilli, M., Chiu, J. J.-S., & Lenardo, M. J. (1993). NFκB and Rel: Participants in a multiform transcriptional regulatory system. *International Reviews in Cytology, 143*, 1–62.

Hatada, E. N., Nieters, A., Wulczyn, F. G., Naumann, M., Meyer, R., Nucifora, G., McKeithan, T. W., & Scheidereit, C. (1992). The ankyrin repeat domains of the NF kappa B precursor p105 and the proto-oncogene bcl-3 act as specific inhibitors of NF kappa B DNA binding. *Proceedings of the National Academy of Sciences of the United States of America, 89*, 2489–2493.

Hayashi, T., Ueno, Y., & Okamoto, T. (1993). Oxidoreductive regulation of nuclear factor kappa B. Involvement of a cellular reducing catalyst thioredoxin. *Journal of Biological Chemistry, 268*, 11380–11388.

Heffetz, D., & Zick, Y. (1989). H_2O_2 potentiates phosphorylation of novel putative substrates for the insulin receptor kinase in intact Fao cells. *Journal of Biological Chemistry, 264*, 10126–10132.

Henkel, T., Zable, U., van Zee, K., Muller, J.,

Fanning, E., & Baeuerle, P. A. (1992). Intramolecular masking of the nuclear location signal and dimmerization domain in the precursor for the p50 nuclear factor kappa B subunit. *Cell, 68*, 1121–1133.

Heydari, A. R., Wu, B., Takahashi, R., Strong, R., & Richardson, A. (1993). Expression of heat shock protein 70 is altered by age and diet at the level of transcription. *Molecular and Cellular Biology, 13*, 2909–2918.

Hibi, M., Lin, A., Smeal, T., Minden, A., & Karin, M. (1993). Identification of an oncoprotein- and UV-responsive protein kinase that binds and potentiates the c-jun activation domain. *Genes and Development, 7*, 2135–2148.

Hoffman-Goetz, L., & Keir, R. (1984). Body temperature responses of aged mice to ambient temperature and humidity stress. *Journal of Gerontology, 39*, 547–551.

Hohmann, H.-P., Remy, R., Scheidereit, C., & VanLoon, A. P. G. M. (1991). Maintenance of NF-Kappa B activity is dependent on protein synthesis and the continuous presence of external stimuli. *Molecular and Cellular Biology, 11*, 259–266.

Holbrook, N. J., & Richardson, A. (1995). Heat-shock protein expression and aging. In Wiley-Liss (Ed.), *Modern Cell Biology Series: Cellular Aging and Cell Death* (pp. 67–80). New York, in press..

Holmgren, A. (1984). Enzymatic reduction-oxidation of protein disulfides by thioredoxin. *Methods in Enzymology, 107*, 295–351.

Holmgren, A. (1985). Thioredoxin. *Annual Review in Biochemistry, 54*, 237–271.

Holmgren, A. (1989). Thioredoxin and glutaredoxin systems. *Journal of Biological Chemistry, 264*, 13963–13966.

Hunter, T., & Karin, M. (1992). The regulation of transcription by phosphorylation. *Cell, 70*, 375–387.

Jakobsen, B. K., & Pelham, H. R. (1991). A conserved heptapeptide restrains the activity of the yeast heat shock transcription factor. *EMBO Journal, 10*, 369–375.

Johnson, P. F., & McKnight, S. L. (1989). Eukaryotic transcriptional regulatory proteins. *Annual Review in Biochemistry, 58*, 799–839.

Johnston, R. N., & Kucey, B. L. (1988). Competitive inhibition of hsp 70 gene expression causes thermosensitivity. *Science, 242*, 1551–1554.

Kaminska, B., & Kaczmarek, L. (1993). Robust induction of AP-1 transcription factor DNA binding activity in the hippocampus of aged rats. *Neuroscience Letters, 153,* 189–191.

Karin, M. (1992). Signal transduction from cell surface to nucleus in development and disease. *FASEB Journal, 6,* 2581–1590.

Karin, M., & Smeal, T. (1992). Control of transcription factors by signal transduction pathways: the beginning of the end. *Trends in Biochemical Science, 17,* 418–422.

Kerppola, T. K., & Curran, T. (1991). Transcription factor interactions: Basics on zippers. *Current Opinion in Structural Biology, 1,* 71–79.

Kerr, L. D., Inoue, J., Davis, N., Link, E., Baeuerle, P. A., Bose, H. R., Jr., & Verma, I. M. (1991). The rel-associated pp40 protein prevents DNA binding of Rel and NF-kappa B: relationship with I kappa B beta and regulation by phosphorylation. *Genes and Development, 5,* 1464–1476.

Kerr, L. D., Duckett, C. S., Wamsley, P., Zhang, Q., Chiao, P., Nabel, G., McKeithan, T. W., Baeuerle, P. A., & Verma, I. M. (1992). The proto-oncogene bcl-3 encodes an I kappa B protein. *Genes and Development, 6,* 2352–2363.

Kieran, M., Blank, V., Logeat, F., Vanderchove, J., Lottspeich, F., LeBail, O., Urban, M. B., Kowilsky, P., Baeuerle, P. A., & Israel, A. (1990). The DNA binding subunit of NF kappa B is identical to factor KBF1 and homologous to the rel oncogene product. *Cell, 62,* 1007–1018.

Kimball, S. R., Vary, T. C., & Jefferson, L. S. (1992). Age-dependent decrease in the amount of eukaryotic initiation factor 2 in various rat tissues. *Biochemical Journal, 286,* 263–268.

Kingston, R. E., Schuetz, T. J., & Larvin, Z. (1987). Heat-inducible human factor that binds to a human hsp 70 promoter. *Molecular and Cellular Biology, 7,* 1530–1534.

Kitrabi, E., Bozas, E., Philippidis, H., & Stylianopoulou, F. (1993). Age-related changes in IGF-II and C-Fos gene expression in the rat brain. *International Journal of Developmental Neuroscience, 11,* 1–9.

Koj, A. (1985). Acute Phase Reactants. In A. C. Allison (Ed.), *Structure and Function of Plasmal Proteins* (Vol. I, pp. 73–125). New York: Plenum Publishing Corp.

Kolesnick, R., & Golde, D. W. (1994). The sphingomyelin pathway in tumor necrosis factor and interleukin-1 signaling. *Cell, 77,* 325–328.

Kouzarides, T., & Ziff, E. (1988). The role of the leucine zipper in the fos-jun interaction. *Nature, 366,* 646–651.

Lamb, P., & McKnight, S. L. (1991). Diversity and specificity in transcriptional regulation: the benefits of heterotypic dimerization. *Trends in Biochemical Science, 16,* 417–423.

Landschulz, W. H., Johnson, P. F., & McKnight, S. L. (1988). The leucine zipper: a hypothetical structure common to a new class of DNA binding proteins. *Science, 240,* 1759–1764.

Lee, W., Mitchell, P., & Tjian, R. (1987). Purified transcription factor AP-1 interacts with TPA-inducible enhancer elements. *Cell, 49,* 741–752.

Lenardo, M. J., & Baltimore, D. (1989). NFκB: a pleiotropic mediator of inducible and tissue-specific gene control. *Cell, 58,* 227–229.

Lenardo, M. J., Fan, C.-m., Maniatis, T., & Baltimore, D. (1989). The involvement of NF kappa B in Beta-Interferon gene regulation reveals its role as widely inducible mediator of signal transduction. *Cell, 57,* 287–294.

Li, G. C., Li, L., Liu, Y.-K., Mak, J. Y., Chen, L., & Lee, W. M. F. (1991). Thermal response of rat fibroblast stably transfected with the human 70-kDa heat shock protein-encoding gene. *Proceedings of the National Academy of Sciences of the United States of America, 88,* 1681–1685.

Li, S. F., & Sedivy, J. M. (1993). Raf-1 protein kinase activates the NF-κB transcription factor by dissociation the cytoplasmic NFκB-IκB complex. *Proceedings of the National Academy of Sciences of the United States of America, 90,* 9247–9251.

Linquist, S. (1986). The heat-shock response. *Annual Review in Biochemistry, 55,* 1151–1191.

Liu, A. Y.-C., Lin, Z., Choi, H. S., Sorhage, F., & Li, B. (1989). Attenuated induction of heat shock gene expression in aging diploid fibroblasts. *Journal of Biological Chemistry, 264,* 12037–12045.

Liu, A. Y.-C., Choi, H. S., Lu, Y.-K., & Chen, K. Y. (1991). Molecular events involved in transcriptional activation of heat shock genes become progressively refractory to heat stimulation during aging of human diploid fibroblasts. *Journal of Cellular Physiology, 149,* 560–566.

Logeat, F., Israel, N., Ten, R., Blank, V., LeBail,

O., Kourilsky, P., & Israel, A. (1991). Inhibition of transcription factors belonging to the rel/NFκB family by a transdominant negative mutant. *EMBO Journal, 10*, 1827–1832.

Lozano, J., Berra, E., Municio, M. M., Diaz-Meco, M. T., Dominguez, I., Sanz, L., & Moscat, J. (1994). Protein kinase C ζ isoform is critical for κB-dependent promoter activation by sphingomyelinase. *Journal of Biological Chemistry, 269*, 19200–19202.

Luce, M. C., & Cristofalo, V. J. (1992). Reduction in heat shock gene expression correlates with increased thermosensitivity in senescent human fibroblast. *Experimental Cell Research, 202*, 9–16.

Lux, S. E., John, K. M., & Bennett, V. (1990). Analysis of cDNA for human erythrocyte ankyrin indicates a repeated structure with homology to tissue-differentiation and cell cycle control proteins. *Nature, 344*, 36–42.

Machleidt, T., Wiegmann, K., Henkel, T., Schutze, S., Baeuerle, P. A., & Kronke, M. (1994). Sphingomyelinase activates proteolytic I kappa B-alpha degradation in a cell-free system. *Journal of Biological Chemistry, 269*, 13760–13765.

Matthews, J. R., Wakasugi, N., Virelizier, J.-L., Yodoi, J., & Hay, R. J. (1992). Thioredoxin regulates the DNA binding activity of NF-Kappa B by reduction of a disulphide bond involving cysteine 62. *Nucleic Acids Research, 20*, 3821–3838.

Meichle, A., Shutze, S., Hansel, G., Brunsing, D., & Kronke, M. (1990). Protein kinase c-independent activation of NFκB by tumor necrosis factor. *Journal of Biological Chemistry, 265*, 8339–8343.

Meister, A. (1991). Glutathione deficiency produced by inhibition of its synthesis, and its reversal, applications in research and therapy. *Pharmacology & Therapeutics, 51*, 155–194.

Meister, A., & Anderson, M. E. (1983). Glutathione. *Annual Review in Biochemistry, 52*, 711–760.

Meyer, R., Hatada, E. N., Hohmann, H.-P., Haiker, M., Bartsch, C., Rothlisberger, U., Lahn, H.-W., Schlaeger, E. J., Van Loon, A. P. G. M., & Scheidereit, C. (1991). Cloning of the DNA-binding subunit of human NFκB: the level of its mRNA is strongly regulated by phorbol ester on tumor necrosis factor alpha. *Proceedings of the National Academy of Sciences of the United States of America, 88*, 966–970.

Minden, A., Lin, A., McMahon, M., Lange-Carter, C., D'erijard, B., Davis, R. J., Johnson, G. L., & Karin, M. (1994). Differential activation of ERK and JNK mitogen-activated protein kinases by Raf-1 and MEKK. *Science, 266*, 1719–1723.

Mizzen, L. A., Chang, C., Garrels, J. I., & Welch, W. J. (1989). Identification, characterization, and purification of two mammalian stress proteins present in mitochondria, grp 75, and a member of the hsp 70 family and hsp 58, a homolog of the bacterial gro EL protein. *Journal of Biological Chemistry, 264*, 20664–20675.

Morimoto, R. I. (1993). Cells in Stress: Transcriptional activation of heat shock genes. *Science, 259*, 1409–1410.

Morimoto, R. I., Tissieres, A., & Georgopoulos, C. (1990). In R. I. Morimoto, A. Tissieres, & C. Georgopoulos (Eds.), *Stress Proteins in Biology and Medicine* (pp. 1–30). Cold Spring Harbor, NY: Cold Spring Harbor Laboratory Press.

Morimoto, R. I., Sarge, K., & Abraya, K. A. (1992). Transcriptional regulation of heat-shock genes. A paradigm for inducible genomic responses. *Journal of Biological Chemistry, 267*, 21987–21990.

Mosialos, G., Hamer, P., Capobianco, A. J., Laursen, R. A., & Gilmore, T. D. (1991). A protein kinase-A recognition sequence is structurally linked to transformation by p59v-rel and cytoplasmic retention of p68c-rel. *Molecular and Cellular Biology, 11*, 5867–5877.

Mosser, D. D., Theodorakis, N. G., & Morimoto, R. I. (1988). Coordinate changes in heat shock element-binding activity and HSP 70 gene transcription rates in human cells. *Molecular and Cellular Biology, 8*, 4736–4744.

Mosser, D. D., Koztbauer, P. T., Sarge, K. D., & Morimoto, R. I. (1990). In vitro activation of heat shock transcription factor DNA-binding Isy calcium and biochemical conditions that affect protein confirmation. *Proceedings of the National Academy of Sciences of the United States of America, 87*, 3748–3752.

Mote, P. L., Grizzle, J. M., Walford, R. L., & Spindler, S. R. (1991). Aging alters hepatic expression of insulin receptor and c-jun mRNA in the mouse. *Mutation Research, 256*, 7–12.

Mueller, C. R., Maire, P., & Shibler, U. (1990). DBP, a liver-enriched transcriptional activator, is expressed late in ontogeny and its tissue specificity is determined posttranscriptionally. *Cell, 61*, 279–291.

Nabel, G. J., & Verma, I. M. (1993). Proposed NFκB/IκB family nomenclature. *Genes and Development, 7*, 2063.

Nakai, A., & Morimoto, R. I. (1993). Characterization of a novel chicken heat shock transcription factor, heat shock factor 3, suggests a new regulatory pathway. *Molecular and Cellular Biology, 13*, 1983–1987.

Nolan, G. P., Ghosh, S., Liou, H.-C., Tempst, P., & Baltimore, D. (1991). DNA binding and IκB inhibition of the cloned p65 subunit of NFκB, a rel-related polypeptide. *Cell, 64*, 961–969.

Nover, L. (1984). In *Heat Shock Response of Eucaryotic Cells*, Leipzig: VEB Georg, Theime.

Oeschsli, F. W., & Buechley, R. W. (1970). Excess mortality associated with three Los Angeles September hot spells. *Environmental Research, 3*, 277–284.

Oh, S. H., Deagen, J. T., Whanger, P. D., & Werving, P. H. (1978). Biological function of metallothionein v. its induction in rats by various stresses. *American Journal of Physiology, 234*, E282–E305.

O'Shea, E. K., Rutkowski, R., Stafford, W. F., III, & Kim, P. S. (1989). Preferential heterodimer formation by isolated leucine zippers from fos and jun. *Science, 245*, 646–648.

Pahlavani, M. A., Denny, M., Moore, S. A., Weindruch, R., & Richardson, A. (1995). The expression of heat shock protein 70 decreases with age in lymphocytes from rats and rhesus monkeys. *Experimental Cell Research*, in press.

Pang, J. W., & Chen, K. Y. (1993). A specific CCAAT-binding protein, CBP/tk, may he involved in the regulation of thymidine kinase gene expression in human IMR-90 diploid fibroblasts during senesence. *Journal of Biological Chemistry, 268*, 2909–2916.

Papaconstantinou, J. (1994). Unifying model of the programmed (intrinsic) and stochastic (extrinsic) theories of aging. *Annals of the New York Academy of Science, 719*, 195–211.

Pardue, S., Groshan, K., Roese, J. D., & Morrison-Bogorad, M. (1992). Hsp70 mRNA induction is reduced in neurons of aged rat hippocampus after thermal stress. *Neurobiology of Aging, 13*, 661–672.

Pare, W. P., & Galvin, G. B. (1986). Restraint stress in biomedical research: a review. *Neuroscience and Biobehavioral Reviews, 10*, 339–370.

Perisic, O., Xiao, H., & Lis, J. T. (1989). Stable binding of *Drosophila* heat shock factor to head-to-head and tail-to-tail repeats of a conserved 5 lsp recognition unit. *Cell, 59*, 797–806.

Post, D. J., Carter, K. C., & Papaconstantinou, J. (1991). The effect of aging on constitutive mRNA levels and LPS inducibility of acute phase genes. *Annals of the New York Academy of Science, 621*, 66–77.

Rabindran, S. K., Giorgi, G., Clos, J., & Wu, C. (1991). Molecular cloning and expression of a human heat shock factor, HSF1. *Proceedings of the National Academy of Sciences of the United States of America, 88*, 6906–6910.

Rabindran, S. K., Haroun, R. I., Clos, J., Wisniewski, J., & Wu, C. (1993). Regulation of heat shock factor trimes formation: role of a conserved leucine zipper. *Science, 259*, 230–234.

Rauscher, F. J., III, Voiulalas, P. J., Franza, B. J., Jr., & Curran, T. (1988). The fos complex and fos-related antigens recognize sequence elements that contain AP-1 binding sites. *Science, 239*, 1150–1153.

Riabowol, K. T. (1992). Transcription factor activity during cellular aging of human diploid fibroblasts. *Biochemistry and Cell Biology, 70*, 1064–1072.

Riabowol, K. T., Mizzen, L. A., & Welch, W. J. (1988). Heat shock is lethal to fibroblasts microinjected with antibodies against hsp 70. *Science, 242*, 433–436.

Riabowol, K., Schiff, J., & Gilman, M. Z. (1992). Transcription factor AP-1 activity is required for initiation of DNA synthesis and is lost during cellular aging. *Proceedings of the National Academy of Sciences of the United States of America, 89*, 157–161.

Rice, N. R., & Ernst, M. K. (1993). In vivo control of NFκB activation by IκBα. *EMBO Journal, 12*, 4685–4695.

Rittling, S. R., Brooks, K. M., Cristofalo, V. J., & Baserga, R. (1986). Expression of cell cycle dependent genes in young and senescent WI-38 fibroblasts. *Proceedings of the Nation-*

al Academy of Sciences of the United States of America, 83, 3316–3320.

Rose, D. W., McCabe, G., Feramisco, J. R., & Adler, M. (1992). Expression of c-fos and AP-1 activity in senescent human fibroblasts is not sufficient for DNA synthesis. Journal of Cell Biology, 119, 1405–1411.

Rosoff, P. M., Savage, N., & Dinarello, C. A. (1988). Interleukin-1 stimulates diacylglyceral production in T lymphocytes by a novel mechanism. Cell, 54, 73–81.

Ruben, S., Dillon, P. J., Schreck, R., Henke, T., Chen, C.-H., Maker, M., Baeuerle, P. A., & Rosen, C. (1991). Isolation of a Rel-related human cDNA that potentially encodes the 65 kD subunit of NF kappa B. Science, 251, 1490–1493.

Ruben, S. M., Narayanan, R., Klement, J. F., Chen, C.-H., & Rosen, C. A. (1992). Functional characterization of the NF-kappa B p65 transcriptional activator and an alternatively spliced derivative. Molecular and Cellular Biology, 12, 444–454.

Ryseck, R.-P., Bull, P., Takamija, M., Bours, V., Seibenlist, U. K., Dobrzanski, P., & Bravo, R. (1992). Molecular and Cellular Biology, 12, 674–684.

Sambucetti, L. C., Cherrington, J. M., Wilkinson, G. W., & Mocarski, E. S. (1989). NF-kappa B activation of the cytomegalovirus enhancer is mediated by a viral transactivator and by T cell stimulation. EMBO Journal, 8, 4251–4258.

Sarge, K. D., Zimarino, V., Holm, K., Wu, C., & Morimoto, R. I. (1991). Cloning and characterization of two mouse heat shock factors with distinct inducible and constitutive DNA binding ability. Genes and Development, 5, 1902–1911.

Sarge, K. D., Murphy, S. P., & Morimoto, R. I. (1993). Activation of heat shock gene transcription by heat shock factor 1 involves oligomerization, acquisition of DNA-binding activity and nuclear localization and can occur in the absences of stress. Molecular and Cellular Biology, 13, 1392–1407.

Schmid, R. M., Perkins, N. D., Duckett, C. S., Andrews, P. C., & Nabel, G. J. (1991). Cloning of an NF-kappa B subunit which stimulates HIV transcription in synergy with p65. Nature, 352, 733–736.

Schmitz, M. L., & Baeuerle, P. A. (1991). The p65 subunit is responsible for the strong transcription activating potential of NF κB. EMBO Journal, 10, 3805–3817.

Schmitz, M. L., Henkel, T., & Baeuerle, P. A. (1991). Rapid characterization of lambda cDNA clones after amplification and radioactive labeling with the PCR technique. Trends in Cell Biology, 1, 130–137.

Schreck, R., Rieber, P., & Baeuerle, P. A. (1991). Reactive oxygen intermediates as apparently widely used messengers in the activation of the NF-κB transcription factor and HIV-1. EMBO Journal, 10, 2247–2258.

Schreck, R., Albermann, K., & Baeuerle, P. A. (1992). Nuclear factor kappa B: an oxidative stress-responsive transcription factor of eukaryotic cells. Free Radical Research Communication, 17, 221–237.

Schutze, S., Nottrott, S., Pfizenmeier, K., & Kronke, M. (1990). Tumor necrosis factor signal transduction: all-type-specific activation and translation of protein kinase C. Journal of Immunology, 144, 2604–2608.

Schutze, S., Potthoff, K., Machleidt, T., Berkovic, D., Wiegmann, K., & Kronke, M. (1992). TNF activates NF-kappa B by phosphatidylcholine-specific phospholipase C-induced "acidic" sphingomyelin breakdown. Cell, 71, 765–776.

Schutze, T. J., Gallo, G. J., Sheldon, L., Tempst, P., & Kingston, R. E. (1991). Isolation of cDNA for HSF2: evidence for two heat shock factor genes in humans. Proceedings of the National Academy of Sciences of the United States of America, 88, 6911–6915.

Schutze-Osthoff, K., Bakker, A. C., Vanhaesebroeck, B., Jacob, W. A., & Fiers, W. (1992). Cytotoxic activity of tumor necrosis factor is mediated by early damage to mitochondrial functions-evidence for the involvement of mitochondrial radical generation. Journal of Biological Chemistry, 267, 5317–5323.

Sen, R., & Baltimore, D. (1986a). Multiple nuclear factors interact with the immunoglobulin enhancer sequences. Cell, 46, 705–716.

Sen, R., & Baltimore, D. (1986b). Inducibility of kappa immunoglobulin enhancer-binding protein NF-kappa B by a posttranslational mechanism. Cell, 47, 921–928.

Shirakawa, F., & Meijel, S. B. (1989). In vitro activation and nuclear translocation of NF κB catalyzed by cyclic AMP-dependent protein kinase and protein kinase C. *Molecular and Cellular Biology, 9,* 2424–2430.

Shock, N. W., Gerulich, R. C., Andres, R., Arenberg, D., Costa, P. T., Lacatta, E. G., & Tobin, J. D. (1984). *Normal Human Aging: The Baltimore Longitudinal Study of Aging.* Washington, DC: U.S. Government Printing Office.

Sierra, F., Fey, G. H., & Guigoz, Y. U. (1989). T-Kininogen gene expression is induced during aging. *Molecular and Cellular Biology, 9,* 5610–5616.

Sikora, E., Kaminska, B., Radziszewska, E., & Kaczmarek, L. (1992). Loss of transcription factor AP-1 DNA binding activity during lymphocyte aging in vivo. *FEBS Letters, 312,* 179–192.

Sikora, E., Radziszewska, E., Kmiec, T., & Maslinska, D. (1993). The impaired transcription factor AP-1 DNA binding activity in lymphocytes derived from subjects with some symptoms of premature aging. *Acta Biochimica Polonica, 40,* 269–272.

Sistonen, L., Sarge, K. D., Phillips, B., Abravaya, K., & Morimoto, R. I. (1992). Activation of heat shock factor 2 during hemin-induced differentiation of human erythroleukemia cells. *Molecular and Cellular Biology, 12,* 4104–4111.

Smeal, T., Binetrug, B., Mercola, D., Birrer, M., & Karin, M. (1991). Oncogenic and transcriptional cooperation with Ha-Ras requires phosphorylation of c-jun on serines 63 and 73. *Nature, 354,* 494–496.

Smeal, T., Binetrug, D., Mercola, D., Gropver-Bardwich, A., Heidecker, G., Rapp, U. R., & Karin, M. (1992). Oncoprotein-mediated signalling cascade stimulates c-jun activity by phosphorylation of serines 63 and 73. *Molecular and Cellular Biology, 12,* 3507–3513.

Song, C. A., Rao, T. R., Demyan, W. F., Mancini, M. A., Chatterjee, B., & Roy, A. K. (1991). *Endocrinology, 128,* 349–356.

Song, L., Stephens, J. M., Kittur, S., Collins, G. D., Nagel, J. E., Pekala, H., & Adler, W. H. (1992). Expression of c-fos, c-jun and jun B in peripheral blood lymphocytes from young and elderly adults. *Mechanisms of Aging and Development, 65,* 149–156.

Sorger, P. K., & Nelson, H. C. M. (1989). Trimerization of a yeast transcriptional activator via coiled-coil motif. *Cell, 59,* 807–813.

Sorger, P. K., & Pelham, H. R. B. (1988). Yeast heat shock factor is an essential DNA-binding protein that exhibits temperature-dependent phosphorylation. *Cell, 54,* 855–864.

Spindler, S. R., Grizzle, J. M., Walford, R. L., & Mote, P. L. (1991). Aging and restriction of dietary calories increases insulin receptor mRNA, and aging increases glucocorticoid receptor mRNA. *Journal of Gerontology, 46,* B233–B237.

Staal, F. J. T., Roederer, M., & Herzenberg, L. A. (1990). Intracellular thiols regulate activation of NF κB and transcription of human immunodeficiency virus. *Proceedings of the National Academy of Sciences of the United States of America, 87,* 9943–9947.

Stein, B., Rahmsdorf, H. J., Steffan, A., Liffin, M., & Herrlich, P. (1989). Cross-coupling of the NF κB p65 and Fos/Jun transcription factors produces potentiated biological function. *Molecular and Cellular Biology, 9,* 5169–5181.

Sun, G.-C., Ganchi, P. A., Ballard, D. W., & Greene, W. C. (1993). NF-kappa B controls expression of inhibitor I kappa B alpha: evidence for an inducible autoregulatory pathway. *Science, 259,* 1912–1915.

Supakar, P. C., Song, C. S., Jung, M. H., Slomczynska, M. A., Kim, J. M., Vellanoweth, R. L., Chatterjee, B., & Roy, A. K. (1993). A novel regulatory element associated with age-dependent expression of the rat androgen receptor. *Journal of Biological Chemistry, 268,* 26400–26408.

Takahashi, T., Schunkert, H., Isoyama, S., Wei, J. Y., Nadal-Ginard, B., Grossman, W., & Izumo, S. (1992). Age-related differences in the expression of proto-oncogene and contractile protein genes in response to pressure overload in rat myocardium. *Journal of Clinical Investigation, 89,* 939–946.

Ten, R. M., Paya, C. V., Israel, N., LeBail, O., Mattei, M.-G., Virelizier, J.-L., Kourilsky, P., & Israel, A. (1992). The characterization of the promoter of the gene encoding the p50 subunit of NFκB indicates that it participates in its own regulation. *EMBO Journal, 11,* 195–203.

Toledano, M. B., & Leonard, W. J. (1991). Modulation of transcription factor NFκB binding activity by oxidation-reduction in vitro. *Proceedings of the National Academy of Sciences of the United States of America, 88,* 4328–4332.

Turner, R., & Tjian, R. (1989). Leucine repeats and an adjacent DNA binding domain mediate the formation of functional c-fos/c-jun heterodimers. *Science, 243*, 1689–1694.

Udelsman, R., Blake, M. J., Stagg, C. A., Li, D., Putney, J., & Holbrook, N. J. (1993). Vascular heat shock expression in response to stress. *Journal of Clinical Investigation, 91*, 465–473.

Van Remmen, H., Ward, W., Sabia, R. V., & Richardson, A. (1994). Effect of age on gene expression and protein degradation. In E. J. Masaro (Ed.), *Handbook of Physiology, Volume on Aging.* New York: Oxford Press.

Visvanathan, K. V., & Goodbourn, S. (1989). Double-Stranded RNA activates binding of NFκB to an inducible element in the human beta-interferon promoter. *EMBO Journal, 8*, 1129–1138.

Welch, W. J. (1993). Heat shock proteins functioning as molecular chaparones: their roles in normal and stressed cells. *Philosophical Transactions of the Royal Society, London, 339*, 327–333.

Westwood, J. T., Clos, J., & Wu, C. (1991). Stress induced oligomerization and chromosomal relocation of heat-shock factor. *Nature, 353*, 822–827.

Wollner, L., & Spalding, J. M. K. (1978). In J. C. Broklehurst (Ed.), *Textbook of Geriatric Medicine and Gerontology* (pp. 245–267). Edinburgh: Livingstone.

Wulczyn, F. F., Naumann, M., & Scheidereit, C. (1992). Candidate pro-oncogene blc-3 encodes a subunit-specific inhibitor of transcription factor NF-kappa B. *Nature, 358*, 597–599.

Xanthoudakis, S., & Curran, T. (1992). Identification and characterization of Ref-1, a nuclear protein that facilitates AP-1 DNA-binding activity. *EMBO Journal, 11*, 653–665.

Xanthoudakis, S., Miao, G., Wang, F., Pan, Y.-C., & Curran, T. (1992). Redox activation of Fos-Jun DNA binding activity is mediated by a DNA repair enzyme. *EMBO Journal, 11*, 3323–3335.

Xiao, H. M., & Lis, J. T. (1988). Germline transformation used to define key features of heat-shock response elements. *Science, 239*, 1139–1142.

Xiao, H., Perisic, O., & Lis, J. T. (1991). Cooperative binding of *Drosophila* heat shock factor to arrays of a conserved 5 bp unit. *Cell, 64*, 585–593.

Zabel, U., & Baeuerle, P. A. (1990). Purified human I kappa B can rapidly dissociate the complex of the NF-kappa B transcriptional factor with its cognate DNA. *Cell, 61*, 255–265.

Zimarino, V., & Wu, C. (1987). Induction of sequence-specific binding of *Drosophila* heat shock activator protein without protein synthesis. *Nature, 327*, 727–730.

Zimarino, V., Tsai, C., Wu, C. (1990). Complex modes of heat shock factor activation. *Molecular and Cellular Biology, 10*, 752–759.

Nine

Protein Modifications with Aging

Rodney L. Levine and Earl R. Stadtman

I. Introduction

Age-dependent changes in the steady-state levels of particular proteins are well-documented, often being considered part of the continuum of developmental biology. These changes in content may be referred to as quantitative alterations in proteins. However, proteins may also exhibit changes in their function, including the alteration of receptors, enzymes, and structural proteins. Changes in function may be referred to as qualitative alterations in proteins, and this chapter focuses on qualitative changes during aging.

A change in function requires a change in shape or conformation. Proteins can often switch between specific conformations, each exhibiting different properties. Conformational switches can be induced through a variety of mechanisms, including the binding of small molecules or simply a change in pH. Covalent modifications also induce conformational changes, often reversibly. Phosphorylation of proteins is a well-known example of a method by which conformation and function are altered. While covalent modifications clearly induce conformational changes, it is traditional to reserve the term "confor-

mational change" for alterations that occur without covalent modification.

Thus, when a change in protein function is observed, one asks whether it is due to a conformational change or a covalent modification. The distinction is important because the underlying mechanisms of alteration are very different, and an understanding of the mechanism provides a basis for rational intervention in the process. Conformational changes can be induced by the binding of small molecules, such as the binding of oxygen or 2,3-diphosphoglycerate to hemoglobin. Such changes may also occur simply with the passage of time, as an equilibrium distribution of the conformer is reached. Suppose that (1) a protein may adopt either conformation A or conformation B, (2) the protein exists completely in conformation A at the time of synthesis, and (3) conformation B is thermodynamically favored so that it would account for 95% of the protein molecules at equilibrium. If this protein turns over much faster than it approaches equilibrium, then the cellular protein would exist predominantly as conformer A. However, if turnover is relatively slow, then conformer B will accumulate and eventually predominate. Thus, the "dwell

Handbook of the Biology of Aging, Fourth Edition

time" within the cell affects the distribution of conformers. A decrease in protein turnover increases the dwell time, providing one mechanism by which altered forms of proteins might accumulate in the cell during aging.

A. Conformational Changes

Changes in conformation or shape can be detected by a variety of techniques, many of which have been used extensively in the study of allosterically induced conformational changes. These include circular dichroism, sedimentation velocity, intrinsic fluorescence, ultraviolet spectroscopy (especially second-derivative spectroscopy), surface hydrophobicity, stability to heating, susceptibility to cleavage or clipping by proteases, affinity of ligands, and catalytic activity. If purified proteins from a young and an old animal differ in one of these properties, then a difference in shape must exist between the two preparations. While one or more of these techniques may establish the existence of a conformational change, it can be difficult to define the nature of that change in detail. To do so requires the determination of the three-dimensional structure of both forms of the protein. Three-dimensional structures can be determined by X-ray diffraction from crystals or by nuclear magnetic resonance spectroscopy in solution. At present there are no age-related changes in protein structure that have been established with these definitive techniques.

Unfortunately, the various available techniques may fail to detect conformational differences between proteins with dramatically different functional characteristics. For example, glutamine synthetase subjected to metal-catalyzed oxidation completely loses its catalytic activity. Yet neither circular dichroism nor sedimentation velocity measurements detected a difference between the native and the oxidized proteins (Rivett & Levine, 1990). Circular dichroism monitors the folding pattern of proteins, while the rate of sedimentation in an ultracentrifuge is particularly sensitive to the shape of the protein.

We must also stress that when a conformational change has been detected, one does not know whether this is a consequence of a simple change in shape or a consequence of a covalent modification.

B. Covalent Modifications

Detection of covalent modifications can be demanding and quite difficult, especially when one does not know the chemical nature of the modification. This is typically the case when comparing proteins from young and old animals. Obviously, the failure to detect a covalent modification with available techniques does not rule out the existence of the modification (Farber & Levine, 1986; Rivett & Levine, 1990).

There is no consensus on the techniques that should be used in the search for covalent modifications. However, the issue is receiving increased attention because of the need to compare natural proteins with those produced by recombinant techniques. One can anticipate that the methods used by pharmaceutical companies to characterize their recombinant products will provide a useful guide for researchers studying age-related changes in proteins.

After one has purified a protein from young and old animals, what methods should be used today in searching for covalent modifications? Obviously if one is interested in a particular modification, then one should use an assay specific for that modification. For example, phosphate analysis or labeling with radioactive phosphate could be used to establish differences in the phosphorylation of a protein. As already mentioned, one usually does not have a specific modification in mind when evaluating the purified proteins. In this case a variety of techniques are again available. Three techniques that are generally useful are (1) isoelectric focusing, (2) accurate determination of molecular weight, and (3) peptide mapping.

Isoelectric focusing determines the pH at which the protein carries no net charge, that is, the pH at which the number of negative charges equals the number of positive charges. Many covalent modifications change the isoelectric point of proteins, almost always making them more acidic. A change of a single charge on a protein is readily detected by isoelectric focusing. The technique is simple, inexpensive, and sensitive.

Advances in mass spectrometry now allow the determination of the molecular weight of proteins with remarkable accuracy (Biemann, 1992). These electrospray spectrometers are often expensive and require considerable expertise to operate, but they provide a mass accuracy of better than 0.02%. One can readily detect the conversion of a single methionine to methionine sulfoxide with confidence. The deamidation of an asparagine to aspartic acid (1-Da difference) or the oxidation of two cysteines to cystine (2-Da difference) would likely still be missed when working with an intact protein, but should be detected in smaller peptides. Nevertheless, it is still reasonable to compare the measured masses of the intact young and old proteins. A reproducible difference of 1 or 2 Da between the young and old forms should suggest such a modification.

Several manufacturers now offer a new class of mass spectrometers that are much cheaper and also much easier to operate. These utilize lasers to induce a charged form of the protein, and they measure the mass of the protein by determining the time required for the protein to strike a target. These instruments are referred to by the acronym MALDI-TOF, which stands for matrix-assisted laser desorption ionization–time of flight. While these instruments do not have the mass accuracy of the more expensive electrospray instruments, they can be used for the determina-

tion of differences in mass between young and old proteins. This should allow the detection of conversion of a single methionine to methionine sulfoxide. The phosphorylation or nitration of a single residue would be easily detected.

Peptide mapping involves cleavage of the protein by chemical or enzymatic means, followed by separation of the peptide mixture by high-pressure liquid chromatography on a reverse-phase column. Peptides are usually detected by their ultraviolet absorption, typically at 210 nm. Covalent modifications are detected by a difference in the elution time of a specific peptide from the young and old proteins. This is a sensitive and useful technique, but important covalent modifications can still be missed (Farber & Levine, 1986). Replacement of the ultraviolet absorption detector with an electrospray mass spectrometer provides a quantum increase in the ability to detect modifications. It is quite possible to detect changes of even 1 Da, so that the conversion of an asparagine to an aspartate could be appreciated.

II. Comparison of Proteins from Young and Old Animals

Analytical techniques for proteins have advanced quickly. As a consequence, there are few published reports that compare purified proteins from young and old animals with the tools mentioned earlier. However, differences in three characteristics have frequently been reported when comparing proteins from young and old animals, and assessment of these characteristics remains an important and simple approach to detecting age-related changes.

A. Specific Activity of Enzymes

First, purified enzymes from young and old animals may demonstrate different specific activities or catalytic efficiencies (Stadtman, 1988). In general the specific activity is lower for the enzyme from older animals, but one can anticipate examples in which it will be increased. Measurement of enzyme activity is usually quite simple, and the finding of a difference in specific activity establishes the existence of a conformational or covalent modification.

B. Altered Heat Stability

Second, proteins from young and old animals may differ in their susceptibility to denaturation by heat (Rothstein, 1984). In the case of a protein that is an enzyme, the assessment of heat denaturation is simple. One incubates the protein solution at an elevated temperature, often between 45 and 60°C. The rate of loss of enzymatic activity establishes the rate of irreversible heat denaturation. One can also determine the rate of heat denaturation for proteins without enzymatic activity, but the assays are more difficult and may require specialized instrumentation such as a calorimeter.

Again, the detection of a difference between the two proteins establishes the existence of a conformational or covalent modification. A homogeneous protein typically follows first-order kinetics during heat denaturation. In other words, a plot of time versus the percentage of native protein remaining will be a straight line when the y-axis is scaled logarithmically (Fig. 1). A change in the rate of heat denaturation will be reflected as a change in the slope of the plotted line. Sometimes the pattern observed in the protein from the older animal is biphasic (Fig. 1). This pattern is consistent with a preparation that contains two forms of the protein rather than one. Often the first phase of denaturation is much faster than the second, and the second may approximate the rate observed for the protein from the young animal. This pattern can be explained by the existence of a "young" form of protein, which is present exclusively in

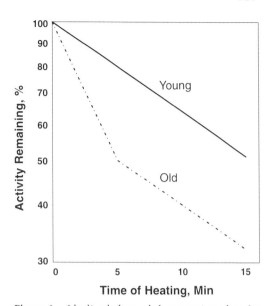

Figure 1. Idealized thermal denaturation plots for an enzyme purified from a young and an old animal (Rothstein, 1984). On this semilogarithmic plot, the loss of activity for the enzyme from the young animal is linear, while that from the old animal is biphasic, implying a molecular heterogeneity.

the preparation from the young animal and which accounts for part of the protein in the preparation from the old animal. The other part is contributed by an "old" form, which is more sensitive to heat denaturation.

C. Carbonyl Content

The third difference between proteins from young and old animals is an increase in the carbonyl content of proteins from older animals (Stadtman, 1992). In this context, carbonyl refers to aldehyde or ketone groups. As discussed in the following, carbonyl groups can be introduced into proteins by reaction with carbohydrates or lipids and by metal-catalyzed oxidation. Unlike specific activity or heat denaturation, the measurement of carbonyl groups usually has been carried out on crude homogenates rather than purified proteins. The carbonyl content of proteins increases dramatically during the last quarter of life

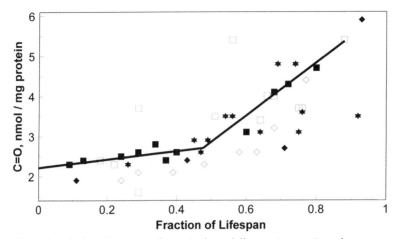

Figure 2. Carbonyl content of protein from different tissues. One observes a dramatic increase in oxidized protein during the last third of the lifespan. The data points were taken from published reports: ■, human dermal fibroblasts in tissue culture (Oliver, Ahn, Moerman, Goldstein, & Stadtman, 1987); ★, human lens (Garland, 1990); □, human brain obtained at autopsy (Smith, Carney, Starke-Reed, et al., 1991); ◆, rat liver (Starke-Reed & Oliver, 1989); and ◇, whole fly (Sohal, Agarwal, Dubey, & Orr, 1993).

span, a finding observed in rat liver, whole fly, human lens and brain, and cultured human fibroblasts (Fig. 2). This pattern implies a global change with age in the covalent modification of proteins.

III. Oxidative Modification of Proteins

The preceding section summarized three biochemical changes that are associated with aging: (1) decreased specific activity of enzymes; (2) altered heat stability of proteins; and (3) increased carbonyl content of proteins. All three of these alterations are also caused by exposing proteins to oxidizing systems *in vitro* (Fucci, Oliver, Coon, & Stadtman, 1983; Rivett & Levine, 1990). This is an important phenomenon that is now well-established experimentally, but that was not expected a priori. On the basis of specific assumptions, one can calculate that the oxidized protein content in an old animal represents at least 30–50% of the total protein content (Starke-Reed & Oliver, 1989; Stadtman, 1992). This estimate is consistent with the finding that the catalytic activity of many enzymes is decreased by 25–50% in old animals, while the level of immunotitratable protein of these enzymes is typically unchanged during aging. Thus, during aging there is quantitative agreement between the levels of less active enzymes and oxidatively modified proteins. At present, we consider oxidative modification to be a unifying concept that facilitates the study and understanding of alterations in proteins during aging. The discussion that follows thus summarizes current information on oxidative modification of proteins.

A. Direct Oxidation of Amino Acid Residues

Some of the more common modifications of proteins elicited by reactive oxygen species are shown in Table I (Stadtman, 1995).

Table I
Oxidative Modification of Protein Amino
Acid Residues

Residue	Oxidation products[a]
Histidine	Aspartic acid, asparagine, 2-oxohistidine
Tyrosine	3,4-Dihydroxyphenylalanine (DOPA), Tyr–Tyr cross-links
Phenylalanine	2-, 3-, and 4-hydroxyphenylalanine
Tryptophan	N-Formylkynurenine, kynurenine, 2-, 4-, 5-, and 6-hydroxytryptophan
Valine	3-Hydroxyvaline
Leucine	3- and 4-hydroxyleucine
Lysine	2-Aminoadipic semialdehyde
Arginine	Glutamic semialdehyde
Proline	Glutamic semialdehyde, pyroglutamic acid, 2-pyrrolidone, 4-hydroxyproline
Glutamic acid	4-Hydroxyglutamic acid, pyruvate α-ketoglutaric acid
Threonine	2-Amino-3-ketobutyric acid
Methionine	Methionine sulfoxide, methionine sulfone
Cysteine	Disulfides Cys-S-S-Cys, Cys-S-S-R

[a]For references, see Stadtman (1990, 1995).

Of these, the conversion of histidine residues to asparagine, aspartic acid, or 2-oxohistidine is of particular importance since histidine residues of proteins are readily oxidized by hydroxyl radical, singlet oxygen, and ozone. Also, because histidine residues are often at the metal-binding sites of proteins, they are among the residues most likely to be modified by metal-catalyzed oxidation systems. Curiously, tryptophan, phenylalanine, tyrosine, and methionine are preferred targets for hydroxyl radical, ozone, and singlet oxygen, but they are not major targets of metal-catalyzed oxidation systems under physiological conditions, presumably because they are not normally present at metal-binding sites.

B. Metal-Catalyzed Oxidation

A significant, and perhaps the most important, source of oxygen free radical damage to proteins is that mediated by metal-catalyzed oxidation systems. These include a number of enzymic and nonenzymic systems capable of catalyzing the reduction of Fe(III) or Cu(II), the reduced forms of which can interact with peroxides to yield reactive oxygen species (OH, ferryl ion, alkoxy radicals) that attack the side chains of amino acid residues at the metal-binding sites. The enzymatic metal-catalyzed oxidation systems include a number of flavoproteins such as xanthine oxidase, cytochrome P_{450}, enzymes, NADH and NADPH oxidases, and other oxidases in combination with nonheme iron proteins (Oliver, Fulks, Levine, et al., 1984; Stadtman, 1990).

Because the substrates for a particular enzyme can protect that enzyme from oxidation by metal-catalyzed oxidation systems, it follows that mutations that affect the concentration, catalytic activity, or regulatory elements of one enzyme in a metabolic pathway may determine the steady-state concentration of the substrates for other enzymes in the pathway and thereby govern their vulnerability to oxidative damage.

In addition to the enzymic metal-catalyzed oxidation systems, any compound capable of reducing Fe(III) or Cu(II) can catalyze the oxidation of proteins in the presence of O_2 and Fe(III) or Cu(II) (Stadtman, 1990, 1992). Ascorbate and mercaptans are such compounds, and they have been widely used in the construction of metal-catalyzed oxidation systems for studies of oxygen free radical damage to protein, lipids, and nucleic acid. To protect themselves from damage by active oxygen species, biological systems have evoked a battery of so-called antioxidant enzymes including superoxide dismutase, glutathione peroxidase, catalase, glutathione *S*-transferases, peroxidases, and the recently identified thiol-specific antioxidant enzyme (Kim, Kim, Lee, Rhee, & Stadtman, 1988). These together with a host of low-molecular-weight compounds, such as ascorbate, glutathione, β-carotene, α-tocopherol, uric acid, quercitin, and bilirubin, serve as scavengers of reactive oxygen species.

Changes in specific proteins observed during aging can be mimicked *in vitro* by the exposure of the purified protein to metal-catalyzed oxidation systems (Fucci, Oliver, Coon, & Stadtman, 1983; Rivett & Levine, 1990). For example, during aging the specific activity of malic enzyme from rat liver decreased by 35% while the number of measurable histidine residues decreased by one (Gordillo, Ayala, F-Lobato, Bautista, & Machado, 1988). Exposure of malic enzyme purified from young animal to metal-catalyzed oxidation caused a decrease of 35% in specific activity and a loss of one histidine residue. Taking another example, during the aging of humans (15–95 years) one can observe a doubling of serum paramagnetic copper content and a tripling of the carbonyl content of serum ceruloplasmin, the major copper-containing protein (Musci, di Patti, Fagiolo, & Calabrese, 1993). Exposure of ceruloplasmin from young individuals to metal-catalyzed oxidation induced both of these changes.

C. Peptide Bond Cleavage

In addition to oxidation of the side chains of amino acid residues, exposure of proteins to oxidizing species leads to the cleavage of some peptide bonds. Peptide bond cleavage occurs by at least four different pathways: (1) the α-amidation pathway, (2) the diamide pathway, (3) the glutamate-specific pathway, and (4) the proline-specific cleavage pathway. The contributions of each type of peptide bond cleavage can be deduced from a quantitative analysis of the products obtained following acid hydrolysis of the protein fragments. Such analyses have not yet been reported during aging, but would be welcome in assessing the impact of oxidative stress during aging. In this context, it is noteworthy that hydrogen peroxide is produced in the α-amidation and glutamate-specific peptide bond cleavage reactions.

D. Glycation and Glycoxidation

Reaction of reducing sugars with proteins creates a variety of modified proteins, many of which have been implicated in diseases associated with aging. This subject was discussed in detail in the previous edition of this Handbook, and that chapter remains a useful reference (Lee & Cerami, 1990). One reaction pathway is initiated by interaction between the sugar and protein molecules. In this process, referred to as glycation (Figure 3), lysine residues and N-terminal amino groups of proteins react with the carbonyl groups of reducing sugars to form Schiff base adducts. Schiff bases readily undergo Amadori rearrangements to yield ketoamines. These Amadori products are highly sensitive to metal-catalyzed glycoxidation, leading to either N^ϵ-carboxymethyllysine derivatives of the protein or to further reactions with arginine residues of proteins to form the pentosidine protein cross-linked derivative (Monnier, 1990). In addition to pentosidine, the Amadori products may undergo dehydration–oxidation to form polycarbonyl derivatives of poorly defined structures. These are referred to collectively as Maillard products or advanced glycosylation end products (AGEs). As shown in the upper pathway of Figure 3, the modifica-

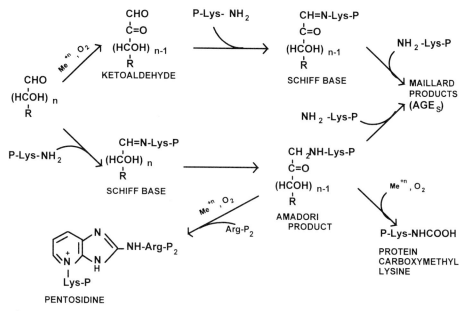

Figure 3. Protein adducts produced by reactions with carbohydrates. Abbreviations: AGE, advanced glycolation end products; Me^{n+}, a metal cation with charge n; P-Lys-NH$_2$, α-amino group of a lysine residue in protein; P$_2$-Arg, arginine residue in another protein molecule.

tion of proteins can also be induced by the metal-catalyzed oxidation of sugars to give ketoaldehydes (Wolff, Jiang, & Hunt, 1991). This reaction emphasizes the interaction of metal-catalyzed oxidations and the Maillard reactions (Wolff, Jiang, & Hunt, 1991; Kristal & Yu, 1992). Advanced glycosylation products may also generate reactive oxygen species in the absence of metal ions (Uchida & Stadtman, 1993).

It is well-established that the levels of advanced glycosylation products increase with aging and are likely implicated in diabetes and eye disorders (Monnier, 1990; Wells-Knecht, Huggins, Dyer, Thorpe, & Baynes, 1993; Makita, Vlassara, Rayfield, et al., 1992; Vlassara, 1994). Studies have also implicated these products in the accumulation of amyloid in Alzheimer's disease (Vitek, Bhattacharya, Glendening, et al., 1994). Circulating AGE-modified hemoglobin doubles in patients with diabetes (Makita, Vlassara, Rayfield, et al., 1992), a process that can be blunted by the

administration of aminoguanidine (Brownlee, Vlassara, Kooney, Ulrich, & Cerami, 1986). In addition to decreasing the formation of AGE-modified proteins, aminoguanidine ameliorates the pathological modifications induced by diabetes in experimental animals (Makita, Vlassara, Rayfield, et al., 1992; Vlassara, 1994). Clinical trials of aminoguanidine in humans are now in progress (Bucala, Makita, Vega, et al., 1994).

E. Modification by Lipid Oxidation Products

Malondialdehyde and α,β-unsaturated aldehydes are produced during the oxidation of polyunsaturated fatty acids. Because it possesses two aldehyde groups, malondialdehyde can react with one or two lysine amino groups of a given protein molecule or just one lysine amino group in each of two different protein molecules to form inter- or intramolecular Schiff base cross-linkages, respectively. Of greater biological interest are the highly cytotoxic α,β-unsaturated aldehydes, such as 4-hydroxy-2-nonenal. As shown in Figure 4, the ε-amino group of lysine residues, the sulfhydryl groups of cysteine residues, and the imidazole moiety of histidine residues may all undergo Michael addition reactions with the α,β-double bond of hydroxynonenal to form the corresponding secondary amine, thioester, and tertiary amine derivatives, respectively (Uchida & Stadtman, 1993; Szweda, Uchida, Tsai, & Stadtman, 1993; Jurgens, Lang, & Esterbauer, 1986). The free aldehyde groups of these Michael addition conjugates can undergo secondary reactions with free amino groups (i.e., ε-amino groups of lysine residues and unblocked N-terminal amino groups) of the same or another protein molecule to form highly fluorescent intra- or intermolecular cross-linkages. Reaction of the Michael addition products with free amino groups of a second protein molecule leads to the formation of either homo- or heterodimers and at high concentrations can yield cross-linked polymers of ever larger size (Uchida & Stadtman, 1993; Friguet, Stadtman, & Szweda, 1994).

IV. Molecular Mechanism of Oxidized Protein Accumulation

While one might hope to identify a single, specific cause of the accumulation of oxidized proteins, at present it seems more reasonable to view this as a phenotype that is expressed by multiple genotypes. A given genotype results from the progressive increase with age of free radical damage that leads randomly, one by one, to impairment in the expression of genes that govern the balance between protein oxidation and oxidized protein degradation. The rate of protein oxidation is a function of the relative concentrations of a multiplicity of prooxidants that mediate the oxidation of proteins on the one hand and the concentrations of antioxidants that scavenge reactive oxygen species or prevent their formation on the other. The combined effects of these factors are balanced against the rates of oxidized protein degradation, which are a function of the relative concentrations of several proteases that degrade oxidized proteins and a multiplicity of factors (inhibitors) that govern their catalytic activities.

It is generally recognized that impair-

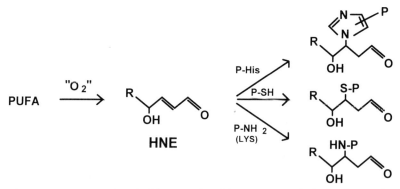

Figure 4. Protein carbonyl adducts produced by reaction with the lipid peroxidation product, 4-hydroxynonenal. Abbreviations: P-HN₂, α-amino group of a lysine residue in protein; PUFA, polyunsaturated fatty acid; HNE, hydroxynonenal; P-SH, sulfhydryl group of a cysteine residue in protein; P-His, imidazole group of a histidine residue in protein.

ment of the normal flow of electrons to oxygen by way of cytochrome C would favor the leakage of electrons from flavoproteins or coenzyme Q directly to oxygen, with the formation of $O_2^{\cdot-}$ and H_2O_2; however, it is not generally appreciated that metabolic defects that alter the steady-state levels of metabolites (such as lactate, pyruvate, crotonyl-CoA, acetoacetyl-CoA, or 3-phosphoglyceraldehyde) involved in oxidation–reduction steps in metabolism can also lead to changes in the redox state of the cell. This can lead to an increase in the steady-state levels of NADH and NADPH and, hence, to increased levels of reduced flavoprotein dehydrogenases, which in the absence of sufficient electron acceptor substrates may undergo the abortive transfer of electrons directly to oxygen to form $O_2^{\cdot-}$ and H_2O_2 or to Fe(III) to form Fe(II). Thus, mutations that affect either the normal flow of electrons in the terminal electron transport chain or the levels of metabolites that serve as substrates in oxidation–reduction steps in metabolism can lead to the production of active oxygen species.

V. Protein Degradation

As already noted, the accumulation of oxidized protein in the cell reflects the relative rates of protein oxidation, as determined by the combined effects of all prooxidant and antioxidant activities in the cell and the rate of degradation of oxidized protein. Unfortunately, knowledge about the latter is very limited. It is known that many oxidized proteins are more susceptible than their native counterparts to degradation by most proteases, and especially by the 19S-multicatalytic cytosolic proteases (Rivett, 1986; Pacifici, Salo, & Davies, 1989; Levine, 1989; Stadtman, 1990; Giulivi & Davies, 1993; Dean, Gieseg, & Davies, 1993). It is also established that the susceptibility of oxidized proteins to proteolytic degradation is influenced by the extent of oxidative damage (Rivett &

Levine, 1990) and that oxidized cross-linked forms of some protein are almost completely resistant to proteolytic degradation (Grant, Jessup, & Dean, 1993). Some investigators have reported an age-dependent decline in protease activity, while others have not observed a change (Starke-Reed & Oliver, 1989; Carney, Starke-Reed, Oliver, et al., 1991; Agarwal & Sohal, 1994; Sahakian, Szweda, Friguet, Kitani, & Levine, 1995). The possibility that an age-related loss in neutral protease activity contributes to the accumulation of damaged protein with age is supported by the results of studies showing that the activity of the neutral protease activity in rat hepatocytes (Starke-Reed & Oliver, 1989) and human brain tissue declines with age (Smith, Carney, Starke-Reed, et al., 1991). In the case of rat hepatocytes, an inverse linear relationship was observed between the amount of abnormal protein that accumulated and the neutral protease activity (Stadtman & Oliver, 1991).

It is not known, however, whether the age-dependent loss of neutral protease activity is due to a decrease in the rate of protease synthesis, a decrease in protease activity as a result of posttranslational modifications (oxidation?), or the age-dependent accumulation of protease inhibitors. Several studies support the hypothesis that intracellular proteolysis declines with age as a consequence of changes in protease inhibitors. First, accumulation of protease inhibitors induces phenotypic changes associated with aging (Ivy, Schottler, Wenzel, Baudry, & Lynch, 1984; Ivy, Ihara, & Kitani, 1991). Administration of the inhibitor leupeptin to young rats caused the accumulation of lipofuscin in liver, brain, and retina and caused the appearance in the brain of immunoreactivity to the abnormal tau protein found in paired helical filaments in Alzheimer's disease. Second, oxidative reactions can give rise to inhibitors of the purified multicatalytic protease (Rivett, 1985; Friguet,

Stadtman, & Szweda, 1994). Oxidation of lipids releases reactive compounds, notably 4-hydroxynonenal, which is known to react with macromolecules, including proteins (Esterbauer, Schaur, & Zollner, 1991). When glucose-6-phosphate dehydrogenase was modified by 4-hydroxynonenal, it became a poor substrate for the multicatalytic protease. However, the modified protein or an early proteolytic product was a potent inhibitor of the degradation of the oxidized glutamine synthetase used in the present studies (Friguet, Stadtman, & Szweda, 1994). Other oxidized proteins appear to be incompletely degraded (Grant, Jessup, & Dean, 1992, 1993), and it is possible that the residual products may be inhibitory. Third, Sierra and colleagues demonstrated dramatic increases in T-kininogen in the serum and liver of old rats. The content of this cysteine protease inhibitor in livers from 24-month-old animals was 6–7 times that found at 10 months (Sierra, Coeytaux, Juillerat, Ruffieux, Gauldie, & Guigoz, 1992). There was also an age-dependent increase in serum T-kininogen, with an extremely steep rise in the few months before death. This dramatic increase during the last 20% of life span is similar to that observed for protein carbonyl groups in several species and organs (Fig. 2). The similarity of the patterns is consistent with a causal relationship, but this possibility has not been tested experimentally. The steep increase that occurs toward the end of life span underscores the point that a modest extension of life span could dramatically affect the results of assays performed at a fixed age, possibly accounting for the differences in measured protease activity reported by different investigators (Sahakian, Szweda, Friguet, Kitani, & Levine, 1995).

VI. Conclusion

It is evident from the preceding considerations that an overwhelming number of factors are potentially involved in determining the accumulation of oxidized proteins. Mutations that affect any one of these factors can contribute to the rate at which proteins and other biomolecules are oxidized. Thus, mutations that affect the expression of enzymes or regulatory proteins that are involved in a multitude of physiological processes may affect the rate at which proteins and other biomolecules are oxidized. Among these processes are (1) oxidation–reduction steps in intermediary metabolism; (2) the transfer of electrons in the respiratory chain; (3) the induction and repression of cytochrome P_{450} enzymes, oxidases, nonheme iron proteins, xanthine oxidase, and NAD(P)H oxidases; (4) the uptake, sequestration, and translocation of iron and copper ions; (5) the synthesis and regulation of antioxidant enzymes (such as superoxide dismutase, glutathione peroxidase, catalase, glutathione-S-transferases, and the thiol-specific antioxidant enzyme); (6) the synthesis, uptake, and metabolism of low-molecular-weight antioxidant, free radical scavengers (such as glutathione, ascorbate, and β-carotene); (7) the activities of enzymes in metabolic pathways that determine the levels of enzyme substrates and, hence, the vulnerability of specific enzymes to oxidation by metal-catalyzed oxidation systems; (8) the synthesis and turnover of intracellular proteinases that catalyze the degradation of oxidized proteins; and (9) the production and destruction of inhibitors or activators of various proteases.

In view of the fact that between 10,000 and 100,000 DNA bases undergo oxygen free radical-mediated modifications per cell per day (Ames, Sigenaga, & Hagen, 1993), it seems reasonable that the failure to repair even a small fraction of this DNA damage over time could lead progressively and in random fashion to the impairment of some of the large number of enzymes and regulatory factors that collectively dictate the rate of protein oxidation and the degradation of oxidized protein. This is the basis of a more generalized concept that the age-related accumulation of oxidized proteins is due to the progressive accumulation of a multiplicity of genetic defects that leads (1) to an increase in the rate of production of reactive oxygen species, (2) to a decrease in the antioxidant defense systems, or (3) to a decrease in the ability to degrade oxidized proteins. The many resultant genotypes yield a common phenotype, namely, the accumulation of oxidatively modified proteins within the cell.

References

Agarwal, S., & Sohal, R. S. (1994). Aging and proteolysis of oxidized proteins. *Archives of Biochemistry and Biophysics, 309*, 24–28.

Ames, B. N., Sigenaga, M. K., & Hagen, T. M. (1993). Oxidants, antioxidants, and the degenerative diseases of aging. *Proceedings of the National Academy of Sciences of the United States of America, 90*, 7915–7922.

Biemann, K. (1992). Mass spectrometry of peptides and proteins. *Annual Review of Biochemistry, 61*, 977–1010.

Brownlee, M., Vlassara, H., Kooney, A., Ulrich, P., & Cerami, A. (1986). Aminoguanidine prevents diabetes-induced arterial wall protein cross-linking. *Science, 232*, 1629–1632.

Bucala, R., Makita, Z., Vega, G., Grundy, S., Koschinsky, T., Cerami, A., & Vlassara, H. (1994). Modification of low density lipoprotein by advanced glycation end products contributes to the dyslipidemia of diabetes and renal insufficiency. *Proceedings of the National Academy of Sciences of the United States of America, 91*, 9441–9445.

Carney, J. M., Starke-Reed, P. E., Oliver, C. N., Landrum, R. W., Cheng, M. S., Wu, J. F., & Floyd, R. A. (1991). Reversal of age-related increase in brain protein oxidation, decrease in enzyme activity, and loss in temporal and spatial memory by chronic administration of the spin-trapping compound N-tert-butyl-α phenylnitrone. *Proceedings of the National Academy of Sciences of the United States of America, 88*, 3633–3636.

Dean, R. T., Gieseg, S., & Davies, M. J. (1993). Reactive species and their accumulation on radical-damaged proteins. *Trends in Biochemical Sciences, 18*, 437–441.

Esterbauer, H., Schaur, R. J., & Zollner, H. (1991). Chemistry and biochemistry of 4-hydroxynonenal, malonaldehyde and related aldehydes. *Free Radical Biology and Medicine, 11*, 81–128.

Farber, J. M., & Levine, R. L. (1986). Sequence of a peptide susceptible to mixed function oxidation: Probable cation binding site in glutamine synthetase. *Journal of Biological Chemistry, 261*, 4574–4578.

Friguet, B., Stadtman, E. R., & Szweda, L. I. (1994). Modification of glucose-6-phosphate dehydrogenase by 4-hydroxy-2-nonenal: Formation of cross-linked protein which inhibits the multicatalytic protease. *Journal of Biological Chemistry, 269*, 21639–21643.

Fucci, L., Oliver, C. N., Coon, M. J., & Stadtman, E. R. (1983). Inactivation of key metabolic enzymes by mixed-function oxidation reactions: Possible implication in protein turnover and ageing. *Proceedings of the National Academy of Sciences of the United States of America, 80*, 1521–1525.

Garland, D. (1990). Role of site-specific, metal-catalyzed oxidation in lens-aging and cataract: a hypothesis. *Experimental Eye Research, 50*, 677–682.

Giulivi, C., & Davies, K. J. A. (1993). Dityrosine and tyrosine oxidation products are endogenous markers for selective proteolysis of oxidatively modified red blood cell hemoglobin by the 19S proteasome. *Journal of Biological Chemistry, 268*, 8752–8759.

Gordillo, E., Ayala, A., F-Lobato, M., Bautista, J., & Machado, A. (1988). Possible involvement of histidine residues in the loss of enzymatic activity of rat liver malic enzyme during aging. *Journal of Biological Chemistry, 263*, 8053–8057.

Grant, A. J., Jessup, W., & Dean, R. T. (1992). Accelerated endocytosis and incomplete catabolism of radical damaged protein. *Biochemica et Biophysica Acta, 1134*, 203–209.

Grant, A. J., Jessup, W., & Dean, R. T. (1993). Inefficient degradation of oxidized regions of protein molecules. *Free Radical Research Communications, 18*, 259–267.

Ivy, G. O., Schottler, F., Wenzel, J., Baudry, M., & Lynch, G. (1984). Inhibitors of lysosomal enzymes: Accumulation of lipofuscin-like dense bodies in the brain. *Science, 226*, 985–987.

Ivy, G. O., Ihara, Y., & Kitani, K. (1991). The protease inhibitor leupeptin induces several signs of aging in brain, retina and internal organs of young rats. *Archives of Gerontology and Geriatrics, 12,* 119–131.

Jurgens, G., Lang, J., & Esterbauer, H. (1986). Modification of human low-density lipoprotein by the lipid peroxidation product 4-hydroxynonenal. *Biochimica et Biophysica Acta, 875,* 103–114.

Kim, K., Kim, I.-H., Lee, K.-Y., Rhee, S. G., & Stadtman, E. R. (1988). The isolation and purification of a specific "protector" protein which inhibits enzyme inactivation by a thiol/Fe(III)/O_2 mixed-function oxidation system. *Journal of Biological Chemistry, 263,* 4704–4711.

Kristal, B. S., & Yu, B. P. (1992). An emerging hypothesis: Synergistic induction of aging by free radicals and Maillard reactions. *Journal of Gerontology Biological Sciences, 47,* B107–B114.

Lee, A. T., & Cerami, A. (1990). Modifications of proteins and nucleic acids by reducing sugars: Possible role in aging. In E. L. Schneider & J. W. Rowe (Eds.), *Handbook of the Biology of Aging* (pp. 116–130). San Diego: Academic Press.

Levine, R. L. (1989). Proteolysis induced by metal-catalyzed oxidation. *Cell Biology Reviews, 21,* 347–360.

Makita, Z., Vlassara, H., Rayfield, E., Cartwright, K., Friedman, E., Rodby, R., Cerami, A., & Bucala, R. (1992). Hemoglobin-AGE: A circulating marker of advanced glycosylation. *Science, 258,* 651–653.

Monnier, V. (1990). Nonenzymatic glycosylation, the Maillard reaction, and the aging process. *Journal of Gerontology Biological Sciences, 45,* B105–B111.

Musci, G., di Patti, M. C. B., Fagiolo, U., & Calabrese, L. (1993). Age-related changes in human ceruloplasmin. Evidence for oxidative modifications. *Journal of Biological Chemistry, 268,* 13388–13395.

Oliver, C. N., Fulks, R., Levine, R. L., Fucci, L., Rivett, A. J., Roseman, J. E., & Stadtman, E. R. (1984). Oxidative inactivation of key metabolic enzymes during aging. In A. K. Roy & B. Chatterjee (Eds.), *Molecular Basis of Aging* (pp. 235–262). New York: Academic Press.

Oliver, C. N., Ahn, B.-W., Moerman, E. J., Goldstein, S., & Stadtman, E. R. (1987). Age-related changes in oxidized proteins. *Journal of Biological Chemistry, 262,* 5488–5491.

Pacifici, R. E., Salo, D. C., & Davies, K. J. A. (1989). Macoxyproteinase (M.O.P.): A 670 kDa proteinase complex that degrades oxidatively denatured proteins in red blood cells. *Free Radical Biology and Medicine, 7,* 521–536.

Rivett, A. J. (1985). The effect of mixed-function oxidation of enzymes on their susceptibility to degradation by a nonlysosomal cysteine proteinase. *Archives of Biochemistry and Biophysics, 243,* 624–632.

Rivett, A. J. (1986). Regulation of intracellular protein turnover: Covalent modification as a mechanism of marking proteins for regulation. *Current Topics in Cellular Regulation, 28,* 291–337.

Rivett, A. J., & Levine, R. L. (1990). Metal-catalyzed oxidation of *Escherichia coli* glutamine synthetase: Correlation of structural and functional changes. *Archives of Biochemistry and Biophysics, 278,* 26–34.

Rothstein, M. (1984). Changes in enzymatic proteins during aging. In A. K. Roy & B. Chatterjee (Eds.), *Molecular Basis of Aging* (pp. 209–232). New York: Academic Press.

Sahakian, J. A., Szweda, L. I., Friguet, B., Kitani, K., & Levine, R. L. (1995). Aging of the liver: Proteolysis of oxidatively modified glutamine synthetase. *Archives of Biochemistry and Biophysics, 318,* 411–417.

Sierra, F., Coeytaux, S., Juillerat, M., Ruffieux, C., Gauldie, J., & Guigoz, Y. (1992). Serum T-kininogen levels increase two to four months before death. *Journal of Biological Chemistry, 267,* 10665–10669.

Smith, C. D., Carney, J. M., Starke-Reed, P. E., Oliver, C. N., Stadtman, E. R., Floyd, R. A., & Markesbery, W. R. (1991). Excess brain protein oxidation and enzyme dysfunction in normal aging and Alzheimer disease. *Proceedings of the National Academy of Sciences of the United States of America, 88,* 10540–10543.

Sohal, R. S., Agarwal, S., Dubey, A., & Orr, W. C. (1993). Protein oxidative damage is associated with life expectancy of houseflies. *Proceedings of the National Academy of Sciences of the United States of America, 90,* 7255–7259.

Stadtman, E. R. (1988). Protein modification in aging. *Journal of Gerontology Biological Sciences, 43,* B112–B120.

Stadtman, E. R. (1990). Metal ion-catalyzed oxidation of proteins: Biochemical mechanism and biological consequences. *Free Radical Biology and Medicine, 9,* 315–325.

Stadtman, E. R. (1992). Protein oxidation and aging. *Science, 257,* 1220–1224.

Stadtman, E. R. (1995). Role of oxidized amino acids in protein breakdown and stability. *Methods in Enzymology,* in press.

Stadtman, E. R., & Oliver, C. N. (1991). Metal-catalyzed oxidation of proteins. Physiological consequences. *Journal of Biological Chemistry, 266,* 2005–2008.

Starke-Reed, P. E., & Oliver, C. N. (1989). Protein oxidation and proteolysis during aging and oxidative stress. *Archives of Biochemistry and Biophysics, 275,* 559–567.

Szweda, L. I., Uchida, K., Tsai, L., & Stadtman, E. R. (1993). Inactivation of glucose-6-phosphate dehydrogenase by 4-hydroxy-2-nonenal. *Journal of Biological Chemistry, 268,* 3342–3347.

Uchida, K., & Stadtman, E. R. (1993). Covalent attachment of 4-hydroxynonenal to glyceral-dehyde-3-phosphate dehydrogenase. *Journal of Biological Chemistry, 268,* 6388–6393.

Vitek, M. P., Bhattacharya, K., Glendening, J. M., Stopa, E., Vlassara, H., Bucala, R., Manogue, K., & Cerami, A. (1994). Advanced glycation end products contribute to amyloidosis in Alzheimer disease. *Proceedings of the National Academy of Sciences of the United States of America, 91,* 4766–4770.

Vlassara, H. (1994). Recent progress on the biologic and clinical significance of advanced glycosylation end products. *Journal of Laboratory and Clinical Medicine, 124,* 19–30.

Wells-Knecht, M. C., Huggins, T. G., Dyer, G., Thorpe, S. R., & Baynes, J. W. (1993). Oxidized amino acids in lens protein with age. *Journal of Biological Chemistry, 268,* 12348–12352.

Wolff, S. P., Jiang, Z. Y., & Hunt, J. V. (1991). Protein glycation and oxidative stress in diabetes mellitus and ageing. *Free Radical Biology and Medicine, 10,* 339–352.

Ten

Genomic and Mitochondrial DNA Alterations with Aging

Kurt Randerath, Erika Randerath, and Charles Filburn

I. Introduction

The basic molecular mechanisms underlying the aging process are poorly understood. Two major types of aging theories have been proposed, namely, damage accumulation theories and genetic theories. Genomic damage, instability, and repair have been the subject of many studies and reviews, including a chapter in an earlier edition of this Handbook (Tice & Setlow, 1985). At that time and from other studies some examples of age-associated increases in damage were reported, but no clear, consistent pattern of increased damage, e.g., chromosomal aberrations, DNA crosslinks, and DNA strand breaks, was found (see Rattan, 1989). Although positive correlations were observed between DNA repair and life span in some studies, there was no general decline in overall DNA repair as a consequence of aging (Tice & Setlow, 1985). Since then, new and improved techniques for detecting altered bases or rearrangements in DNA have changed this picture considerably, particularly with respect to mitochondrial DNA (mtDNA). Clearly, some types of damage or mutations do increase in aging, while other alterations may actually decrease. These changes, particularly those linked to oxidative damage, will be the focus of this chapter. It still remains unclear to what extent changes in DNA repair account for age-associated increases in damage or mutations. The field of DNA repair is developing rapidly, with techniques that allow studies at the level of fine structure, where age-related changes may well emerge (Hanawalt *et al.*, 1992). This chapter will focus on alterations that are now known to occur in nuclear and/or mitochondrial DNA, with only a limited discussion of repair where appropriate.

II. Genomic DNA Alterations with Aging

A. Role of Oxidative Stress in DNA Damage and Aging

For the purpose of this article, two hypotheses in the category of damage accumulation, "the free radical theory of aging" (Harman, 1956) and the "DNA damage hypothesis of aging" (Szilard, 1959), are considered. On the other hand, a number of bulky endogenous DNA modifications (type I I-compounds) that increase with

Handbook of the Biology of Aging, Fourth Edition
Copyright © 1996 Academic Press, Inc. All rights of reproduction in any form reserved.

age cannot be explained in terms of these hypotheses and, therefore, are considered in the context of genetically programmed aging (Section I.E).

The free radical theory of aging is supported by the finding that the metabolic rate of various species (Cutler, 1984) and the formation of free radicals generated during oxygen metabolism (Sohal et al., 1989, 1990b) correlate inversely with lifespan. All aerobic organisms possess antioxidant defense systems (e.g., see Yu, 1993a) that appear to be in dynamic equilibrium with oxygen free radicals. Varying degrees of positive correlation were found between some antioxidant enzymes in some tissues and maximum lifespan potential (MLSP; Sohal et al., 1990), but without a clearcut relationship between overall level of antioxidant defenses and MLSP (Sohal, 1993). However, support for a major role for the defense system is indicated by the observation that overexpression of antioxidant enzymes in transgenic Drosophila increases lifespan (Orr & Sohal, 1994) while retarding age-related oxidative damage and increasing metabolic potential (Sohal et al., 1995). Because of their high reactivity, reactive oxygen species (ROS) are capable of modifying most biological molecules, including membrane lipids and DNA [reviewed in Yu (1993b); Bernstein & Gensler, 1993]. Thus, in 1981 Gensler and Bernstein (see Bernstein & Gensler, 1993) proposed that oxidative DNA damage is the primary cause of aging, on the basis of the two major premises that genomic DNA represents the master code for cellular messages and that only a limited number of DNA copies exist in diploid cells. According to this hypothesis, deterioration of the ability of DNA to be transcribed leads to a decline in cellular function and to lethality associated with aging. Likewise, Ames and Gold (1991) argue that endogenous oxidative DNA damage is a major contributor to aging and the degenerative diseases of aging, such as cancer.

B. Small DNA Oxidation Products

The hypothesis that oxidative DNA damage plays a critical role in aging is supported by experimental evidence, particularly with regard to small oxidative DNA lesions. Oxidized bases generated by intracellular oxidants are quantitatively the most important class of base modifications occurring in mammalian cells [reviewed in Marnett and Burcham (1993)]. Estimates of the total number of oxidized bases formed on a daily basis range from 10^4 to 10^6 per cell (Ames & Gold, 1991). The most likely source of ROS is leakage during oxidations in the mitochondria and the endoplasmic reticulum (see Marnett & Burcham, 1993).

The small DNA oxidation products thymine glycol, thymidine glycol, and hydroxymethyluracil were detected in the urine of both rats and humans, indicating DNA as the source (Ames et al., 1985), and the urinary levels of the two former compounds were found to correlate strongly with metabolic rate in mice, rats, monkeys, and humans (Adelman et al., 1988). 5-Hydroxymethyluracil was also assayed directly in rat liver and mammary gland DNA (Djuric et al., 1992). The level of the DNA oxidation product 8-hydroxydeoxyguanosine (8-OHdG) was reported to amount to eight adducts in 10^6 DNA nucleotides in the liver nuclear DNA of untreated rats (Richter et al., 1988). This oxidation product was found to increase during aging in rat organ DNA (Fraga et al., 1990) and to be enhanced in short-lived species displaying high metabolic rates (Ames & Gold, 1991). Analogous increases were found in the housefly (Agarwal & Sohal, 1994). Furthermore, repair glycosylases, which excise such oxidative DNA lesions, exhibit positive correlations with life span in a number of mammalian species [for references, see Bernstein and Gensler (1993)]. The loss of such a glycosylase specific for 8-OHdG leads to an appreciable increase in the spontaneous mutation rate (Michaels *et al.*, 1992), indicating the intrinsic mutagenic potential of this DNA lesion, which has also been demonstrated by others (e.g., see Marnett and Burcham, 1993). For a review of the experimental evidence documenting the mutagenicity of ROS in prokaryotic and eukaryotic cells, see Marnett and Burcham (1993).

Notably, mitochondrial DNA from rat liver was reported to display more than 10 times the level of oxidative DNA damage compared with nuclear DNA from the same tissue (Richter *et al.*, 1988); possible reasons for this difference are detailed in Section III. In addition to the small DNA oxidation products, oxidative stress induces DNA-reactive lipid peroxidation products, which give rise to DNA modifications, and other bulky DNA modifications (type II I-compounds). These DNA modifications are discussed in Sections II.C and II.D, respectively.

C. Cyclic Endogenous DNA Modifications Resulting from Lipid Peroxidation

Lipid peroxidation increases with age, as evidenced by the progressive accumulation of fluorescent lipofuscin in most tissues [for a review, see Yu (1993b)]. Many lipid peroxidation products, such as aldehydes, are highly reactive and can interact directly with DNA and cause genetic damage. Thus, genotoxic products of lipid peroxidation may be important mediators of oxidative stress. Malondialdehyde (MDA) is the most abundant carbonyl compound and the major mutagenic and carcinogenic product generated by lipid peroxidation [for references, see Chaudhary *et al.* (1994)]. Numerous studies have demonstrated that MDA content and production increase in aged tissues (see Yu, 1993b). The major MDA–DNA adduct 3-β-D-2'-deoxyribofuranosylpyrimido[1,2]-purin-10(3*H*)-one (M_1G-dR) was detected and quantified by a sensitive mass spec-

trometric method in human and rat livers, where it amounts to 1–2 modifications in 10^6 DNA nucleotides (Chaudhary *et al.*, 1994). This level is comparable to that of 8-OHdG in rat liver. Similarly, substituted exocyclic 1,N^2-propanodeoxyguanosine derivatives produced by the lipid peroxidation products acrolein and crotonaldehyde were detected by a combination of HPLC and ^{32}P-postlabeling as common endogenous DNA lesions in the livers of rodents and humans, with levels ranging from 0.2 to 2 modifications in 10^6 DNA nucleotides (Nath & Chung, 1994). Other DNA modifications presumably resulting from lipid peroxidation are exocyclic etheno derivatives of deoxyadenosine, deoxycytidine, and deoxyguanosine (see Marnett & Burcham, 1993). The cyclic nucleic acid adducts arising from lipid peroxidation are efficient premutagenic lesions and are repaired slowly (see Marnett & Burcham, 1993). While the age dependence of the formation of these DNA lesions has not been investigated yet, the increase in lipid peroxidation with age suggests that the adducts may likewise increase with age.

D. Bulky Endogenous DNA Modifications (I-Compounds)

1. Definition, Properties, and Types of I-Compounds

I-compounds are bulky covalent DNA modifications detected as modified deoxyribonucleotides by ^{32}P-postlabeling (K. Randerath *et al.*, 1981, 1992a; Reddy & Randerath, 1986), which accumulate with age in various tissues of unexposed laboratory animals and have, therefore, been termed indigenous (I) compounds (K. Randerath *et al.*, 1986, 1992a, 1993a). These DNA modifications occur in all rodent tissues studied, including liver, kidney, lung, skin, heart, colon, brain, spleen, mammary gland, uterus, ovary, and white blood cells, as well as in human brain (K. Randerath *et al.*, 1986, 1992a, 1993a,b). The number and levels of I-compounds are highest in metabolically active organs, i.e., liver and kidney. For example, total I-compound levels in liver and kidney DNA of 24-month-old male *ad libitum*-fed F344 rats amount to 1.1 and 1.6 modifications, respectively, in 10^7 DNA nucleotides, which exceeds the corresponding 1-month values by 2.3- and 5.2-fold (K. Randerath, *et al.*, 1993c). These findings support the original idea that I-compounds are derived from DNA-reactive intermediates generated during normal nutrient and oxygen metabolism. The wide range of polarities and the complexity of chromatographic profiles indicate that I-modifications represent diverse molecular structures and, hence, may be derived from different types of precursors (K. Randerath *et al.*, 1992a). The formation of I-compounds is determined by both genetic and environmental factors as, in addition to age, their profiles and levels depend on species, strain, tissue, gender, diet, time of day, and exposure to chemicals (K. Randerath *et al.*, 1986, 1992a, 1993b). The characteristic species- and tissue-dependent profiles distinguish I-compounds from exogenous carcinogen–DNA adducts, which almost invariably produce qualitatively identical patterns across tissues and species [reviewed in K. Randerath *et al.* (1992a, 1993a)]. Moreover, a number of I-compounds in rodent liver exhibit circadian variations, which are not observed for carcinogen–DNA adducts (Nath *et al.*, 1992). These findings imply that I-compound formation is primarily related to genetically determined normal metabolic activities rather than to exposure to unidentified environmental carcinogens.

Present knowledge regarding the origins of I-compounds comes largely from indirect experimental evidence, as the structural characterization of these DNA modifications represents a difficult task in view of insufficient sensitivity of available methodology. Two classes of I-compounds, types I and II, have been defined (K. Randerath *et al.*, 1993d, 1995; E. Randerath *et al.*, 1995a,b). Type I-compounds form as a consequence of normal metabolism and display positive linear correlations with median life span, while type II I-compounds represent bulky DNA lesions, which result from oxidative stress (K. Randerath *et al.*, 1991, 1993d, 1995; Chang *et al.*, 1993; E. Randerath *et al.*, 1995a) and also increase with age (K. Randerath, M. Gaeeni, G.-D. Zhou, and E. Randerath, in preparation). These two types of I-compounds can be readily distinguished on the basis of their different chromatographic properties on PEI–cellulose anion-exchange thin layers. While type I I-compounds are resolved by multidirectional PEI–cellulose anion-exchange TLC under standard conditions developed earlier (K. Randerath *et al.*, 1988, 1990, 1992a, 1993d), modified conditions, employing more dilute electrolyte/urea solutions, are utilized for separating type II I-compounds. The nature of type I and type II I-compounds is discussed further in Sections I.D.3 and I.D.4.

2. I-Compounds in Carcinogenesis, Preneoplasia, and Neoplasia

As detailed here, experimental evidence suggests that there is a progressive reduction in type I I-compound levels from the preneoplastic to the neoplastic stage. All carcinogens/tumor promoters studied thus far reduce the levels of most hepatic type I I-compounds [reviewed in K. Randerath *et al.* (1992a, 1993a)], including (i) the nonmutagenic carcinogens 2,3,7,8-tetrachlorodibenzo[*p*]dioxin (TCDD), choline-devoid diet, peroxisome proliferators, and carbon tetrachloride, (ii) the mutagenic carcinogens 2-acetylaminofluorene and 3-methylcholanthrene, and (iii) tumor promoters, such as certain polychlorinated dibenzofurans (PCDFs), Aroclor 1254, and phenobarbital. Reductions in I-compound levels are target organ-specific, as observed for TCDD (K. Randerath *et al.*, 1988, 1990), carbon tetrachloride (Nath *et al.*, 1990), and choline-devoid diet (Li *et al.,* 1990). As levels of individual I-compounds respond differentially to the preceding carcinogens/tumor promoters, the reduction in hepatic I-compound levels apparently is not merely a consequence of tissue proliferation, entailing dilution of modified with unmodified DNA; rather the formation and/or removal of I-compounds appear to be impaired. This idea is further supported by the findings that (i) the reduction in the levels of many I-compounds by carcinogens/tumor promoters is associated with changes in cytochrome P_{450} activities (Moorthy *et al.,* 1993), and (ii) in a series of PCDFs, I-compound-reducing activity parallels Ah receptor agonist activity (E. Randerath *et al.,* 1993). I-compound formation appears to become irreversibly impaired upon chronic carcinogen treatment, as the levels of these DNA modifications are not restored to normal values in rats switched from a choline-devoid diet to a choline-supplemented diet (Li *et al.,* 1990) or in mice after cessation of carbon tetrachloride exposure (Nath *et al.,* 1990). Smaller numbers and lesser amounts of I-compounds are found in target organs of spontaneous carcinogenesis prior to tumor appearance, and I-compounds are weak or undetectable in spontaneous hepatic adenomas of susceptible (C3H) mice and chemically induced rat hepatic tumors [reviewed in K. Randerath (1992a, 1993a)]. A lack of correlation between tumor growth rates and extent of I-compound depletion in Morris hepatomas further implicates impaired I-compound biosynthesis rather than cell proliferation as the primary mechanism underlying the loss of these DNA modifications. Thus, there appears to be an association between the permanent impairment of I-compound formation and malignant transformation.

3. Type I I-Compounds and Effects of Caloric Restriction

Caloric restriction (CR), the most effective measure to date to extend medium and maximum life spans of experimental animals, improve resistance to carcinogenesis, and retard the rate of age-associated degenerative processes [reviewed in Hart and Turturro (1993)], increases rather than decreases I-compound levels when compared to age-matched *ad libitum*-fed (AL) animals (K. Randerath *et al.,* 1993c,d). For example, in 24-month-old male CR F344 rats, total hepatic and renal DNA I-compound levels exceed the values in AL animals by 2.0 and 1.5 times, respectively. Levels of total and many individual I-compounds were found to increase linearly with age in the liver and kidney DNA of CR Brown–Norway (BN) and F344 rats, while I-compound levels in AL animals tend to plateau at an older age (K. Randerath *et al.,* 1993c). A comparative study (K. Randerath *et al.,* 1993d) in three strains of rats (BN, F344, and F344xBN) and two strains of mice (C57BL/6N and B6D2F1) at 24 and 20 months of age, respectively, showed liver and kidney I-compounds in both AL and CR animals to increase in the order F344 < BN < F344xBN and C57BL/6N < B6D2F1, paralleling strain-specific increases in median life span, with the DNA of the longest lived hybrid strains displaying the highest I-compound levels. Likewise, higher I-compound levels were present in the DNA of the longer lived CR animals. Furthermore, as revealed by linear regression analysis, the levels of many individual I-compound fractions in liver and kidney DNA of both rats and mice exhibit significant positive linear correlations with life span.

These results are remarkable; if these DNA modifications (hereafter termed type I I-compounds) were to represent DNA lesions, their formation would have been expected to be decreased rather than increased by CR, as CR reduces the levels of hydroxymethyluracil in rat liver and mammary gland (Djuric *et al.,* 1992) and that of 8-OHdG in rat liver nuclei (Chung *et al.,* 1992) by about 40% and 30%, respectively. Furthermore, measurement of unscheduled DNA synthesis indicates significantly enhanced repair of carcinogen-induced DNA damage in the cells of rodents fed CR diets as compared to cells isolated from AL animals [reviewed in Haley-Zitlin and Richardson (1993)]. Thus, type I I-compounds, being bulky DNA modifications that resemble carcinogen–DNA adducts in their chromatographic properties, do not appear to be amenable to CR-enhanced DNA repair. All results taken together suggest that type I I-compounds represent either innocuous or beneficial DNA modifications. A potential functional role of type I I-compounds is consistent with the observation of circadian rhythms in the regulation of the levels of I-compounds in rat and mouse livers (Nath et al., 1992). Moreover, in view of the opposite effects of carcinogenesis and CR on type I I-compound levels, these DNA modifications may conceivably play a protective role against malignant transformation, possibly via altered cell proliferation and gene expression, while at the same time being linked to normal aging (K. Randerath et al., 1993d).

Preliminary experiments to explore the potential nature of type I I-compounds (K. Randerath and E. Randerath, unpublished) showed that the majority of these DNA modifications do not represent age-dependent advanced glycosylation end products, i.e., derivatives resulting from the non-enzymatic reaction of glucose with DNA (Cerami, 1985). They are also unlikely to contain protein moieties, as their chromatographic properties are not affected by the presence or absence of proteinase K during DNA isolation. Moreover, they do not appear to contain common carbohydrate moieties, since their chromatographic properties are not changed by adding lectins during chromatography. However, in view of the induction of certain specific I-compounds in rat liver by oat lipids (Li et al., 1992) and the bulky/lipophilic properties of these DNA modifications, at least some type I I-compounds appear to be lipid derivatives. Lipid peroxidation, on the other hand, does not appear to be involved in the formation of type I I-compounds, as inferred from the increased levels of these DNA modifications in calorically restricted animals and the ability of CR to reduce lipid peroxidation (e.g., see Yu, 1993b). Furthermore, feeding a diet deficient in the antioxidant vitamin E, which is known to inhibit lipid peroxidation, does not decrease type I I-compound levels (Li et al., 1991). Also, hepatotoxins causing lipid peroxidation, such as carbon tetrachloride, peroxisome proliferators, and diquat, reduce rather than increase type I I-compound levels [reviewed in K. Randerath et al. (1992a, 1993a)].

4. Type II I-Compounds and Effects of Oxidative Stress

In vitro oxidation of DNA by the Fenton reaction (i.e., treatment with H_2O_2 and Fe^{2+} or Ni^{2+}) revealed the induction of two major and a number of minor bulky DNA oxidation products (K. Randerath et al., 1991; Chang et al., 1993), which were shown to represent specific intrastrand cross-links (K. Randerath et al., 1996). Notably, small base oxidation products, such as 8-OHdG and ribonucleotides, generated by the Fenton reaction can also be assayed by ^{32}P-postlabeling, but require different conditions for enzymatic DNA digestion, ^{32}P-labeling, and chromatography of the labeled products (K. Randerath et al., 1992b). Two major kidney I-compounds were found to be intensified severalfold after treatment of mice with the renal carcinogen and prooxidant nickel(II) acetate (Chang et al., 1993). Another renal carcinogen and prooxidant, ferric nitrilotriacetate (Fe-NTA) enhances the same two nonpolar I-compounds in rat kidney, but not in other organs (E. Randerath et al., 1995a; K. Randerath et al., 1995). In addition, Fe-NTA intensifies a polar I-compound, which is also identical to a DNA oxidation product generated by the Fenton reaction. On the other hand, two adducts induced by Fe-NTA were distinct from DNA modifications generated by the Fenton reaction and may have resulted from DNA–protein cross-links (Dizdaroglu, 1991) or the binding of lipid peroxidation products to DNA (e.g., see Marnett & Burcham, 1993). Oxidative enhancement of the various I-compounds amounted to 3.5- to 4.2-fold. However, chromatographic evidence indicates that these compounds are not derived from MDA, which would induce more polar products (Chaudhary et al., 1994). These experiments show that bulky oxidative DNA lesions, which have been termed type II I-compounds, arise by endogenous mechanisms and are intensified by carcinogens that induce oxidative stress in the target organ. In rats, hepatic type II I-compound levels increase by 2- to 3-fold between 1 and 24–36 months of age (E. Randerath, M. Gaeeni, G.-D. Zhou, and K. Randerath, unpublished). Interestingly, Fe-NTA, in addition to intensifying type II I-compounds, reduces the levels of three major type I I-compounds in kidney DNA by 47–78% (E. Randerath et al., 1995a,b). This effect is consistent with the depletion and permanent impairment of I-compound formation during hepatocarcinogenesis.

E. Conclusions

Genomic DNA contains two kinds of endogenous DNA modifications, both of which increase with age and are affected by environmental factors: (i) DNA lesions resulting from oxidative stress, such as small oxidized bases, modifications formed by lipid peroxidation products, and bulky type II I-compounds consisting in part of intrastrand cross-links, and (ii) type I I-compounds, which do not appear to represent DNA damage. Type II I-compounds are considered as DNA lesions since they are induced by prooxidant carcinogens in the target organ in parallel with small base

oxidation products and are presumably premutagenic in view of their bulky character and lack of repair, allowing their accumulation with age. Type I I-compounds appear to represent nondamaging DNA modifications, as CR increases rather than decreases their levels and as a majority of these modifications display positive linear correlations with median life span. The levels of these I-compounds are tightly controlled by an as yet unknown mechanism(s), as indicated by their circadian variation. Thus, it has been proposed (K. Randerath, 1993d) that type I I-compounds may be associated with genetically programmed aging and programmed metabolic and hormonal changes occurring during aging. The hypothesis that type I I-compounds are involved in programmed aging is supported by the irreversible losses of these modifications associated with cellular transformation. On the other hand, type I I-compounds may play a protective role against malignant transformation. Thus, the age-dependent increases in the different types of endogenous DNA modifications are consistent with both the oxidative DNA damage hypothesis of aging and a theory of programmed aging.

III. Mitochondrial DNA Damage

A. Molecular Characteristics

In order to fully appreciate the potential effects of damage to mitochondrial DNA (mtDNA), an awareness of its structure, genetic composition, and modes of transcription and replication is necessary. mtDNA from nematodes to vertebrates is a highly conserved, approximately 16-kb circular molecule that contains genes for 2 ribosomal and 22 transfer RNAs used in the translation of 13 mRNAs. These 13 mRNAs code for subunits of complexes of the electron transport chain and ATP synthase and are essential for oxidative phosphorylation. There are no introns, and less than 1 kb, located mainly in the triple-

et al., 1993). These facts, together with the presumption that mitochondria possessed minimal, if any, ability to repair their DNA, have been used in support of theories that damage to mtDNA and consequent energetic dysfunction play a major role in the aging process [for a thorough discussion of these theories, see DNAging, *Mutation Research*, Vol. 275, Nos. 3–6]. These predictions have been reinforced by the discovery that specific point mutations, in ways similar to deletions, cause mitochondrial myopathies, encephalopathies (Schon *et al.*, 1994), and diabetes (Wallace, 1992). In fact, the list of diseases in which mtDNA mutations of either type have been implicated continues to grow (Shoffner & Wallace, 1994). However, the expectation that point mutations would also increase markedly with age has not been supported consistently in the few studies that have addressed this question. Bodentich *et al.*, (1991) extensively sequenced human mtDNA derived from aged human ocular muscle and found only one base change. Similarly, Gadaleta *et al.* (1992) extensively sequenced clones of mtDNA derived from young and old rat brain and heart and found no base changes. These results are consistent with much earlier findings (Monnat, Maxwell, & Loeb, 1985; Monnat *et al.*, 1985) that mtDNA from various tissues of the same, middle-aged individual showed no differences in sequence. Furthermore, White and Bunn (1985) showed no changes with fibroblast age in a restriction fragment pattern with 19 restriction enzymes.

In contrast to these negative results, studies using PCR techniques to detect myopathic point mutations present a different picture. Munscher *et al.* (1993a) and Zhang *et al.* (1993) detected A to G mutations at nts 8344 and 3243, respectively, in the tissues of older adults, but not infants. These mutations were originally identified in maternally inherited myopathies (see Shoffner & Wallace, 1994). The 8344 mutation was estimated to reach levels of 2.0–2.4% of total mtDNA in extraocular muscles of older individuals (Munscher *et al.*, 1993a), while the 3243 mutation was estimated to reach 0.1% (Zhang *et al.*, 1993). In addition, Munscher *et al.* (1993b) detected various point mutations in tRNA genes of human mtDNA from aged subjects. At present, these contrasting results cannot be reconciled readily. Furthermore, it is not known whether point mutations in aged tissues are present in the mosaic pattern characteristic of deletions. If, in fact, levels of 0.1–2.4% occur at several different positions in the mitochondrial genome, the buildup of a substantial level of point mutations seems possible during aging. Alternatively, these particular mutations may be "hot-spots" where much higher rates of mutation occur due to more damage or less repair. Even more discriminating methods than those used in the latter two studies are needed and must be applied to various species and tissues to resolve this dilemma.

D. DNA Repair and 8-OHdG

It is clear from other studies, however, that considerably more DNA repair occurs in mitochondria than previously had been assumed. Pettepher *et al.* (1991) were the first to show the repair of streptozotocin-induced alkali-labile sites in mtDNA of a rat insulinoma cell line. In contrast, a lower level of repair was found for total nuclear DNA in these same cells. Similarly, LeDoux *et al.* (1992) showed efficient repair of *cis*-platin interstrand cross-links and *N*-methylpurines, but poor repair of pyrimidine dimers, complex alkylation damage, and *cis*-platin intrastrand cross-links in CHO cell mitochondria. Perhaps most importantly, Driggers *et al.* (1993) showed that alloxan-induced oxidative damage, in the form of abasic sites, sugar lesions, formamidopyrimidines, and 8-oxoguanines, was repaired within 4 hr in insulinoma cells. Thus, the dogma that mitochondria lack DNA repair is no longer tenable, particularly regarding oxidative damage.

Despite this clear evidence for repair, the level of 8-OHdG in mtDNA increases with age in rat liver (Ames et al., 1993), human diaphragm muscle (Hayakawa et al., 1992) and brain (Mecocci et al., 1993), and the housefly (Agarwal & Sohal, 1994). In the brain these increases were found almost exclusively in mtDNA, not nuclear DNA, and occurred only in older brains. In the housefly mtDNA was 3 times more susceptible to age-related oxidative damage than nuclear DNA. In addition, a decrease in the physical activity of the flies prolonged life span, while reducing the level of 8-OHdG in both nuclear and mtDNA (Agarwal & Sohal, 1994). I-compounds also increase with age in rat liver mitochondrial DNA (Gupta et al., 1990).

Although estimates of 8-OHdG levels vary significantly in these studies, perhaps due in part to differences in the techniques used and tissues examined, it is clear that marked age-associated increases occur in 8-OHdG in mtDNA. This could result from an age-dependent decrease in the repair of mtDNA or an increase in the rate of damage. In this regard, the studies of Sohal and others [reviewed in Sohal (1993)] are of particular interest. Of the various components studied in aging that contribute to overall oxidative stress, one consistent finding has been an age-dependent increase in the mitochondrial generation of reactive oxygen species (Sohal et al., 1989, 1990c). Since 8-OHdG is considered one of the major byproducts of oxidative damage, age-dependent increases in 8-OHdG in mtDNA may well result from an increase in mitochondrially derived reactive oxygen species without a compensatory increase in repair.

One prediction of theories that propose a major role for mtDNA damage in aging is that damage will enhance the production of oxy radicals, leading to even more damage. At present, no studies of oxy radical generation have been performed on tissues or cells known to harbor either deletions or point mutations. However, it is noteworthy that a strong correlation was reported between 8-OHdG content and deletion levels (Hayakawa et al., 1992), and a substantially greater increase with age of a deletion was observed in diseased hearts, which may be subject to repeated bouts of oxidative stress, versus normal hearts (Corral-Debrinski et al., 1992). One similarity that reports of deletion levels (Sugiyama et al., 1991) and 8-OHdG levels (Mecocci et al., 1993) have in common is the appearance of an exponential increase in levels at advanced ages, as might be expected if damage actually begets more damage.

E. Nuclear–Mitochondrial Interactions

While aberrant expression of mtDNA-encoded genes may play an important role in aging, overall mitochondrial function depends on the expression of a much larger component of nuclear-encoded genes in a coordinated interaction. The importance of potential changes in this interaction in aging was shown by intercellular transfer studies using skin fibroblasts and mtDNA-less (p⁰) HeLa cells (Hayashi et al., 1994). Age-associated decreases in cytochrome oxidase activity could not be attributed to changes in the number of mtDNA molecules or the presence of deletions, but were associated with a decrease in the overall protein synthesis of the mitochondria. Transfer experiments showed that mtDNA from fibroblasts from elderly donors was functionally normal, while HeLa cell nuclei restored cytochrome oxidase activity to deficient fibroblasts. Thus, the age-related phenotype resulted from changes in the nucleus, perhaps in a nuclear-recessive fashion (Hayashi et al., 1994). These surprising results indicate that the whole area of nuclear control of mitochondrial replication, transcription, and translation must now be investigated to adequately understand age-associated changes in energy metabolism.

F. Aging versus Disease

Many of the studies on age changes in mtDNA have attempted to use samples from apparently normal individuals or animals. The assumption that the results actually reflect the aging process and not some disease component is implicit, but not always easy to fully validate. The importance of this is illustrated by differences observed between normal and myopathic hearts (Corral-Debrinski *et al.*, 1992) and by a report on Alzheimer's disease (Corral-Debrinski *et al.*, 1994). In the latter study, levels of the common human deletion in mtDNA appear to show a biphasic response in particular brain regions, with an overall 15-fold increase above age-matched controls in younger Alzheimer's patients, but a subsequent decrease to a level below the now elevated levels in comparably aged controls. These results may reflect a role for oxidative stress in the disease, since levels of 8-OHdG are also elevated in Alzheimer's brains (Beal *et al.*, 1994). It is not clear whether or not the mtDNA damage plays a causal role, but it might if it results in damage that eventually results in the death of the cells involved. In this regard, Wolvetang *et al.* (1994) showed that inhibitors of electron transport complexes can induce apoptotic cell death in cultured cells. Although mutants that are lethal have not, because of their nature, been described in any mitochondrial diseases, it is quite possible that mtDNA damage may be of fundamental importance in tissues where compromised energy metabolism puts cells at risk for death, whether apoptotic or necrotic. The inability at present to prove this, because of the disappearance of the evidence, may remain one of fundamental problems in proving a role for mtDNA mutations in the final end point of the aging process.

G. Conclusion

Increases with age in alterations in mtDNA have been observed across several species. This includes increased levels of oxidized bases, especially 8-OHdG, which increases to a much greater extent in mtDNA than in nuclear DNA. Deletions of major portions of the mitochondrial genome increase with age, are most abundant in postmitotic tissues, and individually may increase by as much as 1000 to 10,000-fold. Despite this remarkable increase, the overall level of a given deletion-containing genome usually accounts for less than 0.1% of the total mtDNA in a tissue. However, histochemical studies suggest that these mutant genomes may be distributed in a mosaic manner and highly concentrated in individual cells in which energy metabolism may be compromised. The frequency of point mutations may increase with age, but at present this remains controversial. The overall mutational load in mtDNA in aged tissues remains unknown, with the possibility that a heterogeneous array of different mutations may exist in small, discrete populations of cells. Repair of oxidative damage to mtDNA occurs, but it is not known whether the age-associated increase in damage and mutations reflects only an increased rate of damage, decreased repair, or both.

References

Adelman, R., Saul, R. L., & Ames, B. N. (1988). Oxidative damage to DNA: Relation to species metabolic rate and lifespan. *Proceedings of the National Academy of Sciences of the United States of America, 85,* 2706–2708.

Agarwal, S., & Sohal, R. S. (1994). DNA oxidative damage and life expectancy in houseflies. *Proceedings of the National Academy of Sciences of the United States of America, 91,* 12332–12335.

Ames, B. N., & Gold, L. S. (1991). Endogenous mutagens and the causes of aging and cancer. *Mutation Research, 250,* 3–16.

Ames, B. N., Saul, R. L., Schwiers, E., Adelman, R., & Cathcart, R. (1985). Oxidative DNA damage as related to cancer and aging: assay of thymine glycol, thymidine glycol and hydroxymethyluracil in human and rat urine. In *Molecular Biology of Aging: Gene Stability and Gene Expression* (pp. 137–144). R. S. Sohal & R. G. Cutler (Eds.), New York: Raven Press.

Ames, B. N., Shigenaga, M. K., & Hagen, T. M. (1993). Oxidants, antioxidants, and the degenerative diseases of aging. *Proceedings of the National Academy of Sciences of the United States of America, 90*, 7915–7922.

Beal, M. F., MacGarvey, U., & Mecocci, P. (1994). Oxidative damage to mitochondrial DNA is increased in Alzheimer's disease. *Society for Neuroscience, Abstracts, 20*, 1675.

Bernstein, H., & Gensler, H. L. (1993). DNA damage and aging. In B. P. Yu (Ed.), *Free Radicals in Aging* (pp. 89–122). Boca Raton, FL: CRC Press.

Bodentich, A., Mitchell, L. G., & Merril, C. R. (1991). A lifetime of retinal light exposure does not appear to increase mitochondrial mutations. *Gene, 108*, 305–309.

Brossas, J. Y., Barreau, E., Courtois, Y., & Treton, J. (1994). Multiple deletions in mitochondrial DNA are present in senescent mouse brain. *Biochemical and Biophysical Research Communications, 202*, 654–659.

Cerami, A. (1985). Hypothesis: Glucose as a mediator of aging. *Journal of the American Geriatric Society, 33*, 626–634.

Chang, J., Watson, W. P., Randerath, E., & Randerath, K. (1993). Bulky DNA-adduct formation induced by Ni(II) in vitro and in vivo as assayed by ^{32}P-postlabeling. *Mutation Research, 291*, 147–159.

Chaudhary, A. K., Nokubo, M., Reddy, G. R., Yeola, S. N., Morrow, J. D., Blair, I. A., & Marnett, L. J. (1994). Detection of endogenous malondialdehde-deoxyguanosine adducts in human liver. *Science, 265*, 1580–1582.

Chen, X., Simonetti, S., DiMauro, S., & Schon, E. A. (1993). Accumulation of mitochondrial DNA deletions in organisms with various lifespans. *Bulletin of Molecular Biology and Medicine, 18*, 57–66.

Chung, M. H., Kasai, H., Nishimura, S., & Yu, B. P. (1992). Protection of DNA damage by dietary restriction. *Free Radical Biology & Medicine, 12*, 523–525.

Corral-Debrinski, M., Stepien, G., Shoffner, J. M., Lott, M. T., Kanter, K., & Wallace, D. C. (1991). Hypoxemia is associated with mitochondrial DNA damage and gene induction. *Journal of the American Medical Association, 266*, 1812–1816.

Corral-Debrinski, M., Horton, T., Lott, M. T., Shoffner, J. M., Beal, M. F., & Wallace, D. C. (1992). Mitochondrial DNA deletions in human brain: regional variability and increase with advanced age. *Nature Genetics, 2*, 324–329.

Corral-Debrinski, M., Horton, T., Lott, M. T., Shoffner, J. M., Mckee, A. C., Beal, M. F., Graham, B. R., & Wallace, D. C. (1994). Marked changes in mitochondrial DNA deletion levels in Alzheimer brains, *Genomics, 23*, 471–476.

Cortopassi, G. A., Shibata, D., Soong, N.-W., & Arnheim, N. (1992). A pattern of accumulation of a somatic deletion of mitochondrial DNA in aging tissues. *Proceedings of the National Academy of Sciences of the United States of America, 89*, 7370–7374.

Cutler, R. G. (1984). Antioxidants, aging and longevity. In *Free Radicals in Biology* (Vol. VI, pp. 371–428). New York: Academic Press.

Dizdaroglu, M. (1991). Chemical determination of free radical-induced damage to DNA. *Free Radical Biology & Medicine, 10*, 225–245.

Djuric, Z., Lu, M. H., Lewis, S. M., Luongo, D. A., Chen, X. W., Heilbrun, L. K., Reading, B. A., Duffy, P. H., & Hart, R. W. (1992). Oxidative DNA damage levels in rats fed low-fat, high-fat, or calorie-restricted diets. *Toxicology and Applied Pharmacology, 115*, 156–160.

Driggers, W. J., LeDoux, S. P., & Wilson, G. L. (1993). Repair of oxidative damage within the mitochondrial DNA of RINr 38 cells. *Journal of Biological Chemistry, 268*, 22042–22045.

Dunbar, D. R., Moonie, P. S., Swingler, R. J., Davidson, D., Roberts, R., & Holt, I. J. (1993). Maternally transmitted partial direct tandem duplication of mitochondrial DNA associated with diabetes mellitus. *Human Molecular Genetics, 2*, 1619–1624.

Edris, W., Burgett, B., Stine, O. C., & Filburn, C. R. (1994). Detection and quantitation of an age-associated increase in a 4.9-kb deletion in rat mitochondrial DNA. *Mutation Research, 316*, 69–78.

Fraga, C. G., Shigenaga, M. K., Park, J. W., Degan, P., & Ames, B. N. (1990). Oxidative damage to DNA during aging: 8-hydroxy-2'-deoxyguanosine in rat organ DNA and urine. *Proceedings of the National Academy of Sciences of the United States of America, 87*, 4533–4537.

Gadaleta, M. N., Rinaldi, G., Lezza, A. M. S., Milella, F., Fracasso, F., & Cantatore, P. (1992). Mitochondrial DNA copy number and mitochondrial DNA deletion in adult and senescent rats. *Mutation Research, 275*, 181–193.

Gupta, K. P., Van Golen, K. L., Randerath, E., & Randerath, K. (1990). Age-dependent covalent DNA alterations (I-compounds) in rat liver mitochondrial DNA. *Mutation Research, 237*, 17–27.

Haley-Zitlin, V., & Richardson, A. (1993). Effect of dietary restriction on DNA repair and DNA damage. *Mutation Research, 295*, 237–245.

Hanawalt, P. C., Gee, M., Ho, L., Hsu, R. K., & Kane, C. J. M. (1992). Genomic heterogeneity of DNA repair. *Annals of the New York Academy of Sciences, 663*, 17–25.

Harman, D. (1956). Aging: a theory based on free radical and radiation biology. *Journal of Gerontology, 11*, 298–300.

Hart, R. W., & Turturro, A. (Eds.) (1993). The Impact of Dietary Restriction on Genetic Stability. Special Issue. *Mutation Research, 295*, 149–292.

Hayakawa, M., Hattori, H., Sugiyama, S., & Ozawa, T. (1992). Age-associated oxygen damage and mutations in mitochondrial DNA in human hearts. *Biochemical and Biophysical Research Communications, 189*, 979–985.

Hayashi, J. I., Ohta, S., Kagawa, Y., Takai, O., Miyabayashi, S., Tada, K., Fukushima, H., Inui, K., Okada, S., Goto, Y., & Nonaka, I. (1994). Functional and morphological abnormalities of mitochondria in human cells containing mitochondrial DNA with pathogenic point mutations in tRNA. *Journal of Biological Chemistry, 269*, 19060–19066.

Katayama, M., Tanaka, M., Yamamoto, H., Ohbayashi, T., Nimura, Y., & Ozawa, T. (1991). Deleted mitochondrial DNA in the skeletal muscle of aged individuals. *Biochemistry International, 25*, 47–56.

Larsson, N. G., Holme, E., Kristiansson, B., Oldfors, A., & Tulinius, M. (1990). Progressive increase of the mutated mitochondrial DNA fraction in Kearns-Sayre syndrome. *Pediatric Research, 28*, 131–136.

LeDoux, S. P., Wilson, G. L., Beecham, E. J., Stevnsner, T., Wassermann, K., & Bohr, V. A. (1992). Repair of mitochondrial DNA after various types of DNA damage in Chinese hamster ovary cells. *Carcinogenesis, 13*, 1967–1973.

Lee, C. M., Eimon, P., Weindruch, R., & Aiken, J. M. (1994). Direct repeat sequences are not required at the breakpoints of age-associated mitochondrial DNA deletions in rhesus monkeys. *Mechanisms of Ageing and Development, 75*, 69–79.

Li, D., Xu, D., Chandar, N., Lombardi, B., & Randerath, K. (1990). Persistent reduction of I-compound levels in liver DNA from male Fischer rats fed choline-devoid diet and in DNA of resulting neoplasms. *Cancer Research, 50*, 7577–7580.

Li, D., Wang, Y.-M., Nath, R. G., Mistry, S., & Randerath, K. (1991). Modulation by dietary vitamin E of I-compounds (putative indigenous DNA modifications) of rat liver and kidney. *Journal of Nutrition, 121*, 65–71.

Li, D., Chen, S., Randerath, E., & Randerath, K. (1992). Oat lipid-induced covalent DNA modifications (I-compounds) in female Sprague-Dawley rats, as determined by ^{32}P-postlabeling. *Chemico–Biological Interactions, 84*, 229–242.

Marnett, L. J., & Burcham, P. C. (1993). Endogenous DNA adducts: Potential and paradox. *Chemical Research in Toxicology, 6*, 771–785.

Mecocci, P., MacGarvey, U., Kaufman, A. E., Koontz, D., Shoffner, J. M., Wallace, D. C., & Beal, M. F. (1993). Oxidative damage to mitochondrial DNA shows marked age-dependent increases in human brain. *Annals of Neurology, 34*, 609–616.

Melov, S., Hertz, G. Z., Stormo, G. D., & Johnson, T. E. (1994). Detection of deletions in the mitochondrial genome of *Caenorhabditis elegans. Nucleic Acids Research, 22*, 1075–1078.

Michaels, M. L., Cruz, C., Grollman, A. P., & Miller, J. H. (1992). Evidence that MutY and MutM combine to prevent mutations by an oxidatively damaged form of guanine in DNA. *Proceedings of the National Academy of Sciences of the United States of America, 89*, 7022–7025.

Monnat, R. J., Jr., & Loeb, L. A. (1985). Nucleotide sequence preservation of human mitochondrial DNA. *Proceedings of the National Academy of Sciences of the United States of America, 82,* 2895–2899.

Monnat, R. J., Jr., Maxwell, C. L., & Loeb, L. A. (1985). Nucleotide sequence preservation of human leukemic mitochondrial DNA. *Cancer Research, 45,* 1809–1814.

Moorthy, B., Chen, S., Li, D., & Randerath, K. (1993). 3-Methylcholanthrene-inducible liver cytochrome P450 in female Sprague-Dawley rats: Possible link between P450 turnover and formation of DNA adducts and I-compounds. *Carcinogenesis, 14,* 879–886.

Moraes, C. T., Ricci, E., Petruzzella, V., Shanske, S., DiMauro, S., Schon, E. A., & Bonilla, E. (1992). Molecular analysis of the muscle pathology associated with mitochondrial DNA deletions. *Nature Genetics, 1,* 359–367.

Muller-Hocker, J. (1989). Cytochrome *c* oxidase deficient cardiomyocytes in the human heart, An age-related phenomenon. *American Journal of Pathology, 134,* 1167–1171.

Muller-Hocker, J., Schneiderbanger, K., Stefani, F. H., & Kadenbach, B. (1992). Progressive loss of cytochrome *c* oxidase in the human extraocular muscles in ageing - a cytochemical–immunohistochemical study. *Mutation Research, 275,* 115–124.

Munscher, C., Muller-Hocker, J., & Kadenbach, B. (1993a). Human aging is associated with various point mutations in tRNA genes of mitochondrial DNA. *Biological Chemistry, Hoppe-Seyler, 374,* 1099–1104.

Munscher, C., Rieger, T., Muller-Hocker, J., & Kadenbach, B. (1993b). The point mutation of mitochondrial DNA characteristic for MERFF disease is found also in healthy people of different ages. *FEBS Letters, 317,* 27–30.

Nath, R. G., & Chung, F.-L. (1994). Detection of exocyclic 1,N^2-propanodeoxyguanosine adducts as common DNA lesions in rodents and humans. *Proceedings of the National Academy of Sciences of the United States of America, 91,* 7491–7495.

Nath, R. G., Li, D., & Randerath, K. (1990). Acute and long-term effects of carbon tetrachloride on DNA modifications (I-compounds) in male mouse liver. *Chemico–Biological Interactions, 76,* 343–357.

Nath, R. G., Vulimiri, S. V., & Randerath, K. (1992). Circadian rhythm of covalent modifications in liver DNA. *Biochemical and Biophysical Research Communications, 189,* 545–550.

Orr, W. C., & Sohal, R. S. (1994). Extension of lifespan by overexpression of superoxide dismutase and catalase in *Drosophila melanogaster. Science, 263,* 1128–1130.

Petruzzella, V., Moraes, C. T., Sano, M. C., Bonilla, E., DiMauro, S., & Schon, E. A. (1994). Extremely high levels of mutant mtDNAs co-localize with cytochrome oxidase-negative ragged-red fibers in patients harboring a point mutation at nt 3243. *Human Molecular Genetics, 3,* 449–454.

Pettepher, C. C., LeDoux, S. P., Bohr, V. A., & Wilson, G. L. (1991). Repair of alkali-labile sites within the mitochondrial DNA of RINr38 cells after exposure to the nitrosourea streptozotocin. *Journal of Biological Chemistry, 266,* 3113–3117.

Piko, L., Hongham, A. J., & Bulpitt, K. J. (1988). Studies of sequence heterogeneity of mitochondrial DNA from rat and mouse tissues: evidence for an increased frequency of deletions/additions with ageing. *Mechanisms of Ageing and Development, 43,* 279–293.

Poulton, J., Deadman, M. E., Bindoff, L., Morten, K., Land, J., & Brown, G. (1993). Families of mtDNA re-arrangements can be detected in patients with mtDNA deletions: duplications may be a transient intermediate form. *Human Molecular Genetics, 2,* 23–30.

Randerath, E., Randerath, K., Reddy, R., Narasimhan, T. R., Wang, X., & Safe, S. (1993). Effects of polychlorinated dibenzofurans on I-compounds in hepatic DNA of female Sprague-Dawley rats. Structure dependence and mechanistic considerations. *Chemico–Biological Interactions, 88,* 175–190.

Randerath, E., Watson, W. P., Zhou, G.-D., Chang, J., & Randerath, K. (1995a). Intensification and depletion of specific bulky renal DNA adducts (I-compounds) following exposure of male F344 rats to the renal carcinogen ferric nitrilotriacetate (Fe-NTA). *Mutation Research, 341,* 265–279.

Randerath, E., Zhou, G.-D., Hart, R. W., & Randerath, K. (1995b). Age-dependent indigenous covalent DNA modifications (I-compounds). In *Dietary Restriction: Implications for the Design and Interpretation of Toxicity and*

Carcinogenicity Studies (in press). Washington, DC: International Life Sciences Institute Press.

Randerath, K., Reddy, M. V., & Gupta, R. C. (1981). ^{32}P-Labeling test for DNA damage. Proceedings of the National Academy of Sciences of the United States of America, 78, 6126–6129.

Randerath, K., Reddy, M. V., & Disher, R. M. (1986). Age- and tissue-related DNA modifications in untreated rats: Detection by ^{32}P-postlabeling assay and possible significance for spontaneous tumor induction and aging. Carcinogenesis, 7, 1615–1617.

Randerath, K., Putman, K. L., Randerath, E., Mason, G., Kelley, M., & Safe, S. (1988). Organ-specific effects of long term feeding of 2,3,7,8-tetrachlorodibenzo-p-dioxin and 1,2,3,7,8-pentachlorodibenzo-p-dioxin on I-compounds in hepatic and renal DNA of female Sprague-Dawley rats. Carcinogenesis, 9, 2285–2289.

Randerath, K., Putman, K. L., Randerath, E., Zacharewski, T., Harris, M., & Safe, S. (1990). Effects of 2,3,7,8-tetrachlorodibenzo-p-dioxin on I-compounds in hepatic DNA of Sprague-Dawley rats: Sex-specific effects and structure-activity relationships. Toxicology and Applied Pharmacology, 103, 271–280.

Randerath, K., Yang, P.-F., Danna, T. F., Reddy, R., Watson, W. P., & Randerath, E. (1991). Bulky adducts detected by ^{32}P-postlabeling in DNA modified by oxidative damage in vitro. Comparison with rat lung I-compounds. Mutation Research, 250, 135–144.

Randerath, K., Li, D., Nath, R., & Randerath, E. (1992a). Exogenous and endogenous DNA modifications as monitored by ^{32}P-postlabeling: Relationships to cancer and aging. Experimental Gerontology, 27, 533–549.
Formation of ribonucleotides in DNA modified by oxidative damage in vitro and in vivo. Characterization by ^{32}P-postlabeling. Mutation Research, 275, 355–366.

Randerath, K., Li, D., Moorthy, B., & Randerath, E. (1993a). I-Compounds - Endogenous DNA markers of nutritional status, aging, tumor promotion and carcinogenesis. In D. H. Phillips, M. Castegnaro, & H. Bartsch (Eds.), Postlabeling Methods for Detection of DNA Adducts (IARC Scientific Publication No. 124, pp. 157–165). Lyon: International Agency for Research on Cancer.

Randerath, K., Putman, K. L., Osterburg, H. H., Johnson, S. A., Morgan, D. G., & Finch, C. E. (1993b). Age-dependent increases of DNA adducts (I-compounds) in human and rat brain DNA. Mutation Research, 295, 11–18.

Randerath, K., Hart, R. W., Zhou, G.-D., Reddy, R., Danna, T. F., & Randerath, E. (1993c). Enhancement of age-related increases in DNA I-compound levels by calorie restriction: Comparison of male B-N and F-344 rats. Mutation Research, 295, 31–46.

Randerath, K., Zhou, G.-D., Hart, R. W., Turturro, A., & Randerath, E. (1993d). Biomarkers of aging: Correlation of DNA I-compound levels with median lifespan of calorically restricted and ad libitum fed rats and mice. Mutation Research, 295, 247–263.

Randerath, K., Chang, J., & Randerath, E. (1995). Age-dependent DNA modifications (I-compounds): Effects of carcinogenesis and oxidative stress. In R. G. Cutler, L. Packer, J. Bertram, & A. Mori (Eds.), Oxidative Stress and Aging (pp. 77–87). Basel, Switzerland: Birkhauser Verlag.

Randerath, K., Randerath, E., Smith, C. V., & Chang, J. (1996). Structural origins of bulky oxidative DNA adducts (Type II I-compounds) as deduced by oxidation of oligonucleotides of known sequence. Chemical Research in Toxicology, in press.

Rattan, S. I. S. (1989). DNA damage and repair during cellular aging. International Reviews in Cytology, 116, 47–88.

Reddy, M. V., & Randerath, K. (1986). Nuclease P1-mediated enhancement of sensitivity of ^{32}P-postlabeling test for structurally diverse DNA adducts. Carcinogenesis, 7, 1543–1551.

Reynier, P., Figarella-Branger, D., Serratrice, G., Charvet, B., & Maltiery, Y. (1994). Association of deletion and homoplasmic point mutation of the mitochondrial DNA in an ocular myopathy. Biochemical and Biophysical Research Communications, 202, 1606–1611.

Richter, C., Park, J.-W., & Ames, B. N. (1988). Normal oxidative damage to mitochondrial and nuclear DNA is extensive. Proceedings of the National Academy of Sciences of the United States of America, 85, 6465–6467.

Schon, E. A., Hirano, M., & DiMauro, S. (1994). Mitochondrial encephalomyopathies: clinical and molecular analysis. Journal of Biomembrane Bioenergetics, 26, 291–299.

Shoffner, J. M., & Wallace, D. C. (1994). Oxidative phosphorylation diseases and mitochondrial DNA mutations: diagnosis and treatment. *Annual Review in Nutrition, 14,* 535–568.

Shoubridge, E. A. (1994). Mitochondrial DNA diseases: histological and cellular studies. *Journal of Biomembrane Bioenergetics, 26,* 301–310.

Shoubridge, E. A., Karpati, G., & Hastings, K. E. M. (1990). Deletion mutants are functionally dominant over wild type mitochondrial genomes in skeletal muscle fiber segments in mitochondrial disease. *Cell, 62,* 43–49.

Simonetti, S. X., Chen, S., DiMauro, & Schon, E. (1992). Accumulation of deletions in human mitochondrial DNA during normal aging: analysis by quantitative PCR. *Biochimica et Biophysica Acta, 1190,* 113–122.

Sohal, R. S. (1993). The free radical hypothesis of aging: an appraisal of the current status. *Aging and Clinical Experimental Research, 5,* 3–17.

Sohal, R. A., Svensson, I., Sohal, B. H., & Brunk, U. T. (1989). Superoxide radical production in different animal species. *Mechanisms of Ageing and Development, 49,* 129–135.

Sohal, R. S., Arnold, L. A., & Sohal, B. H. (1990a). Age-related changes in antioxidant enzymes and prooxidant generation in tissues of the rat with special reference to parameters in two insect species. *Free Radical Biology & Medicine, 9,* 495–500.

Sohal, R. S., Svensson, I., & Brunk, U. T. (1990b). Hydrogen peroxide production by liver mitochondria in different species. *Mechanisms of Ageing and Development, 53,* 209–215.

Sohal, R. S., Sohal, B. S., & Brunk, U. T. (1990c). Relationship between antioxidant defenses and longevity in different mammalian species. *Mechanisms of Ageing and Development, 53,* 217–227.

Sohal, R. S., Agarwal, A., Agarwal, S., & Orr, W. C. (1995). Simultaneous overexpression of copper- and zinc-containing superoxide dismutase and catalase retards age-related oxidative damage and increases metabolic potential in Drosophila melanogaster. *Journal of Biological Chemistry, 270,* 15671–15674.

Sugiyama, S., Hattori, K., Hayakawa, M., & Ozawa, T. (1991). Quantitative analysis of age associated accumulation of mitochondrial DNA with deletion in human hearts. *Biochemical and Biophysical Research Communications, 180,* 894–899.

Szilard, L. (1959). On the nature of the aging process. *Proceedings of the National Academy of Sciences of the United States of America, 45,* 30–45.

Tice, R. R., & Setlow, R. B. (1985). DNA repair and replication in aging organisms and cells. In C. E. Finch & E. L. Schneider (Eds.), *Handbook of the Biology of Aging* (pp. 173–224). New York: Van Nostrand Reinhold.

Wallace, D. C. (1992). Diseases of the mitochondrial DNA. *Annual Review in Biochemistry, 61,* 1175–1212.

Wallace, D. C., Ye, J. H., Neckelmann, S. N., Singh, G., Webster, K. A., & Greenberg, B. D. (1987). Sequence analysis of cDNAs for the human and bovine ATP synthase beta subunit: mitochondrial DNA genes sustain seventeen times more mutations. *Current Genetics, 12,* 81–90.

White, F. A., & Bunn, C. L. (1985). Restriction enzyme analysis of mitochondrial DNA in aging human cells. *Mechanisms of Ageing and Development, 30,* 153–168.

Wolvetang, E. J., Johnson, K. L., Krauer, K., Ralph, S. J., & Linnane, A. W. (1994). Mitochondrial respiratory chain inhibitors induce apoptosis. *FEBS Letters, 339,* 40–44.

Yu, B. P. (Ed.) (1993a). *Free Radicals in Aging.* Boca Raton, FL: CRC Press.

Yu, B. P. (1993b). Oxidative damage by free radicals and lipid peroxidation in aging. In B. P. Yu (Ed.), *Free Radicals in Aging* (pp. 57–88). Boca Raton, FL: CRC Press.

Zhang, C., Linnane, A. W., & Nagley, P. (1993). Occurrence of a particular base substitution (3243 A to G) in mitochondrial DNA of tissues of ageing humans. *Biochemical and Biophysical Research Communications, 195,* 1104–1110.

Part Four

Neurobiology

Edited by
John H. Morrison

Eleven

Neuropsychology of Aging: Findings in Humans and Monkeys

Marilyn S. Albert and Mark B. Moss

I. Introduction

Neuropsychology, the study of structure–function relationships in the brain, is a relatively young specialization in the neurosciences and has begun to focus on the neurobiology of aging. This chapter outlines our current knowledge of the neuropsychology of normal aging based on both human and monkey data. Six cognitive domains are addressed individually (attention, memory, executive function, language, visuospatial processing, and general intelligence), and findings from humans and monkeys are compared wherever possible. This is followed by a brief review of neuroimaging and morpohological findings in humans and monkeys, which point to changes in the brain that may be at least partially responsible for the age-related alterations in cognition described.

Data from the rhesus monkey will be emphasized here because studies in this species are most common and there is considerable information about the life span of the rhesus monkey. There is now general agreement that monkeys 25–29 years old are considered elderly (i.e., comparable to humans at 75–90) and that monkeys 16–23 years old are middle-aged (Tigges *et*

al., 1988). Thus, there is an approximately 3:1 ratio between the age of a human and the age of monkey, and results from young, middle-aged, and elderly monkeys can be compared to comparable data in humans.

A comparison between human and monkey data is instructive for a number of reasons. First, if the pattern of performance within a cognitive domain is similar in both humans and monkeys, then the likelihood that the findings are accurate is strengthened. Second, an examination of carefully selected autopsy tissue in monkeys and humans can likewise serve to address, and potentially reinforce, similar conclusions. Finally, carefully controlled lesion studies in monkeys can shed light on potential structure–function relationships in humans that cannot easily be evaluated by other means.

Before reviewing the data on age-related changes in cognition, it is important to begin by defining what is meant by normal aging, as a number of accepted definitions exist. The emphasis in the current chapter will be on the age-related changes that one sees in the absence of clinical disease. In this context, particular emphasis is placed on excluding subjects in the early stages of

Handbook of the Biology of Aging, Fourth Edition
Copyright © 1996 Academic Press, Inc. All rights of reproduction in any form reserved.

Alzheimer's disease (AD). However, many medical diseases are common in the elderly (hypertension, respiratory or cardiac disease, vitamin deficiency, etc.), all of which may impair intellectual function, and ideally, these disorders should be excluded as well. Subjects selected without evidence of clinical disease will differ greatly from a group of older persons that is chosen to represent the average, because the latter will include many individuals with serious medical illnesses. Although nonrepresentative, the former group can be of heuristic value. It will permit one to differentiate changes related to disease from those related to age. This may make it easier to identify interventions that can minimize age-related change.

II. Domains of Cognitive Function

Although one could fractionate cognitive function into an almost unlimited number of components, most investigators in the field of neuropsychology view higher cortical function as being composed of a relatively small number of major categories. For the purposes of this chapter, we will discuss cognitive function within the following domains: (1) attention, (2) memory, (3) executive function, (4) language, (5) visuospatial processing, and (6) general intelligence. This chapter will discuss all six domains, but will emphasize studies of memory and executive function, since these have been most extensively examined in both humans and monkeys.

III. Attention

The concept of attention has been discussed since the time of William James (1890). It is often thought to encompass at least three interrelated aspects: sustained attention (vigilance), selective attention (the ability to extract relevant from irrelevant information), and attentional capacity (the total attentional resources available to an individual) [see Parasuraman and Davies (1984) and Hasher and Zacks (1979) for reviews]. Some investigators also include within the area of attention the complex set of abilities sometimes referred to as executive functions. For the purposes of the present discussion, the term attention will be used to describe sustained attention only. Executive function ability will be discussed in another section.

Sustained attention assesses the individual's ability to focus on and perform a simple task without losing track of the task objective. Memory demands are minimized in tests of sustained attention by limiting the information that must be remembered to material that falls within a person's immediate memory span (i.e., 7 ± 2). Digit span forward is the most commonly used test of sustained attention and is included in many tests of general intelligence (e.g., WAIS-R and WMS-R). Visual or auditory continuous performance tasks that require the individual to identify a repeating letter (e.g., A) or a repeated letter sequence (I before X) (Mirsky, 1978) are other common means of evaluating sustained attention.

Many studies have demonstrated that sustained attention is well preserved with age. Figure 1 shows the results of seven independent studies of sustained attention across the age range. Of note, there is less than one standard deviation (SD) of change between 20 and 80 years of age.

Simple tests of sustained attention have not been directly assessed in studies of aged monkeys. However, if one assumes that sustained attention is a prerequisite for the ability to learn simultaneous discrimination tasks, then results from this testing paradigm can be used to address this issue. Aged monkeys are as efficient as young adults in their ability to acquire two-choice discrimination problems using either pattern (Moss *et al.*, 1988) or spatial (Lai *et al.*, 1995) stimuli. Thus, it

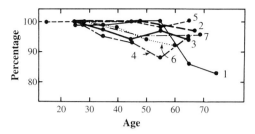

Figure 1. Seven independent studies of sustained attention in subjects 20–75 years old. Performance on this task shows little change with age.

seems reasonable to conclude that, like humans, aging in monkeys does not impair simple or sustained attentional processes.

The neuroanatomical basis and neuronal circuitry of sustained attention point to the brain stem and thalamus (Moruzzi & Magoun, 1949; Stuss & Benson, 1987). The foregoing results would suggest that these regions do not undergo substantial age-related functional change.

IV. Memory

Workers in the field of memory have accepted the conclusion that memory is not a unitary phenomenon, and most models of memory function hypothesize that memory consists of a series of specific yet interactive stores (e.g., Waugh & Norman, 1965; Tulving, 1972). Figure 2 presents an outline of the way in which these aspects

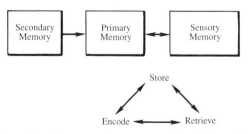

Figure 2. Diagrammatic representation of the model that conceptualizes memory as a series of specific yet interactive stores.

of memory are thought to be related to one another. The aspects of memory presented are briefly discussed in this section.

A. Types of Memory

1. Sensory Memory

Sensory memory, or registration, represents the earliest stage of information processing. It is modality-specific (i.e., visual, auditory, tactile), highly unstable, and characterized by rapid decay.

2. Primary/Immediate Memory

The component of the memory system referred to as primary or immediate memory permits one to hold spans of auditory and/or visual information for relatively long periods of time by active rehearsal. The ability to concentrate on, rehearse, and recall a span of digits, words, or visual features is perhaps the best example of this capacity. Any disruption in the rehearsal process results in the information being lost from immediate memory. Experiments by Petersen and Petersen (1959) have demonstrated that normal subjects forget a significant proportion of new information in less than 1 min when distractions are present. The amount of information that immediate memory can store is limited to about five to seven items, as mentioned earlier. There is not complete consensus among neuropsychologists and memory researchers as to whether immediate memory should be considered a form of memory at all. Primary or immediate memory, as described here, may rely more on attentional skills. Thus, Spitz (1972), among others, has argued that digit span forward is actually a measure of attention rather than memory.

3. Secondary Memory

In order to be retained over a long period of time, information from immediate memory must be assembled into multimodal units to be placed in storage. Storage of information by the memory system appears to take place differentially. As early as 1949, Hebb postulated that two processes were necessary for the brain to retain information. The first process, analogous to what we have termed recent memory, required the continual reverberation of a neural circuit. The second process, equivalent to secondary memory, required an actual structural change in the neural pattern of the central nervous system.

4. Explicit vs Implicit Secondary Memory

Over the past few years, accumulating evidence has suggested that memory functions are composed of at least two distinct types of memory, explicit and implicit memory. Explicit memory pertains to information that is acquired because a person makes a conscious effort to learn and retain it. Implicit memory pertains to information that is acquired without a conscious effort to learn it. Implicit memory therefore is said to refer to "knowing how" or "procedural" or "habit" (Ryle, 1949; Hirsh, 1974; Cohen & Squire, 1980) memory; implicit memory is accessible primarily through the performance of a task or by engaging in the skill in which the knowledge is embedded (Squire, 1986).

B. Explicit Memory Performance and Aging

There is considerable information to indicate that changes in explicit sensory memory are minimal with age. For example, the time necessary to identify a single letter does not change significantly between the late teens and early 70s. When seven-letter strings are used, the rate of letter identification increases with age by a factor of 1.3 (Cerella, Poon, & Fozard, 1982). A partial report paradigm showed that letter

identification latencies change minimally with age when adjusted for the loss of visual discrimination experienced by the elderly. These and other data indicate that there is a minimal decline in sensory memory with age [see Craik, 1977; see Poon (1985) for a detailed review].

Primary explicit memory also shows little decline with age. Most studies report no significant age differences in digit span forward (Drachman & Leavitt, 1972), no age differences in word span (Talland, 1967), and only moderate differences in letter span (Botwinick & Storandt, 1974). Older subjects show as much of a recency effect (i.e., retrieval of the last few items on a list in a word list learning task) as younger subjects (Raymond, 1971).

However, there are substantial changes in explicit secondary memory, in contrast to the minimal age changes in sensory and primary memory [see Craik, 1977; see Poon (1985) for a review]. The age at which changes in secondary memory occur depends upon the methods that are used to test the memory store. Difficult explicit memory tasks (e.g., delayed recall) demonstrate statistically significant differences by subjects in their 50s in comparison to younger individuals (Albert *et al.*, 1987a). Age decrements are greater on recall than recognition tasks. This is true whether words or pictures are used. Cueing during encoding or retrieval also alters the appearance of an age decline. Cueing at both encoding and retrieval produces the smallest age differences, whereas no cueing at either stage of the task maximizes age differences (Craik *et al.*, 1987). However, even with cued recall and recognition, there are often declines. Rabinowitz (1986) reported a 33% age-related decrement in cued recall and an 11% age-related decrement in recognition, when comparing young and old subjects (mean age 19 vs 68).

Figure 3 shows the performance of subjects across the age range on delayed recall of two lengthy paragraphs. That is, each

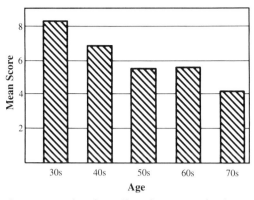

Figure 3. Delayed recall performance of subjects 30–80 years old. The subjects are asked to report what they remember of two lengthy paragraphs after a 15-min delay.

subject is read two lengthy paragraphs, and immediately after hearing each one and then again after 20 min the subject is asked to state what he/she can recall of the paragraphs.

A close examination of these data indicates that the older individuals are not more rapidly forgetting what they learned, but rather they are taking longer to learn the new information. For example, if one compares the difference between immediate and delayed recall over the life span, there are no statistically significant age differences (Petersen *et al.*, 1992). Thus, if one allows older subjects to learn material well (i.e., to the point where few errors are made), they do not forget what they have learned more rapidly than the young (see Fig. 3). However, if older subjects are not given the opportunity to learn material to the same level of proficiency as younger individuals, then after a delay less information will be retained by the average older person.

However, there is considerable variability among older subjects on tasks of this sort. There are many healthy older subjects who have test scores that overlap those of subjects many years younger than themselves [e.g., about one-third of healthy 70-year-old humans have delayed

recall scores that overlap those of 30-year-olds (equated for education)].

Similar findings have emerged from studies in monkeys. Since free recall cannot be easily tested in monkeys, considerable effort has gone into developing a memory task that uses recognition, but determines the quantity of information aging monkeys can retain across varying delay intervals. The delayed nonmatching to sample task (DNMS) is the most widely used method for assessing recognition memory in the nonhuman primate (Bachevalier & Mishkin, 1989; Murray & Mishkin, 1984; 1986; Mishkin, 1978; Mahut *et al.*, 1982; Zola-Morgan & Squire, 1985). This task relies upon a two-alternative forced choice paradigm in which the monkey is required to discriminate which of two objects was recently presented. By using the delayed nonmatching to sample task, many studies have shown that aged monkeys are impaired at learning the nonmatching principle, but are, at best, only mildly impaired across the delay conditions of the test (Moss *et al.*, 1988; Arnsten & Goldman-Rakic, 1990; Bachevalier *et al.*, 1991, Presty *et al.*, 1987; Rapp & Amaral, 1989). Thus, like humans, the old monkeys take longer to learn something new, but do not appear to forget this information more rapidly over lengthening delays than younger monkeys.

Another task, the delayed recognition span test (DRST) (Rehbein, 1983; Moss, 1983), has demonstrated similar findings. This test requires a monkey to identify a novel stimulus from an increasing array of previously presented stimuli. The task has been administered to monkeys with two types of conditions: a spatial version and an object version. In both conditions the monkey first sees a board with 18 positions (food wells) and a stimulus object on one position. A second stimulus is added while the board is obscured from view, and the animal is required to point to the new stimulus. On the first trial of the spatial version, the animal's task is to indicate which of two disks is occupying the new position on the board (i.e., a nonmatching to position task). On the first trial of the object version, the animal's task is to indicate which of the two objects on the board is the new one (i.e., in essence a nonmatching to sample task). However, since new disks/objects are then added in series to the previous ones on the board, the task becomes increasingly difficult. For example, young adult monkeys often achieve a span of five or greater before committing an error.

Middle-aged monkeys (16–23 years) are impaired on the spatial version of the DRST, but not on the color version (Moss et al., 1988, submitted). This finding is similar to the declines in performance on delayed recall seen in middle-aged humans. Aged monkeys (25–27 years) are impaired relative to young adults (5–7 years) under both conditions of the task. This suggests that the performance of monkeys on the spatial version of the DRST may be functionally equivalent to the performance of humans on difficult delayed recall tasks. In addition, the difference between performance on the DNMS and the spatial condition of the DRST appears to be similar to what one sees between recall and recognition paradigms in aging humans.

Longitudinal assessment of memory using the DRST has also been examined (Moss, 1993). Young adult (5–7 years) and aged (23–26 years) monkeys were assessed on the spatial recognition span test after an interval of 4 years. Two of the three young animals showed a slight decline in performance and one showed a slight improvement. In the aged group, two animals showed a very slight decline (as with the young), but the remaining two showed marked declines which, in one case, were severe. Thus, the longitudinal findings confirm the general conclusions of the cross-sectional data.

Like aging humans, there is also considerable variability in the performance of aging monkeys. Among the oldest animals there are subjects who perform within the range of younger animals, even though the mean performance of the group declines significantly. For example, on DNMS, the number of trials to criterion ranges from 50 to 220, and the number of errors ranges from 29 to 60. Among the older monkeys, the trials to criterion range from 200 to 516 and the number of errors ranges from 50 to 115.

Lesion studies in monkeys indicate that the medial temporal region of the brain and/or diencephalic midline structures are essential for normal memory. A lesion of the hippocampus and the amygdala produces profound defects in a monkey's ability to learn the nonmatching to sample principle on the DNMS and to retain correct information over delays of increasing lengths (e.g., Zola-Morgan & Squire, 1985). Likewise, damage to the mediodorsal nucleus of the thalamus produces a striking memory deficit on the DNMS (e.g., Aggleton & Mishkin, 1983). The impairment is present in the monkey's ability to learn (e.g., 140 trials to criterion for controls vs 315 for monkeys with mediodorsal thalamic lesions) and to retain information at long delays (e.g., 80% at 10 min for controls vs 60% for lesioned monkeys). It is noteworthy that the deficits following these lesions are more severe than those seen in age-related declines in monkeys.

Lesion studies in monkeys also indicate that the degree of memory loss following lesions of this type is related to the combination of structures damaged and the location of the lesion within the critical structures. For example, combined damage to the hippocampus and amygdala produces a more severe deficit than a lesion to either structure alone (e.g., Zola-Morgan & Squire, 1985). Similarly, a lesion in the posterior mediodorsal nucleus produces a more severe memory defect than one in the anterior region (Aggleton & Mishkin, 1983). Thus, age-related changes likely produce alterations within this memory network, but the location and extent are not yet clear.

Moreover, several neurotransmitters and hormones can have a modulatory effect on memory performance. For example, the basal forebrain is the primary source of neocortical acetylcholine (Mesulam & Van Hoesen, 1976), and the locus ceruleus is the major source of neocortical norepinephrine (Moore & Bloom, 1979), both of which modulate memory performance. Lesions of the three nuclei within the basal forebrain (the nucleus basalis of Meynert, the medial septal nucleus, and the diagonal band) produce a deficit in DNMS performance in young monkeys, which recovers over time (Aigner et al., 1991). It has been hypothesized that recovery is related to compensatory responses in other neuromodulatory mechanisms; however, if these are also compromised then recovery might not occur. Thus, in order to determine the cause(s) of age-related memory deficits in monkeys, each aspect of the memory network must be evaluated in carefully selected animals, and comparisons must be made to human data. Given the difficulty of this task, the answers are not available.

C. Implicit Memory Performance and Aging

Age-related changes in implicit memory have been examined in a variety of ways. One method uses a priming technique in which learning is inferred by examining the change in the items retained after a single exposure to a set of items (Graf & Schacter, 1985). For example, if one has been asked to read an inverted word once, the speed with which that word will be read a second time increases. Thus, learning is inferred by the change in speed. Commonly used priming paradigms include stem completion and partial word identification. The majority of studies indicate that there is no significant decline

in priming ability with advancing age [see Graf (1990) and Howard (1988) for reviews].

Skill learning is another paradigm used to examine implicit memory. Learning is inferred by examining the change in amount retained after multiple exposures to a procedure (e.g., rotary pursuit, reading inverted words, partial word identification), rather than the change in recall of a specific item. Most of the skill learning studies have examined the improvement in visual skills over time, such as reading inverted words or identifying fragmented pictures. The results published to date indicate that age-related impairments in skill learning appear to depend upon whether or not there is a primary difficulty in processing the information on which training occurs. For example, if inverted words are exposed for a longer duration in the older subjects than in the young, age-related differences are minimal, or if words are degraded by 37%, rather than by 50%, then age-related differences are minimal (Hashtroudi et al., 1991). There is little data on motor skill learning, but those that exist suggest that it is impaired with age (e.g., Harrington & Haaland, 1992).

Classical conditioning, on the other hand, demonstrates significant declines with age (Solomon et al., 1989). This is typically examined by observing the change in response to stimulus 1 that comes after coupling stimulus 1 and stimulus 2 together, (e.g., eye blink in response to a tone, after the tone has been coupled with a puff of air to the eye). It has been hypothesized that these declines are related to alterations in neurotransmitter levels in subcortical nuclei (see the following).

In monkeys, initial evidence suggests that procedural learning, at least with respect to motor skill learning, is only minimally affected by age. The performance of aged monkeys on a timed task in which a lifesaver is moved along a metal form, varying in number and angle of curves, did not differ significantly either in latency or trials to criterion, as compared with young adult monkeys (Ronald, 1992).

Lesion studies in monkeys and findings in humans with brain damage indicate that the brain regions responsible for implicit memory are different from those responsible for explicit memory performance. Monkeys with lesions of the medial temporal lobe (i.e., hippocampus and amygdala) perform in the normal range on motor skill tasks, including the lifesaver task described earlier (Zola-Morgan & Squire, 1984). Likewise, humans with extensive lesions of the medial temporal lobe that produce a dramatic explicit memory deficit can learn new motor skills (e.g., Corkin, 1968). By contrast, monkeys with lesions of the nucleus accumbens are impaired on the lifesaver task, but not on tests of explicit memory, including the DNMS task (Killiany & Mahut, 1992). The nucleus accumbens is continuous with the caudate and putamen in the monkey; thus, these findings implicate the striatum in motor skill learning. On the basis of data from patients with Huntington's disease, it has also been hypothesized that the striatal network is involved in motor skill learning (Heindel et al., 1989). Since an impairment in motor skill learning with age has been reported, its origin may be related to alterations in the striatum.

V. Executive Function

The complex set of abilities sometimes referred to as executive functions include concurrent manipulation of information (e.g., cognitive flexibility), concept formation, and cue-directed behavior. The wide variety of abilities that are sometimes included under the term executive function is therefore striking.

Tests evaluating concept formation and set shifting uniformly show significant changes with age, primarily when subjects are in their late 60s or 70s. For example, the similarities subtest of the Wechsler Adult Intelligence Scale (WAIS), which asks subjects to identify how two objects (e.g., a table and a chair) are similar to each other, is the subtest on the verbal scale of the WAIS that shows the greatest decline with age (Heaton et al., 1986). Education appears to be a modifier of this decline, in that subjects with lower amounts of education demonstrate declines at younger ages; however, all subjects in the oldest group (mean age 68 years), regardless of educational level, show significant declines in performance.

Series completion tests also show substantial age declines. These tests generally require the subject to examine a series of letters or numbers and determine the rule that governed the sequencing of the items in the series. Cross-sectional and longitudinal data demonstrate age-related declines on tasks of this sort (e.g., Lachman & Jelalian, 1984; Schaie, 1983).

Proverb interpretation tests, which require the subject to provide the general meaning of a proverb (e.g., barking dogs seldom bite), also demonstrate age-related declines (Albert et al., 1990). This is true whether subjects are asked to provide the meaning of the proverb themselves or are given alternate choices among which to choose. Similarly, set shifting tasks, such as the Visual–Verbal task (in which subjects are asked to look at a series of cards and indicate how three of the four objects on each card are alike in one way and then how three of the objects are alike in another way), also show substantial age-related declines. These changes appear to be related to the fact that older subjects have difficulty switching from one abstract answer to another (i.e., they tend to get the first item in the set correct but the second one wrong). Slowness in establishing mental set (i.e., getting the first item in the set wrong but the second one right) and failure to establish set (i.e., getting both items in the set wrong) did not increase differentially with age (Albert *et al.*, 1990).

Changes in executive function in monkeys have been examined primarily by using reversal learning paradigms (Bartus *et al.*, 1979; Rapp, 1990; Lai *et al.*, 1995). Reversal learning involves responding to a change in reinforcement contingencies by first "unlearning" or breaking the initial stimulus–reinforcement bond and then acquiring or "shifting" to a new one. In this way, reversal learning can be considered a measure of executive function. Data have accumulated to suggest that aged monkeys have difficulty in reversing established stimulus–reward contingencies, particularly when based on spatial location. Thus, compared to young adult monkeys, aged monkeys, as a group, are impaired on spatial, but not object, reversal learning. Moreover, aged monkeys tend to make more perseverative responses than young adults on both spatial and object reversal learning.

Lesion studies in monkeys indicate that reversal learning ability is related to frontal lobe function. Pohl administered object and spatial ("place") reversal tasks to monkeys that underwent surgical ablation of the dorsolateral prefrontal region. Compared to monkeys with lesions of either the inferior temporal or the parietal cortex, monkeys with frontal lesions were markedly impaired on spatial, but not object, reversal learning. Classically, damage to the dorsolateral prefrontal cortex (DLPC) results in a spatial working memory deficit demonstrated by monkeys on spatial delayed response performances. Like the spatial delayed response, the spatial reversal test may preferentially engage DLPC function since (1) internal, vs external, informative stimuli serve as cues for the correct response, and (2) this informative stimulus must be held "on line" for brief periods of time and continuously updated. Thus, the age-related changes seen in spatial reversal learning suggest that prefrontal regions are altered with age and are responsible for executive function changes.

Direct behavioral support implicating the prefrontal region in age-related change is provided by Rapp and Amaral's finding that the spatial delayed response performance by aged monkeys was impaired relative to young adults and that spatial reversal learning showed larger age-related declines than did performance on delayed nonmatching to sample (Rapp & Amaral, 1991). Bachevalier *et al.* (1991) corroborated these results and reported declines on spatial delayed reversal tasks in earlier age groups than those for delayed nonmatching to sample in a cross-sectional primate study.

VI. Visuospatial Function

Visuospatial function is characterized by the ability to produce and recognize figures and to form relationships among spatial locations. Specific visual functions include the ability to recognize familiar faces, the ability to copy or match objects or pictures, and the ability to translate spatial elements from one mode to another. Translation of mirror image spatial arrangements into self-oriented positions is an example of a task that requires intact and efficient visuospatial abilities. Visuospatial ability therefore can be assessed by (1) constructional tasks, such as the assembly of blocks, sticks, or puzzles, (2) drawing tasks that involve copying, or (3) matching tasks that require the subject to identify pictures with similar elements.

The most complex three-dimensional construction task in common use is the Block Design subtest of the WAIS. The subject is presented with a two-dimensional drawing in red and white of a target design and a set of blocks (some sides of the blocks are all red, some are all white, and some are half red and half white). The subject is asked to arrange the blocks, which are of course three-dimensional, so that they mimic the two-dimensional design. To receive credit, the subject must assemble the blocks correctly within a specified time limit. This task shows substantial declines with age (Doppelt & Wallace, 1955).

Performance on figure drawing tasks is also affected by age. Older subjects are impaired, in comparison to the young, in depicting and perceiving three-dimensional drawings. Plude *et al.* (1986) asked a group of young and old adults (mean ages 21 and 67, respectively, and equated for static visual acuity) to draw a cube to command. The cubes were then rated by 10 independent raters, with an inter-rater reliability of 0.98. The drawings of the young adults were rated as significantly better than those of the old. The older subjects were also less accurate than the young in judging the adequacy of drawings of cubes that were distorted to varying degrees. The elderly were less accurate than the young in discriminating between distorted and undistorted cubes. They were, however, equally able to copy a cube when landmarks were provided regarding the size of the lines. Comparable reports of the depiction and perception of two-dimensional drawings are not available.

Spatial abilities in monkeys also evidence change with age, and, like humans, the presence or degree of impairment appears to be related to the demand characteristics of the task. Lai *et al.* (1995) showed that aged monkeys were impaired on a spatial task that required the ability of animals to use allocentric rather than egocentric spatial cues. Monkeys were first required to learn a simple two-choice spatial discrimination by displacing, on a small table top, one of two identical plaques set either to the left or to the right of the animal to a 90% learning criterion. Once the criterion was reached, the animals were wheeled to the other side of the table so that, with respect to the animal's body position, the previously correct plaque was now reversed. Thus, an animal

that first learned to displace the plaque to its left to obtain a reward now had to displace the plaque to its right. Unlike young monkeys, aged monkeys (23–26 years old) evidenced a strong tendency to choose the plaque that retained the same location with reference to body position (egocentric cue), rather than to choose the plaque that retained the same location with reference to other external cues in the environment (allocentric cues). In contrast, there was no significant difference between young and aged monkeys in initially learning to choose the left or right plaque.

VII. Language

Linguistic ability is thought to encompass at least four domains: phonological, lexical, syntactic, and semantic. It previously was assumed that linguistic ability is preserved into very old age, primarily because performance on the vocabulary subtest of the WAIS, the best general estimate of verbal intelligence, is well-maintained until the individuals are in their 80s (Schaie, 1983). However, within the last decade, a number of studies have shown that some aspects of linguistic knowledge decline with age, although not until relatively late in the life span (i.e., >70).

A. Phonology

Phonological knowledge refers to the use of the sounds of language and the rules for their combination. Phonological capabilities are well-preserved with age (Bayles & Kaszniak, 1987).

B. Lexicon

Psycholinguists distinguish between the lexical representation of a word, i.e., the name of an item, and its semantic representation, i.e., the meaning of a word (Clark & Clark, 1977). The lexicon of healthy older individuals appears to be intact, as are the semantic relationships of the lexicon.

C. Syntax

Syntactic knowledge refers to the ability to meaningfully combine words. A large number of studies have shown that age has little effect on syntax. Obler *et al.* (1985) found that syntactic forms that were difficult for older individuals were also difficult for younger ones.

D. Semantic Knowledge

Older individuals appear to have difficulty with the semantic aspects of word retrieval. Several groups of investigators have reported that scores on a test of confrontation naming decrease with age (Borod *et al.*, 1980; LaBarge *et al.*, 1986; Albert *et al.*, 1987b). However, declines in naming ability do not become statistically significant until subjects are in their 70s (Albert *et al.*, 1987b). When subjects could not correctly name an item, the most common error they committed was semantic in nature, i.e., they produced semantically related associates, circumlocutions, and nominalizations. The nature of these semantic errors suggests that older individuals have a great deal of knowledge about the target word. For example, a semantically related associate ("dice" for "dominoes") can only be produced if the subject apprehends the general category associated with the stimulus item.

Verbal fluency also assesses semantic ability. In a verbal fluency task a subject is asked to name as many examples of a category (e.g., animals or vegetables) as possible in a specified period of time (e.g., 1 min) or as many words beginning with a particular letter (e.g., F) within a specified period of time. Several studies report a decline in verbal fluency with age (Obler *et al.*, 1985; Albert *et al.*, 1987b). These changes also occur relatively late in the life span (>70). Thus, semantic linguistic

ability appears to change with advancing age, while other aspects of linguistic ability are relatively well-preserved.

VIII. General Intelligence

Although intelligence tests measure most of the abilities previously discussed, they do so in a complex way. Intelligence tests were designed to predict, with a reasonable degree of certainty, how a person would function in an academic environment, not to provide a complete assessment of cognitive function. Thus, intelligence tests do not assess all aspects of cognitive ability. For example, the Wechsler Adult Intelligence Scale does not include an evaluation of memory. In addition, IQ tests do not assess cognitive abilities in relative isolation from one another. Many of the tasks require a complex interaction of abilities and often depend upon speed for an adequate level of performance. Nevertheless, intelligence testing has been one of the most widely explored topics in the psychology of aging.

There is widespread agreement that there are changes in intelligence test performance with age. There has, however, been considerable debate about the point at which declines occur and the magnitude of the declines. The age at which declines are observed appears to depend upon the methodology employed. There is some consensus that relatively little decline in performance occurs prior to the time that people are in their 50s (Schaie & Labouvie-Vief, 1974). After this age, results differ depending upon whether cross-sectional or longitudinal testing designs were employed. The cross-sectional method shows declines of 1 SD or more beginning about age 60 (Doppelt & Wallace, 1955; Schaie, 1983); over the age of 70 scores drop sharply. The longitudinal method shows declines beginning in the late 60s. Both methods find substantial declines after individuals are in their mid-70s. Thus, the major difference between cross-sectional and longitudinal investigations is observed between subjects in their late 50s and early 60s. In this age range, the cross-sectional method shows greater age declines than the longitudinal method.

IX. Changes in Brain Structure and Function

There is substantial evidence that, as people age, they show significant increases in cerebrospinal fluid (CSF) and decreases in brain tissue (Stafford *et al.*, 1988; Zatz *et al.*, 1982). That is, there is increasing atrophy with age. This alteration becomes statistically significant when subjects are in their 70s (Stafford *et al.*, 1988).

However, studies in humans suggest that the decrease in brain tissue observed is primarily the result of decreases in white matter with age ($p \leq 0.001$). Decreases in gray matter are only marginally statistically significant; approximately 48% of brain tissue consists of gray matter among both 30-year-olds and 70-year-olds (Albert *et al.*, submitted). These findings are consistent with data in humans (Haug, 1984; Terry *et al.*, 1987; Leuba & Garey, 1989), indicating that with advancing age neuronal loss in the cortex is either not significant or not as extensive as earlier reports (i.e., reports prior to 1984) had suggested (Brody, 1955, 1970; Colon, 1972; Shefer, 1973; Henderson *et al.*, 1980; Anderson *et al.*, 1983).

There are comparable data in monkeys. Minimal neuronal cortical loss with age in monkeys has now been demonstrated in the striate cortex (Vincent *et al.*, 1989), motor cortex (Tigges *et al.*, 1992), frontal cortex (Peters *et al.*, 1994), and entorhinal cortex (Amaral, 1993). Likewise, data in monkeys and humans indicate that neuronal loss is highly selective within the hippocampal formation. For example, the subiculum shows a significant age-related

loss in humans and a similar trend in monkeys; however, the CA1, CA2, and CA3 fields show no evidence of age-related neuronal loss (Amaral, 1993; Rosene, 1993; West *et al.*, 1994). These general conclusions have been reached not only on the basis of a comparison of counts of neurons in young (5–6 years) and old (over 25 years of age) monkeys but also on the basis of an examination of the cortices by electron microscopy (Peters *et al.*, 1994). Beyond an accumulation of lipofuscin granules in the perikarya of some neurons in the older animals, there is very little evidence of changes with age in the neurons, although the neuroglial cells do show significant accumulation of cellular debris (Peters *et al.*, 1991).

On the other hand, there is substantial neuronal loss in selected subcortical regions responsible for the production of neurotransmitters important for memory function, such as the basal forebrain and the locus ceruleus (e.g., Chan-Palay & Asan, 1989; Rosene, 1993). For example, in humans and monkeys there is approximately a 50% neuronal loss with age in the basal forebrain and a 35–40% loss in the locus ceruleus and dorsal raphe (Kemper, 1993). This compares with an approximate loss of 5% in CA1 of the hippocampus. Although neuronal loss appears to be minimal in the hippocampus with age, reports suggest alterations in specific receptor types (e.g., NMDA receptors) that may play a role in memory function (Gazzaley *et al.*, 1995).

In addition, there is an age-related decrease in dopaminergic binding sites in the caudate nucleus (Severson *et al.*, 1982) and the substantia nigra and a loss of neurons in the substantia nigra of about 6% per year (McGeer *et al.*, 1977). This loss of dopamine is thought to be responsible for many neurological symptoms that increase in frequency with age, such as decreased arm swing and increased rigidity (Odenheimer *et al.*, 1994). Changes in dopamine levels may also cause age-related changes in cognitive flexibility. This is suggested by the fact that patients with Parkinson's disease (a disorder associated with a loss of cells in the substantia nigra and a severe decline in dopamine levels) have cognitive deficits that have variably been described as "mental inflexibility" (Lees & Smith, 1983), a disorder of the "shifting attitude" (Cools *et al.*, 1984), an "instability of cognitive set" (Flowers & Robertson, 1985), and difficulty with "set formation, maintenance and shifting" (Taylor *et al.*, 1987). An age-related functional loss of dopamine has been demonstrated in monkeys (Arnsten *et al.*, 1994), making it possible to study this hypothesis in nonhuman primates.

X. Conclusion

Significant age-related changes in mental abilities occur in both healthy humans and monkeys. The age at which these changes are evident differs with the ability being evaluated and the method of evaluation. There is considerable variability among both elderly humans and monkeys; some subjects show minimal changes with age and others show substantial declines. These alterations in ability appear to be, at least in part, related to changes in brain structure and function. The ability to alter these cognitive changes in a long-lasting and generalized manner, and/or the brain alterations associated with them, remains to be determined.

References

Aggleton, J., & Mishkin, M. (1983). Memory impairments following restricted medial thalamic lesions in monkeys. *Experiments in Brain Research, 21*, 199–209.

Aigner, T., Mitchell, S., Aggleton, J., DeLong, M., Struble, R., Price, D., Wenk, G., Pettigrew, K., & Mishkin, M. (1991). Transient impairment of recognition memory following ibotenic-acid lesions of the basal fore-brain in macaques. *Experiments in Brain Research, 86*, 18–26.

Albert, M., Duffy, F., & Naeser, M. (1987a). Non-linear changes in cognition with age and neurophysiological correlates. *Canadian Journal of Psychology, 41*, 141–157.

Albert, M., Heller, H., & Milberg, W. (1987b). Changes in naming ability with age. *Psychology & Aging, 41*, 141–157.

Albert, M., Wolfe, J., & Lafleche, G. (1990). Differences in abstraction ability with age. *Psychology & Aging, 5*, 94–100.

Amaral, D. (1993). Morphological analyses of the brains of behaviorally characterized aged nonhuman primates. *Neurobiology of Aging, 14*, 671–672.

Anderson, J., Hubbard, B., Coghill, G., & Slidders, W. (1983). The effect of advanced old age on the neuron content of the cerebral cortex. Observations with an automatic image analyser point counting method. *Journal of Neurological Science, 58*, 233–244.

Arnsten, A., & Goldman-Rakic, P. (1990). Analysis of alpha-2 adrenergic agonist effects on the delayed non-matching-to-sample performance of aged rhesus monkeys. *Neurobiology of Aging, 11*, 583–590.

Arnsten, A., Cai, J., Steere, J., & Goldman-Rakic, P. (1994). Dopamine D2 receptor mechanisms in the cognitive performance of young adult and aged monkeys. *Psychopharmacology, 116*, 143–151.

Bachevalier, J., & Mishkin, M. (1989). Mnemonic and neuropathological effects of occluding the posterior cerebral artery in *Macaca mulatta. Neuropsychologia, 27*, 83–105.

Bachevalier, J., Landis, L., Walker, M., Brickson, M., Mishkin, M., Price, D., & Cork, L. (1991). Aged monkeys exhibit behavioral deficits indicative of widespread cerebral dysfunction. *Neurobiology of Aging, 12*, 99–111.

Bartus, R., Dean, R., & Fleming, D. (1979). Aging in the rhesus monkey: effects on visual discrimination learning and reversal learning. *Journal of Gerontology, 34*, 209–219.

Bayles, K., & Kaszniak, A. (1987). *Communication and Cognition in Normal Aging and Dementia.* Boston: Little Brown.

Borod, J., Goodglass, H., & Kaplan, E. (1980). Normative data on the Boston Diagnostic Aphasia Examination, parietal lobe battery, and Boston Naming Test. *Journal of Clinical Neuropsychology, 2*, 209–215.

Botwinick, J., & Storandt, M. (1974). *Memory, Related Functions and Age.* Springfield, IL: Charles C. Thomas.

Brody, H. (1955). Organization of cerebral cortex III. A study of aging in the human cerebral cortex. *Journal of Comparative Neurology, 102,* 511–556.

Brody, H. (1970). Structural changes in the aging nervous system. *Interdisciplinary Topics in Gerontology, 7,* 9–21.

Cerella, J., Poon, L., & Fozard, J. (1982). Age and iconic read-out. *Journal of Gerontology, 37,* 197–202.

Chan-Palay, V., & Asan, E. (1989). Quantitation of catecholamine neurons in the locus ceruleus in human brains of normal young and older adults in depression. *Journal of Comparative Neurology, 287,* 357–372.

Clark, H., & Clark, E. (1977). *Psychology and Language: An Introduction to Psycholinguistics.* New York: Harcourt, Brace, Jovanovich.

Cohen, N., & Squire, L. (1980). Preserved learning and retention of pattern analyzing skill in amnesia: Dissociation of knowing how and knowing that. *Science, 210,* 207–210.

Colon, E. (1972). The elderly brain. A quantitative analysis of the cerebral cortex in two cases. *Psychiatria, Neurologia, Neurochirurgia, 75,* 261–270.

Cools, A., Van Den Bercken, J., Horstink, M., & Van Spaendonck, H. (1984). Cognitive and motor shifting aptitude disorder in Parkinson's disease. *Journal of Neurology, Neurosurgery and Psychiatry, 4,* 443–453.

Corkin, S. (1968). Acquisition of motor skill after bilateral medial temporal lobe excision. *Neuropsychologia, 6,* 225–265.

Craik, F. (1977). Age differences in human memory. In J. Birren & K. Schaie (Eds.), *Handbook of the Psychology of Aging* (pp. 384–420). New York: Van Nostrand Reinhold.

Craik, F., Byrd, M., & Swanson, J. (1987). Patterns of memory loss in three elderly samples. *Psychology & Aging, 2,* 79–86.

Doppelt, J., & Wallace, W. (1955). Standardization of the Wechsler Adult Intelligence Scale for older persons. *Journal of Abnormal Social Psychology, 51,* 312–330.

Drachman, D., & Leavitt, J. (1972). Memory impairment in the aged: Storage versus retrieval deficit. *Journal of Experimental Psychology, 93,* 302–308.

Flowers, K., & Robertson, C. (1985). The effect of Parkinson's disease on the ability to maintain mental set. *Journal of Neurology, Neurosurgery and Psychiatry, 48,* 517–529.

Gazzaley, A., Siegel, S., Kordower, J., Mufson, E., & Morrison, J. (1995). Circuit-specific alterations of NMDA receptors in the hippocampus of aged monkeys. *Society of Neuroscience, Abstracts,* in press.

Graf, P. (1990). Life-span changes in implicit and explicit memory. *Bulletin of the Psychonomic Society, 28,* 353–358.

Graf, P., & Schacter, D. (1985). Implicit and explicit memory for new associations in normal and amnesic subjects. *Journal of Experimental Psychology: Learning, Memory and Cognition, 11,* 501–518.

Harrington, D., & Haaland, K. (1992). Skill learning in the elderly: Diminished implicit and explicit memory for a motor sequence. *Psychology & Aging, 7,* 425–434.

Hasher, L., & Zacks, R. (1979). Automatic and effortful processes in memory. *Journal of Experimental Psychology, 108,* 356–388.

Hashtroudi, S., Chrosniak, L., & Schwartz, B. (1991). Effects of aging on priming and skill learning. *Psychology & Aging, 6,* 605–615.

Haug, H. (1984). Macroscopic and microscopic morphometry of the human brain and cortex. A survey in the light of new results. *Brain Pathology, 1,* 123–149.

Heaton, R., Grant, I., & Matthes, C. (1986). Differences in neuropsychological function test performance associated with age, education, and sex. In I. Grant & K. Adams (Eds.), *Neuropsychological Assessment of Neuropsychiatric Disorders* (pp. 100–120). New York: Oxford University Press.

Hebb, D. O. (1949). *The Organization of Behavior.* New York: Wiley.

Heindel, W., Salmon, D., Shults, C., Wallicke, P., & Butters, N. (1989). Neuropsychological evidence for multiple implicit memory systems: A comparison of Alzheimer's, Huntington's, and Parkinson's disease. *Journal of Neuroscience, 9,* 582–587.

Henderson, G., Tomlinson, B., & Gibson, P. (1980). Cell counts in human cerebral cortex in normal adults throughout life, using an image analysing computer. *Journal of Neurological Science, 46,* 113–136.

Hirsh, R. (1974). The hippocampus and contextual retrieval of information from memory. A theory. *Behavioral Biology, 12,* 421–444.

Howard, D. (1988). Implicit and explicit assessment of cognitive aging. In C. Brainerd & M. Howe (Eds.), *Cognitive Development in Adulthood* (pp. 3–37). New York: Springer-Verlag.

James, W. (1890). *The Principles of Psychology.* New York: Holt.

Kemper, T. (1993). The relationship of cerebral cortical changes to nuclei in the brainstem. *Neurobiology of Aging, 14,* 659–660.

Killiany, R., & Mahut, M. (1992). Lesions of the nucleus accumbens in adult rhesus monkeys result in a deficit of motor learning but not in S-R associative learning or memory. *Society of Neuroscience, Abstracts, 18,* 1063.

LaBarge, E., Edwards, D., & Knesevich, J. (1986). Performance of normal elderly on the Boston Naming Test. *Brain & Language, 27,* 380–384.

Lachman, M., & Jelalian, E. (1984). Self-efficacy and attributions for intellectual performance in young and elderly adults. *Journal of Gerontology, 39,* 577–582.

Lai, Z., Moss, M., Killiany, R., & Rosene, D. (1995). Executive system dysfunction in the aged monkeys: Spatial and object reversal learning. *Neurobiology of Aging,* in press.

Lees, A., & Smith, E. (1983). Cognitive deficits in the early stages of Parkinson's disease. *Brain, 106,* 257–270.

Leuba, G., & Garey, L. (1989). Comparison of neuronal and glial numerical density in primary and secondary visual cortex. *Experiments in Brain Research, 77,* 31–38.

Mahut, H., Zola-Morgan, S., & Moss, M. (1982). Hippocampal resections impair associative learning and recognition memory in the monkey. *Journal of Neuroscience, 2,* 1214–1229.

McGeer, P., McGeer, E., & Suzuki, J. (1977). Aging and extrapyramidal function. *Archives of Neurology, 34,* 33–35.

Mesulam, M.-M., & Van Hoesen, G. (1976). Acetylcholinesterase-rich projections from the basal forebrain of the rhesus monkey to neocortex. *Brain Research, 109,* 152–157.

Mirsky, A. (1978). Attention: A neuropsychological perspective. In J. Chall & A. Mirsky (Eds.), *Education and the Brain. Seventy-seventh Yearbook of the Study of Aging, Part II.* Chicago: Chicago Univ. Press.

Mishkin, M. (1978). Memory in monkeys severely impaired by combined but not separate removal of amygdala and hippocampus. *Nature, 273,* 297–298.

Moore, R., & Bloom, F. (1979). Central catecholamine neuron systems: anatomy and physiology of the dopamine systems. *Annual Review in Neuroscience, 2,* 113–168.

Moruzzi, B., & Magoun, H. (1949). Brain stem reticular formation and activation of the EEG. *Electroencephalography and Clinical Neurophysiology, 1,* 459–473.

Moss, M. (1983). Assessment of memory in amnesic and dementia patients: Adaptation of behavioral tests used with non-human primates. *INSA Bulletin, 5,* 15.

Moss, M. (1993). The longitudinal assessment of recognition memory in aged rhesus monkeys. *Neurobiology of Aging, 14,* 635–636.

Moss, M., Rosene, D., & Peters, A. (1988). Effects of aging on visual recognition memory in the rhesus monkey. *Neurobiology of Aging, 9,* 495–502.

Murray, E., & Mishkin, M. (1984). Severe tactual as well as visual memory deficits follow combined removal of the amygdala and hippocampus in monkeys. *Journal of Neuroscience, 4,* 2565–2580.

Murray, E., & Mishkin, M. (1986). Visual recognition in monkeys following rhinal cortical ablations combined with either amygdalectomy or hippocampectomy. *Journal of Neuroscience, 6,* 1991–2003.

Obler, L., Nicholas, M., Albert, M. L., & Woodward, S. (1985). On comprehension across the adult life span. *Cortex, 21,* 273–280.

Odenheimer, G., Funkenstein, H., Beckett, L., Chown, M., Pilgrim, D., Evans, D., & Albert, M. (1994). Comparison of neurologic changes in successfully aging persons vs the total aging population. *Archives in Neurology, 51,* 573–580.

Parasuraman, R., & Davies, R. (1984). *Varieties of Attention.* New York: Academic Press.

Peters, A., Josephson, K., & Vicent, S. (1991). Effects of aging on the neuroglial cells and pericytes within area 17 of the rhesus monkey (*Macaca mulatta*). *Anatomical Record, 229,* 384–398.

Peters, A., Leahu, D., Moss, M., & McNally, K. (1994). The effects of aging on Area 46 of the frontal cortex of the rhesus monkey. *Cerebral Cortex, 6*, 621–635.

Petersen, L., & Petersen, M. (1959). Short term retention of individual items. *Journal of Experimental Psychology, 91*, 341–343.

Petersen, R., Smith, G., Kokmen, E., Ivnik, R., & Tangalos, E. (1992). Memory function in normal aging. *Neurology, 42*, 396–401.

Plude, D., Milberg, W., & Cerella, J. (1986). Age differences in depicting and perceiving tridimensionality in simple line drawings. *Experiments in Aging Research, 12*, 221–225.

Poon, L. (1985). Differences in human memory with aging. In J. E. Birren & K. W. Schaie (Eds.), *Handbook of the Psychology of Aging* (pp. 427–462). New York: Van Nostrand Reinhold.

Presty, S., Bachevalier, J., Walker, L., Struble, R., Price, D., Mishkin, M., & Cork, L. (1987). Age differences in recognition memory of the Rhesus monkey (*Macaca mulatta*). *Neurobiology of Aging, 8*, 435–440.

Rabinowitz, J. (1986). Priming in episodic memory. *Journal of Gerontology, 41*, 204–213.

Rapp, P. (1990). Visual discrimination and reversal learning in the aged monkey (*Macaca mulatta*). *Behavioral Neuroscience, 104*, 876–888.

Rapp, P., & Amaral, D. (1989). Evidence for task-dependent memory dysfunction in the aged monkey. *Journal of Neuroscience, 9*, 3568–3576.

Rapp, P., & Amaral, D. (1991). Recognition memory deficits in a subpopulation of aged monkeys resemble the effects of medial temporal lobe damage. *Neurobiology of Aging, 12*, 481–486.

Raymond, B. (1971). Free recall among the aged. *Psychological Reports, 29*, 1179–1182.

Rehbein, L. (1983). Long-term effects of early hippocampectomy in the monkey. Doctoral Thesis, Northeastern University.

Ronald, P. (1992). Motor skill learning, performance, and handedness in aged rhesus monkeys. Master's Dissertation, Boston University School of Medicine.

Rosene, D. (1993). Comparing age-related changes in the basal forebrain and hippocampus of the rhesus monkey. *Neurobiology of Aging, 14*, 669–670.

Ryle, G. (1949). *The Concept of Mind.* London: Hitchinson.

Schaie, K. (1983). The Seattle longitudinal study: A 21 year exploration of psychometric intelligence in adulthood. In K. W. Schaie (Ed.), *Longitudinal Studies of Adult Psychological Development* (pp. 64–135). New York: Guilford.

Schaie, K., & Labouvie-Vief, G. (1974). Generational vs ontogenetic changes in adult cognitive behavior: a fourteen year cross-sequential study. *Developmental Psychology, 10*, 305–320.

Severson, J., Marcusson, J., Winblad, B., & Finch, C. (1982). Age-correlated loss of dopaminergic binding sites in human basal ganglia. *Journal of Neurochemistry, 39*, 1623–1631.

Shefer, V. (1973). Absolute number of neurons and thickness of the cerebral cortex during aging, senile and vascular dementia, and Pick's and Alzheimer's diseases. *Neuroscience Behavioral Physiology, 6*, 319–324.

Solomon, P., Pomerleau, D., Bennett, L., James, J., & Morse, D. (1989). Acquisition of the classically conditioned eyeblink response in humans over the lifespan. *Psychology & Aging, 4*, 34–41.

Spitz, H. (1972). Note on immediate memory for digits: Invariance over the years. *Psychology Bulletin, 78*, 183–185.

Squire, L. (1986). Mechanisms of memory. *Science, 232*, 1612–1619.

Stafford, J., Albert, M., Naeser, M., Sandor, T., & Garvey, A. (1988). Age-related differences in computed tomographic scan measurements. *Archives in Neurology, 45*, 405–419.

Stuss, D., & Benson, F. (1987). The frontal lobes and control of cognition and memory. In E. Perecman (Ed.), *The Frontal Lobes Revisited* (pp. 141–158). New York: IBRN Press.

Talland, G. (1967). Age and the immediate memory span. *The Gerontologist, 7*, 4–9.

Taylor, A., Saint-Cyr, J., & Lang, A. (1987). Parkinson's disease: Cognitive changes in relation to treatment response. *Brain, 110*, 35–51.

Terry, R., Deteresa, R., & Hansen, L. (1987). Neocortical cell counts in normal human adult aging. *Annals of Neurology, 21*, 530–539.

Tigges, J., Gordon, T., McClure, H., Hall, E., & Peters, A. (1988). Survival rate and life span of rhesus monkeys at the Yerkes Regional Primate Research Center. *American Journal of Primatology, 15,* 263–273.

Tigges, J., Herndon, J., & Peters, A. (1992). Neuronal population of area 4 during life span of rhesus monkeys. *Neurobiology of Aging, 11,* 201–208.

Tulving, E. (1972). Episodic and semantic memory. In E. Tulving & W. Donaldson (Eds.), *Organization of Memory* (pp. 381–403). New York: Academic Press.

Vincent, S., Peters, A., & Tigges, J. (1989). Effects of aging on neurons within area 17 of rhesus monkey cerebral cortex. *Anatomical Record, 223,* 329–341.

Waugh, N., & Norman, D. (1965). Primary memory. *Psychology Reviews, 72,* 89–104.

West, M., Coleman, P., Flood, D., & Troncoso, J. (1994). Differences in the pattern of hippocampal neuronal loss in normal ageing and Alzheimer's disease. *Lancet, 344,* 769–772.

Zatz, L., Jernigan, T., & Ahumada, A. (1982). Changes in computed cranial tomography with aging: Intracranial fluid volume. *American Journal of Neuroradiation, 3,* 1–11.

Zola-Morgan, S., & Squire, L. (1984). Preserved learning in monkeys with medial temporal lesions: Sparing of motor and cognitive skills. *Journal of Neuroscience, 4,* 1072–1085.

Zola-Morgan, S., & Squire, L. (1985). Medial temporal lesions in monkeys impair memory in a variety of tasks sensitive to amnesia. *Behavioral Neuroscience, 17,* 558–564.

Twelve

Neuroendocrinology of Aging

Charles V. Mobbs

I. Introduction

Neuroendocrine systems sense and integrate humoral and sensory information to maintain appropriate endocrine (and neural) output. Neuroendocrine systems operate in two domains, the homeostatic and the homeodynamic. The main function of the homeostatic domain is to determine and regulate average physiological set points (like body weight, temperature, and glucose levels), which are functions of the sensitivity of the neural components to humoral signals. The main function of the homeodynamic domain is to regulate the temporal organization of physiological systems, largely by coordinating the phase, amplitude, and period of the rhythms or pulses in these systems. Although each gland (pituitary, adrenal, pancreas, and gonads) possesses independent regulatory mechanisms, the major neural locus for coordinated regulation of these systems is in the hypothalamus. Some hypothalamic neurons sense circulating levels of hormones and respond like a thermostat through a negative feedback system to increase or decrease levels of the cognate hormones appropriately, producing a generally constant average. Other hy-

pothalamic neurons regulate rhythms. However, other neural loci, such as the hippocampus, may also play a modulatory role.

A major motivation to study neuroendocrine systems during aging is the observation that small changes in the small number of (mostly) hypothalamic neurons can have broad physiological effects. Numerous studies over the last 20 years have suggested that changes in homeostatic and homeodynamic neuroendocrine parameters occur during aging, with deleterious physiological consequences. An important early influence on the development of this field were proposals by Finch (1969), who suggested that impairments in neuroendocrine regulation could have broad, cascading pathological consequences during aging, and by Dilman (1971), who proposed that the sensitivity of the hypothalamus to homeostatic negative feedback of hormones decreases during aging. This concept of decreased neuroendocrine sensitivity to hormones appeared to be supported by numerous studies indicating that receptors to hormones generally decrease during aging, as well as extensive evidence that responses to neurotransmitters and growth factors

Handbook of the Biology of Aging, Fourth Edition
Copyright © 1996 Academic Press, Inc. All rights of reproduction in any form reserved.

are attenuated with age (Roth, 1995). Therefore, this concept has dominated the study of neuroendocrinology of aging until the present time. Another early influence was that of Pittendrigh and Daan, who in 1974 showed that circadian periodicity decreases with age. A further important development occurred in 1978, when Landfield *et al.* suggested that a mechanism causing a change in neuroendocrine sensitivity to glucocorticoids could be the cumulative deleterious effect of exposure to glucocorticoids. The concept of persistent cumulative effects referred to as "hysteresis" (Mobbs, 1994), with its potential as a primary mechanism driving age-correlated impairments, has been broadened to include other humoral substances, including estrogen and glucose. Changing hypothalamic (or hippocampal) sensitivity to hormones, especially due to persistent effects of these hormones, and changing rhythms are the dominant themes of the research of the neuroendocrinology of aging in the last 5 years and therefore will be the main focus of this chapter.

Since neuroendocrinology is mainly concerned with functional systems, this review will be organized largely according to these systems (reproductive, stress response, rhythms, etc.). However, since hypothalamic neurons constitute the main locus of neuroendocrine regulation, some studies focusing on hypothalamic properties with age will be discussed outside the context of specific functional systems. In such studies, as with all descriptive studies which compose the bulk of the gerontological literature, it is important to appreciate that during aging many impairments and pathologies develop, so biological changes may be secondary to these pathologies. For this reason, studies which manipulate age-related changes, for example, by manipulating chronic exposure to hormones or through dietary restriction, are more informative regarding the basic causes of age-related changes.

A general result that has appeared in several studies over the last 5 years, especially in humans, is that in some aged individuals peripheral levels of target hormones (testosterone, estrogen, thyroid hormone, and glucocorticoids) decrease, but levels of stimulating hormones (LH, TSH, and ACTH, respectively) remain constant. A common interpretation of these results is that peripheral hormone levels fall due to glandular impairments, but that the older animal exhibits increased sensitivity to negative feedback, leading to constant levels of stimulating hormones in the face of falling levels of target hormones. This surprising result is corroborated by other studies directly examining the effects of hormones on molecular and electrical responses. Thus, the decrease in neuroendocrine receptors during aging must now be considered in the light of evidence of increased neuroendocrine responsiveness in some individuals.

A related theme is the role of activation of neuroendocrine systems in the development of age-related impairments. One of the oldest concepts in the neuroendocrinology of aging is that activation of neuroendocrine systems drives age-related impairments, a concept which might be called "use-it-and-lose-it." Such a concept is closely allied with the rate of living theory, as well as the simpler metaphor of "wear-and-tear." For example, removal of individual glands (pituitary, gonads, or adrenal gland) is reported to prevent various age-related impairments and, in some cases, extend lifespan (Everitt, 1988). This perhaps unexpected effect of normally functioning neuroendocrine systems leading to age-related impairments and even death can be rationalized in an evolutionary context, that late-life dysfunction is essentially a side-effect of optimal early life reproductive success (Mobbs and Finch, 1995). In any case, the physiological consequences of changing neuroendocrine sensitivity, and the possible role of persistent effects of hormone exposure in contributing to changes in neuroendocrine sensitivity, are emerging as important themes for the next generation of studies in the neuroendocrinology of aging.

Although it is easy to get the impression that aging is accompanied by a kind of universal degeneration, in fact careful studies have shown that most neuroendocrine functions change only minimally with age. Indeed, there is considerable evidence of increased functionality, or at least activity, during aging. It is a major goal of gerontology to explicate the specificity of changes which do occur during aging. For example, the hypothalamic areas most pertinent to neuroendocrinology are the arcuate nucleus, ventromedial nucleus, dorsomedial nucleus, paraventricular nucleus, supraoptic nucleus, and suprachiasmatic nucleus. Generally included in the analysis of hypothalamic neurons are neurons in the preoptic area, which include the sexually dimorphic nucleus and the medial preoptic area. All of these nuclei have been implicated in the regulation of metabolism and reproduction. The most thorough single analysis of age-correlated changes in these areas in rodents, based purely on cell counts and anatomically defined boundaries, is the study of Sartin and Lamperti (1985) who reported that of these nuclei, only the ventromedial nucleus and arcuate nucleus exhibited progressive age-related decrease in neuronal number. Thus this study demonstrated that for most hypothalamic nuclei in rats, neuron number is relatively stable during aging.

In humans a somewhat different and possibly more meaningful method of analyzing hypothalamic neurons, defining neurons by their peptide products, indicated that while neurons in two hypothalamic areas show some evidence of degeneration, other hypothalamic areas, far from degenerating, actually exhibited hypertrophy (Swaab, 1995; Rance et al., 1993; Rance, 1992) (Table I). For example,

numbers of neurons in the sexual dimorphic and suprachiasmatic nuclei in humans appear to decrease with age (Swaab, 1995). On the other hand, in the paraventricular nucleus neurons which express vasopressin increase in size and show increased nucleolar size as well, indicating hypertrophy of these neurons (Hoogendijk et al., 1985). Furthermore, the number of neurons in the paraventricular nucleus which express both vasopressin and corticotropin-releasing hormone increases dramatically during aging, also indicating an age-related activation of these neurons (Raadsheer et al., 1993). Similarly, numbers of hypothalamic neurons which express oxytocin were also stable with age (Wierda et al., 1991).

A fascinating phenomenon which is possibly related to hyperactivity of vasopression neurons with age is the observation that in the homozygous Brattleboro rat, whose genetic diabetes insipidus is due to a frame-shift mutation in the vasopressin gene, there is a gradual increase in expression of wild-type vasopressin during aging (van Leeuwen et al., 1989). This increase in wild-type vasopressin in rats with homozygous mutant genes was apparently due to replacement codons in two hot spots (Evans et al., 1994). Furthermore, chronic vasopressin infusion for 40 weeks reduced the incidence of the codon substitution. These data suggest that changes in neuroendocrine gene sequences can develop with age, and that these molecular changes can be influenced by chronic exposure to hormones. These precisely identified molecular phenomena may constitute a precedent for the study of the persistent effects of hormones in other neuroendocrine systems, as described below.

II. Female Reproductive System

Fertility in females exhibits the earliest and most robust age-correlated failure among mammalian physiological systems

Table I
Hypertrophy of Some Hypothalamic Neurons with Age

Crespo, D., Fernandez-Viadero, C., & Gonzalez, C. (1992). The influence of age on supraoptic nucleus neurons of the rat: morphometric and morphologic changes. *Mechanisms of Ageing and Development, 62,* 223–228.

Evans, D. A. P., van der Kleu, A. A. M., Sonnemans, M. A. F., Burbach, J. P. H., & van Leeuwen, F. W. V. (1994). Frameshift mutations of two hotspots in vasopressin transcripts in post-mitotic neurons. *PNAS 91,* 6059–6063.

Hoogendijk, J. E., Fliers, E., Swaab, D. F., & Verwer, R. W. (1985). Activation of vasopressin neurons in the human supraoptic and paraventricular nucleus in senescence and senile dementia. *Journal of the Neurological Sciences, 69*(3), 291–299.

Raadsheer, F. C., Oorschot, D. E., Verwer, R. W., Tilders, F. J., & Swaab, D. F. (1994). Age-related increase in the total number of corticotropin-releasing hormone neurons in the human paraventricular nucleus in controls and Alzheimer's disease: Comparison of the disector with an unfolding method. *Journal of Comparative Neurology, 339,* 447–457.

Raadsheer, F. C., Sluiter, A. A., Ravid, R., Tilders, F. J., & Swaab, D. F. (1993). Localization of corticotropin-releasing hormone (CRH) neurons in the paraventricular nucleus of the human hypothalamus; age-dependent colocalization with vasopressin. *Brain Research, 615,* 50–62.

Rance, N. E., Uswandi, S. V., & McMullen, N. T. (1993). Neuronal hypertrophy in the hypothalamus of older men. *Neurobiology of Aging, 14,* 337–342.

Rance, N. E., McMullen, N. T., Smialek, J. E., Price, D. L., Young, W. S., III (1990). Postmenopausal hypertrophy of neurons expressing the estrogen receptor gene in the human hypothalamus. *Journal of Clinical Endocrinology and Metabolism, 71*(1), 79–85.

Silverman, W. F., & Sladek, J. R., Jr. (1991). Ultrastructural changes in magnocellular neurons from the supraoptic nucleus of aged rats. *Brain Research, 58,* 25–34.

Sturrock, R. R. (1991). Stability of neuronal glial number in the aging mouse supraoptic nucleus. *Anatomischer Anzeiger, 172,* 123–128.

Sturrock, R. R. (1992). Stability of neuron number in the ageing mouse paraventricular nucleus. *Anatomischer Anzeiger, 174,* 337–340.

Swaab, D. F. (1993). Neurohypophysial peptides in the human hypothalamus in relation to development, sexual differentiation, aging and disease. *Regulatory Peptides, 45,* 143–147.

Swaab, D. F. (1995). Ageing of the human hypothalamus, *Hormone Research, 43,* 8–11.

Swaab, D. F., Goudsmit, E., Kremer, H. P., Hofman, M. A., & Ravid, R. (1992). The human hypothalamus in development, sexual differentiation, aging and Alzheimer's disease. *Progress in Brain Research, 91,* 465–472.

Swaab, D. F., Grundke-Iqbal, I., Iqbal, K., Kremer, H. P., Ravid, R., & van de Nes, J. A. (1992). Tau and ubiquitin in the human hypothalamus in aging and Alzheimer's disease. *Brain Research, 590,* 239–249.

Swaab, D. F., Hofman, M. A., Lucassen, P. J., Purba, J. S., Raadsheer, F. C., & van de Nes, J. A. (1993). Functional neuroanatomy and neuropathology of the human hypothalamus. *Anatomy and Embryology, 187,* 317–330.

Terwel, D., Markerink, M., & Jolles, J. (1992). Age-related changes in concentrations of vasopressin in the central nervous system and plasma of the male Wistar rat. *Mechanisms of Ageing and Development, 65,* 127–136.

van Leeuwen, F., van der Beek, E., Seger, M., Burbach, P., & Ivell, R. (1989). Age-related development of a heterozygous phenotype in solitary neurons of the homozygous Brattleboro rat. *PNAS, 86,* 6417–6420.

van Leeuwen, F. W., & van der Beek, E. M. (1991). The amount of mutant vasopressin precursor in the supraoptic and paraventricular nucleus of Brattleboro rats increases with age. *Brain Research, 542,* 163–166.

Wierda, M., Goudsmit, E., Van der Woude, P. F., Purba, J. S., Hofman, M. A., Bogte, H., & Swaab, D. F. (1991). Oxytocin cell number in the human paraventricular nucleus remains constant with aging and in Alzheimer's disease. *Neurobiology of Aging, 12,* 511–516.

---

and therefore has been the subject of extensive analysis. As a model system for the study of neuroendocrine senescence, it has the experimental advantage that the target gland, the ovary, can be removed with little effect on other physiological functions. Therefore, the specifically neuroendocrine components (hypothalamic and pituitary) can be more precisely studied. In humans, the main cause of decreased fertility is ovarian failure; at menopause, neuroendocrine impairments are difficult to demonstrate in women (Richardson, 1993). However, after menopause occurs and gonadotropins are released from ovarian inhibition, impairments in the hypothalamic regulation of gonadotropins may progressively develop (Rossmanith, 1995). Nevertheless, loss of fertility in female rodents is characterized by more robust neuroendocrine impairments, which in the context of a model system have been the subject of extensive studies (Table II).

Reproductive cycles in female rodents become regular by 3 months of age, begin to lengthen and become less regular by 8 months of age, and generally cease completely between 12 and 14 months of age; these age-correlated changes entail neuroendocrine impairments (Wise, 1993). On the other hand, ovarian impairments also occur in rodents, as in humans. Reciprocal ovarian grafts between young and middle-aged mice indicate that the majority of mice actually stop cycling because of ovarian impairments, whereas a minority stop cycling because of neuroendocrine impairments (Mobbs & Finch, 1992). The simultaneous impairment in both hormone-sensitive neurons and the gland producing the hormone is a ubiquitous feature of aging. To specifically assess changes in neuroendocrine sensitivity during aging, the ovaries are generally removed, and estrogen is supplemented to equal levels in animals of each age. By using this approach, the surge of luteinizing hormone (LH, the normal signal for ovulation) that occurs in ovariectomized animals with estrogen replacement is dramatically impaired in middle-aged rodents (but not, apparently, in humans), and this impairment is correlated with the age-correlated loss in estrous cycles and in the ability to support estrous cycles with young ovarian

grafts (Lu et al., 1981; Wise and Parsons, 1984; Mobbs et al., 1984a). Because the LH surge is a robust neuroendocrine response to a hormone and is dramatically impaired early during aging, even before cycles are lost or other impairments are demonstrable, this neuroendocrine impairment has been the subject of intense study. For example, studies have shown that aging is associated with a dramatic reduction in the activation (or at least expression of c-fos) in hypothalamic neurons of rats ovariectomized and given estrogen replacement to stimulate an LH surge (Lloyd, Hoffman, & Wise, 1994).

Impairments in the estrogen-induced LH surge are characterized by a decrease in hypothalamic estrogen receptors and, in particular, by a slower translocation of estrogen receptors to the nucleus (Wise and Parsons, 1984). In ovariectomized animals, estrogen receptors are primarily in a state considered to be cytosolic or "loose-nuclear," and the number of hypothalamic receptors in this state clearly decreases with age. However, the relevance of cytosolic receptors is unclear, since receptors must be translocated, or at least transformed, upon binding to the steroid before effecting biological responses. In the classic study by Wise and Parsons (1984), 2 days after estrogen replacement, the estrogen-induced translocation of the hypothalamic estrogen receptor to the nucleus was greatly attenuated in middle-aged female rats, concomitant with impaired production of the LH surge and induction of progesterone receptors. However, 4 days after replacement the nuclear translocation in the older animals was much less attenuated, and at this time the estrogen-induced responses were also much less attenuated. Age-correlated retardation of estrogen receptor translocation has also been demonstrated in mouse hypothalamus (Belisle et al., 1989), and similar results were obtained by Brown et al. (1990) in rats. However, an interesting difference between the study by Brown et al. and that by Wise and Parsons is that

Brown *et al.* examined receptors 3 days after estrogen replacement. At this time, translocation was still attenuated, as had been observed by Wise and Parsons at 2 days, but interestingly the induction of progesterone receptors was normal in the older rats, despite the decreased nuclear estrogen receptors. The major impairment in responsiveness to estradiol appears to be manifested within the first 2 days after estrogen replacement, when the slower nuclear translocation is most significant. After this time, impairments in estradiol-induced responses generally have not been demonstrated, despite the observation that in the ovariectomized state the older animals exhibit lower levels of estradiol receptors. These studies therefore have clearly indicated the importance of the changes in dynamic properties of neuroendocrine systems with age and, thus, the importance of distinguishing between the kinetic and steady-state responses to hormones during aging.

Studies that examined responses induced by steady-state (or at least longer term) exposure to estrogen generally have not indicated impaired responsiveness to estrogen, and in fact possibly the contrary. An early study indicated that estrogen-induced female sexual behavior (in rats given chronic estrogen over many days) actually increases in older female rats (Cooper, 1977). By using a similar design involving chronic estrogen replacement, these results have been replicated (Kleopoulos *et al.*, 1992). Similarly, induction of prolactin in response to estradiol increases with age (Mobbs *et al.*, 1985). When older female rodents were exposed to steady-state levels of estradiol for 4 days or more, pituitary dopamine (Telford *et al.*, 1986) and glucose-6-phosphate-dehydrogenase (G6PDH) were at least as responsive in older mice as in younger mice. Similarly, when 3-, 10-, and 15-month-old female rats were ovariectomized for 2 weeks and then given estradiol implants for 4 days, the induction of hypothalamic oxytocin receptors, pre-proenkephalin, neurotensin, LHRH, and progesterone receptor mRNAs, and the increase in serum prolactin and lordosis behavior, were at least as great in older rats as in younger rats (Funabashi *et al.*, 1993; Mobbs, 1994).

On the other hand, responses that are inhibited by estradiol appear, by one analysis, to be less sensitive to estradiol in older animals. The most robust example of such a result is that, in aging female rodents, estrogen generally fails to significantly decrease hypothalamic pre-opiomelanocorticotropin (POMC) mRNA and its associated peptide β-endorphin during reproductive senescence (Weiland, Scarbrough, & Wise, 1992; Karelus & Nelson, 1992; Tomimatsu *et al.*, 1993). Similarly, in aging female rats estrogen fails to inhibit hypothalamic estrogen receptor mRNA (Funabashi *et al.*, 1993). However, because estradiol-inhibited parameters tend to decrease with age (as opposed to estradiol-stimulated parameters, which tend to increase with age; Mobbs, 1994), and because there is a minimum below which these parameters cannot be further suppressed by estradiol, the interpretation of sensitivity of estradiol-inhibited parameters can be problematic. In particular, an apparent loss of negative feedback sensitivity could actually be due to a floor effect (the mRNAs could already be maximally inhibited even in ovariectomized animals). Further studies will be required in order distinguish between decreased sensitivity and persistent inhibition or even increased sensitivity.

A similar phenomenon is apparent in studies examining suppression of LH by estradiol. In the absence of ovarian secretion (after ovariectomy or ovarian exhaustion such as menopause), LH levels in older female rats and humans are lower than those in their younger counterparts. However, LH is very sensitive to ovarian steroids, so when steroids are replaced in young and old females, LH is usually suppressed to the same baseline, which represents maximum inhibition. Since young and old females exhibit the same level of

LH after steroid replacement, but old animals exhibit lower levels of LH before steroid replacement, the percentage of inhibition is lower in older females; therefore, some investigators have concluded that the older female is less sensitive to estrogen. However, these results probably reflect a floor effect, and do not really address the sensitivity to estrogen. A more rigorous examination of sensitivity requires a dose–response curve at steady-state, at doses of estradiol which do not produce maximum inhibition. When such a study was carried out in female mice, the dose–response curve was shifted to the left, which indicated possibly increased sensitivity to estrogen (Mobbs, 1994). Such a result is consistent with results in aging male rats and humans, who exhibit increased sensitivity to inhibition of LH by testosterone (Gray & Wexler, 1980b). Clarification of the question of changing neuroendocrine sensitivity to estrogen will require more such dose–response curves at steady-state.

Age-correlated neuroendocrine impairments in the female reproductive system may be due in part to persistent effects of previous exposure to ovarian steroids (Lu et al., 1981; Aschheim, 1983; Felicio et al., 1983; Mobbs et al., 1984a; Wise et al., 1988b). For example, the removal of ovaries from young rodents would delay some reproductive neuroendocrine impairments (Aschheim, 1983) and even reverse some impairments (Lu et al., 1981). It should be noted that some impairments developed even in the absence of the ovaries, but these impairments developed later than if the ovaries had been present during aging (Mobbs et al., 1984a; Felicio et al., 1983). More extensive characterization indicated that, while both amplitude and frequency of LH pulsatile release decrease with age, it is primarily the amplitude decrease that is ovary-dependent, while the frequency decrease appears to develop independent of the ovary (Wise et al., 1988b). Such results suggest that

ovary-dependent neuroendocrine impairments during aging are due, at least in part, to ovary-dependent impairments in the pituitary regulation of LH, as was demonstrated directly by Collins and Parkening (1991). It remains unproven whether normal estrous cycles can cause cumulative irreversible damage or whether neuroendocrine impairments during aging occur only after estradiol levels become relatively elevated during regular cycles. However, when progesterone implants, which decrease estradiol secretion, were given to rats from 4 to 6 months of age, reproductive impairments were delayed, and the delay was partially counteracted by estradiol implants (LaPolt et al., 1986, 1988). These studies suggest that even during normal cycles, well before age-related changes in steroid levels, persistent deleterious effects of estradiol can occur.

While, as discussed earlier, removal of the ovaries delays some age-correlated neuroendocrine impairments, elevated estradiol in young animals can accelerate the onset of such impairments (Kawashima, 1960; Brawer et al., 1978; Lu et al., 1981; Mobbs et al., 1984b). Prolonged exposure of young ovariectomized rats to estradiol implants impaired the steroid-induced LH surge as dramatically as the impairments exhibited by old acyclic rats (Lu et al., 1981). Similarly in mice, priming the LH surge with estradiol only twice as high as the optimal priming dose blocks the LH surge (Gee et al., 1984). Furthermore, a single injection of 2 mg estradiol valerate (EV), as well as estradiol implants producing high physiological levels of estradiol, in young cycling mice caused persistent neuroendocrine impairments similar in many respects to impairments exhibited during aging (Mobbs et al., 1984b; Simard et al., 1987). In a subsequent study, a series of E_2 implants that produced increasing amounts of estradiol in the physiological range caused persistent reproductive impairments monotonically related to the dose of estradiol

(Mobbs & Finch, 1992). Similar persistent impairments (demonstrable many months after treatment with estradiol) could be induced by oral estradiol in the high physiological range (Kohama et al., 1989) or by implants in the supraphysiological (Jesionowska et al., 1990) range, although this latter study also reported a persistent facilitatory effect at lower doses of estradiol (humoral hormesis). This latter result suggests that, while persistent hormonal effects may produce facilitated physiological function in young animals, cumulative effects may eventually lead to impaired function.

The mechanism by which elevated estradiol impairs reproductive function remains unknown, but current hypotheses involve either estrogen-induced toxicity or persistent (and possibly facilitatory) effects of estrogen on gene expression. The earliest studies suggested that estrogen was toxic to specific cells in the arcuate nucleus (Brawer et al., 1978). This hypothesis has been elegantly confirmed and extended by several studies of Desjardins and colleagues, who have determined that neurons which produce β-endorphin are particularly sensitive to the toxic effects of estradiol (Desjardins et al., 1993). These results are particularly intriguing, in view of the observation that among neurons in the arcuate nucleus, neurons which synthesize β-endorphin are particularly sensitive to aging (Weiland, Scarborough, & Wise, 1992; Karelus & Nelson, 1992). Furthermore, the effect of estradiol to reduce β-endorphin neurons can be attenuated with anti-oxidants (Desjardins et al., 1992; Schipper et al., 1994). This latter result suggests that the effects of estradiol on β-endorphin neurons may not be mediated by classic estrogen receptors, a hypothesis consistent with the observation that loss of β-endorphin neurons is no greater in neurons which express the estrogen receptor than in neurons which do not express the estrogen receptor (Miller et al., 1995). However, the relevance to aging of the

sensitivity to β-endorphin neurons to estradiol still remains unclear, since long-term ovariectomy, which delays some reproductive impairments, including gliosis during aging (Schipper et al., 1981), has no appreciable effect on the loss of β-endorphin neurons during aging (Miller et al., 1995). Indeed, Miller et al. suggested that "the presence of the ovary is somehow helpful in maintaining certain neuronal populations, since in L-OVX females there were inevitably fewer neuron populations, regardless of cell type" (Miller et al., 1995). Such a result is consistent with data suggesting that several products which are induced by estradiol in young animals become increasingly elevated during aging in female rodents, and several parameters, such as lordosis, exhibit increasing responsiveness to estrogen during aging (Mobbs, 1994). Although physiological impairment resulting from increased responsiveness to hormones during aging seems paradoxical, several mechanisms could mediate such a result (Mobbs, 1994).

While the estrogen-dependent component of female reproductive senescence may be related to persistent effects of estrogen on estrogen-regulated gene expression (Mobbs, 1994) or toxicity, the estrogen-independent component appears to be related to more general age-related changes in biological rhythms (Wise, 1994). The first clear evidence of this hypothesis was the study by Wise, Dueker, and Wittke (1988b), which demonstrated that long-term ovariectomy delayed the age-related decrease in LH pulse amplitude, but had no effect on the age-related decrease in LH pulse frequency. As will be described later, many studies have demonstrated changes in circadian rhythms during aging. The LH surge is a highly constrained temporal event and thus is particularly dependent on the neural components that regulate circadian rhythms. Indeed, it is possible that this particular sensitivity to the diurnal rhythm accounts

Table II
Female Reproductive Senescence

Aschheim, P. (1983). Relation of neuroendocrine system to reproductive decline in female rats. In J. Meites (Ed.), *Neuroendocrinology of Aging* (pp. 73–102). New York: Plenum Press.

Bourguignon, J. P., Gerard, A., Alvarez Gonzalez, M. L., & Franchimont, P. (1993). Acute suppression of gonadotropin-releasing hormone secretion by insulin-like growth factor I and subproducts: An age-dependent endocrine effect. *Neuroendocrinology, 58,* 525–530.

Brawer, J. R., Naftolin, F., Martin, J., & Sonnenschein, C. (1978). Effects of a single injection of EV on the hypothalamic arcuate nucleus and on reproductive function in the female rat. *Endocrinology, 103,* 501–512.

Brown, T. J., Maclusky, N. J., Shanabrough, M., & Naftolin, F. (1990). Comparison of age- and sex-related changes in cell nuclear estrogen-binding capacity and progestin receptor induction in the rat brain. *Endocrinology, 126,* 2965–2972.

Burch, J. B. E., & Evans, M. I. (1986). Chromatin structural transitions and the phenomenon of vitellogenin gene memory in chickens. *Molecular and Cellular Biology, 6,* 1886–1893.

Carriere, P. D., Farookhi, R., & Brawer, J. R. (1989). The role of abberant hypothalamic opiatergic function in generating polycystic ovaries in the rat. *Canadian Journal of Physiology and Pharmacology, 67,* 896–901.

Ceresini, G., Merchenthaler, A., Negro-Vilar, A., & Merchenthaler, I. (1994). Aging impairs galanin expression in luteinizing hormone-releasing hormone neurons: Effect of ovariectomy and/or estradiol treatment. *Endocrinology, 134,* 324–330.

Chambers, K. C., Thornton, J. E., & Roselli, C. E. (1991). Age-related deficits in brain androgen binding and metabolism, testosterone, and sexual behavior of male rats. *Neurobiology of Aging, 12,* 123–130.

Collins, T. J., & Parkening, T. A. (1991). Exposure to estradiol impairs luteinizing hormone function during aging. *Mechanisms in Ageing and Development, 58,* 207–220.

Cooper, R. L. (1977). Sexual receptivity in aged female rats. Behavioral evidence for increased sensitivity to estrogen. *Hormones and Behavior, 9,* 321

Desjardins, G. C., Beaudet, A., Meaney, M. J., & Brawer, J. R. (1995). Estrogen-induced hypothalamic beta-endorphin neuron loss: A possible model of hypothalamic aging. *Experimental Gerontology, 30,* 253–267.

Desjardins, G. C., Beaudel, A., Schipper, H. M., & Brawer, J. R (1992). Vitamin E protects beta-endorphin neurons from estradiol toxicity. *Endocrinology, 131,* 2481–2482.

Felicio, L. S., Nelson, J. F., Gosden, R. G., & Finch, C. E. (1983). Restoration of ovulatory cycles by young ovarian grafts in aging mice; Potentiation by long-term ovariectomy decreases with age. *Proceedings of the National Academy of Sciences of the United States of America, 80,* 6076.

Funabashi, T., Kleopoulos, S. P., Brooks, P. J., Kato, J., Kimura, F., Pfaff, D. W., & Mobbs, C. V. (1993). Regulation of estrogen receptor mrna and progesterone receptor mrna by estrogen in female rat hypothalamus during aging. *Society of Neuroscience, Abstracts,* in press.

Gee, D. M., Flurkey, K., Mobbs, C. V., Sinha, Y. N., & Finch, C. E. (1984). The regulation of luteinizing hormone and prolactin in C57BL/6J mice: Effects of E2 implant size, ovariectomy, and aging. *Endocrinology, 114,* 685–693.

Gordon, M. N., Mobbs, C. V., & Finch, C. E. (1988). Pituitary and hypothalamic glucose-6-phosphate dehydrogenase: Effects of estradiol and age in C57BL/6J mice. *Endocrinology, 122,* 726–733.

Gray, G. D., & Wexler, B. C. (1980). Estrogen and testosterone sensitivity of middle-aged female rats and the regulation of LH. *Experimental Gerontology, 15,* 201.

Jesionowska, H., Karelus, K., & Nelson, J. F. (1990). Effects of chronic exposure to estradiol on ovarian cyclicity in C57Bl/6J mice: Potentiation at low doses and only partial suppression at high doses. *Biology of Reproduction, 43,* 312–317.

Karelus, K., & Nelson, J. F. (1992). Aging impairs estrogenic suppression of hypothalamic proopiomelanocortin messenger ribonucleic acid in the mouse. *Neuroendocrinology, 55,* 627–633.

Kawashima, S. (1960). Influence of continued injections of sex steroids on the estrous cycle in the female rat. *Annotationes Zoologicae Japonenses, 33,* 226.

Kleopoulos, S. P., Krey, L., & Mobbs, C. V. (1992). Regulation of hypothalamic oxytocin receptors and lordosis reflex during reproductive senescence of female Fisher rats. *Society of Neuroscience, Abstracts, 18,* 1485.

(continued)

Table II *(Continued)*

Kohama, S. G., Anderson, C. P., Osterburg, H. H., May, P. C., & Finch, C. E. (1989). Oral administration of estradiol to young C57Bl/6J mice induces age-like neuroendocrine dysfunctions in the regulation of estrous cycles. *Biology of Reproduction, 41,* 227–232.

LaPolt, P. S., Matt, D. W., Judd, H. L., & Lu, J. K. H. (1986). The relation of ovarian steroid levels in young female rats to subsequent estrous cyclicity and reproductive function during aging. *Biology of Reproduction, 35,* 1131–1139.

LaPolt, P. S., Yu, S. M., & Lu, J. K. H. (1988). Early treatment of young female rats with progesterone delays the aging-associated reproductive decline: A counteraction by estradiol. *Biology of Reproduction, 38,* 987–995.

Lloyd, J. M., Scarbrough, K., Weiland, N. G., & Wise, P. M. (1991). Age-related changes in proopiomelanocortin (POMC) gene expression in the periarcuate region of ovariectomized rats. *Endocrinology, 129,* 1896–1902.

Lu, J. H. K., Gilman, D. P., Meldrum, D. R., Judd, H. L., & Sawyer, C. H. (1981). Relationship between circulating estrogens and the central mechanisms by which ovarian steroids stimulate luteinizing hormone secretion in aged and young female rats. *Endocrinology, 108,* 836–841.

Miller, M. M., Tousignant, P., Yang, U., Pedvis, S., & Billiar, R. B. (1995). Effects of age and long-term ovariectomy on the estrogen-receptor containing sub-populations of beta-endorphin immunoreactive neurons in the arcuate nucleus of female C57Bl/6J mice. *Neuroendocrinology, 6,* 542–551.

Miller, M. M., & Zhu, L. (1992). Aging changes in the beta-endorphin neuronal system in the preoptic area of the C57BL/6J mouse: ultrastructural analysis. *Neurobiology of Aging, 13,* 773–781.

Miller, M. M., Joshi, D., Billiar, R. B., & Nelson, J. F. (1991). Loss during aging of beta-endorphinergic neurons in the hypothalamus of female C57BL/6J mice. *Neurobiology of Aging, 12,* 239–244.

Mobbs, C. V., & Finch, C. E. (1992). Estrogen-induced impairments as a mechanism in reproductive senescence of female C57Bl/6J mice. *Journal of Gerontology, 47,* B48–B51.

Mobbs, C. V., Gee, D. M., & Finch, C. E. (1984a). Reproductive senescence in female C57BL/6J mice: Ovarian impairments and neuroendocrine impairments that are partially reversible and delayable by ovariectomy. *Endocrinology, 115,* 1653–1662.

Mobbs, C. V., Flurkey, K., Gee, D. M., Yamamoto, K., Sinha, Y. N., & Finch, C. E. (1984b). Estradiol-induced adult anovulatory syndrome in female C57BL/6J mice: Age-like neuroendocrine, but not ovarian, impairments. *Biology of Reproduction, 30,* 556–563.

Mobbs, C. V., Cheyney, D., Sinha, Y. N., & Finch, C. E. (1985). Age-correlated and ovary-dependent changes in relationships between plasma estradiol and luteinizing hormone, prolactin, and growth hormone in female C57BL/6J mice. *Endocrinology, 116,* 813–820.

Mohankumar, P. S., Thyagarajan, S., & Quadri, S. K. (1994). Correlations of catecholamine release in the medial preoptic area with proestrous surges of luteinizing hormone and prolactin: effects of aging. *Endocrinology, 135,* 119–126.

Neafsey, P. J., Boxenbaum, H., Ciraulo, D. A., & Fournier, D. J. (1988). A gompertz age-specific mortality-rate model of aging, hormesis, and toxicity: Fixed-dose studies. *Drug Metabolism Reviews, 19,* 369–401.

Nelson, J. F., Bender, M., & Schacter, B. S. (1988). Age-related changes in preopiomelanocortin messenger ribonucleic acid levels in hypothalamus and pituitary of female C57Bl/6J mice. *Endocrinology, 123,* 340–344.

Rance, N. E., McMullen, N. T., Smialek, J. E., Price, D. L., & Young, W. S., III (1990). Postmenopausal hypertrophy of neurons expressing the estrogen receptor gene in the human hypothalamus. *Journal of Clinical Endocrinology and Metabolism, 71*(1), 79–85.

Richardson, S. J. (1993). The biological basis of the menopause. *Baillieres Clinical Endocrinological Metabolism, 7,* 1–16.

Rossi, G. L., Bestetti, G. E., & Reymond, M. J. (1992). Tuberoinfundibular dopaminergic neurons and lactotropes in young and old female rats. *Neurobiology of Aging, 13,* 275–281.

Rossmanith, W. G. (1995). Gonadotropin secretion during aging in women. Review article. *Experimental Gerontology, 30,* 369–381.

Rossmanith, W. G., Reichelt, C., & Scherbaum, W. A. (1994). Neuroendocrinology of aging in humans: Attenuated sensitivity to sex steroid feedback in elderly post-menopausal women. *Neuroendocrinology, 59,* 355.

(continued)

Table II *(Continued)*

Rossmanith, W. G., Scherbaum, W. A., & Lauritzen, C. (1991). Gonadotropin secretion during aging in post-menopausal women. *Neuroendocrinology, 54,* 211–218.

Rubin, B. S. (1992). Isolated hypothalami from aging female rats do not exhibit reduced basal or potassium-stimulated secretion of luteinizing hormone-releasing hormone. *Biology of Reproduction, 47,* 254–261.

Rubin, B. S. (1993). Naloxone stimulates comparable release of luteinizing hormone-releasing hormone from tissue fragments from ovariectomized, estrogen-treated young and middle-aged female rats. *Brain Research, 601,* 246–254.

Schipper, H., Brawer, J. R., Nelson, J. F., Felicio, L. S., & Finch, C. E. (1981). The role of the gonads in the histologic aging of the hypothalamic arcuate nucleus. *Biology of Reproduction, 25,* 413–418.

Schipper, H. M., Desjardins, G. C., Beaudet, A., & Brawer, J. (1994). The 21-aminosteroid antioxidant, U743-89F, prevents estradiol-induced depletion of hypothalamic beta-endorphin neurons in adult female rats. *Brain Research, 652,* 161–163.

Telford, N., Mobbs, C. V., Sinha, Y. N., & Finch, C. E. (1986). The increase of anterior pituitary dopamine in aging C57BL/6J mice is caused by ovarian steroids, not intrinsic pituitary aging. *Neuroendocrinology, 43,* 135–142.

Tomimatsu, N., Hashimoto, S., & Akasofu, K. (1993). Effects of oestrogen on hypothalamic beta-endorphin in ovariectomized and old rats. *Maturitas, 17,* 5–16.

Wise, P. M. (1993). Neuroendocrine ageing: its impact on the reproductive system of the female rat. *Journal of Reproduction and Fertility, Supplement, 46,* 35–46.

Wise, P. M., Dueker, E., & Wuttke, W. (1988b). Age-related alterations in pulsatile luteinizing hormone release: Effects of long-term ovariectomy, repeated pregnancies, and naloxone. *Biology of Reproduction, 39,* 1060–1066.

Wise, P. M., Scarbrough, K., Weiland, N. G., & Larson, G. H. (1990). Diurnal pattern of pro-opiomelanocorticotropin gene expression in the arcuate nucleus of proestrous, ovariectomized, and steroid-treated rats: Possible role in cyclic luteinizing hormone secretion. *Molecular Endocrinology, 4,* 886–892.

Witkin, J. W. (1992). Increased synaptic input to gonadotropin-releasing hormone neurons in aged, virgin, male Sprague-Dawley rats. *Neurobiology of Aging, 13,* 681–686.

in part for the relatively young age at which the LH surge is impaired in females compared, for example, to impairments in LH regulation during aging in males. A particularly elegant and rich demonstration of the relative roles of changing circadian rhythms vs persistent changes in gene expression is a study by Cai and Wise (1994). In this study, transplantation of fetal suprachiasmatic nuclei (which generally regulate circadian rhythms) into old rats restored the amplitude of the POMC mRNA rhythm in the pituitary gland (which was not, apparently, a function of rhythmic transcription, but apparently one of rhythmic changes in mRNA degradation), but did not restore the age-related impairments in POMC transcription. The studies by Cai and Wise (1994) and Wise, Dueker, and Wittke (1988b) should serve as models in coming years for the crucial

analysis of the relationship between changing biological rhythms and persistent effects of hormones on gene expression in aging neuroendocrine systems.

III. Male Reproductive System

In aging male humans and rats, neuroendocrine responses to testosterone appear to increase with age (Winters et al., 1984; Pirke et al., 1978; Gray et al., 1980; Gruenewald & Matsumoto, 1991a,b) (Table III). In particular, plasma LH appears to decrease largely because of increased sensitivity to the negative feedback effects of testosterone (Winters et al., 1984; Gray et al., 1980; Pirke et al., 1978). For example, even though testosterone decreases with age (due at least in part to testicular failure), serum gonadotropins and LHRH mRNA (which are suppressed by testosterone and therefore should increase as testosterone decreases) also decrease with age (Gruenewald *et al.*, 1991b). Furthermore, the age-related decreases in serum gonadotropins and LHRH mRNA are largely reversed after orchidectomy, which largely eliminates testosterone (Gruenewald & Matsumoto, 1991b). To explain their data, Gruenewald *et al.* suggest that "chronic lifelong exposure to testicular factors (e.g., sex steroids) in old rats results in a neural defect. . . ." Such a neural defect could plausibly involve a residual, persistent effect of testosterone to inhibit LHRH mRNA, which would facilitate the acute suppression of LHRH mRNA (and subsequent inhibition of LH and FSH) by testosterone (Mobbs, 1994). The relevance of hypothalamic impairments to age-correlated impairments in

male reproductive physiological function was demonstrated in a remarkable study by Huang and colleagues (1987), which reported that transplantation of fetal hypothalamic tissue into old male rats restored sexual behavior in these rats. However, the role of decreased LHRH in age-correlated decreases in sexual behavior remains to be elucidated.

IV. Circadian Rhythms and Aging

Age-correlated changes in circadian rhythms are increasingly appreciated as playing a critical role in neuroendocrine impairments, as, for example, in female reproductive senescence (Wise, 1994) (Table IV). Like all rhythms, circadian rhythms are characterized by an average value (mesor), amplitude (difference between maximum and minimum; usually, for

Table III
Male Reproductive Senescence

Gray, G. D., Smith, E. R., & Davidson, J. M. (1980). Gonadotropin regulation in middle-aged male rats. *Endocrinology, 107,* 2021.

Gruenewald, D. A., & Matsumoto, A. M. (1991a). Age-related decrease in proopiomelanocortin gene expression in the arcuate nucleus of the male rat brain. *Neurobiology of Aging, 12,* 113–121.

Gruenewald, D. A., & Matsumoto, A. M. (1991b). Age-related decreases in serum gonadotropin levels and gonadotropin-releasing hormone gene expression in the medial preoptic area of the male rat are dependent upon testicular feedback. *Endocrinology, 129,* 2442–2450.

Gruenewald, D. A., Naai, M. A., Marck, B. T., & Matsumoto, A. M. (1994). Age-related decrease in neuropeptide-Y gene expression in the arcuate nucleus of the male rat brain is independent of testicular feedback. *Endocrinology, 134,* 2383–2389.

Huang, H. H., Kissane, J. Q., & Hawrylewicz, E. J. (1987). Restoration of sexual function and fertility by fetal hypothalamic transplant in impotent aged male rats. *Neurobiology of Aging, 8*(5), 465–72.

Pirke, K. M., Geiss, M., & Sintermann, R. (1978). A quantitative study on feedback control of LH by testosterone in young adult and old male rats. *Acta Endocrinologica (Copenhagen), 89,* 798–795.

Piva, F., Celotti, F., Dondi, D., Limonta, P., Maggi, R., Messi, E., Negri-Cesi, P., Zanisi, M., Motta, M., & Martini, L. (1993). Ageing of the neuroendocrine system in the brain of male rats: receptor mechanisms and steroid metabolism. *Journal of Reproduction and Fertility, Supplement, 46,* 47 59.

Roselli, C. E., Thornton, J. E., & Chambers, K. C. (1993). Age-related deficits in brain estrogen receptors and sexual behavior of male rats. *Behavioral Neuroscience, 107,* 202–209.

Vermeulen, A., & Kaufman, J. M. (1992). Role of the hypothalamo-pituitary function in the hypoandrogenism of healthy aging [editorial] [corrected and republished editorial originally printed in *Journal of Clinical Endocrinological Metabolism,* (1992) 74(6), 1226-A–1226C] [comment]. *Journal of Clinical Endocrinological Metabolism, 75,* 704–706.

Winters, S. J., Sherins, R. J., & Troen, P. (1984). The gonadotropin-suppressing activity of androgen is increased in elderly men. *Metabolism, 33,* 1052–1059.

circadian rhythms, 12 hr apart), phase (time at which maximum value occurs), and period (length of the rhythm; for circadian rhythms, by definition, "about" 24 hr). Virtually all rhythms that have been examined (in well over 100 studies) have reported that the amplitude of the rhythm decreases with age (Brock, 1991). Of particular interest, the amplitudes of rhythms in hypothalamic 2-deoxyglucose, receptors, and gene expression decrease with age [reviewed in Wise (1994)]. In most studies the average value, or mesor, also decreases with age (Brock, 1991). However, the mesor and the amplitude are, in principle, independent and do not always both decrease with age. Of the two parameters, amplitude probably more fundamentally reflects the function of the central pacemaker.

In about one-fourth of all studies that have examined the phase of the circadian rhythm, phase has been reported to advance with age (Brock, 1991); in other words, maximum activity (as well as onset of sleep) occurs earlier during aging. It must be considered, however, that to demonstrate a change in phase the parameter of interest usually must be measured very frequently (for circadian rhythms, at least every 20 min or so). Therefore, phase shifts usually can only be demonstrated for behaviors or body temperature, although a few studies have sampled hormones frequently enough to demonstrate a phase advance, especially for glucocorticoids (Sherman, Wysham, & Pfohl, 1985). The majority of studies with high-frequency sampling have reported a phase advance with age.

Age-related phase advance could be related to a shortening of the circadian period. A shortening of the period of activity rhythms in animals under free-running (constant dark) conditions was first reported by Pittendrigh and Daan (1974), and several investigators have reported similar results (Brock, 1991). However, recent studies in mice have indicated that in this

species, period may increase with age (Possidente et al., 1995). The age-correlated shortening of the period of circadian rhythms is an interesting contrast to the age-correlated increase in the period (or, equivalently, a decrease in frequency) of many ultradian endocrine rhythms (e.g, Wise et al., 1988a). It could be argued that aging animals are less sensitive to the entraining stimulus (usually light; see the following), raising the possibility that aging (possibly light-insensitive) individuals become, in effect, unentrained. However, when six different activities were measured continuously under entrained conditions, and the phase of the specifically 24-hr rhythm of each behavior was calculated by Fourier analysis, the phase of the 24-hr rhythm in old animals, compared to the 24-hr rhythm in young animals, was advanced during aging (by about 2 hr) for all behaviors (Wenzel & Randall, 1982). Therefore, regardless of whether the summation of rhythms (which is reflected by the acrophase of total activity) exhibits a shortening of period, the specifically 24-hr component still appears to exhibit a phase advance. The relationship of age-related changes in circadian rhythms to age-related changes in responses to entrainment stimuli has been the subject of a particularly interesting series of studies (Turek et al., 1995). Other aspects of changing neuroendocrine rhythms have also been recently reviewed (Copinschi and van Cauter, 1995; Touitou, 1995).

Since the hypothalamic suprachiasmatic nucleus (SCN) has been established as the primary locus for the regulation of circadian rhythms, it has been hypothesized that changes in circadian rhythms with age are related to age-correlated impairments in the SCN (Wise, 1994). The age-correlated decrease in the free-running period, while of unclear physiological importance, provides important (although circumstantial) support for this hypothesis since incomplete lesions of the SCN lead to a shortening of the free-running period, with the degree of shortening correlated with the degree of damage to the SCN (Pickard & Turek, 1983; Davis & Gorski, 1984). Direct assessment of oscillations in the SCN, as assessed by 2-deoxyglucose uptake (Wise *et al.*, 1988a), and physiological measurements (Satinoff *et al.*, 1993), clearly indicates changes in these oscillations during aging. Similarly, some (although not all) studies have reported morphological evidence of damage in the SCN of extremely old rodents [reviewed in Brock (1991)]. Studies using c-fos as a marker have suggested that light is relatively less effective in activating the SCN of aging rats (Sutin *et al.*, 1993). An obvious hypothesis is that the ability to detect light decreases with age, leading to a relative weakening in entrainment. Nevertheless, the bulk of the data suggests that the SCN incurs damage during aging, leading to changes in circadian rhythms during aging. The study by Cai and Wise (1994) reported that at least some age-correlated changes in circadian rhythms can be corrected by fetal transplants of the SCN. Similarly, Van Reeth *et al.* (1994) reported that fetal transplants of the SCN restore the responsiveness of the aging circadian system to a phase-setting stimulus. If such studies are extended to hormonal rhythms, the role of SCN impairments in causing other age-correlated impairments should be clarified dramatically.

Another potentially fundamental pacemaker, the rhythm of melatonin from the pineal gland, has recently become of considerable interest (reviewed by Reiter, 1995). The amplitude of the rhythm of plasma levels of melatonin, derived from the pineal gland, decreases with age in humans and other species (Reiter, 1995). The changing rhythm of melatonin, however, is of particular interest because melatonin itself entrains activity rhythms, possibly by an action on the suprachiasmatic nucleus (Cassone *et al.*, 1986). Therefore, a decrease in the rhythm of melatonin could account for, or at least amplify, changes in other rhythms. Furthermore, dietary restriction, which extends life span, also attenuates the age-related impairment in melatonin rhythms (Stokkan *et al.*, 1991). Perhaps most provocative is the report that injections of melatonin, as well as pineal transplants, extend lifespan in aging mice (Pierpaoli and Regelson, 1994). Recent reports that melatonin is an even more potent free radical scavenger than glutathione (Tan *et al.*, 1993a), and that melatonin is particularly effective in blocking oxidative damage to DNA (Tan *et al.*, 1993b), provide a potential mechanism by which melatonin might amelioriate age-related impairments. Therefore, the hypothesis that enhancement of the melatonin rhythm during aging, to an amplitude exhibited in young individuals, certainly deserved further study. However, it should be realized that while there are many reports claiming an extension of lifespan by various treatments, with equally compelling potential mechanisms, to date the only manipulation for which these effects have been reliably replicated is dietary restriction (Masoro, 1993). Thus a key question will be whether effects of melatonin replacement on age-related impairments can be replicated and extended.

V. Stress and Aging

There has been much speculation concerning the relationship between "stress," which intuitively seems unpleasant and does not seem like a good thing, and aging, about which the same could be said. In general, stress has been hypothesized to be a cause of the impairments that occur during aging, and aging has been hypothesized to impair the ability to respond to stress. These hypotheses have stimulated much fascinating research in the neuroendocrinology of aging, which will be discussed below. However, to place this

Table IV
Neuroendocrine Rhythms and Aging

Cai, A., & Wise, P. M. (1994). Effects of age and suprachiasmatic nucleus (SCN) transplants on the diurnal rhythm on pituitary proopiomelanocorticotropin (POMC) gene expression. *Society of Neuroscience, Abstracts, 20* (Part 1), 49.

Cincotta, A. H., Schiller, B. C., Landry, R. J., Herbert, S. J., Miers, W. R., & Meier, A. H. (1993). Circadian neuroendocrine role in age-related changes in body fat stores and insulin sensitivity of the male Sprague-Dawley rat. *Chronobiology International, 10,* 244–258.

Copinschi, G., & van Cauter, E. (1995). Effects of aging on modulation of hormonal secretions by sleep and circadian rhythmicity. *Hormone Research, 43,* 20–24.

Davis, F. C., & Gorski, R. A. (1984). Unilateral lesions of the hamster suprachiasmatic nuclei: evidence for redundant control of circadian rhythms. *Journal of Comparative Physiology, A154,* 221.

Mirmiran, M., Swaab, D. F., Kok, J. H., Hofman, M. A., Witting, W., & Van Gool, W. A. (1992). Circadian rhythms and the suprachiasmatic nucleus in perinatal development, aging and Alzheimer's disease. *Progress in Brain Research, 93,* 151–62.

Pickard, G. E., & Turek, F. W. (1983). The suprachiasmatic nuclei: Two circadian clocks? *Brain Research, 268,* 201.

Pierpaoli, W., & Regelson, W. (1994). Pineal control of aging: Effect of melatonin and pineal grafting in aging mice. *PNAS, 91,* 781–791.

Pittendrigh, C. S., & Daan, S. (1974). Circadian oscillations in rodents: A systematic increase of their frequency with age. *Science, 186,* 548–551.

Possidente, B., McEldowney, S., & Pabon, A. (1995). Aging lengthens circadian period for wheel-running activity in C57Bl/6J mice. *Physical Behavior, 57,* 575–580.

Reiter, R. J. (1995). The pineal gland and melatonin in relation to aging: A summary of the theories and of the data. *Experimental Gerontology, 30,* 199–212.

Reymond, F., Denereaz, N., & Lemarchand-Beraud, T. (1992). Thyrotropin action is impaired in the thyroid gland of old rats. *Acta Endocrinologica (Copenhagen), 126,* 55–63.

Romero, M. T., Lehman, M. N., & Silver, R. (1993). Age of donor influences ability of suprachiasmatic nucleus grafts to restore circadian rhythmicity. *Brain Research: Developments in Brain Research, 71,* 45–52.

Satinoff, E., Li, H., Tcheng, T. K., Liu, C., McArthur, A. J., Medanic, M., & Gillette, M. U. (1993). Do the suprachiasmatic nuclei oscillate in old rats as they do in young ones? *American Journal of Physiology, 265,* R1216–R1222.

Stokkan, K. A., Reiter, R. J., Nonaka, K. O., Lerchel, A., Yu, B. P., & Vaughan, M. K. (1991). Food restriction retards aging of the pineal gland. *Brain Research, 545,* 66–72.

Sutin, E. L., Dement, W. C., Heller, H. C., & Kilduff, T. S. (1993). Light-induced gene expression in the suprachiasmatic nucleus of young and aging rats. *Neurobiology of Aging, 14,* 441–446.

Tan, D. X., Chen, D. X., Poeggleler, B., Manchester, L. C., & Reiter, R. J. (1993a). Melatonin: A potent, endogenous hydroxyl radical scavenger. *Endocrine Journal, 1,* 57–60.

Tan, D. X., Poeggleler, B., Reiter, R. J., Chen, L. D., Chen, S., & Manchester, L. C. (1993a). The pineal hormone melatonin inhibits DNA-adduct formation induced by the chemical carcinogen safrole in vivo. *Cancer Letters, 70,* 65–71.

Touitou, Y. (1995). Effects of ageing on endocrine and neuroendocrine rhythms in humans. *Hormone Research, 43,* 12–19.

Touitou, Y., & Haus, E. (1994). Aging of the human endocrine and neuroendocrine time structure. *Annals of the New York Academy of Science, 719,* 378–397.

Turek, F. W., Penev, P., Zhang, Y., van Reeth, O., & Zee, P. (1995). Effects of age on the circadian system. *Neuroscience and Biobehavioral Review, 19,* 53–58.

van der Zee, E. A., Streefland, C., Strosberg, A. D., Schroder, H., & Luiten, P. G. (1991). Colocalization of muscarinic and nicotinic receptors in cholinoceptive neurons of the suprachiasmatic region in young and aged rats. *Brain Research, 542,* 348–352.

Van Reeth, O., Zhang, Y., Zee, P. C., & Turek, F. W. (1994). Grafting fetal suprachiasmatic nuclei in the hypothalamus of old hamsters restores responsiveness of the circadian clock to a phase shifting stimulus. *Brain Research, 643,* 338–342.

(continued)

Table IV   (*Continued*)

Van Reeth, O., Zhang, Y., Reddy, A., Zee, P., & Turek, F. W. (1993). Aging alters the entraining effects of an activity-inducing stimulus on the circadian clock. *Brain Research, 607*, 286–292.

Weiland, N. G., Scarbrough, K., & Wise, P. M. (1992). Aging abolishes the estradiol-induced suppression and diurnal rhythm of proopiomelanocortin gene expression in the arcuate nucleus. *Endocrinology, 131*, 2959–2964.

Wenzel, Z. M., & Randall, P. K. (1982). Phase changes of eating and activity circadian rhythms in young and old female rats. *Society for Neuroscience, Abstracts, 8*, 544.

Whealin, J. M., Burwell, R. D., & Gallagher, M. (1993). The effects of aging on diurnal water intake and melatonin binding in the suprachiasmatic nucleus. *Neuroscience Letters, 154*, 149–152.

Wise, P. M. (1994). Nathan Shock Memorial Lecture 1991. Changing neuroendocrine function during aging: impact on diurnal and pulsatile rhythms. *Experimental Gerontology, 29*, 13–19.

Wise, P. M., Cohen, I. R., Weiland, N. G., *et al.* (1988a). Aging alters the circadian rhythm of glucose utilization in the suprachiasmatic nucleus. *Proceedings of the National Academy of Sciences of the United States of America, 85*, 5305.

Woods, W. H., Powell, E. W., Andrews, A., & Ford, C. W., Jr. (1993). Light and electron microscopic analysis of two divisions of the suprachiasmatic nucleus in the young and aged rat. *Anatomical Record, 237*, 71–88.

research in its proper context, it is essential to clarify more rigorously what is meant by stress, and why stress is an important concept in physiology.

The most important concept in considering the physiology of stress is not the nature of the stress (that is, the stimulus), but rather that of the stress response. A remarkable biological fact is that there is a complex but *stereotypic* response to a wide variety of stimuli, which have in common that they can be perceived as potentially deleterious. It is largely unknown how such a wide variety of stimuli can be sensed as potentially threatening and give rise to such a highly constrained stereotypic response. There are three well-characterized "stress" responses: neuroendocrine, molecular, and immune. The most salient features of the neuroendocrine stress response are activation of the sympathetic nervous system (most subjectively familiar) and elevation of plasma glucocorticoid levels. As it became clear that these stereotypic responses could be activated by a wide variety of stimuli, the stimuli began to be considered under the aggregate rubric of "stress." Stress stimuli that activate the neuroendocrine stress response are sensory, including pain, restraint, and dramatic changes in sensory input (loud noises, etc.), and generally can be understood as proxies for threatening environments. Considering the huge variety of sensory stimuli with which the nervous system is constantly inundated, it is remarkable that the stress response is activated generally only by stimuli that can be understood to be threatening. The basis by which stimuli are sorted into "stress" and "non-stress" is quite mysterious and constitutes one of the most fascinating questions in neurobiology. Not surprisingly, however, the stereotypic stress response is sometimes activated by stimuli that are not, in reality, threatening, such as restraint (especially in rodents). Furthermore, as more is understood about the stress response, it becomes clearer that the response is not as stereotypic as originally thought, that is, different "stressors" actually give rise to different patterns of stress response. These variations from the ideal stress response may relate to some age-correlated pathologies, as described below.

In addition to the neuroendocrine stress response, stereotypic molecular and immune responses have also been characterized. The most salient feature of the molecular stress response is the induction of a small number of cellular heat-shock or stress gene products. Stress stimuli that activate the molecular response are biophysical, including hyperthermia, ischemia, and metabolic toxins. The most salient feature of the immune stress response is the activation of the inflammatory process (edema and cytokine production). Stress stimuli that activate the inflammation response are generally mechanical, including scratches or bruises, but they may also include biological agents such as antigens or lipopolysaccharides.

Several studies have indicated that basal activity of the neuroendocrine stress response systems, that is, sympathetic nervous system and plasma glucocorticoid levels, may increase with age. However, it has been difficult to demonstrate that this apparently increased basal activity of the stress response systems is actually related to the stress response. In fact, the increased basal levels of plasma catecholamines and glucocorticoids may be related more to decreased clearance and uptake of these hormones, and in the presence of stress the neuroendocrine response may be attenuated during aging (see below).

Although the function of specific aspects of the stress response are not always clear (for example, glucocorticoid elevations), it may be assumed that these responses are generally adaptive under circumstances that are ordinarily encountered. Therefore, activation of the stress response might, up to a point, actually minimize age-related impairments. Such a result has been reported by Brodish and Odio (1989). Similarly, dietary restriction, which is well-established to increase longevity in rodents, concomitantly activates at least one element of the stress response by causing an elevation of glucocorticoids (Stewart et al., 1988; Sabatino et al., 1991). Thus, it is plausible to hypothesize that an optimum activation of the stress response might actually increase longevity (Leakey et al., 1994).

A. Glucocorticoids and Aging

Because elevated levels of adrenal hormones produce acute impairments similar to some impairments exhibited during aging, cumulative deleterious effects of adrenal hormones have long been proposed as contributing to the aging process (Findley, 1949; Solez, 1952; Robertson et al., 1961; Selye & Tuchweber, 1976; Wexler, 1976; Landfield et al., 1978; Landfield, 1980; Sapolsky et al., 1986). A seminal discovery in this field was that in male rats a gradual rise in glucocorticoid levels can be detected and correlated with evidence of morphological damage to the hippocampus, which expresses high levels of glucocorticoid receptors (Landfield et al., 1978). This discovery led Landfield to propose that a cumulative exposure of glucocorticoids causes the gradual erosion of hippocampal neurons (Landfield, 1980). Landfield also speculated that the loss of hippocampal inhibition of glucocorticoid secretion during aging could lead to a gradual increase in glucocorticoids. This "adrenocortical hypothesis of brain and somatic aging" was strengthened by the demonstration that adrenalectomy attenuates the development of specific age-correlated impairments in the hippocampus, and elevated glucocorticoid levels can accelerate these impairments (Landfield et al., 1981).

The hypothesis was extended by reports that older animals fail to terminate the secretion of glucocorticoids after stress, leading (along with other experiments) to the hypothesis that neuroendocrine sensitivity to the negative feedback effects of glucocorticoids after stress is impaired with age (Sapolsky et al., 1983). These investigators further proposed that the reported impairments in negative feedback during aging were specifically linked to a down-regulation of glucocorticoid receptors in the CA3 region of the hippocampus (Sapolsky et al., 1985). Thus, these investigators proposed a "glucocorticoid cascade hypothesis," postulating that stress-induced glucocorticoid secretion damages CA3 neurons, leading to a loss of negative feedback after stress, leading to increased glucocorticoid secretion, and so on in a recursive destructive cycle. This hypothesis differed from Landfield's initial proposal by focusing on the effects of stress to down-regulate hippocampal receptors (especially in the CA3 region), rather than the cumulative effects of normal, nonstress levels. It was further suggested that the increased glucocorticoid levels that thus occur during aging could account for a wide range of age-correlated impairments, including impaired immune responses and diabetes. The remarkable specificity of these results (the specific impairments in negative feedback only during the recovery phase after stress and the specific vulnerability of the CA3 neuronal field) and the simultaneous description of how stress could accelerate aging and how older animals are impaired in their ability to respond to stress stimulated much research in this field. While Landfield's original hypothesis continues to be of great interest, the more ambitious "cascade" hypothesis has been much more controversial.

Probably the best-established element of the adrenocortical hypothesis is that glucocorticoids potentiate damage in some hippocampal neurons [reviewed by Landfield (1994)]. Two lines of investigation have been of particular interest. First, several studies by Sapolsky and colleagues have reported that glucocorticoid-potentiated damage can be demonstrated in hippocampal primary neuronal cultures (Chou, Lin, & Sapolsky, 1994; Elliott & Sapolsky, 1992, 1993; Stein-Behrens, Elliott, et al., 1992; Stein-Behrens, Lin, & Sapolsky, 1994; Tombaugh & Sapolsky, 1992; Tombaugh et al., 1992). This line of investigation shows great promise in clarifying the mechanism by which glucocorticoids potentiate damage to hippocampal neurons. A second line of investigation

has focused on assessing the effects of elevated glucocorticoid levels on hippocampal damage in vivo (Kerr et al., 1991; Levy et al., 1994). Of particular interest is that the damaging effects of glucocorticoids in vivo appear to be most (or only) evident in older animals (Kerr et al., 1991; Levy et al., 1994). These results were corroborated by direct electrophysiological evidence that effects of glucocorticoids on hippocampal neurons increase with age (Kerr et al., 1989, 1991).

Nevertheless, the relationship between glucocorticoids and hippocampal damage is highly sensitive to anatomy. For example, studies have demonstrated that the removal of adrenal steroids by adrenalectomy, far from protecting neurons from damage, actually causes dramatic neuronal loss in the dentate gyrus of the hippocampus (Sloviter, Dean, & Neubort, 1993; Sloviter et al., 1993; Armstrong et al., 1993). In fact, the hippocampal neuronal loss produced by the removal of glucocorticoids in the dentate gyrus is far more robust and dramatic than the neuronal loss in hippocampal pyramidal cells produced by excess glucocorticoids. Landfield's original data suggested that the CA1 region of the hippocampus is the most sensitive to damage by glucocorticoids and aging (Landfield et al., 1981). In contrast, a later study suggested that the CA3 region was more vulnerable to glucocorticoids and aging (Sapolsky et al., 1985). Subsequently, another study reported that CA1 neurons exhibited more damage during aging, in correlation with elevated glucocorticoid levels (Issa et al., 1990). Subsequent clarification of the distribution of subtypes of the glucocorticoid receptors suggests that CA1 neurons, whose main receptor subtype is maximally occupied only at elevated glucocorticoid levels, are the most plausibly vulnerable to elevated glucorticoid levels. In contrast, the main receptor subtype in CA3 neurons is maximally occupied at basal levels of glucocorticoids and so presumably would not be particularly sensitive to an elevation of glucocorticoid levels (Landfield, 1994).

While the hypothesis that a cumulative effect of glucocorticoids potentiates hippocampal damage during aging, as hypothesized by Landfield (1980), has been supported by subsequent studies, the "glucocorticoid cascade hypothesis" that this damage leads to a self-amplifying cycle of elevated glucocortoids with further hippocampal damage, has not been supported. Although self-amplifying destructive feedback cycles, such as that envisioned by the glucocorticoid cascade hypothesis or the similar "run-away positive feedback" cycle of Orgel's error hypothesis, are appealing as theories of aging, the data do not generally support such mechanisms. In contradiction to the glucocorticoid cascade hypothesis, glucocorticoids generally do not increase with age in humans or other species. Most studies report a decrease in plasma glucocorticoids during aging in humans (Sherman et al., 1985), although a thorough study examining only very healthy men demonstrated no age-related changes in the levels or turnover of plasma glucocorticoids (Barton et al., 1993). Furthermore, dietary restriction increases glucocorticoid levels, yet delays many age-correlated impairments (Sabatino et al., 1991). On the basis of these and other results, Sabatino (1991) et al. concluded that "the Glucocorticoid Cascade Hypothesis does not describe a major aspect of the aging process." Since these investigators did not examine hippocampal function, it is possible that dietary restriction may have accelerated age-correlated hippocampal damage. However, dietary restriction attenuated the age-related increase in GFAP, a marker of neuronal damage in the hippocampus (Major et al., 1995) and the hypothalamus (Nichols et al., 1995), thus suggesting that if glucocorticoids do damage neurons during aging, the effect is much smaller than the protective effect of dietary restriction.

Furthermore, few studies suggest an impaired neuroendocrine sensitivity to glucocorticoids during aging; in fact, an increased sensitivity is reported by several studies. Most of the early studies used glucocorticoid levels as the primary indicator of neuroendocrine negative feedback sensitivity. Such studies assume that the rest of the system (adrenal responsiveness to ACTH, neural processing of stress, etc.) does not change with age. Faced with similar confounds, researchers in the reproductive system use as a standard paradigm removal of the end-organ gland (the ovaries) and examine the effects of steroid replacement on neuroendocrine output (LH). The equivalent design, removal of adrenal glands and examination of the effects of steroid replacement on ACTH, is more difficult in the adrenocortical system and until recently has been rarely used. Several studies have demonstrated the importance of measuring ACTH levels.

In rats, the many studies of potential age-correlated impairments in the neuroendocrine regulation of glucocorticoids in rats have not yielded consistent results. While most studies have reported an increase in the basal secretion of glucocorticoids, many of these have reported that the change is not significant. The complexity of this literature is exemplified by reports in a single journal issue of both decreased (Cizza et al., 1994) and increased (Hauger et al., 1994) glucocorticoid levels in aging male Fischer rats. A review (Sapolsky, 1992) pointed out that, in studies reporting relatively low basal levels in young rats, the basal levels in old rats are likely to be significantly higher, whereas when the basal levels in young rats are relatively higher, the age-related differences tend not to be significant. The higher levels of glucocorticoids in young rats in some studies presumably were due to relatively stressful environments or protocols in those studies. Interestingly, these apparently stressful environments tended to increase glucocorticoid levels in young rats, but not in old rats since glucocorticoid levels in the older rats of different studies were equivalent, regardless of whether the young rats exhibited elevated levels of glucocorticoids. This raises the possibility that, in the presence of stress, age-correlated differences in glucocorticoids are minimized, a result that was directly demonstrated by Brodish and Odio (1989). Such a result might be expected if older rats demonstrated less responsiveness to stress or if the negative feedback sensitivity during stress was in fact greater in the older rats.

When ACTH is used as the indicator of stress responsiveness, several studies have indicated that suppression of ACTH by glucocorticoids is greater in older rats and dogs than in younger animals. Although early studies in rats reported that the return of glucocorticoids to baseline after stress is delayed in older animals (Sapolsky et al., 1983), other studies have shown the opposite, that glucocorticoids return earlier to baseline after stress in older rats (Stewart et al., 1988; van den Berg et al., 1991). However, since glucocorticoid clearance may decrease during aging (Romanoff et al., 1961), a more valid measurement is ACTH. In those studies that measured ACTH, suppression of ACTH after stress was greater in older rats (van den Berg et al., 1991; Gilad et al., 1993; van Eekelen et al., 1992) and dogs (Reul et al., 1991; Rothuizen et al., 1991, 1993). Taken together, these studies suggest that basal levels of glucocorticoids do increase during aging in rats and dogs, but that the sensitivity to negative feedback associated with stress may increase during aging. Furthermore, glucocorticoids increase calcium flux in hippocampal neurons, and hippocampal neurons become increasingly sensitive to this glucocorticoid-induced calcium flux during aging (Landfield et al., 1992).

Nevertheless, basal glucocorticoid levels have been reported to increase in many studies (Sapolsky, 1992). In studies of the aging dog (whose glucocorticoid physiol-ogy is more similar to that in humans than that in rats), the age-correlated increase in basal glucocorticoid secretion appears to be related to a specific decrease in mineralcorticoid receptors in both the hippocampus and the hypothalamus, but there is no change in glucocorticoid receptors (Reul et al., 1991; Rothuizen et al., 1991, 1993). Mineralcorticoid receptors appear to mediate the basal feedback of glucocorticoids, whereas glucocorticoid receptors appear to mediate feedback during stress (de Kloet et al., 1991a,b). In rats, glucocorticoid receptors (as opposed to mineralcorticoid receptors) have been reported to decrease with age (Sapolsky et al., 1986). However, careful analysis indicates that, in the presence of glucocorticoids, glucocorticoid receptors are not downregulated in the older animal as they are in the younger animal (Eldridge et al., 1989b). This lack of down-regulation could lead to relatively elevated levels of receptors in the older animal after stress (Landfield, 1994). This rather surprising phenomenon has also been observed with the estrogen receptor, whose mRNA estradiol fails to down-regulate in the hypothalamus of older animals (Funabashi et al., 1993), thus leading to relatively elevated levels of the receptor mRNA in the presence of hormone. These new data suggest that an effective increase in some receptors in the presence of hormone (due to impaired down-regulation in the older animal) may mediate the apparently greater responses to hormones exhibited in some parameters in the older animals. Taken together, these studies suggest that it is the basal, mineralcorticoid-receptor-mediated glucocorticoid regulation that is most affected by aging in rats and dogs, in both the hippocampus and the hypothalamus. In contrast, the negative feedback suppression of glucocorticoids after stress and the electrophysiological response of hippocampal neurons to glucocorticoids appear to be, if anything, more sensitive during aging (Table V).

Table V
Glucorticoids and Aging

Arbel, I., Kadar, T., Silberman, M., & Levy, A. (1994). The effects of long-term corticosterone administration on hippocampal morphology and cognitive performance of middle-aged rats. *Brain Research, 657,* 227–235.

Armanini, D., Scali, M., Vittadello, G., Ribecco, M., Zampollo, V., Pratesi, C., Orlandini, E., Zovato, S., Zennaro, C. M., & Karbowiak, I. (1993). Corticosteroid receptors and aging. *Journal of Steroid Biochemistry and Molecular Biology, 45,* 191–194.

Armstrong, J. N., McIntyre, D. C., Neubort, S., & Sloviter, R. S. (1993). Learning and memory after adrenalectomy-induced hippocampal dentate granule cell degeneration in the rat. *Hippocampus, 3,* 359–371.

Ashworth, J. B., Reuben, D. B., & Benton, L. A. (1994). Functional profiles of healthy older persons. *Age and Ageing, 23,* 34–39.

Barton, R. N., Horan, M. A., Weijers, J. W., Sakkee, A. N., Roberts, N. A., & van Bezooijen, C. F. (1993). Cortisol production rate and the urinary excretion of 17-hydroxycorticosteroids, free cortisol, and 6-beta-hydroxycortisol in healthy elderly men and women. *Journal of Gerontology, 48,* M213–M218.

Brandtstadter, J., Baltes-Gotz, B., Kirschbaum, C., & Hellhammer, D. (1991). Developmental and personality correlates of adrenocortical activity as indexed by salivary cortisol: observations in the age range of 35 to 65 years. *Journal of Psychosomatic Research, 35,* 173–185.

Brodish, A., & Odio, M. (1989). Age-dependent effects of chronic stress on ACTH and corticosterone responses to an acute novel stress. *Neuroendocrinology, 49,* 496–501.

Chou, Y. C., Lin, W. J., & Sapolsky, R. M. (1994). Glucocorticoids increase extracellular [^{3}H]D-aspartate over-flow in hippocampal cultures during cyanide-induced ischemia. *Brain Research, 654,* 8–14.

Cizza, G., Calogero, A. E., Brady, L. S., Bagdy, G., Bergamini, E., Blackman, M. R., Chrousos, G. P., & Gold, P. W. (1994). Male Fischer 344/N rats show a progressive central impairment of the hypothalamic-pituitary-adrenal axis with advancing age. *Endocrinology, 134,* 1611–1620.

Cocchi, D. (1992). Age-related alterations in gonadotropin, adrenocorticotropin and growth hormone secretion. *Aging (Milano), 4,* 103–113.

Cugini, P., Lucia, P., Di Palma, L., Re, M., Canova, R., Gasbarrone, L., & Cianetti, A. (1992). The circadian rhythm of atrial natriuretic peptide, vasoactive intestinal peptide, beta-endorphin and cortisol in healthy young and elderly subjects. *Clinical Autonomic Research, 2,* 113–118.

de Kloet, E. R. (1992). Corticosteroids, stress, and aging. *Annals of the New York Academy of Science, 663,* 357–371.

de Kloet, E. R., Sutanto, W., Rots, N., van Haarst, A., van den Berg, D., Oitzl, M., van Eekelen, A., & Voorhuis, D. (1991a). Plasticity and function of brain corticosteroid receptors during aging. *Acta Endocrinologica (Copenhagen), 125 (Suppl. 1),* 65–72.

de Kloet, E. R., Joels, M., Oitzl, M., & Sutanto, W. (1991b). Implication of brain corticosteroid receptor diversity for the adaptation syndrome concept. In G. Jasmin & M. Cantin (Eds.), Stress Revisited. 1. Neuroendocrinology of Stress, *Methods and Achievements in Experimental Pathology, 14,* 104–132.

Eldridge, J. C., Fleenor, D. G., Kerr, D. S., & Landfield, P. W. (1989a). Impaired up-regulation of type II corticosteroid receptors in hippocampus of aging rats. *Brain Research,* 248–256.

Eldridge, J C., Kute, T., Brodish, A., & Landfield, P. W. (1989b). Apparent age-related resistance of hippocampal type II corticoid receptors to downregulation by chronic escape training. *Journal of Neuroscience, 9,* 3237–3242.

Elliott, E. M., & Sapolsky, R. M. (1992). Corticosterone enhances kainic acid-induced calcium elevation in cultured hippocampal neurons. *Journal of Neurochemistry, 59,* 1033–1040.

Elliott, E. M., & Sapolsky, R. M. (1993). Corticosterone impairs hippocampal neuronal calcium regulation—possible mediating mechanisms. *Brain Research, 602,* 84–90.

Fukushima, M., Nakai, Y., Tsukada, T., Naito, Y., Nakaishi, S., Tominaga, T., Murakami, N., Kawamura, H., Fukata, J., & Ikeda, H. (1992). Immunoreactive corticotropin-releasing hormone levels in the hypothalamus of female Wistar fatty rats. *Neuroscience Letters, 138,* 245–248.

Gilad, G. M., Li, R., Wyatt, R. J., & Tizabi, Y. (1993). Effects of genotype on age-related alterations in the concentrations of stress hormones in plasma and hypothalamic monoamines in rats. *Journal of Reproduction and Fertility, Supplement, 46,* 119.

(continued)

Table V   *(Continued)*

Goya, R. G., Brooks, K., & Meites, J. (1991a). A comparison between hormone levels and T lymphocyte function in young and old rats. *Mechanisms in Ageing and Development, 61,* 275–285.

Greenspan, S. L., Rowe, J. W., Maitland, L. A., McAloon-Dyke, M., & Elahi, D. (1993). The pituitary-adrenal glucocorticoid response is altered by gender and disease. *Journal of Gerontology, 48,* M72–M77.

Hakkinen, K., & Pakarinen, A. (1993). Muscle strength and serum testosterone, cortisol and SHBG concentrations in middle-aged and elderly men and women. *Acta Physiologica Scandinavica, 148,* 199–207.

Hauger, R. L., Thrivikraman, K. V., & Plotsky, P. M. (1994). Age-related alterations of hypothalamic-pituitary-adrenal axis function in male Fischer 344 rats. *Endocrinology, 134,* 1528–1536.

Heuser, I. J., Wark, H. J., Keul, J., & Holsboer, F. (1991). Hypothalamic-pituitary-adrenal axis function in elderly endurance athletes. *Journal of Clinical Endocrinological Metabolism, 73,* 485–488.

Honma, K.-I., Honma, S., & Hiroshige, T. (1983). Critical role of food amount for prefeeding corticosterone peak in rats. *American Journal of Physiology, 245,* R339–R344.

Horan, M. A. (1994). Aging, injury and the hypothalamic-pituitary-adrenal axis. *Annals of the New York Academy of Science, 719,* 285–290.

Irwin, M., Hauger, R., & Brown, M. (1992). Central corticotropin-releasing hormone activates the sympathetic nervous system and reduces immune function: increased responsivity of the aged rat. *Endocrinology, 131,* 1047–1053.

Issa, A. M., Rowe, W., Gauthier, S., & Meaney, M. J. (1990). Hypothalamic-pituitary-adrenal activity in aged, cognitively impaired and cognitively unimpaired rats. *Journal of Neuroscience, 10,* 3247–3254.

Jaarsma, D., Postema, F., & Korf, J. (1992). Time course and distribution of neuronal degeneration in the dentate gyrus of rat after adrenalectomy: a silver impregnation study. *Hippocampus, 2,* 143–150.

Kerr, D. S., Campbell, L. W., Hao, S.-Y., & Landfield, P. W. (1989). Corticosteroid modulation of hippocampal potentials: Increased effect with age. *Science, 245,* 1505–1509.

Kerr, D. S., Campbell, L. W., Applegate, M. D., Brodish, A., & Landfield, P. W. (1991). Chronic stress-induced acceleration of electrophysiological and morphometric biomarkers of hippocampal aging. *Journal of Neuroscience, 11,* 1316–1324.

Landfield, P. (1980). Adrenocortical hypothesis of brain and somatic aging. In R. T. Shimke (Ed.), *Biological Mechanisms in Aging* (Publication No. 81–2194, pp. 658–672). Washington, DC: NIH.

Landfield, P. W. (1994). Nathan Shock Memorial Lecture 1990. The role of glucocorticoids in brain aging and Alzheimer's disease: an integrative physiological hypothesis. *Experimental Gerontology, 29,* 3–11.

Landfield, P. W., & Eldridge, J. C. (1991). The glucocorticoid hypothesis of brain aging and neurodegeneration: recent modifications. *Acta Endocrinologica (Copenhagen), 125 (Suppl. 1),* 54–64.

Landfield, P. W., & Eldridge, J. C. (1994). Evolving aspects of the glucocorticoid hypothesis of brain aging: Hormonal modulation of neuronal calcium homeostasis. *Neurobiology of Aging, 15,* 579–588.

Landfield, P., Waymire, J., & Lynch, G. (1978). Hippocampal aging and adrenocorticoids: A quantitative correlation. *Science, 202,* 1098–1102.

Landfield, P. W., Baskin, R. K., & Pitler, T. A. (1981). Brain-age correlates: Retardation by hormonal pharmacological manipulations. *Science, 214,* 581–584.

Landfield, P. W., Thibault, O., Mazzanti, M. L., Porter, N. M., & Kerr, D. S. (1992). Mechanisms of neuronal death in brain aging and Alzheimer's disease: role of endocrine-mediated calcium dyshomeostasis. *Journal of Neurobiology, 23,* 1247–1260.

Lawrence, M. S., & Sapolsky, R. M. (1994). Glucocorticoids accelerate ATP loss following metabolic insults in cultured hippocampal neurons. *Brain Research, 646,* 303–306.

Leakey, J. E., Chen, S., Manjgaladze, M., Turturro, A., Duffy, P. H., Pipkin, J. L., & Hart, R. W. (1994). Role of glucocorticoids and caloric stress in modulating the effects of caloric restriction in rodents. *Annals of the New York Academy of Science, 719,* 171–194.

Levy, A., Dachir, S., Arbel, I., & Kadar, T. (1994). Aging, stress, and cognitive function. *Annals of the New York Academy of Science, 717,* 79–88.

Lombardi, G., Merola, B., Savastano, S., Tommaselli, A. P., Valentino, R., Rossi, R., Ghiggi, M. R., & Cataldi, M. (1991). Hypothalamus-pituitary-adrenal (HPA) axis in physiological and pathological aging brain. *Acta Neurologica (Napoli), 13,* 368–373.

(continued)

Table V (*Continued*)

Major, D. E., Kesslack, J. P., Cotman, C. W., Finch, C. E., & Day, J. R. (1994). Life-long dietary restriction attenuates age-related increases in glial fibrillary acidic protein (GFAP) mRNA in the rat hippocampus. *Society for Neurosciences Abstracts, 28.19*, 50.

Marchetti, B., Peiffer, A., Morale, M. C., Batticane, N., Gallo, F., & Barden, N. (1994). Transgenic animals with impaired type II glucocorticoid receptor gene expression. A model to study aging of the neuroendocrine-immune system. *Annals of the New York Academy of Science, 719*, 308–327.

McEwen, B. S. (1992). Re-examination of the glucocorticoid hypothesis of stress and aging. *Progress in Brain Research, 93*, 365–81.

Meaney, M. J., Aitken, D. H., Bhatnagar, S., & Sapolsky, R. M. (1991). Postnatal handling attenuates certain neuroendocrine, anatomical, and cognitive dysfunctions associated with aging in female rats. *Neurobiology of Aging, 12*, 31–38.

Meaney, M. J., Aitken, D. H., Sharma, S., & Viau, V. (1992). Basal ACTH, corticosterone and corticosterone-binding globulin levels over the diurnal cycle, and age-related changes in hippocampal type I and type II corticosteroid receptor binding capacity in young and aged, handled and nonhandled rats. *Neuroendocrinology, 55*, 204–213.

Muneoka, K., Mikuni, M., Ogawa, T., Kitera, K., & Takahashi, K. (1994). Periodic maternal deprivation-induced potentiation of the negative feedback sensitivity to glucocorticoids to inhibit stress-induced adrenocortical response persists throughout the animal's life-span. *Neuroscience Letters, 168*, 89–92.

Nichols, N. R., Finch, C. E., & Nelson, J. F. (1995). Food restriction delays the age-related increase in GFAP mRNA in rat hypothalamus. *Neurobiology of Aging, 16*, 105–110.

Nolan, C. J., Bestervelt, L. L., Mousigian, C. A., Maimansomsuk, P., Cai, Y., & Piper, W. N. (1991). Chronic ethanol consumption depresses hypothalamic-pituitary-adrenal function in aged rats. *Life Science, 49*, 1923–1928.

Okamoto, M., Kita, T., Okuda, H., Tanaka, T., & Nakashima, T. (1992). Effects of acute administration of nicotine on convulsive movements and blood levels of corticosterone in old rats. *Japanese Journal of Pharmacology, 60*, 381–384.

Reul, J. M., Rothuizen, J., & de Kloet, E. R. (1991). Age-related changes in the dog hypothalamic-pituitary-adrenocortical system: neuroendocrine activity and corticosteroid receptors, *Journal of Steroid Biochemistry and Molecular Biology, 40*, 63–69.

Robertson, O. H., Wexler, B. C., & Miller, B. F. (1961). Degenerative changes in the cardiovascular system of spawning Pacific salmon. *Circulation Research, 9*, 826–834.

Romanoff, L. P., Morris, C. W., Welch, P., Roderiguez, R. M., & Pincus, G. (1961). The metabolism of corticol-4-C14 in young and elderly men. I. Secretion rate of cortisol and daily excretion of tetrahydrocorticol, allotetrahydrocorticol, tetrahydrocortisone and cortolone (20α and 20β). *Journal of Clinical Endocrinological Metabolism, 21*, 1413–1425.

Rothuizen, J., Reul, J. M., Rijnberk, A., Mol, J. A., & de Kloet, E. R. (1991). Aging and the hypothalamus-pituitary-adrenocortical axis, with special reference to the dog. *Acta Endocrinologica (Copenhagen), 125* (Suppl. 1), 73–76.

Rothuizen, J., Reul, J. M., van Sluijs, F. J., Mol, J. A., Rijnberk, A., & de Kloet, E. R. (1993). Increased neuroendocrine reactivity and decreased brain mineralocorticoid receptor-binding capacity in aged dogs. *Endocrinology, 132*, 161–168.

Sabatino, F., Masoro, E. J., McMahan, C. A., & Kuhn, R. W. (1991). Assessment of the role of the glucocorticoid system in aging processes and in the action of food restriction. *Journal of Gerontology, 46*, B171–B179.

Sapolsky, R. M. (1992). Do glucocorticoid concentrations rise with age in the rat? *Neurobiology of Aging, 13*, 171–174.

Sapolsky, R. M., & Altmann, J. (1991). Incidence of hypercortisolism and dexamethasone resistance increases with age among wild baboons. *Biological Psychiatry, 30*, 1008–1016.

Sapolsky, R. M., Krey, L., & McEwen, B. S. (1983). The adrenocortical stress-response in the aged male rat: impairment of recovery from stress. *Experimental Gerontology, 18*, 55.

Sapolsky, R. M., Krey, L., & McEwen, B. S. (1985). Prolonged glucocorticoid exposure reduces hippocampal neuron number: Implications for aging. *Journal of Neuroscience, 5*, 1222–1227.

(continued)

Table V *(Continued)*

Sapolsky, R. M., Krey, L., & McEwen, B. S. (1986). The neuroendocrinology of stress and aging: The glucocorticoid cascade hypothesis. *Endocrine Reviews, 7,* 284–301.

Schlaghecke, R., Beuscher, D., Kornely, E., & Specker, C. (1994). Effects of glucocorticoids in rheumatoid arthritis. *Arthritis and Rheumatism, 37,* 1127–1131.

Schwartz, A. G., & Pashko, L. L. (1994). Role of adrenocortical steroids in mediating cancer-preventive and age-retarding effects of food restriction in laboratory rodents. *Journal of Gerontology, 49,* B37–B41.

Secki, J. R., & Olsson, T. (1995). Glucocorticoid hypersecretion and the age-impaired hippocampus: cause or effect? *Journal of Endocrinology, 145,* 201–211.

Seeman, T. E., & Robbins, R. J. (1994). Aging and hypothalamic-pituitary-adrenal response to challenge in humans. *Endocrine Reviews, 15,* 233–260.

Selye, H., & Tuchweber, B. (1976). Stress in relation to aging and disease. In A. V. Everitt & J. A. Burgess (Eds.), *Hypothalamus, Pituitary, and Aging* (pp. 553–569). Springfield: Charles C. Thomas.

Servatius, R. J., Ottenweller, J. E., Bergen, M. T., Sodan, S., & Natelson, B. H. (1994). Persistent stress-induced sensitization of adrenocortical and startle responses. *Physiology and Behavior, 56,* 945–954.

Sherman, B., Wysham, C., & Pfohl, B. (1985). Age-related changes in the circadian rhythm of plasma cortisol in man. *Journal of Clinical Endocrinological Metabolism, 61,* 439–443.

Sloviter, R. S., Dean, E., & Neubort, S. (1993a). Electron microscopic analysis of adrenalectomy-induced hippocampal granule cell degeneration in the rat: apoptosis in the adult central nervous system. *Journal of Comparative Neurology, 330,* 337–351.

Sloviter, R. S., Sollas, A. L., Dean, E., & Neubort, S. (1993b). Adrenalectomy-induced granule cell degeneration in the rat hippocampal dentate gyrus: characterization of an in vivo model of controlled neuronal death. *Journal of Comparative Neurology, 330,* 324–336.

Solez, C. (1952). Aging and adrenal cortical hormones. *Geriatrics, 7,* 241–245.

Stein-Behrens, B. A., Elliott, E. M., Miller, C. A., Schilling, J. W., Newcombe, R., & Sapolsky, R. M. (1992). Glucocorticoids exacerbate kainic acid-induced extracellular accumulation of excitatory amino acids in the rat hippocampus. *Journal of Neurochemistry, 58,* 1730–1735.

Stein-Behrens, B. A., Lin, W. J., & Sapolsky, R. M. (1994). Physiological elevations of glucocorticoids potentiate glutamate accumulation in the hippocampus. *Journal of Neurochemistry, 63,* 596–602.

Stewart, J., Meaney, M. J., Aitken, D., Jensen, L., Kalant, N. (1988). The effects of acute and life-long food restriction on basal and stress-induced serum corticosterone levels in young and aged rats. *Endocrinology, 123,* 1934–1941.

Tanaka, H., Akama, H., Ichikawa, Y., Homma, M., & Oshima, H. (1991). Glucocorticoid receptors in normal leukocytes: effects of age, gender, season, and plasma cortisol concentrations. *Clinical Chemistry, 37,* 1715–1719.

Tombaugh, G. C., & Sapolsky, R. M. (1992). Corticosterone accelerates hypoxia- and cyanide-induced ATP loss in cultured hippocampal astrocytes. *Brain Research, 588,* 154–158.

Tombaugh, G. C., Yang, S. H., Swanson, R. A., & Sapolsky, R. M. (1992). Glucocorticoids exacerbate hypoxic and hypoglycemic hippocampal injury in vitro: biochemical correlates and a role for astrocytes. *Journal of Neurochemistry, 59,* 137–146.

Tsuchiya, T., Nakayama, Y., & Sato, A. (1992). Somatic afferent stimulation-plasma corticosterone, luteinizing hormone (LH), and testosterone responses in aged male rats under anesthetization. *Japanese Journal of Physiology, 42,* 793–804.

van den Berg, H., Mocking, J. A., & Seifert, W. F. (1991). The effect of immobilization and insulin-induced hypoglycemia on ACTH and corticosterone release in aging Brown-Norway rats. *Acta Endocrinologica (Copenhagen), 125 (Suppl. 1),* 104–106.

van Eekelen, J. A., Rots, N. Y., Sutanto, W., & de Kloet, E. R. (1992). The effect of aging on stress responsiveness and central corticosteroid receptors in the brown Norway rat. *Neurobiology of Aging, 13,* 159–170.

Waltman, C., Blackman, M. R., Chrousos, G. P., Riemann, C., & Harman, S. M. (1991). Spontaneous and glucocorticoid-inhibited adrenocorticotropic hormone and cortisol secretion are similar in healthy young and old men. *Journal of Clinical Endocrinological Metabolism, 73,* 495–502.

(continued)

Table V (*Continued*)

Wexler, B. C. (1976). Comparative aspects of hyperadrenocorticism and aging. In A. V. Everitt & J. A. Burgess (Eds.), *Hypothalamus, Pituitary, and Aging* (pp. 333–361). Springfield: Charles C. Thomas.

White-Gbadebo, D., & Hamm, R. J. (1993). Chronic corticosterone treatment potentiates deficits following traumatic brain injury in rats: implications for aging. *Journal of Neurotrauma, 10*, 297–306.

Yau, J. L., Morris, R. G. M., & Seckl, J. R. (1994). Hippocampal corticosteroid receptor mRNA expression and spatial learning in the aged Wistar rat. *Brain Research, 657*, 59–64.

Zoli, M., Ferraguti, F., Gustafsson, J. A., Toffano, G., Fuxe, K., & Agnati, L. F. (1991). Selective reduction of glucocorticoid receptor immunoreactivity in the hippocampal formation and central amygdaloid nucleus of the aged rat. *Brain Research, 545*, 199–207.

B. Sympathetic Nervous System

Compared to the subtle age-related changes in glucocorticoid secretion in humans, age-related increases in sympathetic nervous system tone are quite robust in humans and other species (Rowe and Troen, 1980). The reasons that plasma catecholamine levels increase with age are not known, but they probably include increased sympathetic nerve activity (Ng *et al.*, 1994), as well as impaired reuptake and clearance of plasma catecholamines (Elser *et al.*, 1995). In any case, in both humans (Ng *et al.*, 1994b) and animals (Cizza *et al.*, 1995), basal activity of the sympathetic system appears to be elevated, but response of the sympathetic system to stress is probably attenuated. The age-related changes in the sympathetic system are perhaps broadly similar to those exhibited by the hypothalamic–pituitary axis. In any case, since elevated catecholamines are directly related to cardiovascular disease (Haskin *et al.*, 1986), the mechanisms which underlie the age-related increase in catecholamines are obviously of great interest and clearly merit further study (Table VI).

C. Neuroendocrine Heat-Shock Response

One of the most interesting developments in the neuroendocrinology of stress has been the studies by Holbrook and colleagues that psychological stress induces heat-shock protein gene expression in adrenal cortex and heart and that this induction is more attenuated in aging rats (Blake *et al.*, 1991; Udelsman *et al.*, 1993) (Table VII). These groups demonstrated that the induction was mediated by neuroendocrine systems, thus providing a link between the neuroendocrine and the molecular stress responses. Similarly, the induction of the heat-shock protein in the hippocampus by thermal stress was impaired with age (Pardue *et al.*, 1992).

VI. Neuroendocrinology of Glucose Metabolism and Aging

Metabolism must play an integral role in the aging process, both as a direct cause of age-related changes (e.g., through free radicals and glycation) and by virtue of the age-related impairments in metabolic activity. Furthermore, dietary restriction, which retards aspects of the aging process, exerts its most obvious effects on metabolism. Age-related changes in metabolism are reflected in part by age-related changes in glucose disposal (Poehlman, 1993; Young, 1992; McCarter and Palmer, 1992) and appetite (Rolls, 1992; Rammohan *et al.*, 1989; Morley and Silver, 1988; Pich *et al.*, 1992; Van Reemen and Ward, 1994), both

Table VI
Sympathetic Nervous System and Aging

Andrews, T., Lincoln, J., Milner, P., Burnstock, G., & Cowen, T. (1993). Differential regulation of tyrosine hydroxylase protein and activity in rabbit sympathetic neurones after long-term cold exposure: altered responses in ageing. *Brain Research, 624,* 69–74.

Blandini, F., Martignoni, E., Melzi, E., Biasio, L., Sances, G., Lucarelli, C., Rizzo, V., Costa, A., & Nappi, G. (1992). Free plasma catecholamine levels in healthy subjects: a basal and dynamic study. The influence of age. *Scandinavian Journal of Clinical and Laboratory Investigation, 52,* 9–17.

Cizza, G., Pacak, K., Kvetnansky, R., Palkovits, M., Goldstein, D. S., Brady, L. S., Fukuhara, K., Bergamini, E., Kopin, I. J., Blackman, M. R., Chrousos, G. P., & Gold, P. W. (1995). Decreased stress responsivity of central and peripheral catecholaminergic systems in aged 344/N Fischer rats. *Journal of Clinical Investigation, 95,* 1217–1224.

Esler, M.D., Turner, A. G., Kaye, D. M., Thompson, J. M., Kingwell, B. A., Morris, J., Lamdert, G. W., Jennings, G. L., Cox, H. S., & Seals, D. R. (1995). Aging effects on humans sympathetic neuronal function. *American Journal of Physiology, 268,* R278–R285.

Haigh, R. A., Harper, G. D., Burton, R., Macdonald, I. A., & Potter, J. F. (1991). Possible impairment of the sympathetic nervous system response to postprandial hypotension in elderly hypertensive patients. *Journal of Human Hypertension, 5,* 83–89.

Irwin, M. (1993). Stress-induced immune suppression. Role of the autonomic nervous system. *Annals of the New York Academy of Science, 697,* 203–218.

Landsberg, L., & Young, J. B. (1978). Fasting, feeding, and regulation of the sympathetic nervous system. *New England Journal of Medicine, 298,* 195–1301.

Morrow, L. A., Rosen, S. G., & Halter, J. B. (1991). Beta-adrenergic regulation of insulin secretion: evidence of tissue heterogeneity of beta-adrenergic responsiveness in the elderly. *Journal of Gerontology, 46,* M108–M113.

Morrow, L. A., Morganroth, G. S., Herman, W. H., Bergman, R. N., & Halter, J. B. (1993). Effects of epinephrine on insulin secretion and action in humans. Interaction with aging. *Diabetes, 42,* 307–315.

Ng, A. V., Callister, R., Johnson, D. G., & Seals, D. R. (1993). Age and gender influence muscle sympathetic nerve activity at rest in healthy humans. *Hypertension, 21,* 498–503.

Ng, A. V., Callister, R., Johnson, D. G., & Seals, D. R. (1994). Sympathetic neural reactivity to stress does not increase with age in healthy humans. *American Journal of Physiology, 267,* H344–H353.

Qualy, J. M., & Westfall, T. C. (1993). Age-dependent overflow of endogenous norepinephrine from paraventricular hypothalamic nucleus of hypertensive rats. *American Journal of Physiology, 265,* H39–H46.

Rowe, J. W., & Troen, B. R. (1980). Sympathetic nervous system and aging in man. *Endocrine Reviews, 1,* 167–178.

Rowe, J. W., Young, J. B., Minaker, K. L., Stevens, A. L., Pallotta, J., & Landsberg, L. (1981). Effect of insulin and glucose infusions on sympathetic nervous system activity in normal man. *Diabetes, 30,* 219–225.

Supiano, M. A., Hogikyan, R. V., Morrow, L. A., Ortiz-Alonso, F. J., Herman, W. H., Bergman, R. N., & Halter, J. B. (1992). Hypertension and insulin resistance: role of sympathetic nervous system activity. *American Journal of Physiology, 263,* E935–E942.

Supiano, M. A., Hogikyan, R. V., Morrow, L. A., Ortiz-Alonso, F. J. Herman, W. H., Galecki, A. T., & Halter, J. B. (1993). Aging and insulin sensitivity: role of blood pressure and sympathetic nervous system activity. *Journal of Gerontology, 48,* M237–M243.

Young, J. B., Rowe, J. W., Pallotta, J. A., Sparrow, D., & Landsberg, L. (1980). Enhanced plasma norepinephrine response to upright posture and oral glucose administration in elderly human subjects. *Metabolism, 29,* 477–482.

Young, J. B., Troisi, R. J., Weiss, S. T., Parker, D. R., Sparrow, D., & Landsberg, L. (1992). Relationship of catecholamine excretion to body size, obesity, and nutrient intake in middle-aged and elderly men. *American Journal of Clinical Nutrition, 56,* 827–834.

of which are regulated by neuroendocrine systems (Table VIII).

Possibly pertinent to the decreased food intake with age is that in general aging animals appear less sensitive to effects of fasting. In particular, when young rodents are

Table VII
Stress and Aging—Other

Azaryan, A., Dovanjyan, G., & Lajtha, A. (1991). Stress-induced change in cerebral ATP + ubiquitin-dependent proteinase activity vary with age. *Acta Biologica Hungarica, 42,* 297–300.

Barnhill, J. G., Miller, L. G., Greenblatt, D. J., Thompson, M. L., Ciraulo, D. A., & Shader, R. I. (1991). Benzodiazepine receptor binding response to acute and chronic stress is increased in aging animals. *Pharmacology, 42,* 181–187.

Blake, M. J., Udelsman, R., Feulner, G. J., Norton, D. D., & Holbrook, N. J. (1991). Stress-induced heat shock protein 70 expression in adrenal cortex: an adrenocorticotropic hormone-sensitive, age-dependent response. *Proceedings of the National Academy of Sciences of the United States of America, 88,* 9873–9877.

Calza, L., Giardino, L., & Ceccatelli, S. (1993). NOS mRNA in the paraventricular nucleus of young and old rats after immobilization stress. *Neuroreport, 4,* 627–630.

Clevenger, F. W., Rodriguez, D. J., Demarest, G. B., Osler, T. M., Olson, S. E., & Fry, D. E. (1992). Protein and energy tolerance by stressed geriatric patients. *Journal of Surgical Research, 52,* 135–139.

Findley, T. (1949). Role of the neurohypophysis in the pathogenesis of hypertension and some allied disorders associated with aging. *American Journal of Medicine, 7,* 70–84.

Frolkis, V. V. (1993). Stress-age syndrome. *Mechanisms in Ageing and Development, 69,* 93–107.

Handa, R. J., Cross, M. K., George, M., Gordon, B. H., Burgess, L. H., Cabrera, T. M., Hata, N., Campbell, D. B., & Lorens, S. A. (1993). Neuroendocrine and neurochemical responses to novelty stress in young and old mate F344 rats: effects of d-fenfluramine treatment. *Pharmacology, Biochemistry and Behavior, 46,* 101–109.

Jeevanandam, M., Petersen, S. R., & Shamos, R. F. (1993). Protein and glucose fuel kinetics and hormonal changes in elderly trauma patients. *Metabolism, 42,* 1255–1262.

Korte, S. M., Buwalda, B., Bouws, G. A., Koolhaas, J. M., Maes, F. W., & Bohus, B. (1992). Conditioned neuroendocrine and cardiovascular stress responsiveness accompanying behavioral passivity and activity in aged and in young rats. *Physiology & Behavior, 51,* 815–822.

Natelson, B. H., Ottenweller, J. E., Servatius, R. J., Drastal, S., Bergen, M. T., & Tapp, W. N. (1992). Effect of stress and food restriction on blood pressure and lifespan of Dahl salt-sensitive rats. *Journal of Hypertension, 10,* 1457–1462.

Odio, M., & Brodish, A. (1991). Decreased plasticity of glucoregulatory responses in aged rats: effects of chronic stress. *Journal of Gerontology, 46,* B188–B196.

Pardue, S., Groshan, K., Raese, J. D., & Morrison-Bogorad, M. (1992). Hsp70 mRNA induction is reduced in neurons of aged rat hippocampus after thermal stress. *Neurobiology of Aging, 13,* 661–672.

Perego, C., Vetrugno, G. C., De Simoni, M. G., & Algeri, S. (1993). Aging prolongs the stress-induced release of noradrenaline in rat hypothalamus. *Neuroscience Letters, 157,* 127–130.

Taylor, G. T., Bardgett, M., Farr, S., Womack, S., Komitowski, D., & Weiss, J. (1993). Steroidal interactions in the ageing endocrine system: absence of suppression and pathology in reproductive systems of old males from a mixed-sex socially stressful rat colony. *Journal of Endocrinology, 137,* 115–122.

Udelsman, R., Blake, M. J., Stagg, C. A., Li, D. G., Putney, D. J., & Holbrook, N. J. (1993). Vascular heat shock protein expression in response to stress. Endocrine and autonomic regulation of this age-dependent response. *Journal of Clinical Investigation, 91,* 465–473.

fasted overnight, they exhibit a compensatory hyperphagia when allowed access to food. However, compared with young rodents, older rats (Pich *et al.*, 1992), and mice (Silver *et al.*, 1988) show greatly attenuated hyperphagia in response to fasting.

Decreased appetite with age, and in particular impaired fasting-induced hyperphagia during aging, could be related to impairments in expression of hypothalamic neuropeptide Y (NPY). NPY synthesized in the arcuate nucleus (ARC) of the hypothalamus and secreted into the paraventricular nucleus (PVN) appears to be a major regulator energy homeostasis, insulin secretion, and feeding behavior (White, 1993; Schwartz et al., 1993; Leibowitz, 1991). NPY is a potent stimulator of feeding behavior (White, 1993), with the PVN the site most sensitive to these effects (Stanley et al., 1993). When infused into the hypothalamus, NPY also produces other anabolic effects such as increased insulin secretion (White, 1993). Conversely, attenuating NPY synthesis by infusing into the hypothalamus anti-sense oligonucleotides complementary to NPY mRNA decreases food intake and decreases insulin (Akabayashi et al., 1994).

Hypothalamic NPY mRNA (Gruenewald et al., 1994) and peptide (Kowalski et al., 1992; Kalra et al., 1993) decrease with age. Of particular interest, NPY mRNA in the arcuate nucleus increases after prolonged fasting in young rodents, but this induction is greatly attenuated during aging (Chua et al., 1991; Jhanawar-Uniyal & Chua, 1993; Mobbs et al., 1993). When NPY is infused into young and old rats after an overnight fast, NPY has no effect in the younger rats (who are already exhibiting maximal hyperphagia), but NPY increases the food intake of the older rats to levels of hyperphagia exhibited by the young rats (Pich et al., 1992). On the other hand, NPY is equally effective in young and old rats if they were not fasted before testing (Pich et al., 1992). These data are consistent with the hypothesis that impaired production of NPY in the older rats may contribute to impaired feeding after fasting. Analogous with the hypothesized persistent effects of estrogen and glucocorticoids during aging, it has been hypothesized that glucose also exerts long-term effects on the neuroendocrine loci which regulate glucose, which possibly entail long-term effects on gene expression (Mobbs, 1994). For example, since glucose appears to inhibit NPY gene expression in the arcuate nucleus, persistent or enhanced effects of glucose to inhibit NPY

mRNA during aging could contribute to the impaired induction of NPY by fasting (Mobbs, 1994). The phenomenon of persistent effects of humoral substances on gene expression, called "molecular hysteresis" (Mobbs, 1994), remains a speculative but promising mechanism to explicate the persistent effects of estrogen (Burch & Evans, 1986), glucocorticoids, glucose (Roy et al., 1990), and other humoral substances during aging. Although it is clear that elevated glucose can produce long-term changes and impairments in neuroendocrine function, just as elevated glucocorticoids and estrogen can produce long-term impairments in their cognate neuroendocrine regulatory cells, it is far from clear if these effects contribute to a quantitatively significant degree to the impairments which actually do occur during aging. For example, impairments in the arcuate nucleus and hippocampus develop during aging independent of estrogen, glucose, or glucocorticoids; therefore, a challenge for the next generation of studies is to determine the degree to which these changes actually depend on hysteretic effects.

VII. Growth Hormone and Aging

Plasma growth hormone (GH) decreases between maturity and middle age, in both sexes, in several species including humans (Table IX). The earliest convincing study that accounted for the pulsatility of GH secretion reported that about 60% of 3-month-old rats exhibited large pulses of GH (greater than 300 ng/ml), whereas only about 10% of the 18-month-old rats exhibited these large pulses (Sonntag et al., 1980). These results were confirmed and extended in female mice, in which average GH levels (1 hr after subjective night began) declined by about 50% between 6 and 12 months of age and declined even further by 18 months (Mobbs et al., 1985). Numerous subsequent studies in humans have

Table VIII
Neuroendocrinology of Glucose Metabolism and Aging

Akabayashi, A., Wahlestedt, C., Alexander, J. T., & Leibowitz, S. F. (1994). Specific inhibition of endogenous neuropeptide Y synthesis in arcuate nucleus by anti-sense oligonucleotides suppresses feeding behavior and insulin secretion. *Brain Research, 21,* 55–61.

Bergen, H., & Mobbs, C. V. (1992). Hypothalamic lesion by gold-thio-glucose (GTG) leads to hyperglycemia in mice. *Endocrine Society, Abstracts,* 91.

Bergen, H., Kleopoulos, S. P., Pfaus, J., & Mobbs, C. V. (1992). Effect of gold-thio-glucose (GTG) on hypothalamic oxytocin receptors and neuropeptide Y (NPY) mRNA. *Society for Neuroscience, Abstracts, 18,* 1485.

Campillo, B., Bories, P. N., Devanlay, M., Pornin, B., Le Parco, J. C., Gaye-Bareyt, E., & Fouet, P. (1992). Aging, energy expenditure and nutritional status: evidence for denutrition-related hypermetabolism. *Annals of Nutrition & Metabolism, 36,* 265–272.

Chua, S. C., Jr., Leibel, R. L., & Hirsch, J. (1991). Food deprivation and age modulate neuropeptide gene expression in the murine hypothalamus and adrenal gland. *Brain Research: Molecular Brain Research, 9,* 95–101.

Gruenewald, D. A., Naai, M. A., Marck, B. T., & Matsumoto, A. M. (1994). Age-related decrease in neuropeptide-Y gene expression in the arcuate nucleus of the male rat brain is independent of testicular feedback. *Endocrinology. 134,* 2383–2389.

Jhanwar, M., & Chua, S. C. (1993). Critical effects of aging and nutritional state on hypothalamic neuropeptide Y and galanin gene expression in lean and genetically obese Zucker rats. *Brain Research, 19*(3), 195–202.

Kalra, S. P., Sahu, A., & Kalra, P. S. (1993). Ageing of the neuropeptidergic signals in rats. *Journal of Reproduction and Fertility, Supplement, 46,* 11–19.

Kowalski, C., Micheau, J., Corder, R., Gaillard, R., & Conte-Devolx, B. (1992). Age-related changes in cortico-releasing factor, somatostatin, neuropeptide Y, methionine enkephalin and beta-endorphin in specific rat brain areas. *Brain Research, 582,* 38–46.

Masoro, E. J. (1992). Potential role of the modulation of fuel use in the antiaging action of dietary restriction. *Annals of the New York Academy of Science, 663,* 403–411.

Masoro, E. J. (1993). Dietary restriction and aging. *Journal of the American Geriatric Society, 41,* 994–999.

Masoro, E. J., Katz, M. S., & McMahan, C. A. (1989). Evidence for the glycation hypothesis of aging from the food-restricted rodent model. *Journal of Gerontology, 44,* B20–B22.

Masoro, E. J., Shimokawa, I., & Yu, B. P. (1991). Retardation of the aging processes in rats by food restriction, *Annals of the New York Academy of Science, 621,* 337–352.

Masoro, E. J., McCarter, R. J., Katz, M. S., & McMahan, C. A. (1992). Dietary restriction alters characteristics of glucose fuel use [published erratum appears in *J. Gerontol.* (1993) 48(2); B73]. *Journal of Gerontology, 47,* B202–B208.

McCarter, R. J., & Palmer, J. (1992). Energy metabolism and aging: a lifelong study of Fischer 344 rats. *American Journal of Physiology, 263,* E448–E452.

Mobbs, C. V. (1990). Neurotoxic effects of estrogen, glucose, and glucocorticoids: Neurohumoral hysteresis and its pathological consequences during aging. *Reviews of Biological Research on Aging, 4,* 201–228.

Mobbs, C. V. (1993). Genetic influences on glucose neurotoxicity, aging, and diabetes: A possible role for glucose hysteresis. *Genetica, 91,* 239–253.

Mobbs, C. V. (1994). Molecular hysteresis: Age-related impairments due to residual effects of hormones and glucose on gene expression. *Neurobiology of Aging, 15,* 523–534.

Mobbs, C. V., & Bergen, H. (1992). Glucose metabolism during aging in mice: Hypoglycemia and hyperinsulinemia. *Endocrine Society, Abstracts,* 370.

Mobbs, C. V., & Kleopoulos, S. P. (1992). Regulation of hypothalamic neuropeptide Y (NPY) by fasting during aging in male rats. *Society for Neuroscience, Abstracts, 18,* 1485.

Mobbs, C. V., Kleopoulos, S. P., & Bergen, H. (1993a). Hypoglycemia precedes hyperglycemia during aging: effect of dietary enhancement and dietary restriction. *Endocrine Society, Abstracts,* 367.

(continued)

Table VIII   *(Continued)*

Mobbs, C. V., Kleopoulos, S. P., & Funabashi, T. (1993). A glucokinase/AP-1 glucose transduction mechanism in the ventromedial hypothalamic satiety center. *Society for Neuroscience, Abstracts, 19,* in press.

Morley, J. E., & Silver, A. J. (1988). Anorexia in the elderly. *Neurobiology of Aging, 9,* 9–16.

Pich, E. M., Messori, B., Zoli, M., Ferraguti, F., Marrama, P., Biagini, G., Fuxe, K., & Agnati, L. F. (1992). Feeding and drinking responses to neuropeptide Y injections in the paraventricular hypothalamic nucleus of aged rats. *Brain Research, 575,* 265–271.

Poehlman, E. T. (1993). Regulation of energy expenditure in aging humans. *Journal of the American Geriatric Society, 41,* 552–559.

Rammohan, M., Juan, D., & Jung, D. (1989). Hypophagia among hospitalized elderly. *Journal of the American Dietetic Association, 89,* 1774–1779.

Rolls, B. J. (1992). Aging and appetite. *Nutrition Reviews, 50,* 422–426.

Roy, S., Sala, R., Cagliero, E., & Lorenzi, M. (1990). Overexpression of fibronectin induced by diabetes or high glucose: Phenomenon with a memory. *Proceedings of the National Academy of Sciences, 87,* 404–408.

Schwartz, M. W., Figlewicz, D. P., Woods, S. C., Porte, D., Jr., & Baskin, D. G. (1993). Insulin, neuropeptide Y, and food intake. *Annals of the New York Academy of Science, 692,* 60–71.

Silver, A. J., Flood, J. F., & Morley, J. E. (1988). Effect of gastrointestinal peptides on ingestion in old and young mice. *Peptides, 9,* 221–225.

Somani, S. M., Buckenmeyer, P., Dube, S. N., Mandalaywala, R. H., Verhulst, S. J., & Knowlton, R. G. (1992). Influence of age on caloric expenditure during exercise. *International Journal of Clinical Pharmacology, Therapy and Toxicology, 30,* 1–6.

Stanley, B. G., Magdalin, W., Seirafi, A., Thomas, W. J., & Leibowitz, S. F. (1993). The perifonical area: The major focus of (a) patchily distributed hypothalamic neuropeptide Y-sensitive feeding system. *Brain Research, 604,* 304–317.

Surwit, R. S., Kuhn, C. M., Cochrane, C., McCubbin, J. A., & Feinglos, M. N. (1988). Diet-induced Type II diabetes in C57Bl/6J mice. *Diabetes, 37,* 1163–1167.

Surwit, R. S., Seldin, M. F., Kuhn, C. M., Cochrane, C., & Feinglos, M. N. (1990). Control of expression of insulin resistance and hyperglycemia by different genetic factors in diabetic C57BL/6J mice. *Diabetes, 40,* 82–87.

Van Remmen, H., & Ward, W. F. (1994). Effect of age on induction of hepatic phosphoenolpyruvate carboxykinase by fasting. *American Journal of Physiology, 267,* G195–G200.

White, J. D. (1993). Neuropeptide Y: a central regulator of energy homeostasis. *Regulatory Peptides, 49,* 93–107.

Young, V. R. (1992). Energy requirements in the elderly. *Nutrition Reviews, 50,* 95–101.

Young, V. R., Yu, Y. M., & Fukagawa, N. K. (1991). Protein and energy interactions throughout life. Metabolic basis and nutritional implications. *Acta Paediatrica (Stockholm), Supplement, 373,* 5–24.

consistently reported a steady decline in plasma GH after about 20 years of age, primarily in the 3–4 hr of nighttime [reviewed in Corpas *et al.* (1993a,b)]. Similarly, numerous studies have reported that plasma insulin-like growth factor I (IGFI), which is induced by and mediates many effects of GH, also decreases with age by about 50% in 70- vs 30-year-old humans [reviewed in Corpus *et al.* (1993a,b).

In adults, GH, either directly or through its mediators such as IGFI, may be the most important protein anabolic agent in the body (Everitt & Meites, 1989). GH enhances protein synthesis (Riggs & Walker, 1960), immune function [Nagy *et al.* (1983) and see the following], and bone metabolism (Rasmussen, 1974). Since these impairments in these functions and others are associated with both GH deficiency and aging, GH deficiency has been hypothesized to account for numerous age-correlated pathologies in humans and other species (Sonntag et al., 1983; Corpas et al., 1993a,b). Major support for this hypothesis came from studies showing that GH replacement in older humans resulted in improvements in protein synthesis, an increase in lean body mass, and a decrease in adiposity (Rudman et al., 1990; Marcus et al., 1990). Even more striking are several reports that examined the effect of GH replacement on immune function in older animals [reviewed in Kelley et al. (1992)] and on longevity (Khansari & Gustad, 1991). Other studies showed that direct injection of recombinant human growth hormone into old mice (Knyszynski et al., 1992), bovine growth hormone into old dogs (Goff et al., 1987; Monroe et al., 1987), and ovine growth hormone into 12-month-old mice (Goya et al., 1992) increases thymic weight and other indices of immune function. However, the most robust effects seem to be produced by GH3 cells, which also secrete prolactin, so that further studies are needed. Furthermore, the idea of treating older patients with GH must be viewed with considerable caution, since studies have indicated that chronic overexpression of GH can be even more deleterious to longevity than underexpression (Steger et al., 1993).

Several studies have examined the cause of decreased plasma GH with age. GH mRNA in the pituitary gland was reported to decrease by about 25% between 7 and 12 months of age in male rats, although this decrease was not evident in female rats (Martinoli et al., 1991). Between 12 and 20 months, GH mRNA in both males and females declined further (Martinoli et al., 1991). Gene expression of hypothalamic somatostatin, which inhibits GH secretion, decreases with age (Sonntag et al., 1990; Martinoli et al., 1991), so that increased somatostatin mRNA would not appear to cause the age-related decline in GH, although in vitro secretion of one form of somatostatin from hypothalamus has been reported to increase in old rats

(Sonntag et al., 1986). However, mRNA and the immunoreactivity of hypothalamic growth-hormone-releasing factor (GHRF), which is the main stimulus for secretion of GH (Plotsky & Vale, 1985), were reported to decrease by about 50% between 3 and 24 months of age (de Gennaro Collona et al., 1989). Since GHRF appears to be the main regulator of synthesis and release of GH and stimulates the proliferation of somatotropes (Billestrup et al., 1986), and since the age-related decrease in GH mRNA is plausibly due to a decrease in somatotropes (Takahashi et al., 1988), it was proposed that the decrease in GH mRNA and GH secretion during aging could be secondary to the decrease in GHRF (de Gennaro Collona et al., 1989). In a follow-up study, de Gennaro Collona et al. (1993) reported that the negative feedback effects of GH on GHRF mRNA could no longer be demonstrated in aging rodents. However, since GHRF mRNA is even, without GH supplementation, as low in aging rats as it is in young rats with GH supplementation, it must be considered that GHRF mRNA is already maximally inhibited in aging rats. Therefore, the apparent loss of negative feedback could, as with POMC or LH in female reproductive aging described earlier, be due to a floor effect or even to increased negative feedback sensitivity to the lower levels of GH exhibited in the older rats. The decrease in GHRF mRNA during aging in rats has been replicated using in situ hybridization in a study that also demonstrated that the inhibition of GHRF by fasting is also impaired during aging (Kleopoulos & Mobbs, 1993), possibly, again, due to a floor effect.

VIII. Thyroid Hormone and Aging

Generally, plasma T3 decreases gradually during aging (Cizza et al., 1992; Lewis et al., 1991) (Table X). In young individuals, this decrease in T3 should be accompanied

Table IX
Growth Hormone and Aging

Bando, H., Zhang, C., Takada, Y., Yamasaki, R., & Saito, S. (1991). Impaired secretion of growth hormone-releasing hormone, growth hormone and IGF-I in elderly men. *Acta Endocrinologica (Copenhagen), 124,* 31–36.

Borst, S. E., Millard, W. J., & Lowenthal, D. T. (1994). Growth hormone, exercise, and aging: the future of therapy for the frail elderly. *Journal of the American Geriatric Society, 42,* 528–535.

Cella, S. G., Arce, V. M., Pieretti, F., Locatelli, V., Settembrini, B. P., & Muller, E. E. (1993). Combined administration of growth-hormone-releasing hormone and clonidine restores defective growth hormone secretion in old dogs. *Neuroendocrinology, 57,* 432–438.

Cianfarani, S., Vaccaro, F., Pasquino, A. M., Marchione, S. A., Passeri, F., Spadoni, G. L., Bernardini, S., Spagnoli, A., & Boscherini, B. (1994). Reduced growth hormone secretion in Turner syndrome: is body weight a key factor? *Hormone Research, 41,* 27–32.

Corpas, E., Harman, S. M., Pineyro, M. A., Roberson, R., & Blackman, M. R. (1992). Growth hormone (GH)-releasing hormone-(1–29) twice daily reverses the decreased GH and insulin-like growth factor-I levels in old men. *Journal of Clinical Endocrinological Metabolism, 75,* 530–535.

Corpas, E., Harman, S. M., Pineyro, M. A., Roberson, R., & Blackman, M. R. (1993a). Continuous subcutaneous infusions of growth hormone (GH) releasing hormone 1–44 for 14 days increase GH and insulin-like growth factor-I levels in old men. *Journal of Clinical Endocrinological Metabolism, 76,* 134–138.

Corpas, E., Harman, S. M., & Blackman, M. R. (1993b). Human growth hormone and human aging. *Endocrine Reviews, 14,* 20–39.

D'Costa, A. P., Ingram, R. L., Lenham, J. E., & Sonntag, W. E. (1993). The regulation and mechanisms of action of growth hormone and insulin-like growth factor 1 during normal ageing. *Journal of Reproduction and Fertility. Supplement, 46,* 87–98.

de Gennaro Colonna, V., Fidone, F., Cocchi, D., & Muller, E. E. (1993). Feedback effects of growth hormone on growth hormone-releasing hormone and somatostatin are not evident in aged rats. *Neurobiology of Aging, 14,* 503–507.

Florio, T., Ventra, C., Postiglione, A., & Schettini, G. (1991). Age-related alterations of somatostatin gene expression in different rat brain areas. *Brain Research, 557,* 64–68.

Flyvbjerg, A., Dorup, I., Everts, M. E., & Orskov, H. (1991). Evidence that potassium deficiency induces growth retardation through reduced circulating levels of growth hormone and insulin-like growth factor I. *Metabolism, 40,* 769–775.

Goya, R. G., Castelletto, L., & Sosa, Y. E. (1991). Plasma levels of growth hormone correlate with the severity of pathologic changes in the renal structure of aging rats. *Laboratory Investigations, 64,* 29–34.

Goya, R. G., Gagnerault, M. C., De Moraes, M. C., Savino, W., & Dardenne, M. (1992). In vivo effects of growth hormone on thymus function in aging mice. *Brain, Behavior, and Immunity, 6,* 341–354.

Goya, R. G., Castro, M. G., Saphier, P. W., Sosa, Y. E., & Lowry, P. J. (1993a). Thymus-pituitary interactions during ageing. *Age and Ageing, 22,* S19–S25.

Goya, R. G., Gagnerault, M. C., Sosa, Y. E., Bevilacqua, J. A., & Dardenne, M. (1993b). Effects of growth hormone and thyroxine on thymulin secretion in aging rats. *Neuroendocrinology, 58,* 338–343.

Horikawa, R., Tanaka, T., Katsumata, N., Satoh, M., Nagashima, A., Watanabe, T., Kokai, Y., Tanae, A., & Hibi, I. (1994). Clinical significance of growth hormone-binding protein measurements in children. *Proceedings of the Society for Experimental Biology and Medicine, 206,* 320–323.

Iranmanesh, A., & Veldhuis, J. D. (1992). Clinical pathophysiology of the somatotropic (GH) axis in adults. *Endocrinology and Metabolism Clinics of North America, 21,* 783–816.

Iranmanesh, A., Lizarralde, G., & Veldhuis, J. D. (1991). Age and relative adiposity are specific negative determinants of the frequency and amplitude of growth hormone (GH) secretory bursts and the half-life of endogenous GH in healthy men. *Journal of Clinical Endocrinological Metabolism, 73,* 1081–1088.

Kelley, K. W., Arkin, S., & Li, Y. M. (1992). Growth hormone, prolactin, and insulin-like growth factors: New jobs for old players. *Brain, Behavior, and Immunity, 6,* 317–326.

Khansari, D. N., & Gustad, T. (1991). Effects of long-term, low-dose growth hormone therapy on immune function and life expectancy. *Mechanisms of Ageing and Development, 57,* 87–100.

(continued)

Table IX *(Continued)*

Kleopoulos, S. P., & Mobbs, C. V. (1993). Hypothalamic growth-hormone releasing hormone mRNA levels, and response to fasting, decrease with age in male rats. *Society for Neuroscience, Abstracts, 19,* in press.

Marcus, R., Butterfield, G., Holloway, L., Gilliland, L., Baylink, D. J., Hintz, R. L., & Sherman, B. M. (1990). Effects of short-term administration of recombinant human growth hormone to elderly people. *Journal of Clinical Endocrinological Metabolism, 70,* 519–527.

Martinoli, M. G., Ouellet, J., Rheaume, E., & Pelletier, G. (1991). Growth hormone and somatostatin gene expression in adult and aging rats as measured by quantitative in situ hybridization. *Neuroendocrinology, 54,* 607–615.

Parenti, M., Cocchi, D., Ceresoli, G., Marcozzi, C., & Muller, E. E. (1991). Age-related changes of growth hormone secretory mechanisms in the rat pituitary gland. *Journal of Endocrinology, 131,* 251–257.

Rosen, T., Hohannsson, G., Hoansson, J.-O., & Begtsson, B.-A. (1995). Consequences of growth hormone deficiency in adults and the benefits and risks of recombinant human growth hormone treatment. *Hormone Research, 43,* 93–99.

Rudman, D., & Shetty, K. R. (1994). Unanswered questions concerning the treatment of hyposomatotropism and hypogonadism in elderly men. *Journal of the American Geriatric Society, 42,* 522–527.

Rudman, D., Feller, A. G., Nagraj, H. S., Gerfans, G. A., Lalitha, P. Y., Goldberg, A. F., Schlenker, R. A., Cohn, L., Rudman, I. W., & Mattson, D. E. (1990). Effect of human growth hormone in men over 60 years old. *New England Journal of Medicine, 323,* 1–6.

Rudman, D., Feller, A. G., Cohn, L., Shetty, K. R., Rudman, I. W., & Draper, M. W. (1991). Effects of human growth hormone on body composition in elderly men. *Hormone Research, 36, (Suppl. 1),* 73–81.

Sato, M., & Frohman, L. A. (1993). Differential effects of central and peripheral administration of growth hormone (GH) and insulin-like growth factor on hypothalamic GH-releasing hormone and somatostatin gene expression in GH-deficient dwarf rats. *Endocrinology, 133,* 793–799.

Sohmiya, M., & Kato, Y. (1992). Renal clearance, metabolic clearance rate, and half-life of human growth hormone in young and aged subjects. *Journal of Clinical Endocrinological Metabolism, 75,* 1487–1490.

Spik, K. W., Boyd, R. L., & Sonntag, W. E. (1991). Effect of aging on GHRF-induced growth hormone release from anterior pituitary cells in primary culture. *Journal of Gerontology, 46,* B72–B77.

Steger, R. W., Bartke, A., & Cecim, M. (1993). Premature ageing in transgenic mice expressing different growth hormone genes. *Journal of Reproduction and Fertility, Supplement, 46,* 61–75.

Tanaka, K., Inoue, S., Shiraki, J., Shishido, T., Saito, M., Numata, K., & Takamura, Y. (1991). Age-related decrease in plasma growth hormone: response to growth hormone-releasing hormone, arginine, and L-dopa in obesity. *Metabolism, 40,* 1257–1262.

Weltman, A., Weltman, J. Y., Hartman, M. L., Abbott, R. D., Rogol, A. D., Evans, W. S., & Veldhuis, J. D. (1994). Relationship between age, percentage body fat, fitness, and 24-hour growth hormone release in healthy young adults: effects of gender. *Journal of Clinical Endocrinological Metabolism, 78,* 543–548.

Wolf, E., Kahnt, E., Ehrlein, J., Hermanns, W., Brem, G., & Wanke, R. (1993). Effects of long-term elevated serum levels of growth hormone on life expectancy of mice: lessons from transgenic animal models. *Mechanisms of Ageing and Development, 68,* 71–87.

by a rise in TSH, since T3 exerts a negative feedback effect on TSH. However, in at least a subpopulation of humans and rats, TSH remains at normal levels despite a decrease in T3. Extensive analysis of such a subpopulation in humans has suggested that this persistently suppressed TSH in the presence of falling T3 indicates a "re-setting of thresh-hold" of the negative feedback, in the direction of increased sensitivity to T3 (Lewis *et al.,* 1991). Similar results have been found in rats (Cizza *et al.,* 1992). Although persistent effects of thyroid hormones on gene expression have not been reported, the exposure of neonatal rats to elevated T3 appears to perma-

Table X
Thyroid Hormone and Aging

Bakke, J. L., Lawrence, N., & Robinson, S. (1972). Late effects of thyroxine injected into the hypothalamus of the neonatal rat. *Neuroendocrinology, 10,* 183–195.

Bakke, J. L., Lawrence, N. L., Bennett, J., & Robinson, S. (1974). The late effects of neonatal hyperthyroidism upon the feedback regulation of TSH secretion in rats. *Endocrinology, 97,* 659–664.

Cizza, G., Grady, L. S., Calogero, A. E., Bagdy, G., Lynn, A. B., Kling, M. A., Blackman, M. R., Chrousos, G. P., & Gold, P. W. (1992). Central hypothyroidism is associated with advanced age in male Fischer 344/N rats: in vivo and in vitro studies. *Endocrinology, 131,* 2672–2680.

Fabris, N., Mocchegiani, E., & Procinciali, M. (1995). Pituitary-hormone axis and immune system: A reciprocal neuroendocrine-immune interaction. *Hormone Research, 43,* 29–38.

Florini, J. R. (1989). Limitations of interpretation of age-related changes in hormone levels: illustration by effects of thyroid hormones on cardiac and skeletal muscle. *Journal of Gerontology, 44,* B107–B109.

Impallomeni, M., Kaufman, B. M., & Palmer, A. J. (1994). Do acute diseases transiently impair anterior pituitary function in patients over the age of 75? A longitudinal study of the TRH test and basal gonadotrophin levels. *Postgraduate Medical Journal, 70,* 86–91.

Langer, P., Balazova, E., Vician, M., Martino, E., Jezova, D., Michalikova, S., & Moravec, R. (1992). Acute development of low T3 syndrome and changes in pituitary-adrenocortical function after elective cholecystectomy in women: some differences between young and elderly patients. *Scandinavian Journal of Clinical and Laboratory Investigation, 52,* 215–220.

Lewis, G. F., Alessi, C. A., Imperial, J. G., & Refetoff, S. (1991). Low serum free thyroxine index in ambulating elderly is due to a resetting of the threshold of thyrotropin feedback suppression. *Journal of Clinical Endocrinological Metabolism, 73,* 843–849.

nently increase the sensitivity of TSH to thyroxine feedback (Bakke *et al.,* 1974), apparently acting through a ventromedial hypothalamic locus (Bakke *et al.,* 1972). These results suggest the possibility that thyroid hormone, like other hormones, might exert a persistent effect on hypothalamic function which accumulates during aging. Several effects of thyroid hormone replacement in aging animals have been reported (reviewed by Fabris *et al.,* 1995). However, like all hormone replacement studies, these studies deserve attention but must be replicated to determine how robust the effects are and if there are untoward pharmacological effects (Table X).

IX. Conclusion

In conclusion, aging generally entails the development of glandular impairments, often leading to decreased levels of peripheral hormone, accompanied by a normal level of stimulating hormone. This has led several investigators to suggest that in some respects the neuroendocrine sensitivity to these hormones actually increases, rather than decreases, with age. The apparent impairments in response to some hormones, such as the estrogen-induced LH surge in female rodents, may involve temporal impairments, rather than a decreased sensitivity to the hormone per se. Some evidence suggests that changing sensitivity to hormones may involve a cumulative effect of hormones on neuroendocrine loci. However, while it is clear that hormones can cause persistent changes in neuroendocrine responses, the quantitative relevance of these changes to age-related impairments remains to be determined. These recent results indicate that the neuroendocrinology of aging is a quickly developing field, and many longstanding hypotheses, such as a general decrease in sensitivity during aging, require new analysis. Nevertheless, that the field is now in a position to test quantitative hypotheses of aging is an indication of dramatic progress.

References

Akabayashi, A., Wahlestedt, C., Alexander, J. T., & Leibowitz, S. F. (1994). Specific inhibition of endogenous neuropeptide Y synthesis in arcuate nucleus by anti-sense oligonucleotides suppresses feeding behavior and insulin secretion. *Brain Research: Molecular Brain Research, 21,* 55–61.

Arbel, I., Kadar, T., Silberman, M., & Levy, A. (1994). The effects of long-term corticosterone administration on hippocampal morphology and cognitive performance of middle-aged rats. *Brain Research, 657,* 227–235.

Armanini, D., Scali, M., Vittadello, G., Ribecco, M., Zampollo, V., Pratesi, C., Orlandini, E., Zovato, S., Zennaro, C. M., & Karbowiak, I. (1993). Corticosteroid receptors and aging. *Journal of Steroid Biochemistry and Molecular Biology, 45,* 191–194.

Armstrong, J. N., McIntyre, D. C., Neubort, S., & Sloviter, R. S. (1993). Learning and memory after adrenalectomy-induced hippocampal dentate granule cell degeneration in the rat. *Hippocampus, 3,* 359–371.

Aschheim, P. (1983). Relation of neuroendocrine system to reproductive decline in female rats. In J. Meites (Ed.), *Neuroendocrinology of Aging* (pp. 73–102). New York: Plenum Press.

Bakke, J. L., Lawrence, N., & Robinson, S. (1972). Late effects of thyroxine injected into the hypothalamus of the neonatal rat. *Neuroendocrinology, 10,* 183–195.

Bakke, J. L., Lawrence, N. L., Bennett, J., & Robinson, S. (1974). The late effects of neonatal hyperthyroidism upon the feedback regulation of TSH secretion in rats. *Endocrinology, 97,* 659–664.

Bando, H., Zhang, C., Takada, Y., Yamasaki, R., & Saito, S. (1991). Impaired secretion of growth hormone-releasing hormone, growth hormone and IGF-I in elderly men. *Acta Endocrinologica (Copenhagen), 124,* 31–36.

Barnhill, J. G., Miller, L. G., Greenblatt, D. J., Thompson, M. L., Ciraulo, D. A., & Shader, R. I. (1991). Benzodiazepine receptor binding response to acute and chronic stress is increased in aging animals. *Pharmacology, 42,* 181–187.

Barton, R. N., Horan, M. A., Weijers, J. W., Sakkee, A. N., Roberts, N. A., & van Bezooijen, C. F. (1993). Cortisol production rate and the urinary excretion of 17-hydroxycorticosteroids, free cortisol, and 6-beta-hydroxycortisol in healthy elderly men and women. *Journal of Gerontology, 48,* M213–M218.

Belisle, S., Bellabarba, D., & Lehoux, J. G. (1990). Hypothalamic–pituitary axis during reproductive aging in mice. *Mechanisms of Ageing Development, 52,* 207–217.

Bergen, H., & Mobbs, C. V. (1992). Hypothalamic lesion by gold-thio-glucose (GTG) leads to hyperglycemia in mice. *Endocrine Society Abstracts,* 91.

Bergen, H., Kleopoulos, S. P., Pfaus, J., & Mobbs, C. V. (1992). Effect of gold-thioglucose (GTG) on hypothalamic oxytocin receptors and neuropeptide Y (NPY) mRNA. *Society of Neuroscience, Abstracts, 18,* 1485.

Billestrup, N., Swanson, L. W., & Vale, W. (1986). Growth-hormone-releasing factor stimulates proliferation of somatotrophs in vitro. *Proceedings of the National Academy of Science, 83,* 6854–6857.

Blake, M. J., Udelsman, R., Feulner, G. J., Norton, D. D., & Holbrook, N. J. (1991). Stress-induced heat shock protein 70 expression in adrenal cortex: an adrenocorticotropic hormone-sensitive, age-dependent response. *Proceedings of the National Academy of Sciences of the United States of America, 88,* 9873–9877.

Blandini, F., Martignoni, E., Melzi, E., Biasio, L., Sances, G., Lucarelli, C., Rizzo, V., Costa, A., & Nappi, G. (1992). Free plasma catecholamine levels in healthy subjects: a basal and dynamic study. The influence of age. *Scandinavian Journal of Clinical and Laboratory Investigation, 52,* 9–17.

Brawer, J. R., Naftolin, F., Martin, J., & Sonnenschein, C. (1978). Effects of a single injection of EV on the hypothalamic arcuate nucleus and on reproductive function in the female rat. *Endocrinology, 103,* 501–512.

Brock, M. A. (1991). Chronobiology and aging. *Journal of the American Geriatrics Society*, 39, 74–91.

Brodish, A., & Odio, M. (1989). Age-dependent effects of chronic stress on ACTH and corticosterone responses to an acute novel stress. *Neuroendocrinology*, 49, 496–501.

Brown, T. J., Maclusky, N. J., Shanabrough, M., & Naftolin, F. (1990). Comparison of age- and sex-related changes in cell nuclear estrogen-binding capacity and progestin receptor induction in the rat brain. *Endocrinology*, 126, 2965–2972.

Burch, J. B. E., & Evans, M. I. (1986). Chromatin structural transitions and the phenomenon of vitellogenin gene memory in chickens. *Molecular and Cellular Biology*, 6, 1886–1893.

Cai, A., & Wise, P. M. (1994). Effects of age and suprachiasmatic nucleus (SCN) transplants on the diurnal rhythm on pituitary pro-opiomelanocorticotropin (POMC) gene expression. *Society of Neuroscience, Abstracts*, 20(1), 49.

Calza, L., Giardino, L., & Ceccatelli, S. (1993). NOS mRNA in the paraventricular nucleus of young and old rats after immobilization stress. *Neuroreport*, 4, 627–630.

Campillo, B., Bories, P. N., Devanlay, M., Pornin, B., Le Parco, J. C., Gaye-Bareyt, E., & Fouet, P. (1992). Aging, energy expenditure and nutritional status: evidence for denutrition-related hypermetabolism. *Annals of Nutrition & Metabolism*, 36, 265–272.

Chambers, K. C., Thornton, J. E., & Roselli, C. E. (1991). Age-related deficits in brain androgen binding and metabolism, testosterone, and sexual behavior of male rats. *Neurobiology of Aging*, 12, 123–130.

Chou, Y. C., Lin, W. J., & Sapolsky, R. M. (1994). Glucocorticoids increase extracellular [3H]D-aspartate overflow in hippocampal cultures during cyanide-induced ischemia. *Brain Research*, 654, 8–14.

Chua, S. C., Jr., Leibel, R. L., & Hirsch, J. (1991). Food deprivation and age modulate neuropeptide gene expression in the murine hypothalamus and adrenal gland. *Brain Research: Molecular Brain Research*, 9, 95–101.

Cizza, G., Brady, L. S., Calogero, A. E., Bagdy, G., Lynn, A. B., Kling, M. A., Blackman, M. R., Chrousos, G. P., & Gold, P. W. (1992). Central hypothyroidism is associated with advanced age in male Fischer 344/N rats: in vivo and in vitro studies. *Endocrinology*, 131, 2672–2680.

Cizza, G., Calogero, A. E., Brady, L. S., Bagdy, G., Bergamini, E., Blackman, M. R., Chrousos, G. P., & Gold, P. W. (1994). Male Fischer 344/N rats show a progressive central impairment of the hypothalamic-pituitary-adrenal axis with advancing age. *Endocrinology*, 134, 1611–1620.

Cocchi, D. (1992). Age-related alterations in gonadotropin, adrenocorticotropin and growth hormone secretion. *Aging (Milano)*, 4, 103–113.

Collins, T. J., & Parkening, T. A. (1991). Exposure to estradiol impairs luteinizing hormone function during aging. *Mechanisms in Ageing and Development*, 58, 207–220.

Cooper, R. L. (1977). Sexual receptivity in aged female rats. Behavioral evidence for increased sensitivity to estrogen. *Hormones and Behavior*, 9, 321.

Copinschi, G., & van Cauter, E. (1995). Effects of aging on modulation of hormonal secretions by sleep and circadian rhythmicity. *Hormone Research*, 43, 20–24.

Corpas, E., Harman, S. M., Pineyro, M. A., Roberson, R., & Blackman, M. R. (1992). Growth hormone (GH)-releasing hormone-(1–29) twice daily reverses the decreased GH and insulin-like growth factor-I levels in old men. *Journal of Clinical Endocrinological Metabolism*, 75, 530–535.

Corpas, E., Harman, S. M., & Blackman, M. R. (1993a). Human growth hormone and human aging. *Endocrinology Reviews*, 14, 20–39.

Corpas, E., Harman, S. M., Pineyro, M. A., Roberson, R., & Blackman, M. R. (1993b). Continuous subcutaneous infusions of growth hormone (GH) releasing hormone 1–44 for 14 days increase GH and insulin-like growth factor-I levels in old men. *Journal of Clinical Endocrinological Metabolism*, 76, 134–138.

Crespo, D., Fernandez-Viadero, C., & Gonzalez, C. (1992). The influence of age on supraoptic nucleus neurons of the rat: morphometric and morphologic changes. *Mechanisms in Ageing and Development*, 62, 223–228.

Davis, F. C., & Gorski, R. A. (1984). Unilateral lesions of the hamster suprachiasmatic nuclei: evidence for redundant control of circadian rhythms. *Journal of Comparative Physiology, A154*, 221.

D'Costa, A. P., Ingram, R. L., Lenham, J. E., & Sonntag, W. E. (1993). The regulation and mechanisms of action of growth hormone and insulin-like growth factor 1 during normal ageing. *Journal of Reproduction and Fertility, Supplement, 46*, 87–98.

de Gennaro Colonna, V., Fidone, F., Cocchi, D., & Muller, E. E. (1993). Feedback effects of growth hormone on growth hormone-releasing hormone and somatostatin are not evident in aged rats. *Neurobiology of Aging, 14*, 503–507.

de Gennaro Colonna, V. G., Zoli, M., Cocchi, D., Maggi, A., Marrama, P., Agnati, L. F., & Muller, E. E. (1989). Reduced growth hormone releasing factor (GHRF)-like immunoreactivity and GHRF gene expression in the hypothalamus of aged rats. *Peptide, 10*, 705–708.

de Kloet, E. R. (1992). Corticosteroids, stress, and aging. *Annals of the New York Academy of Science, 663*, 357–371.

de Kloet, E. R., Sutanto, W., Rots, N., van Haarst, A., van den Berg, D., Oitzl, M., van Eekelen, A., & Voorhuis, D. (1991a). Plasticity and function of brain corticosteroid receptors during aging. *Acta Endocrinologica (Copenhagen), 125 (Suppl. 1)*, 65–72.

de Kloet, E. R., Joels, M., Oitzl, M., & Sutanto, W. (1991b). Implication of brain corticosteroid receptor diversity for the adaptation syndrome concept. In G. Jasmin & M. Cantin (Eds.), Stress Revisited. 1. Neuroendocrinology of Stress, *Methods and Achievements in Experimental Pathology, 14*, 104–132.

de Lacalle, S., Iraizoz, I., & Gonzalo, L. M. (1993). Cell loss in supraoptic and paraventricular nucleus in Alzheimer's disease. *Brain Research, 609*, 154–158.

Desjardins, G. C., Beaudet, A., Meaney, M. J., & Brawer, J. R. (1995). Estrogen-induced hypothalamic beta-endorphin neuron loss: A possible model of hypothalamic aging. *Experimental Gerontology, 30*, 253–267.

Desjardins, G. C., Beaudet, A., Schipper, H. M., & Brawer, J. R. (1992). Vitamin E protects beta-endorphin neurons from estradiol toxicity. *Endocrinology, 131*, 2481–2482.

Dilman, V. M. (1971). Age-associated elevation of hypothalamic threshold to feedback control, and its role in development, aging and disease. *Lancet, 1*, 1211–1218.

Eldridge, J. C., Fleenor, D. G., Kerr, D. S., & Landfield, P. W. (1989a). Impaired upregulation of type II corticosteroid receptors in hippocampus of aging rats. *Brain Research*, 248–256.

Eldridge, J. C., Kute, T., Brodish, A., & Landfield, P. W. (1989b). Apparent age-related resistance of hippocampal type II corticoid receptors to down-regulation by chronic escape training. *Journal of Neuroscience, 9*, 3237–3242.

Elliott, E. M., & Sapolsky, R. M. (1992). Corticosterone enhances kainic acid-induced calcium elevation in cultured hippocampal neurons. *Journal of Neurochemistry, 59*, 1033–1040.

Elliott, E. M., & Sapolsky, R. M. (1993). Corticosterone impairs hippocampal neuronal calcium regulation—possible mediating mechanisms. *Brain Research, 602*, 84–90.

Esler, M. D., Thompson, J. M., Kaye, D. M., Andrea, G. T., Jennings, G. L., Cox, H. S., Lambert, G. W., & Seals, D. R. (1995). Effects of aging on the responsiveness of the human cardiac sympathetic nerves to stressors. *Circulation, 91*, 351–358.

Evans, D. A. P., van der Kleu, A. A. M., Sonnemans, M. A. F., Burbach, J. P. H., & van Leeuwen, F. W. V. (1994). Frameshift mutations at two hotspots in vasopressin transcripts in post-mitotic neurons. *Proceedings of the National Academy of Science, 91*, 6059–6063.

Everitt, A. V. (1988). Hormonal basis of aging: antiaging action of hypophysectomy. In A. V. Everitt & J. R. Walton, (Eds.), *Regulation of neuroendocrine aging* (pp. 51–60). Basel: Kargcr.

Felicio, L. S., Nelson, J. F., Gosden, R. G., & Finch, C. E. (1983). Restoration of ovulatory cycles by young ovarian grafts in aging mice: Potentiation by long-term ovariectomy decreases with age. *Proceedings of the National Academy of Sciences of the United States of America, 80*, 6076.

Finch, C. E., Foster, J. R., & Mirsky, A. E. (1969). Aging and the regulation of cell activities during exposure to cold. *Journal of General Physiology, 54*, 690–712.

Findley, T. (1949). Role of the neurohypophysis in the pathogenesis of hypertension and some allied disorders associated with aging. *American Journal of Medicine, 7,* 70–84.

Florini, J. R. (1989). Limitations of interpretation of age-related changes in hormone levels: illustration by effects of thyroid hormones on cardiac and skeletal muscle. *Journal of Gerontology, 44,* B107–B109.

Florio, T., Ventra, C., Postiglione, A., & Schettini, G. (1991). Age-related alterations of somatostatin gene expression in different rat brain areas. *Brain Research, 557,* 64–68.

Frolkis, V. V. (1993). Stress-age syndrome. *Mechanisms in Ageing and Development, 69,* 93–107.

Funabashi, T., Kleopoulos, S. P., Brooks, P. J., Kato, J., Kimura, F., Pfaff, D. W., & Mobbs, C. V. (1993). Regulation of estrogen receptor mrna and progesterone receptor mRNA by estrogen in female rat hypothalamus during aging. *Society of Neuroscience, Abstracts, 20,* 817.

Gee, D. M., Flurkey, K., Mobbs, C. V., Sinha, Y. N., & Finch, C. E. (1984). The regulation of luteinizing hormone and prolactin in C57BL/6J mice: Effects of E2 implant size, ovariectomy, and aging. *Endocrinology, 114,* 685–693.

Goff, B. L., Roth, J. A., Arp, L. H., & Icefy, G. S. (1987). Growth hormone treatment stimulates thymulin production in aged dogs. *Clinical and Experimental Immununology, 68,* 580–587.

Gordon, M. N., Mobbs, C. V., & Finch, C. E. (1988). Pituitary and hypothalamic glucose-6-phosphate dehydrogenase: Effects of estradiol and age in C57BL/6J mice. *Endocrinology, 122,* 726–733.

Goya, R. G., Brooks, K., & Meites, J. (1991a). A comparison between hormone levels and T lymphocyte function in young and old rats. *Mechanisms in Ageing and Development, 61,* 275–285.

Goya, R. G., Castelletto, L., & Sosa, Y. E. (1991b). Plasma levels of growth hormone correlate with the severity of pathologic changes in the renal structure of aging rats. *Laboratory Investigation, 64,* 29–34.

Goya, R. G., Gagnerault, M. C., De Moraes, M. C., Savino, W., & Dardenne, M. (1992). In vivo effects of growth hormone on thymus function in aging mice. *Brain, Behavior, and Immunity, 6,* 341–354.

Goya, R. G., Castro, M. G., Saphier, P. W., Sosa, Y. E., & Lowry, P. J. (1993a). Thymus-pituitary interactions during ageing. *Age and Ageing, 22,* S19–S25.

Goya, R. G., Gagnerault, M. C., Sosa, Y. E., Bevilacqua, J. A., & Dardenne, M. (1993b). Effects of growth hormone and thyroxine on thymulin secretion in aging rats. *Neuroendocrinology, 58,* 338–343.

Gray, G. D., & Wexler, B. C. (1980). Estrogen and testosterone sensitivity of middle-aged female rats and the regulation of LH. *Experimental Gerontology, 15,* 201.

Gray, G. D., Smith, E. R., & Davidson, J. M. (1980). Gonadotropin regulation in middle-aged male rats. *Endocrinology, 107,* 2021.

Greenspan, S. L., Rowe, J. W., Maitland, L. A., McAloon-Dyke, M., & Elahi, D. (1993). The pituitary-adrenal glucocorticoid response is altered by gender and disease. *Journal of Gerontology, 48,* M72–M77.

Gruenewald, D. A., & Matsumoto, A. M. (1991a). Age-related decrease in pro-opiomelanocortin gene expression in the arcuate nucleus of the male rat brain. *Neurobiology of Aging, 12,* 113–121.

Gruenewald, D. A., & Matsumoto, A. M. (1991b). Age-related decreases in serum gonadotropin levels and gonadotropin-releasing hormone gene expression in the medial preoptic area of the male rat are dependent upon testicular feedback. *Endocrinology, 129,* 2442–2450.

Haigh, R. A., Harper, G. D., Burton, R., Macdonald, I. A., & Potter, J. F. (1991). Possible impairment of the sympathetic nervous system response to postprandial hypotension in elderly hypertensive patients. *Journal of Human Hypertension, 5,* 83–89.

Hakkinen, K., & Pakarinen, A. (1993). Muscle strength and serum testosterone, cortisol and SHBG concentrations in middle-aged and elderly men and women. *Acta Physiologica Scandinavica, 148,* 199–207.

Hauger, R. L., Thrivikraman, K. V., & Plotsky, P. M. (1994). Age-related alterations of hypothalamic-pituitary-adrenal axis function in male Fischer 344 rats. *Endocrinology, 134,* 1528–1536.

Heuser, I. J., Wark, H. J., Keul, J., & Holsboer, F. (1991). Hypothalamic-pituitary-adrenal axis function in elderly endurance athletes. *Journal of Clinical Endocrinological Metabolism, 73,* 485–488.

Honma, K.-I., Honma, S., & Hiroshige, T. (1983). Critical role of food amount for prefeeding corticosterone peak in rats. *American Journal of Physiology, 245,* R339–R344.

Hoogendijk, J. E., Fliers, E., Swaab, D. F., & Verwer, R. W. (1985). Activation of vasopressin neurons in the human supraoptic and paraventricular nucleus in senescence and senile dementia. *Journal of Neurological Science, 69,* 291–299.

Horan, M. A. (1994). Aging, injury and the hypothalamic-pituitary-adrenal axis. *Annals of the New York Academy of Science, 719,* 285–290.

Huang, H. H., Kissane, J. Q., & Hawrylewicz, E. J. (1987). Restoration of sexual function and fertility by fetal hypothalamic transplant in impotent aged male rats. *Neurobiology of Aging, 8*(5), 465–72.

Irwin, M. (1993). Stress-induced immune suppression. Role of the autonomic nervous system. *Annals of the New York Academy of Science, 697,* 203–218.

Irwin, M., Hauger, R., & Brown, M. (1992). Central corticotropin-releasing hormone activates the sympathetic nervous system and reduces immune function: increased responsivity of the aged rat. *Endocrinology, 131,* 1047–1053.

Issa, A. M., Rowe, W., Gauthier, S., & Meaney, M. J. (1990). Hypothalamic-pituitary-adrenal activity in aged, cognitively impaired and cognitively unimpaired rats. *Journal of Neuroscience, 10,* 3247–3254.

Jaarsma, D., Postema, F., & Korf, J. (1992). Time course and distribution of neuronal degeneration in the dentate gyrus of rat after adrenalectomy: a silver impregnation study. *Hippocampus, 2,* 143–150.

Jeevanandam, M., Petersen, S. R., & Shamos, R. F. (1993). Protein and glucose fuel kinetics and hormonal changes in elderly trauma patients. *Metabolism, 42,* 1255–1262.

Jesionowska, H., Karelus, K., & Nelson, J. F. (1990). Effects of chronic exposure to estradiol on ovarian cyclicity in C57Bl/6J mice: Potentiation at low doses and only partial suppression at high doses. *Biology of Reproduction, 43,* 312–317.

Jhanwar, M., & Chua, S. C. (1993). Critical effects of aging and nutritional state on hypothalamic neuropeptide Y and galanin gene expression in lean and genetically obese Zucker rats. *Brain Research: Molecular Brain Research, 19*(3), 195–202.

Kalra, S. P., Sahu, A., & Kalra, P. S. (1993). Ageing of the neuropeptidergic signals in rats. *Journal of Reproduction and Fertility, Supplement, 46,* 11–19.

Karelus, K., & Nelson, J. F. (1992). Aging impairs estrogenic suppression of hypothalamic proopiomelanocortin messenger ribonucleic acid in the mouse. *Neuroendocrinology, 55,* 627–633.

Kawashima, S. (1960). Influence of continued injections of sex steroids on the estrous cycle in the female rat. *Annotations Zoologicae Japonenses, 33,* 226.

Kelley, K. W., Arkin, S., & Li, Y. M. (1992). Growth hormone, prolactin, and insulin-like growth factors: New jobs for old players. *Brain, Behavior, and Immunity, 6,* 317–326.

Kerr, D. S., Campbell, L. W., Hao, S.-Y., & Landfield, P. W. (1989). Corticosteroid modulation of hippocampal potentials: Increased effect with age. *Science, 245,* 1505–1509.

Kerr, D. S., Campbell, L. W., Applegate, M. D., Brodish, A., & Landfield, P. W. (1991). Chronic stress-induced acceleration of electrophysiological and morphometric biomarkers of hippocampal aging. *Journal of Neuroscience, 11,* 1316–1324.

Khansari, D. N., & Gustad, T. (1991). Effects of long-term, low-dose growth hormone therapy on immune function and life expectancy. *Mechanisms of Ageing and Development, 57,* 87–100.

Kleopoulos, S. P., & Mobbs, C. V. (1993). Hypothalamic growth-hormone releasing hormone mRNA levels, and response to fasting, decrease with age in male rats. *Society of Neuroscience, Abstracts, 19,* 898.

Kleopoulos, S. P., Krey, L., & Mobbs, C. V. (1992). Regulation of hypothalamic oxytocin receptors and lordosis reflex during reproductive senescence of female Fisher rats. *Society of Neuroscience, Abstracts, 18,* 1485.

Knyszynski, A., Adler-Kunin, S., & Globerson, A. (1992). Effects of growth hormone on thymocyte development from progenitor cells in bone marrow. *Brain Behavior and Immunology, 6*, 327–338.

Kohama, S. G., Anderson, C. P., Osterburg, H. H., May, P. C., & Finch, C. E. (1989). Oral administration of estradiol to young C57Bl/6J mice induces age-like neuroendocrine dysfunctions in the regulation of estrous cycles. *Biology of Reproduction, 41*, 227–232.

Landfield, P. (1980). Adrenocortical hypothesis of brain and somatic aging. In R. T. Shimke (Ed.) *Biological Mechanisms in Aging* (Publication No. 81–2194, pp. 658–672) Washington, DC: NIH.

Landfield, P. W. (1994). Nathan Shock Memorial Lecture 1990. The role of glucocorticoids in brain aging and Alzheimer's disease: an integrative physiological hypothesis. *Experimental Gerontology, 29*, 3–11.

Landfield, P. W., & Eldridge, J. C. (1991). The glucocorticoid hypothesis of brain aging and neurodegeneration: recent modifications. *Acta Endocrinologica (Copenhagen), 125 (Suppl. 1)*, 54–64.

Landfield, P. W., & Eldridge, J. C. (1994). Evolving aspects of the glucocorticoid hypothesis of brain aging: Hormonal modulation of neuronal calcium homeostasis. *Neurobiology of Aging, 15*, 579–588.

Landfield, P., Waymire, J., & Lynch, G. (1978). Hippocampal aging and adrenocorticoids: A quantitative correlation. *Science, 202*, 1098–1102.

Landfield, P. W., Baskin, R. K., & Pitler, T. A. (1981). Brain-age correlates: Retardation by hormonal pharmacological manipulations. *Science, 214*, 581–584.

Landfield, P. W., Thibault, O., Mazzanti, M. L., Porter, N. M., & Kerr, D. S. (1992). Mechanisms of neuronal death in brain aging and Alzheimer's disease: role of endocrine-mediated calcium dyshomeostasis. *Journal of Neurobiology, 23*, 1247–1260.

Landsberg, L., & Young, J. B. (1978). Fasting, feeding, and regulation of the sympathetic nervous system. *New England Journal of Medicine, 298*, 195–1301.

Langer, P., Balazova, E., Vician, M., Martino, E., Jezova, D., Michalikova, S., & Moravec, R. (1992). Acute development of low T3 syndrome and changes in pituitary-adreno-

cortical function after elective cholecystectomy in women: some differences between young and elderly patients. *Scandinavian Journal of Clinical and Laboratory Investigation, 52*, 215–220.

LaPolt, P. S., Matt, D. W., Judd, H. L., & Lu, J. K. H. (1986). The relation of ovarian steroid levels in young female rats to subsequent estrous cyclicity and reproductive function during aging. *Biology of Reproduction, 35*, 1131–1139.

LaPolt, P. S., Yu, S. M., & Lu, J. K. H. (1988). Early treatment of young female rats with progesterone delays the aging-associated reproductive decline: A counteraction by estradiol. *Biology of Reproduction, 38*, 987–995.

Lawrence, M. S., & Sapolsky, R. M. (1994). Glucocorticoids accelerate ATP loss following metabolic insults in cultured hippocampal neurons. *Brain Research, 646*, 303–306.

Leakey, J. E., Chen, S., Manjgaladze, M., Turturro, A., Duffy, P. H., Pipkin, J. L., & Hart, R. W. (1994). Role of glucocorticoids and caloric stress in modulating the effects of caloric restriction in rodents. *Annals of the New York Academy of Science, 719*, 171–194.

Levy, A., Dachir, S., Arbel, I., & Kadar, T. (1994). Aging, stress, and cognitive function. *Annals of the New York Academy of Science, 717*, 79–88.

Lewis, G. F., Alessi, C. A., Imperial, J. G., & Refetoff, S. (1991). Low serum free thyroxine index in ambulating elderly is due to a resetting of the threshold of thyrotropin feedback suppression. *Journal of Clinical Endocrinological Metabolism, 73*, 843–849.

Lloyd, J. M., Hoffman, G. E., & Wise, P. M. (1994). Decline in immediate early gene expression in gonadotropin-releasing hormone neurons during proestrus in regularly cycling, middle-aged rats. *Endocrinology, 134*, 1800–1805.

Lloyd, J. M., Scarbrough, K., Weiland, N. G., & Wise, P. M. (1991). Age-related changes in proopiomelanocortin (POMC) gene expression in the periarcuate region of ovariectomized rats. *Endocrinology, 129*, 1896–1902.

Lu, J. H. K., Gilman, D. P., Meldrum, D. R., Judd, H. L., & Sawyer, C. H. (1981). Relationship between circulating estrogens and the

central mechanisms by which ovarian steroids stimulate luteinizing hormone secretion in aged and young female rats. *Endocrinology, 108,* 836–841.

Major E. E., Kesslack, J. P., Cotman, C. W.,
Finch, C. E., & Day, J. R. (1994). Life-long
dietary restriction attenuates age-related
increases in glial fibrillary acidic protein
(GFAP) mRNA in the rat hippocampus. *Society for Neurosciences Abstracts, 28.19,* 50.

Marcus, R., Butterfield, G., Holloway, L., Gilliland, L., Baylink, D. J., Hintz, R. L., & Sherman, B. M. (1990). Effects of short-term administration of recombinant human growth
hormone to elderly people. *Journal of Clinical Endocrinological Metabolism, 70,* 519–
527.

Martinoli, M. G., Ouellet, J., Rheaume, E., &
Pelletier, G. (1991). Growth hormone and somatostatin gene expression in adult and
aging rats as measured by quantitative in
situ hybridization. *Neuroendocrinology, 54,*
607–615.

McCarter, R. J., & Palmer, J. (1992). Energy metabolism and aging: a lifelong study of
Fischer 344 rats. *American Journal of Physiology, 263,* E448–E452.

McEwen, B. S. (1992). Re-examination of the
glucocorticoid hypothesis of stress and aging.
Progress in Brain Research, 93, 365–81.

Meaney, M. J., Aitken, D. H., Bhatnagar, S., &
Sapolsky, R. M. (1991). Postnatal handling
attenuates certain neuroendocrine, anatomical, and cognitive dysfunctions associated
with aging in female rats. *Neurobiology of
Aging, 12,* 31–38.

Meaney, M. J., Aitken, D. H., Sharma, S., &
Viau, V. (1992). Basal ACTH, corticosterone
and corticosterone-binding globulin levels
over the diurnal cycle, and age-related
changes in hippocampal type I and type II
corticosteroid receptor binding capacity in
young and aged, handled and nonhandled
rats. *Neuroendocrinology, 55,* 204–213.

Miller, M. M., & Zhu, L. (1992). Aging changes
in the beta-endorphin neuronal system in the
preoptic area of the C57BL/6J mouse: ultrastructural analysis. *Neurobiology of Aging,
13,* 773–781.

Miller, M. M., Joshi, D., Billiar, R. B., & Nelson,
J. F. (1991). Loss during aging of beta-
endorphinergic neurons in the hypo-

thalamus of female C57BL/6J mice. *Neurobiology of Aging, 12,* 239–244.

Mirmiran, M., Swaab, D. F., Kok, J. H., Hofman,
M. A., Witting, W., & Van Gool, W. A. (1992).
Circadian rhythms and the suprachiasmatic
nucleus in perinatal development, aging and
Alzheimer's disease. *Progress in Brain Re-
search, 93,* 151–62.

Mobbs, C. V. (1989). Neurohumoral hysteresis
as a mechanism for senescence; Comparative aspects. In C. G. Scanes & M. P. Schrieb-
man (Eds.), *Development, Maturation, and
Senescence of the Neuroendocrine System*
(pp. 223–252). Academic Press.

Mobbs, C. V. (1990). Neurotoxic effects of estrogen, glucose, and glucocorticoids: Neurohumoral hysteresis and its pathological
consequences during aging. *Reviews of Biological Research on Aging, 4,* 201–228.

Mobbs, C. V. (1993). Genetic influences on glucose neurotoxicity, aging, and diabetes: A
possible role for glucose hysteresis. *Genetica, 91,* 239–253.

Mobbs, C. V. (1994). Molecular hysteresis: Age-
related impairments due to residual effects of
hormones and glucose on gene expression.
Neurobiology of Aging, 15, 523–534.

Mobbs, C. V., & Bergen, H. (1992). Glucose metabolism during aging in mice: Hypoglycemia and hyperinsulinemia. *Endocrine
Society, Abstracts, 74,* 370.

Mobbs, C. V., & Finch, C. E. (1992). Estrogen-
induced impairments as a mechanism in reproductive senescence of female C57Bl/6J
mice. *Journal of Gerontology, 47,* B48–B51.

Mobbs, C. V., & Finch, C. E. (1996). Not wisely
but too well: Mortality and senescence as
costs of neuroendocrine activation. *Frontiers
in Neuroendocrinology* (submitted for publication).

Mobbs, C. V., & Kleopoulos, S. P. (1992). Regu-
lation of hypothalamic neuropeptide Y
(NPY) by fasting during aging in male rats.
Society of Neuroscience, Abstracts, 18, 1485.

Mobbs, C. V., Gee, D. M., & Finch, C. E.
(1984a). Reproductive senescence in female
C57BL/6J mice: Ovarian impairments and
neuroendocrine impairments that are partially reversible and delayable by ovariectomy. *Endocrinology, 115,* 1653–1662.

Mobbs, C. V., Flurkey, K., Gee, D. M.,
Yamamoto, K., Sinha, Y. N., & Finch, C. E.

(1984b). Estradiol-induced adult anovulatory syndrome in female C57BL/6J mice: Age-like neuroendocrine, but not ovarian, impairments. *Biology of Reproduction, 30,* 556–563.

Mobbs, C. V., Cheyney, D., Sinha, Y. N., & Finch, C. E. (1985). Age-correlated and ovary-dependent changes in relationships between plasma estradiol and luteinizing hormone, prolactin, and growth hormone in female C57BL/6J mice. *Endocrinology, 116,* 813–820.

Mobbs, C. V., Kleopoulos, S. P., & Bergen, H. (1993a). Hypoglycemia precedes hyperglycemia during aging: effect of dietary enhancement and dietary restriction. *Endocrine Society, Abstracts, 75,* 367.

Mobbs, C. V., Kleopoulos, S. P., & Funabashi, T. (1993b). A glucokinase/AP-1 glucose transduction mechanism in the ventromedial hypothalamic satiety center. *Society of Neuroscience, Abstracts, 19,* 583.

Monroe, W. E., Roth, J. A., Grier, R. L., Arp, L. H., & Naylor, P. H. 91987). Effects of growth hormone in the adult canine thymus. *Thymus, 9,* 173–187.

Morley, J. E., & Silver, A. J. (1988). Anorexia in the elderly. *Neurobiology of Aging, 9,* 9–16.

Morrow, L. A., Rosen, S. G., & Halter, J. B. (1991). Beta-adrenergic regulation of insulin secretion: evidence of tissue heterogeneity of beta-adrenergic responsiveness in the elderly. *Journal of Gerontology, 46,* M108–M113.

Morrow, L. A., Morganroth, G. S., Herman, W. H., Bergman, R. N., & Halter, J. B. (1993). Effects of epinephrine on insulin secretion and action in humans. Interaction with aging. *Diabetes, 42,* 307–315.

Muneoka, K., Mikuni, M., Ogawa, T., Kitera, K., & Takahashi, K. (1994). Periodic maternal deprivation-induced potentiation of the negative feedback sensitivity to glucocorticoids to inhibit stress-induced adrenocortical response persists throughout the animal's lifespan. *Neuroscience Letters, 168,* 89–92.

Nagy, E., Berczi, I., & Friesen, H. G. (1983). Regulatin of immunity in rats by lactogenic and growth hormones. *Acta Endocrinology, 102,* 351–357.

Natelson, B. H., Ottenweller, J. E., Servatius, R. J., Drastal, S., Bergen, M. T., & Tapp, W. N. (1992). Effect of stress and food restriction on blood pressure and lifespan of Dahl salt-sensitive rats. *Journal of Hypertension, 10,* 1457–1462.

Neafsey, P. J., Boxenbaum, H., Ciraulo, D. A., & Fournier, D. J. (1988). A gompertz age-specific mortality-rate model of aging, hormesis, and toxicity: Fixed-dose studies. *Drug Metabolism Reviews, 19,* 369–401.

Nelson, J. F., Bender, M., & Schacter, B. S. (1988). Age-related changes in preopiomelanocortin messenger ribonucleic acid levels in hypothalamus and pituitary of female C57Bl/6J mice. *Endocrinology, 123,* 340–344.

Ng, A. V., Callister, R., Johnson, D. G., & Seals, D. R. (1993). Age and gender influence muscle sympathetic nerve activity at rest in healthy humans. *Hypertension, 21,* 498–503.

Ng, A. V., Callister, R., Johnson, D. G., & Seals, D. R. (1994). Sympathetic neural reactivity to stress does not increase with age in healthy humans. *American Journal of Physiology, 267,* H344–H353.

Nichols, N. R., Finch, C. E., & Nelson, J. F. (1995). Food restriction delays the age-related increase in GFAP mRNA in rat hypothalamus. *Neurobiology of Aging, 15,* 105–110.

Odio, M., & Brodish, A. (1991). Decreased plasticity of glucoregulatory responses in aged rats: effects of chronic stress. *Journal of Gerontology, 46,* B188–B196.

Okamoto, M., Kita, T., Okuda, H., Tanaka, T., & Nakashima, T. (1992). Effects of acute administration of nicotine on convulsive movements and blood levels of corticosterone in old rats. *Japanese Journal of Pharmacology, 60,* 381–384.

Pardue, S., Groshan, K., Raese, J. D., & Morrison-Bogorad, M. (1992). Hsp70 mRNA induction is reduced in neurons of aged rat hippocampus after thermal stress. *Neurobiology of Aging, 13,* 661–672.

Parenti, M., Cocchi, D., Ceresoli, G., Marcozzi, C., & Muller, E. E. (1991). Age-related changes of growth hormone secretory mechanisms in the rat pituitary gland. *Journal of Endocrinology, 131,* 251–257.

Perego, C., Vetrugno, G. C., De Simoni, M. G., & Algeri, S. (1993). Aging prolongs the stress-induced release of noradrenaline in rat hypothalamus. *Neuroscience Letters, 157,* 127–130.

Pich, E. M., Messori, B., Zoli, M., Ferraguti, F., Marrama, P., Biagini, G., Fuxe, K., & Agnati, L. F. (1992). Feeding and drinking responses to neuropeptide Y injections in the paraventricular hypothalamic nucleus of aged rats. *Brain Research, 575,* 265–271.

Pickard, G. E., & Turek, F. W. (1983). The suprachiasmatic nuclei: Two circadian clocks? *Brain Research, 268,* 201.

Pierpaoli, W., & Regelson, W. (1994). Pineal control of aging: Effect of melatonin and pineal grafting in aging mice. *Proceedings of the National Academy of Science USA, 91,* 781–791.

Pirke, K. M., Geiss, M., & Sintermann, R. (1978). A quantitative study on feedback control of LH by testosterone in young adult and old male rats. *Acta Endocrinologica (Copenhagen), 89,* 789–795.

Pittendrigh, C. S., & Daan, S. (1974). Circadian oscillations in rodents: A systematic increase of their frequency with age. *Science, 186,* 548–551.

Piva, F., Celotti, F., Dondi, D., Limonta, P., Maggi, R., Messi, E., Negri-Cesi, P., Zanisi, M., Motta, M., & Martini, L. (1993). Ageing of the neuroendocrine system in the brain of male rats: receptor mechanisms and steroid metabolism. *Journal of Reproduction and Fertility, Supplement, 46,* 47–59.

Plotsky, P. M., & Vale, W. (1985). Patterns of growth-hormone releasing factor and somatostatin secretion into the hypophysial–portal circulation of the rat. *Science, 230,* 461–463.

Poehlman, E. T. (1993). Regulation of energy expenditure in aging humans. *Journal of the American Geriatric Society, 41,* 552–559.

Possidente, B., McEldowney, S., & Pabon, A. (1995). Aging lengthens circadian period for wheel-running activity in C57Bl/6J mice. *Physiology and Behavior, 57,* 575–580.

Raadsheer, F. C., Sluiter, A. A., Ravid, R., Tilders, F. J., & Swaab, D. F. (1993). Localization of corticotropin-releasing hormone (CRH) neurons in the paraventricular nucleus of the human hypothalamus; age-dependent colocalization with vasopressin. *Brain Research, 615,* 50–62.

Raadsheer, F. C., Oorschot, D. E., Verwer, R. W., Tilders, F. J., & Swaab, D. F. (1994).

Age-related increase in the total number of corticotropin-releasing hormone neurons in the human paraventricular nucleus in controls and Alzheimer's disease: comparison of the disector with an unfolding method. *Journal of Comparative Neurology, 339,* 447–457.

Rammohan, M., Juan, D., & Jung, D. (1989). Hypophagia among hospitalized elderly. *Journal of the American Dietetic Association, 89,* 1774–1779.

Rance, N. E., McMullen, N. T., Smialek, J. E., Price, D. L., & Young, W. S. (1990). Postmenopausal hypertrophy of neurons expressing the estrogen receptor gene in the human hypothalamus. *Journal of Clinical Endocrinology and Metabolism, 71,* 79–85.

Rance, N. E., Uswandi, S. V., & McMullen, N. T. (1993). Neuronal hypertrophy in the hypothalamus of older men. *Neurobiology of Aging, 14,* 337–342.

Rasmussen, H. (1974). Parathyroid hormone, calcitonin, and the calciferols, In *Textbook for Endocrinology,* pp. 660–773.

Reiter, R. J. (1995). The pineal gland and melatonin in relation to aging: A summary of the theories and of the data. *Experimental Gerontology, 30,* 199–212.

Reul, J. M., Rothuizen, J., & de Kloet, E. R. (1991). Age-related changes in the dog hypothalamic-pituitary-adrenocortical system: neuroendocrine activity and corticosteroid receptors. *Journal of Steroid Biochemistry and Molecular Biology, 40,* 63–69.

Reymond, F., Denereaz, N., & Lemarchand-Beraud, T. (1992). Thyrotropin action is impaired in the thyroid gland of old rats. *Acta Endocrinologica (Copenhagen), 126,* 55–63.

Richardson, S. J. (1993). The biological basis of the menopause. *Baillieres Clinical Endocrinological Metabolism, 7,* 1–16.

Riggs, T. R., & Walker, L. M. (1960). Growth hormone stimulation of amino acid transport into rat tissues in vivo. *Journal of Biological Chemistry, 235,* 3603–3607.

Robertson, O. H., Wexler, B. C., & Miller, B. F. (1961). Degenerative changes in the cardiovascular system of spawning Pacific salmon. *Circulation Research, 9,* 826–834.

Rolls, B. J. (1992). Aging and appetite. *Nutritional Reviews, 50,* 422–426.

Romanoff, L. P., Morris, C. W., Welch, P., Roderiguez, R. M., & Pincus, G. (1961). The metabolism of cortical-4-C^{14} in young and elderly men. I. Secretion rate of cortisol and daily excretion of tetrahydrocortical, allotetralrydrocortical, tetrahydrocortisone and cortalone (20α and 20β). *Journal of Clinical Endocrinological Metabolism, 21*, 1413–1425.

Romero, M. T., Lehman, M. N., & Silver, R. (1993). Age of donor influences ability of suprachiasmatic nucleus grafts to restore circadian rhythmicity. *Brain Research: Developments in Brain Research, 71*, 45–52.

Roselli, C. E., Thornton, J. E., & Chambers, K. C. (1993). Age-related deficits in brain estrogen receptors and sexual behavior of male rats. *Behavioral Neuroscience, 107*, 202–209.

Rosen, T., Hohannssson, G., Hoansson, J.-O., & Begtsson, B.-A. (1995). consequences of growth hormone deficiency in adults and the benefits and risks of recombinant human growth hormone treatment. *Hormone Research, 43*, 93–99.

Rossi, G. L., Bestetti, G. E., Galbiati, E., Muller, E. E., & Cocchi, D. (1991). Sexually dimorphic effects of aging on rat somatotropes and lactotropes. *Journal of Gerontology, 46*, B152–B158.

Rossi, G. L., Bestetti, G. E., & Reymond, M. J. (1992). Tuberoinfundibular dopaminergic neurons and lactotropes in young and old female rats. *Neurobiology of Aging, 13*, 275–281.

Rossi, G. L., Bestetti, G. E., & Neiger, R. (1993). Sexually dimorphic effects of aging on tuberoinfundibular dopaminergic neurons and lactotropes of rats. *Mechanisms in Ageing and Development, 72*, 129–143.

Rossmanith, W. G. (1995). Gonadotropin secretion during aging in women: Review article. *Experimental Gerontology, 30*, 369–381.

Rossmanith, W. G., Scherbaum, W. A., & Lauritzen, C. (1991). Gonadotropin secretion during aging in postmenopausal women. *Neuroendocrinology, 54*, 211–218.

Roth, G. S. (1995). Changes in tissue responsiveness to hormones and neurotransmitters during aging. *Experimental Gerontology, 30*, 361–368.

Rothuizen, J., Reul, J. M., Rijnberk, A., Mol, J. A., & de Kloet, E. R. (1991). Aging and the hypothalamus-pituitary-adrenocortical axis, with special reference to the dog. *Acta Endo-

crinologica (Copenhagen), 125 (Suppl. 1)*, 73–76.

Rothuizen, J., Reul, J. M., van Sluijs, F. J., Mol, J. A., Rijnberk, A., & de Kloet, E. R. (1993). Increased neuroendocrine reactivity and decreased brain mineralocorticoid receptor-binding capacity in aged dogs. *Endocrinology, 132*, 161–168.

Rowe, J. W., & Troen, B. R. (1980). Sympathetic nervous system and aging in man. *Endocrine Reviews, 1*, 167–178.

Rowe, J. W., Young, J. B., Minaker, K. L., Stevens, A. L., Pallotta, J., & Landsberg, L. (1981). Effect of insulin and glucose infusions on sympathetic nervous system activity in normal man. *Diabetes, 30*, 219–225.

Roy, S., Sala, R., Cagliero, E., & Lorenzi, M. (1990). Overexpression of fibronectin induced by diabetes or high glucose: Phenomenon with a memory. *Proceedings of the National Academy of Sciences of the United States of America, 87*, 404–408.

Rudman, D., & Shetty, K. R. (1994). Unanswered questions concerning the treatment of hyposomatotropism and hypogonadism in elderly men. *Journal of the American Geriatric Society, 42*, 522–527.

Rudman, D., Feller, A. G., Nagraj, H. S., Gerfans, G. A., Lalitha, P. Y., Goldberg, A. F., Schlenker, R. A., Cohn, L., Rudman, I. W., & Mattson, D. E. (1990). Effect of human growth hormone in men over 60 years old. *New England Journal of Medicine, 323*, 1–6.

Rudman, D., Feller, A. G., Cohn, L., Shetty, K. R., Rudman, I. W., & Draper, M. W. (1991). Effects of human growth hormone on body composition in elderly men. *Hormone Research, 36 (Suppl. 1)*, 73–81.

Sabatino, F., Masoro, E. J., McMahan, C. A., & Kuhn, R. W. (1991). Assessment of the role of the glucocorticoid system in aging processes and in the action of food restriction. *Journal of Gerontology, 46*, B171–B179.

Sapolsky, R. M. (1992). Do glucocorticoid concentrations rise with age in the rat? *Neurobiology of Aging, 13*, 171–174.

Sapolsky, R. M., & Altmann, J. (1991). Incidence of hypercortisolism and dexamethasone resistance increases with age among wild baboons. *Biological Psychiatry, 30*, 1008–1016.

Sapolsky, R. M., Krey, L., & McEwen, B. S. (1983). The adrenocortical stress-response in the aged male rat: impairment of recovery from stress. *Experimental Gerontology, 18,* 55.

Sapolsky, R. M., Krey, L., & McEwen, B. S. (1985). Prolonged glucocorticoid exposure reduces hippocampal neuron number: Implications for aging. *Journal of Neuroscience, 5,* 1222–1227.

Sapolsky, R. M., Krey, L., & McEwen, B. S. (1986). The neuroendocrinology of stress and aging: The glucocorticoid cascade hypothesis. *Endocrine Reviews, 7,* 284–301.

Sartin, J. L., & Lamperti, A. A. (1985). Neuron numbers in hypothalamic nuclei of young, middle-aged and aged male rats. *Experientia, 41,* 109–111.

Satinoff, E., Li, H., Tcheng, T. K., Liu, C., McArthur, A. J., Medanic, M., & Gillette, M. U. (1993). Do the suprachiasmatic nuclei oscillate in old rats as they do in young ones? *American Journal of Physiology, 265,* R1216–R1222.

Sato, M., & Frohman, L. A. (1993). Differential effects of central and peripheral administration of growth hormone (GH) and insulin-like growth factor on hypothalamic GH-releasing hormone and somatostatin gene expression in GH-deficient dwarf rats. *Endocrinology, 133,* 793–799.

Schipper, H., Brawer, J. R., Nelson, J. F., Felicio, L. S., & Finch, C. E. (1981). The role of the gonads in the histologic aging of the hypothalamic arcuate nucleus. *Biology of Reproduction, 25,* 413–418.

Schipper, H. M., Desjardins, G. C., Beaudet, A., & Brawer, J. (1994). The 21-aminosteroid antioxidant, U743-89F, prevents estradiol-induced depletion of hypothalamic beta-endorphin neurons in adult female rats. *Brain Research, 652,* 616–163.

Schwartz, M. W., Figlewicz, D. P. Woods, S. C., Porte, D., Jr., & Baskin, D. G. (1993). Insulin, neuropeptide Y, and food intake. *Annals of the New York Academy of Science, 692,* 60–71.

Schwartz, A. G., & Pashko, L. L. (1994). Role of adrenocortical steroids in mediating cancer-preventive and age-retarding effects of food restriction in laboratory rodents. *Journal of Gerontology, 49,* B37–B41.

Seeman, T. E., & Robbins, R. J. (1994). Aging and hypothalamic-pituitary-adrenal response to challenge in humans. *Endocrine Reviews, 15,* 233–260.

Selye, H., & Tuchweber, B. (1976). Stress in relation to aging and disease. In A. V. Everitt, & J. A. Burgess (Eds.), *Hypothalamus, Pituitary, and Aging* (pp. 553–569). Springfield: Charles C. Thomas.

Sherman, B., Wysham, C., & Pfohl, B. (1985). Age-related changes in the circadian rhythm of plasma cortisol in man. *Journal of Clinical Endocrinological Metabolism, 61,* 439–443.

Silver, A. J., Flood, J. F., & Morley, J. E. (1988). Effect of gastrointestinal peptides on ingestion in old and young mice. *Peptides, 9,* 221–225.

Silverman, W. F., & Sladek, J. R., Jr. (1991). Ultrastructural changes in magnocellular neurons from the supraoptic nucleus of aged rats. *Brain Research: Developments in Brain Research, 58,* 25–34.

Simard, M., Brawer, J. R., & Farookhi, R. (1987). An intractable, ovary independent impairment in hypothalamo-pituitary function in the E_2-valerate-induced polycystic ovarian condition in the rat. *Biology of Reproduction, 36,* 1229–1237.

Sloviter, R. S., Dean, E., & Neubort, S. (1993a). Electron microscopic analysis of adrenalectomy-induced hippocampal granule cell degeneration in the rat: apoptosis in the adult central nervous system. *Journal of Comparative Neurology, 330,* 337–351.

Sloviter, R. S., Sollas, A. L., Dean, E., & Neubort, S. (1993b). Adrenalectomy-induced granule cell degeneration in the rat hippocampal dentate gyrus: characterization of an in vivo model of controlled neuronal death. *Journal of Comparative Neurology, 330,* 324–336.

Solez, C. (1952). Aging and adrenal cortical hormones. *Geriatrics, 7,* 241–245.

Somani, S. M., Buckenmeyer, P., Dube, S. N., Mandalaywala, R. H., Verhulst, S. J., & Knowlton, R. G. (1992). Influence of age on caloric expenditure during exercise. *International Journal of Clinical Pharmacology, Therapy and Toxicology, 30,* 1–6.

Sonntag, W. E., Boyd, R. L., & Booze, R. M. (1990). Somatostatin gene expression in the hypothalamus and cortex of aging male rats. *Neurobiology of Aging, 1,* 409–416.

Sonntag, W. E., Forman, L. J., & Meites, J. (1983). Changes in growth hormone secretion in aging rats and man, and its possible relation to diminished physiological functions. In J. Meites (Ed.), *Neuroendocrinology of Aging* (pp. 275–308). New York, NY: Plenum.

Sonntag, W. E., Steger, R. W., Forman, L. J., & Meites, J. (1980). Decreased pulsatile release of growth hormone in old male rats. *Endocrinology, 107,* 1875–1880.

Spik, K. W., Boyd, R. L., & Sonntag, W. E. (1991). Effect of aging on GHRF-induced growth hormone release from anterior pituitary cells in primary culture. *Journal of Gerontology, 46,* B72–B77.

Stanley, B. G., Magdalin, W., Seirafi, A., Thomas, W. J., & Leibowitz, S. F. (1993). The perifonical area: The major focus of (a) patchily distributed hypothalamic neuropeptide Y-sensitive feeding system. *Brain Research, 604,* 304–317.

Steger, R. W., Bartke, A., & Cecim, M. (1993). Premature ageing in transgenic mice expressing different growth hormone genes. *Journal of Reproduction and Fertility, Supplement, 46,* 61–75.

Stein-Behrens, B. A., Elliott, E. M., Miller, C. A., Schilling, J. W., Newcombe, R., & Sapolsky, R. M. (1992). Glucocorticoids exacerbate kainic acid-induced extracellular accumulation of excitatory amino acids in the rat hippocampus. *Journal of Neurochemistry, 58,* 1730–1735.

Stein-Behrens, B. A., Lin, W. J., & Sapolsky, R. M. (1994). Physiological elevations of glucocorticoids potentiate glutamate accumulation in the hippocampus. *Journal of Neurochemistry, 63,* 596–602.

Stewart, J., Meaney, M. J., Aitken, D., Jensen, L., & Kalant, N. (1988). The effects of acute and life-long food restriction on basal and stress-induced serum corticosterone levels in young and aged rats. *Endocrinology, 123,* 1934–1941.

Stokkan, K. A., Reiter, R. J., Nonaka, K. O., Lerchel, A., Yu, B. P., & Vaughan, M. K. (1991). Food restriction retards aging of the pineal gland. *Brain Research, 545,* 66–72.

Sturrock, R. R. (1991). Stability of neuronal glial number in the aging mouse supraoptic nucleus. *Anatomischer Anzeiger, 172,* 123–128.

Sturrock, R. R. (1992). Stability of neuron number in the ageing mouse paraventricular nucleus. *Anatomischer Anzeiger, 174,* 337–340.

Supiano, M. A., Hogikyan, R. V., Morrow, L. A., Ortiz-Alonso, F. J., Herman, W. H., Bergman, R. N., & Halter, J. B. (1992). Hypertension and insulin resistance: role of sympathetic nervous system activity. *American Journal of Physiology, 263,* E935–E942.

Supiano, M. A., Hogikyan, R. V., Morrow, L. A., Ortiz-Alonso, F. J., Herman, W. H., Galecki, A. T., & Halter, J. B. (1993). Aging and insulin sensitivity: role of blood pressure and sympathetic nervous system activity. *Journal of Gerontology, 48,* M237–M243.

Sutin, E. L., Dement, W. C., Heller, H. C., & Kilduff, T. S. (1993). Light-induced gene expression in the suprachiasmatic nucleus of young and aging rats. *Neurobiology of Aging, 14,* 441–446.

Swaab, D. F. (1993). Neurohypophysial peptides in the human hypothalamus in relation to development, sexual differentiation, aging and disease. *Regulatory Peptides, 45,* 143–147.

Swaab, D. F. (1995). Ageing of the human hypothalamus. *Hormone Research, 43,* 8–11.

Swaab, D. F., Goudsmit, E., Kremer, H. P., Hofman, M. A., & Ravid, R. (1992a). The human hypothalamus in development, sexual differentiation, aging and Alzheimer's disease. *Progress in Brain Research, 91,* 465–472.

Swaab, D. F., Grundke-Iqbal, I., Iqbal, K., Kremer, H. P., Ravid, R., & van de Nes, J. A. (1992b). Tau and ubiquitin in the human hypothalamus in aging and Alzheimer's disease. *Brain Research, 590,* 239–249.

Swaab, D. F., Hofman, M. A., Lucassen, P. J., Purba, J. S., Raadsheer, F. C., & van de Nes, J. A. (1993). Functional neuroanatomy and neuropathology of the human hypothalamus. *Anatomy and Embryology, 187,* 317–330.

Takahashi, S., Nomura, K., & Kawashima, S. (1988). Age-related changes in growth-hormone secretion in the rat. *International Congress of Endocrinology, 8,* 118.

Tan, D. X., Chen, D. X., Poeggleler, B., Manchester, L. C., and Reiter, R. J. (1993a). Melatonin: A potent, endogenous hydroxyl radical scavenger. *Endocrine Journal, 1,* 57–60.

Tan, D. X., Poeggleler, B., Reiter, R. J., Chen, L. D., Chen, S., & Manchester, L. C. (1993b). The pineal hormone melatonin inhibits DNA-adduct formation induced by the chemical carcinogen safrole in vivo. *Cancer Letters, 70,* 65–71.

Tanaka, H., Akama, H., Ichikawa, Y., Homma, M., & Oshima, H. (1991a). Glucocorticoid receptors in normal leukocytes: effects of age, gender, season, and plasma cortisol concentrations. *Clinical Chemistry, 37,* 1715–1719.

Tanaka, K., Inoue, S., Shiraki, J., Shishido, T., Saito, M., Numata, K., & Takamura, Y. (1991b). Age-related decrease in plasma growth hormone: response to growth hormone-releasing hormone, arginine, and L-dopa in obesity. *Metabolism, 40,* 1257–1262.

Telford, N., Mobbs, C. V., Sinha, Y. N., & Finch, C. E. (1986). The increase of anterior pituitary dopamine in aging C57BL/6J mice is caused by ovarian steroids, not intrinsic pituitary aging. *Neuroendocrinology, 43,* 135–142.

Terwel, D., Markerink, M., & Jolles, J. (1992). Age-related changes in concentrations of vasopressin in the central nervous system and plasma of the male Wistar rat. *Mechanisms in Ageing and Development, 65,* 127–136.

Tombaugh, G. C., & Sapolsky, R. M. (1992). Corticosterone accelerates hypoxia- and cyanide-induced ATP loss in cultured hippocampal astrocytes. *Brain Research, 588,* 154–158.

Tombaugh, G. C., Yang, S. H., Swanson, R. A., & Sapolsky, R. M. (1992). Glucocorticoids exacerbate hypoxic and hypoglycemic hippocampal injury in vitro: biochemical correlates and a role for astrocytes. *Journal of Neurochemistry, 59,* 137–146.

Tomimatsu, N., Hashimoto, S., & Akasofu, K. (1993). Effects of oestrogen on hypothalamic beta-endorphin in ovariectomized and old rats. *Maturitas, 17,* 5–16.

Touitou, Y., & Haus, E. (1994). Aging of the human endocrine and neuroendocrine time structure. *Annals of the New York Academy of Science, 719,* 378–397.

Turek, F. W., Penev, P., Zhang, Y., van Reeth, O., & Zee, P. (1995). Effects of age on the circadian system. *Neuroscience and Biobehavioral Reviews, 19,* 53–58.

Udelsman, R., Blake, M. J., Stagg, C. A., Li, D. G., Putney, D. J., & Holbrook, N. J. (1993). Vascular heat shock protein expression in response to stress. Endocrine and autonomic regulation of this age-dependent response. *Journal of Clinical Investigation, 91,* 465–473.

van den Berg, H., Mocking, J. A., & Seifert, W. F. (1991). The effect of immobilization and insulin-induced hypoglycemia on ACTH and corticosterone release in aging Brown-Norway rats. *Acta Endocrinologica (Copenhagen) 125 (Suppl. 1),* 104–106.

van Eekelen, J. A., Rots, N. Y., Sutanto, W., & de Kloet, E. R. (1992). The effect of aging on stress responsiveness and central corticosteroid receptors in the brown Norway rat. *Neurobiology of Aging, 13,* 159–170.

van Leeuwen, F. W., & van der Beek, E. M. (1991). The amount of mutant vasopressin precursor in the supraoptic and paraventricular nucleus of Brattleboro rats increases with age. *Brain Research, 542,* 163–166.

van Reeth, O., Zhang, E. Y., Reddy, A., Zee, P., & Turhk, F. W. (1993). Aging alters the entraining effects of an activity-inducing stimulus on the circadian clock. *Brain Research, 607,* 286–292.

van Reeth, O., Zhang, Y., Zee, P. C., & Turek, F. W. (1994). Grafting fetal suprachiasmatic nuclei in the hypothalamus of old hamsters restores responsiveness of the circadian clock to a phase shifting stimulus. *Brain Research, 643,* 338–342.

van Remmen, H., & Ward, W. F. (1994). Effect of age on induction of hepatic phosphoenolpyruvate carboxykinase by fasting. *American Journal of Physiology, 267,* G195–G200.

Vermeulen, A., & Kaufman, J. M. (1992). Role of the hypothalamo-pituitary function in the hypoandrogenism of healthy aging. *Journal of Clinical Endocrinological Metabolism, 75,* 704–706.

Waltman, C., Blackman, M. R., Chrousos, G. P., Riemann, C., & Harman, S. M. (1991). Spontaneous and glucocorticoid-inhibited adrenocorticotropic hormone and cortisol secretion are similar in healthy young and old men. *Journal of Clinical Endocrinological Metabolism, 73,* 495–502.

Weiland, N. G., Scarbrough, K., & Wise, P. M. (1992). Aging abolishes the estradiol-induced suppression and diurnal rhythm of pro-opiomelanocortin gene expression in the arcuate nucleus. *Endocrinology, 131,* 2959–2964.

Weltman, A., Weltman, J. Y., Hartman, M. L., Abbott, R. D., Rogol, A. D., Evans, W. S., & Veldhuis, J. D. (1994). Relationship between age, percentage body fat, fitness, and 24-hour growth hormone release in healthy young adults: effects of gender. *Journal of Clinical Endocrinological Metabolism, 78,* 543–548.

Wenzel, Z. M., & Randall, P. K. (1982). Phase changes of eating and activity circadian rhythms in young and old female rats. *Society for Neuroscience, Abstracts, 8,* 544.

Wexler, B. C. (1976). Comparative aspects of hyperadrenocorticism and aging. In A. V. Everitt & J. A. Burgess (Eds.), Hypothalamus, Pituitary, and Aging (pp. 333–361). Springfield: Charles C. Thomas.

Whealin, J. M., Burwell, R. D., & Gallagher, M. (1993). The effects of aging on diurnal water intake and melatonin binding in the suprachiasmatic nucleus. *Neuroscience Letters, 154,* 149–152.

White, J. D. (1993). Neuropeptide Y: A central regulator of energy homeostasis. *Regulatory Peptides, 49,* 93–107.

Wierda, M., Goudsmit, E., Van der Woude, P. F., Purba, J. S., Hofman, M. A., Bogte, H., & Swaab, D. F. (1991). Oxytocin cell number in the human paraventricular nucleus remains constant with aging and in Alzheimer's disease. *Neurobiology of Aging, 12,* 511–516.

Winters, S. J., Sherins, R. J., & Troen, P. (1984). The gonadotropin-suppressing activity of androgen is increased in elderly men. *Metabolism, 33,* 1052–1059.

Wise, P. M. (1993). Neuroendocrine ageing: its impact on the reproductive system of the female rat. *Journal of Reproduction and Fertility, Supplement, 46,* 35–46.

Wise, P. M. (1994). Nathan Shock Memorial Lecture 1991. Changing neuroendocrine function during aging: impact on diurnal and pulsatile rhythms. *Experimental Gerontology, 29,* 13–19.

Wise, P. M., Cohen, I. R., Weiland, N. G., *et al.,* (1988a). Aging alters the circadian rhythm of glucose utilization in the suprachiasmatic nucleus. *Proceedings of the National Academy of Sciences of the United States of America, 85,* 5305.

Wise, P. M., Dueker, E., & Wuttke, W. (1988b). Age-related alterations in pulsatile luteinizing hormone release: Effects of long-term ovariectomy, repeated pregnancies, and naloxone. *Biology of Reproduction, 39,* 1060–1066.

Wise, P. M., and Parsons, B. (1994). Nuclear estradiol and cytosol progestin receptor concentrations in the brain and pituitary gland and sexual behavior in ovariectomized estradiol-treated middle-aged rats. *Endocrinology, 115,* 810–816.

Wise, P. M., Scarbrough, K., Weiland, N. G., & Larson, G. H. (1990). Diurnal pattern of pro-opiomelanocorticotropin gene expression in the arcuate nucleus of proestrous, ovariectomized, and steroid-treated rats: Possible role in cyclic luteinizing hormone secretion. *Molecular Endocrinology, 4,* 886–892.

Wolf, E., Kahnt, E., Ehrlein, J., Hermanns, W., Brem, G., & Wanke, R. (1993). Effects of long-term elevated serum levels of growth hormone on life expectancy of mice: lessons from transgenic animal models. *Mechanisms in Ageing and Development, 68,* 71–87.

Woods, W. H., Powell, E. W., Andrews, A., & Ford, C. W., Jr. (1993). Light and electron microscopic analysis of two divisions of the suprachiasmatic nucleus in the young and aged rat. *Anatomical Record, 237,* 71–88.

Yau, J. L., Morris, R. G. M., & Seckl, J. R. (1994). Hippocampal corticosteroid receptor mRNA expression and spatial learning in the aged Wistar rat. *Brain Research, 657,* 59–64.

Young, J. B., Rowe, J. W., Pallotta, J. A., Sparrow, D., & Landsberg, L. (1980). Enhanced plasma norepinephrine response to upright posture and oral glucose administration in elderly human subjects. *Metabolism, 29,* 477–482.

Young, J. B., Troisi, R. J., Weiss, S. T., Parker, D. R., Sparrow, D., & Landsberg, L. (1992). Relationship of catecholamine excretion to body size, obesity, and nutrient intake in middle-aged and elderly men. *American Journal of Clinical Nutrition, 56,* 827–834.

Young, V. R. (1992). Energy requirements in the elderly. *Nutrition Reviews, 50,* 95–101.

Young, V. R., Yu, Y. M., & Fukagawa, N. K. (1991). Protein and energy interactions throughout life. Metabolic basis and nutritional implications. *Acta Paediatrica (Stockholm), Supplement, 373*, 5–24.

Zoli, M., Ferraguti, F., Gustafsson, J. A., Toffano, G., Fuxe, K., & Agnati, L. F. (1991). Selective reduction of glucocorticoid receptor immunoreactivity in the hippocampal formation and central amygdaloid nucleus of the aged rat. *Brain Research, 545*, 199–207.

Thirteen

Activity-Dependent Plasticity and the Aging Brain

Carl W. Cotman and Shawne Neeper

In the course of aging, the brain is subjected to a variety of insults, often leading to functional loss and dementia. One of the major goals of future research is the development of rational strategies to prevent decline and promote successful aging.

The aging brain has several natural mechanisms to respond to insult and promote recovery. If understood, it may be possible to draw upon these mechanisms to preserve circuitry and maintain functioning at higher levels during aging. For example, after neuronal injury, surviving fibers grow (sprout) and can form new, functional connections. This means of replacing lost connections can stem functional decline and rebuild neural systems following minor losses. Less severe forms of stimulation, which do not cause neuronal injury, also appear to be capable of inducing growth and vitality in neuronal circuitry. Indeed, various types of behavior can influence neuronal structure and functionality in the brain. Thus, the architecture of the brain is responsive to a variety of environmental and behavioral influences that can remodel and rebuild it. Accordingly, it is essential to identify the fundamental mechanisms underlying synaptic growth and remodeling, and interventions that stimulate such effects, in order to utilize these intrinsic promoters of central nervous system (CNS) function to fight age-related declines. At present, most studies have addressed activity-dependent neuronal plasticity at the cellular or structural level and describe phenomena, but do not define the underlying molecular regulatory pathways. There is a great need to identify the key systems and molecules at the molecular level of resolution. In this way it should be possible to identify earlier activity-dependent changes, find more sensitive indices of the stimuli that promote plasticity, and elucidate principles for interventions that support it.

In this chapter, we suggest that some behaviors that appear to promote the health of the individual (e.g., exercise) can induce the expression of neurotrophic factors, which may benefit participating neurons. In the first section we discuss current data suggesting that select families of neurotrophic factors may be critical in the regulation of neuronal plasticity, growth, and function and in providing neurons with greater resilience against insult and degeneration. In the next section we discuss

Handbook of the Biology of Aging, Fourth Edition
Copyright © 1996 Academic Press, Inc. All rights of reproduction in any form reserved.

evidence that some behaviors (e.g., exercise) can influence the function and health of the human brain, particularly during aging. We go on to examine new data that indicate that one simple behavior, exercise, can influence the availability of neurotrophic factors in the brain, providing evidence for a molecular mechanism by which activity and environment may influence neuronal function and health. In the final section we discuss the significance of this finding in the context of the literature addressing influences of activity and environment on brain structure and transmitter systems. Taken together, these data suggest that select behaviors that benefit the individual organism as a whole may also improve the vitality, function, and resilience of neurons involved in the behavior. In other words, some activities can induce neurons to provide themselves with factors needed for their health. We suggest that the effects of such activity-dependent plasticity on the brain may be a critical factor in the achievement of successful aging.

I. Neurotrophic Factors, Neuronal Health, and Brain Function

Neurotrophic factors, such as those of the neurotrophin and fibroblast growth factor (FGF) families, protect neurons from damage, promote their growth and function, and serve in the long-term maintenance and plasticity of the nervous system. Their expression has been linked to neuronal activity following seizure or application of exogenous neurotransmitter substances. If their expression can be regulated by physiological levels of neuronal activity, these molecules may provide a molecular link between an animal's activities and CNS plasticity.

Brain-derived neurotrophic factor (BDNF) and nerve growth factors (NGF) are the best-defined members of the neurotrophin family of growth factors. Both are expressed at high levels in the cerebral cortex and hippocampus, areas important to cognitive and memory functions (Ayer et al., 1988; Ernfors et al., 1990). These factors aid the differentiation, function, and survival of several types of neurons in vitro and in vivo, including the cholinergic (ACh) neurons of the basal forebrain (Alderson et al., 1990; Ghosh et al., 1994; Hefti & Will, 1987; Morse et al., 1993; Nonomura & Hatanaka, 1992; Widmer et al., 1993), which atrophy in aging and Alzheimer's disease, and the dopaminergic neurons of the mesencephalon (Altar et al., 1992; Sauer et al., 1993), which degenerate in Parkinson's disease. BDNF and NGF increase the activity of several free radical scavengers, thus increasing protection against oxidative injury (Nistico et al., 1992; Spina et al., 1992). Both BDNF and NGF are target-derived growth factors for specific neuronal populations, most notably forebrain ACh cells, and a sustained supply may be essential for the survival and/or function of these neurons (DiStefano et al., 1992; Morse et al., 1993; Widmer et al., 1993).

There is considerable evidence that CNS expression of BDNF and NGF is regulated by neuronal activity in vitro and in vivo (Boatell et al., 1992; Cosi et al., 1993; Follesa & Mocchetti, 1993; Gall et al., 1991; Gall & Isackson, 1989; Kokaia et al., 1993; Lapchak et al., 1993; Okazawa et al., 1992; Yakovlev et al., 1990; Zafra et al., 1990, 1991, 1992). BDNF and NGF mRNA expression is increased following seizure, which involves extremely heightened neuronal activity and sensory stimulation in vivo (Castren et al., 1992; Isackson et al., 1991). Excitatory neurotransmitter exposure increases their production in vivo and in vitro, while exposure to inhibitory substances decreases it (Zafra et al., 1991, 1992). NGF and BDNF mRNA are also increased with the induction of long-term potentiation, a likely mechanism of learning, in the hippocampus in vivo (Castren et al., 1993), linking neurotrophin expression with neuroplasticity.

The FGF family is another important class of growth factors found in the brain and regulated in an activity-dependent manner. FGF-2, or basic FGF, can support the survival and growth of a wide variety of neurons *in vitro* and *in vivo* (Anderson *et al.*, 1988; Cummings *et al.*, 1992; Mattson *et al.*, 1989). FGF-2, like the neurotrophins, is up-regulated after injury and as a function of neural activity (Follesa *et al.*, 1994; Follesa & Mocchetti, 1993; Gomez-Pinilla *et al.*, 1989; Mocchetti & Isackson, 1994; Riva *et al.*, 1992; Van Der Wal *et al.*, 1994). We and others have shown that seizures induce FGF-2 mRNA and protein, as measured immunocytochemically, in astrocytes and select neurons (Gall *et al.*, 1994; Van Der Wal *et al.*, 1994). The induction in astrocytes is surprising and suggests that neuronal activity can have an effect on these cells. FGF-2 is associated with angiogenesis and has been shown to promote vessel growth in the brain (Chen *et al.*, 1994; Gall & Isackson, 1989; Puumala *et al.*, 1990). Thus, it is important to examine the regulation of select members of the FGF family, as they could have a role in the maintenance of cerebral blood flow in aging, in addition to influencing neuronal and astrocytic vitality.

During the course of aging it would be anticipated that growth factors would have an increasingly important role, given their importance to neuronal growth and function. Yet levels of NGF mRNA and NGF protein, as well as the NGF receptor, are decreased in the aging brain (Gomez-Pinilla *et al.*, 1989; Larkfors *et al.*, 1987, 1988; Nishizuka *et al.*, 1991). Moreover, infusion of NGF protein can ameliorate age-related deficits in cognitive and memory functions in rats (Fischer *et al.*, 1991; Markowska *et al.*, 1994; Scott *et al.*, 1994). There is also evidence that BDNF levels are decreased in the brains of patients with Alzheimer's disease. Thus, interventions that increase neurotrophin levels, or prevent their decline, may be helpful in preventing age-related declines in CNS function.

In exploring factors that may be important to functional support in the aging brain, it is useful to identify specific challenges to CNS health in aging. The aging brain shows patterns of neuronal atrophy and functional decline, in addition to cell death. In the basal forebrain, there is a decline in cholinergic transmitter production and receptor density in aging (Sherman & Friedman, 1990). Neurotrophin infusion causes hypertrophy and increased transmitter production in these cells, indicating one potential direct benefit of increased neurotrophin levels in the aging brain (Fischer *et al.*, 1987; Sherman & Friedman, 1990).

During aging, neurons die by one of two pathways, necrosis or programmed cell death. Necrosis occurs when the cell's physical integrity has been overcome. Programmed cell death is a natural form of deliberate, selective cell death, important during developmental "pruning" of neuronal populations and thought to be operative in age-related neuronal loss and progressive degenerative diseases such as Alzheimer's disease (Cotman, 1994; Forloni *et al.*, 1993; Mattson, 1994). Programmed cell death may be initiated by several potentially age-associated events, including withdrawal of growth factors (Kondo *et al.*, 1994; Rich, 1992), loss of metabolic support, i.e., ischemia or hypoglycemia (Crumrine *et al.*, 1994; Linnik *et al.*, 1993), and oxidative insult (Buttke & Sandstrom, 1994; Richter, 1993). Oxidative tissue damage, in turn, has been shown to increase in the course of normal aging (Floyd & Carney, 1992; Oliver *et al.*, 1990; Smith *et al.*, 1991) and can lead to neuronal dysfunction and, eventually, cell death (Wyllie *et al.*, 1980). It is implicated in cell death due to Alzheimer's disease (Cotman, 1994; Mattson, 1994) and stroke (ischemia and hypoglycemia) (Floyd & Carney, 1992; Mattson *et al.*, 1993; Oliver *et al.*, 1990).

Neurotrophic factors can protect neurons against several causes of neuronal death associated with injury, aging, and degenerative diseases. FGF-2 and NGF tect cultured neurons against hypo-glycemia (Cheng & Mattson, 1991) and ex-citotoxicity (Mattson et al., 1993), which may be involved in stroke- and injury-related neurodegeneration. Application of neurotrophins can also protect cells from several forms of oxidative damage, possibly by increasing the activity of free radical scavengers (Jackson et al., 1990; Nistico et al., 1992; Oppenheim et al., 1992; Pechan et al., 1991; Richter, 1993; Sampath et al., 1994; Spina et al., 1992). Neurotrophic factors thus may have the potential to slow or prevent neuronal loss, as well as functional decline, in aging. Interventions that increase the availability of these important, plasticity-related molecules could protect and possibly improve brain functions and resilience in aging.

Thus, it is an emerging principle that the maintenance of proper levels of neuro-trophic factors may be important to neuronal function and survival and, thus, brain health. In the following sections, we discuss current literature that examines the involvement of specific behavioral activity on brain function across the life span. We build the case that behavioral activity, in principle, may regulate key brain neuro-trophic factors, that this might underlie some of the reported changes evoked in the brain by environment and activity, and importantly that neurotrophic factor up-regulation should be beneficial, and possibly crucial, to the maintenance and plasticity of the brain.

II. Human Studies Show That Activity Can Influence Performance and May Aid in the Maintenance of Function with Aging

Studies are defining ways in which experience and activity can influence mental health and alter the function, and even the survival, of several populations of CNS neurons. Such effects may be particularly evident in aging. To help elucidate factors that promote health and high function in aging, one large epidemiological study examined relationships between life experience and activities and physical and mental function in men and women aged 70–79 years. Education and regular, strenuous physical activity, such as gardening, emerged as predictors of significantly higher scores on five separate measures of cognitive and memory functions (Berkman et al., 1993). Another epidemiological study found that regular physical activity was related to both survival and cognitive capacity in aging men and women (Schroll et al., 1993).

Physical activity may have a positive effect on several aspects of CNS function. Research in humans has generally shown improvements in psychiatric status, such as reductions in depression and anxiety (Blumenthal et al., 1991; Hill et al., 1993; Labbe et al., 1988; Lichtman & Poser, 1983; Simons & Birkimer, 1988; Valliant & Asu, 1985; Young, 1979), following long-term aerobic training. Cross-sectional studies report quicker reaction times (Berkman et al., 1993; Clarkson-Smith & Hartley, 1989; Gleser & Mendelberg, 1990; Lupinacci et al., 1993) and better cognitive and memory functions in physically fit men and women relative to sedentary peers, particularly in aging populations (Clarkson-Smith et al., 1989; Dustman et al., 1990; Emmerson et al., 1989; Gleser & Mendelberg, 1990; Lupinacci et al., 1993). Several longitudinal studies of aging subjects also report better cognitive and memory functions in exercise program participants relative to sedentary controls (Berkman et al., 1993; Blomquist & Danner, 1987; Hill et al., 1993; Rogers et al., 1990). Group differences in these studies were primarily due to functional decline in aging sedentary controls, with concomitant preservation in aging exercisers. Some longitudinal studies that report no changes in cognitive or memory functions with exercise participation may be limited by ceiling effects in tests of mental function (Blumenthal *et al.*, 1991; Blumenthal & Madden, 1988) or by exercise programs that may be of insufficient duration and/or vigor to produce an effect or prevent functional decline in particular (Madden *et al.*, 1989; Molloy *et al.*, 1988).

The evidence suggests that regular exercise improves affect and could have a protective influence against declines in CNS function, such as those often seen with aging. One 4-year prospective study also begins to address possible biological effects of exercise in the brain that correlate with functional preservation. This study showed that aging (ages 65–69) individuals who remain active score better on cognitive tests and do not show the declines in cerebral blood flow seen in sedentary peers (Rogers *et al.*, 1990). This is consistent with other studies demonstrating a relationship between cerebral blood flow and cognitive capacity in aging (de la Torre *et al.*, 1992; Goldstein & Reivich, 1991; Kawamura *et al.*, 1991). Thus, a simple behavior (e.g., exercise) emerges as a potential factor in the maintenance of brain health.

III. Exercise and Voluntary Wheel Running Up-Regulates Brain Neurotrophic Factors

Can exercise influence key molecular systems that serve the maintenance and plasticity of the brain? In order to evaluate the influence of exercise on brain growth factors, we sought a method that, in so far as possible, parallels aspects of human studies, can be delivered or monitored in a quantitative manner, and allows exercise to be isolated as the central variable. For this we selected voluntary wheel running. This allows the animal to choose whether or not to run, as people decide when and

how much to exercise. Self-selected wheel running is also quantifiable and avoids possible confounding variables associated with investigator handling and the potential stress of forced treadmill running.

Rats appear to find physical activity inherently rewarding, and most will voluntarily run several kilometers during the night if given unlimited access to a running wheel. Once acclimated to running, each rat tends to maintain a characteristic activity level by running a similar total distance each night (unpublished observations). In our studies, wheel running was monitored by using software that summed wheel revolutions, measured by magnetic switches on the wheels, for each rat per 24-hr period, noon to noon. All rats, including controls, were given a 3-day training period in the wheel cages to reduce the effect of novelty or learning during the treatment running period. After training, rats were put in standard (no wheel) cages for 10 days to attenuate any physiological effect of the training period and then given 0 (control), 2, 4, or 7 nights in the wheel cages before sacrifice. Hybridization of radiolabeled antisense probe to rat BDNF mRNA was measured in specific areas of the brain using nuclease protection assays or *in situ* hybridization.

As we have reported previously (Neeper *et al.*, 1995), nuclease protection assays (Fig. 1A) revealed that exercise induced significant increases in BDNF mRNA hybridization in the hippocampus and the caudal one-third of the neocortex. The increase in hippocampal BDNF mRNA was significant after 2 nights with exercise and was sustained at a similar level after 4 and 7 nights (Fig. 1B). In the caudal neocortex, BDNF mRNA was also significantly increased after 2 nights of exercise and remained significantly higher than the control level after 4 and 7 nights (Fig. 1C).

Autoradiograms of *in situ* hybridization in control rats (Fig. 2A) show the greatest BDNF mRNA hybridization in the hippocampus, including the pyramidal cell layer

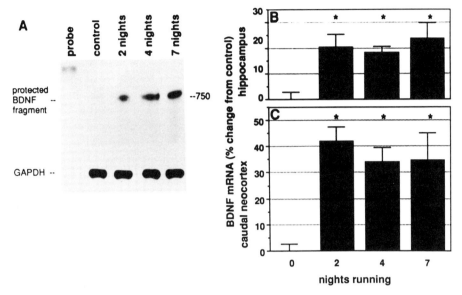

Figure 1. (A) Nuclease protection assay for BDNF mRNA in caudal neocortex. A BDNF cRNA 1077-base BDNF cRNA probe was used which resulted in a 750-base protected fragment. Hybridization was also performed with a 367-base cRNA probe to glyceraldehyde-phosphate dehydrogenase (GAPDH; Ambion, TX) to confirm that all samples contained equivalent total RNA. Protected mRNA fragments were separated by electrophoresis on a 5% polyacrylamide, 7 *M* urea gel. The gel was subsequently dried, and the protected fragment was visualized by autoradiography on β-max film (Amersham Labs, IL). BDNF mRNA content was estimated by computer densitometry using a Microcomputer Imaging Device (MCID) (Imaging Inc., St. Catherines, Ontario, Canada). The hippocampus (B) and caudal $\frac{1}{3}$ of neocortex (C) show significantly (*$P \leq 0.05$, analysis of variance (ANOVA), Fischer test) increased hybridization in 2 (n = 3), 4 (n = 4), and 7 (n = 4) night exercise groups compared to controls (n = 3). Bars represent standard error.

of Ammon's horn, fields 1–4 (CA1–4), and the granule cell layer of the dentate gyrus. Clear hybridization appears in layers II–III and V–VI of the neocortex. This distribution is consistent with previous reports (Ernfors *et al.*, 1990; Phillips *et al.*, 1990).

BDNF mRNA is notably increased in several cell layers following exercise (Fig. 2B). Within the hippocampus, the pyramidal cells of CA1 showed increases in labeling, reaching up to 190% of sedentary control values (Fig. 3A). Hybridization in these areas was significantly higher than that in the control after 2 nights with exercise and thereafter. In the caudal neocortex, layers II–III and V–VI also exhibited progressive increases in BDNF mRNA hybridization (Fig. 3B), which were signifi-

cantly higher than those of the control. Layers II–III increased more dramatically to 185% of control levels after 7 nights, compared to 142% of control in layers V–VI.

Small but significant ($P \leq 0.05$) increases in BDNF mRNA were detected in the cerebellum and frontal cerebral cortex at the later time points using both nuclease protection assay and *in situ* hybridization (data not shown). No significant changes in BDNF mRNA were detected in the middle one-third of the neocortex with nuclease protection assay.

To further test the hypothesis that physical activity can influence BDNF mRNA expression, we examined the relationship between BDNF mRNA measures from nuclease protection and the mean

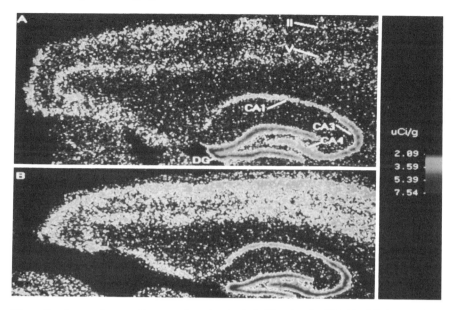

Figure 2.   Image of autoradiograms from *in situ* hybridization for BDNF mRNA in rat fore-brain (sagittal plane). (A) Control. (B) Following 7 nights with exercise. Increased BDNF mRNA expression in the exercised animal (B) is apparent in neocortical layers II and V, hippocampal subfields CA1–4, and the dentate gyrus (DG).

distance run by each rat per night. A significant positive correlation was found between mean distance run/night and BDNF mRNA in hippocampus and caudal neocortex (Fig. 4A, B) for all running groups. One rat in these studies chose not to run at all. This rat was in the 2-night running group shown in Fig. 4A. The BDNF mRNA measures for this rat were the lowest in that group and are close to the control levels.

We have only begun to examine NGF expression in response to running. Nuclease protection for NGF mRNA revealed significant increases in the hippocampus and the caudal one-third of the cerebral cortex with exercise. Hippocampal NGF mRNA increased to over 130% of control values after 2 nights with exercise. The increase was highest in field CA1, as determined by *in situ* hybridization.

We have demonstrated that a simple behavior, wheel running, can increase the expression of neurotrophic factors. This effect may illustrate one molecular mechanism by which an animal's activities can influence CNS structure and function and may underlie some previously observed forms of activity-dependent CNS plasticity.

IV. Studies on Animals Show That Activity Can Influence Brain Structure and Chemistry

Animal studies support the conclusion that exercise can have a positive effect on the brain. Aerobic training leads to an increase in the density of blood vessels in the cerebellum (molecular layer) in young adult male (Black *et al.*, 1990) and female (Isaacs *et al.*, 1992) rats. This parallels the observation that physical activity prevents declines in cerebral blood flow in aging humans (Rogers *et al.*, 1990). Other evidence from animal studies indicates that the effects of exercise in the brain go beyond the support of cerebral blood flow. In rats, treadmill running produces changes in high-affinity choline uptake

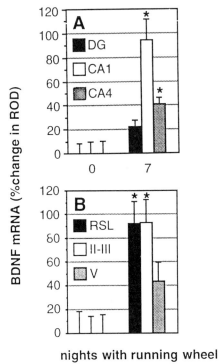

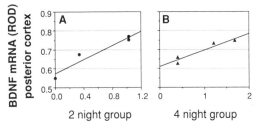

Figure 4. Correlation between BDNF mRNA expression [relative optical density (ROD) measures from nuclease protection assay] and the rats' mean activity levels. Mean distance run per night and BDNF mRNA within the caudal ⅓ of cerebral cortex were significantly correlated in the (A) 2-night ($r = 0.96$, $P = 0.05$) and (B) 4-night ($r = 0.995$, $P = 0.05$) exercise groups. Plots show best-fit linear functions from Cricket Graph 1.3 (Cricket Software, PA).

Figure 3. *In situ* hybridization for BDNF mRNA in specific cell populations in sedentary controls ($n = 6$) and rats allowed 7 ($n = 6$) nights with free access to running wheels. Relative optical density (ROD) values for each target area minus background ROD level (corpus callosum), expressed as percentage change from control values, show (A) a 90% increase in the pyramidal layer of CA1 of the hippocampus after 7 nights, a 40% increase in CA4. The dentate gyrus granular layer (DG) showed an increasing trend which did not reach significance. (B) Layers II–III of the caudal neocortex (ccx II–III) and retrosplenial cortex (RSL) showed significantly increased BDNF mRNA hybridization, which reached 90% elevation over control values after 7 nights. Caudal neocortex layers V–VI (ccx V–VI) showed a nonsignificant increasing trend. ($*P \leq 0.05$)

a marker of cholinergic function, in the hippocampus and parietal cortex and increases muscarinic ACh receptor density relative to sedentary controls (Fordyce & Farrar, 1991a,b). Moreover, daily treadmill running prevents age-related declines in hippocampal muscarinic receptor density (Cartee & Farrar, 1987; Dustman *et al.*, 1990; Fordyce *et al.*, 1991). This is particularly interesting considering the signifi-

cant atrophy and loss of cholinergic function seen with aging and Alzheimer's disease (Sherman *et al.*, 1990). Physical exercise may also support the dopaminergic neurons of the mesencephalon, which are targets of Parkinson's disease. Exercise increases dopamine receptor density in the striatum of adult rats (Gilliam *et al.*, 1984) and attenuates age-related declines in dopamine function (MacRae *et al.*, 1987). Exercise thus has been shown to promote the resilience of vulnerable neuronal systems. These effects on ACh and dopamine neurons are consistent with the actions of neurotrophic factors on these neurons, supporting the hypothesis that neurotrophic factors may be mediating such activity-dependent CNS plasticity.

Observations that regular mental activity, such as puzzle-solving, can support CNS function underscore the role of environment and activity in mental functioning. Rats raised in enriched conditions, which include toys, exercise wheels, and mazes for exploration, perform better on spatial learning tasks as adults than rats raised in impoverished conditions, which generally include housing in smaller, plain cages (Escorihuela *et al.*, 1994; Falkenberg *et al.*, 1992; Mohammed *et al.*, 1990; Murtha *et al.*, 1990; Nilsson *et al.*, 1993; Park *et al.*, 1992; Ryan & Pappas, 1990). Exposure to enriched conditions following brain injury (lesion, ectopia, or prenatal ethanol or monosodium glutamate exposure) also appears to increase compensation for damage, as demonstrated by enhanced performance on learning and motor tasks (Fisher *et al.*, 1991; Hannigan *et al.*, 1993; Rose *et al.*, 1993; Schrott *et al.*, 1992). The behavioral effects of environmental enrichment are complemented by physical changes in the brain. Rats exposed to enriched conditions for 30 days show increases in the thickness of the occipital and frontal cortices relative to rats kept in impoverished conditions (Diamond *et al.*, 1987). Enrichment produces synaptogenesis, angiogenesis, and increased dendritic branching in the visual cortex (Black *et al.*, 1990; Greenough *et al.*, 1985; Greenough & Volkmar, 1973; Volkmar & Greenough, 1972). This type of environmentally induced plasticity has been seen in humans. Educational level has been correlated with length and branching of dendrites within areas of the cerebral cortex associated with language in men and women (Jacobs *et al.*, 1993). These effects are consistent with the actions of neurotrophic factors.

The aging brain also responds to environmental enrichment. Aging rats (aged 25–30 months) housed in enriched conditions for 138 days showed a 4–10% increase in the thickness of the occipital and frontal cortices relative to rats housed in plain cages (Diamond *et al.*, 1985). However, enriched-condition-induced increases in cortical thickness and angiogenesis in the rat visual cortex have been shown to be considerably reduced in aged (24 month) relative to young adult animals (Black *et al.*, 1989). The data indicate that activity-dependent plasticity is present, but perhaps decreased, in the aging brain. It is conceivable that the decrease in spontaneous activity level as rats age (unpublished observations) may contribute to the decreased production of neurotrophic factors and age-related decreases in brain plasticity.

We suggest that the ability of behavioral activity to regulate neurotrophic factors may underlie much of the inherent, activity-dependent plasticity in the brain. This is supported by the observation that young adult rats exposed to an enriched environment for 30 days express more NGF protein and NGF1A mRNA in the hippocampus than rats housed in plain cages (Mohammed *et al.*, 1993). As discussed earlier, exercise can increase neurotrophin levels in the adult rat brain in 2–7 days (Neeper *et al.*, 1995). It remains to be shown whether these effects can be induced in the aging brain, but the evidence of other activity-dependent changes present in both the young adult and aging rat brain gives reason to believe that it is possible. The evidence that neurotrophic factors not only support neuronal growth and sprouting but also increase survival and resilience to withstand insult suggests that activity-dependent increases in brain neurotrophic factors could be of considerable benefit to the health of the aging brain.

V. Increases in Neurotrophic Factors May Stimulate Neural Growth

The ability of activity to regulate neurotrophic factors may stimulate the regenerative capacity of the brain after cell loss. Neurotrophic factors are one of the fundamental mechanisms that regulate growth or sprouting after injury (Cotman *et al.*, 1994). Since growth factors stimulate neuronal growth, higher levels driven by activity-dependent mechanisms should enhance reactive sprouting and the richness of connectivity as the brain ages. As a function of aging, some brain regions show very minor neuronal losses, whereas others show major losses. Despite these neuronal losses, however, the functional capacity of central nervous system circuits may be better preserved than might be predicted from cell loss alone. It has been suggested that the loss of neurons triggers the surviving cells to sprout and replace lost connections. This view is consistent with studies of reactive synaptogenesis in the injured aged brain (Cotman & Anderson, 1988). In brain regions that show partial neuronal loss, dendritic arbors actually continue to grow between middle and old age (Coleman & Flood, 1986). Surviving neurons increase their dendritic branching to fill in the area vacated by the dead neuron. Astrocytes may increase their production of growth-promoting agents as they become reactive. Thus, during aging, compensatory mechanisms of growth and remodeling, such as dendritic hypertrophy and synaptic growth, may be part of the lifelong program to maintain and adapt brain function. Only in very old age does the dendritic tree in humans appear to regress to that of mature younger adults (Coleman & Flood, 1986). Perhaps certain types of behavioral activities can help to offset declines in dendritic branching.

VI. Conclusion

As discussed in this chapter, activity-dependent plasticity mechanisms may play a central role in the achievement of successful aging. For example, exercise, a behavior known to be beneficial to health, could increase the expression of key neurotrophic factors, molecules known to be beneficial to neurons. This enhancement in neurotrophic factors requires only a few days and occurs in some of the brain areas serving higher cognitive function, for example, the hippocampus. Thus the exercise-dependent increase in these factors may provide a fundamental molecular mechanism for use-dependent changes in cellular structure of the brain, such as those that have been previously described for animals placed in enriched environments.

It is possible that activity-dependent changes in neurotrophic factors and other plasticity-related molecules may provide common mechanisms for the effects of diverse types of physical and mental activity on the maintenance of brain function with aging. For example, as discussed earlier in this chapter, a certain level of strenuous physical activity appears to correlate with the maintenance of high cognitive function in healthy elderly people. Perhaps more neurotrophic factors are produced in the brains of active individuals, preserving brain function. Exercise is of course not the only type of behavioral stimulation that can in principle benefit the brain. Other types of behavior or behavioral combinations including learning or learning and physical activity can protect and strengthen participating brain cells.

On the basis of our findings and those of others in the field, we suggest that some types of behaviors selectively reward the neurons serving those behaviors. Such a theory is in line with the current concepts of the activity-dependent control of neurotrophic factors and brain plasticity. As discussed previously in this chapter, it is now clear that neurotrophic factor expression is controlled by the level and type of synaptic activity. When neurotrophic factors such as BDNF are produced and released from neurons, they can act back on the same neurons through their receptors (via autocrine mechanisms) and/or act on nearby neurons also expressing these receptors (via paracrine mechanisms). With the increased level of particular factors the affected neurons may be more competitive in terms of growth potential, metabolic functions, and thus their ability to remain healthy and resilient (Fig. 5A). In this way any specific behavior accessing growth factor regulatory mechanisms could contribute to brain health and in turn reinforce the capacity to perform that specific behavior. In other words, particular behaviors (e.g., exercise) strengthen neurons by increasing the expression of neurotrophic factors or other plasticity-related mole-

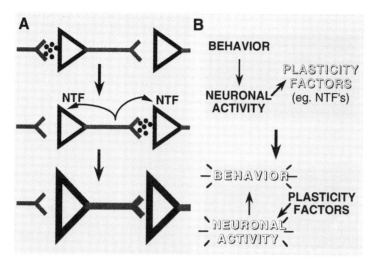

Figure 5. (A) Excitatory stimulation of a neuron causes it to increase production of neurotrophic factors (NTF), which in turn enhance neuronal growth, function, and viability. (B) A behavior increases the activity of specific neurons, inducing production of factors that mediate activity-dependent plasticity. These plasticity factors strengthen the activated neural pathways, improving the vitality of the behavioral system that activated them.

cules. In turn, stronger, healthier neurons strengthen the behavior(s) they serve (Fig. 5B). In the context of successful aging these data highlight the fundamental need to maintain and perhaps even increase brain stimulation in aging. Further studies using animal models will help refine the exact conditions that maximize access to the growth factor expression mechanisms and thereby aid in the prediction and rationale of new interventions for successful aging.

References

Alderson, R. F., Alterman, A. L., Barde, Y. A., & Lindsay, R. M. (1990). Brain-derived neurotrophic factor increases survival and differentiated functions of rat septal cholinergic neurons in culture. *Neuron, 5,* 297–306.

Altar, C. A., Boylan, C. B., Jackson, C., Hershenson, S., Miller, J., Wiegand, S. J., Lindsay, R. M., & Hyman, C. (1992). Brain-derived neurotrophic factor augments rotational behavior and nigrostriatal dopamine turnover in vivo. *Proceedings of the National Academy of Sciences of the United States of America, 89,* 11347–51.

Anderson, K. J., Dam, D., Lee, S., & Cotman, C. W. (1988). Basic fibroblast growth factor prevents death of lesioned cholinergic neurons in vivo. *Nature, 332,* 360–1.

Ayer, L. C., Olson, L., Ebendal, T., Seiger, A., & Persson, H. (1988). Expression of the beta-nerve growth factor gene in hippocampal neurons. *Science, 240,* 1339–41.

Berkman, L. F., Seeman, T. E., Albert, M., Blazer, D., Kahn, R., Mohs, R., Finch, C., Schneider, E., Cotman, C., McClearn, G., *et al.* (1993). High, usual and impaired functioning in community-dwelling older men and women: findings from the MacArthur Foundation Research Network on Successful Aging. *Journal of Clinical Epidemiology, 46,* 1129–40.

Black, J. E., Polinsky, M., & Greenough, W. T. (1989). Progressive failure of cerebral angiogenesis supporting neural plasticity in aging rats. *Neurobiology of Aging, 10,* 353–8.

Black, J. E., Isaacs, K. R., Anderson, B. J., Alcantara, A. A., & Greenough, W. T. (1990). Learning causes synaptogenesis, whereas motor activity causes angiogenesis, in cerebellar cortex of adult rats. *Proceedings of the National Academy of Sciences of the United States of America, 87,* 5568–72.

Blomquist, K. B., & Danner, F. (1987). Effects of physical conditioning on information-processing efficiency. *Perception and Motor Skills, 65,* 175–86.

Blumenthal, J. A., & Madden, D. J. (1988). Effects of aerobic exercise training, age, and physical fitness on memory-search performance. *Psychology of Aging, 3,* 280–5.

Blumenthal, J. A., Emery, C. F., Madden, D. J., Schniebolk, S., Walsh, R. M., George, L. K., McKee, D. C., Higginbotham, M. B., Cobb, F. R., & Coleman, R. E. (1991). Long-term effects of exercise on psychological functioning in older men and women. *Journal of Gerontology, 46,* P352–61.

Boatell, L. L., Lindefors, N., Ballarin, M., Ernfors, P., Mahy, N., & Persson, H. (1992). Activation of basal forebrain cholinergic neurons differentially regulates brain-derived neurotrophic factor mRNA expression in different projection areas. *Neuroscience Letters, 136,* 203–8.

Buttke, T. M., & Sandstrom, P. A. (1994). Oxidative stress as a mediator of apoptosis. *Immunology Today, 15,* 7–10.

Cartee, G. D., & Farrar, R. P. (1987). Muscle respiratory capacity and VO2 max in identically trained young and old rats. *Journal of Applied Physiology, 63,* 257–61.

Castren, E., Zafra, F., Thoenen, H., & Lindholm, D. (1992). Light regulates expression of brain-derived neurotrophic factor mRNA in rat visual cortex. *Proceedings of the National Academy of Sciences of the United States of America, 89,* 9444–8.

Castren, E., Pitkanen, M., Sirvio, J., Parsadanian, A., Lindholm, D., Thoencn, H., & Riekkinen, P. J. (1993). The induction of LTP increases BDNF and NGF mRNA but decreases NT-3 mRNA in the dentate gyrus. *Neuroreport, 4,* 895–8.

Chen, H. H., Chien, C. H., & Liu, H. M. (1994). Correlation between angiogenesis and basic fibroblast growth factor expression in experimental brain infarct. *Stroke, 25,* 1651–7.

Cheng, B., & Mattson, M. P. (1991). NGF and bFGF protect rat hippocampal and human cortical neurons against hypoglycemic dam-

age by stabilizing calcium homeostasis. *Neuron, 7,* 1031–41.

Clarkson-Smith, L., & Hartley, A. A. (1989). Relationships between physical exercise and cognitive abilities in older adults. *Psychology of Aging, 4,* 183–9.

Coleman, P. D., & Flood, D. G. (1986). Dendritic proliferation in the aging brain as a compensatory repair mechanism. *Progress in Brain Research, 70,* 227–37.

Cosi, C., Spoerri, P. E., Comelli, M. C., Guidolin, D., & Skaper, S. D. (1993). Glucocorticoids depress activity-dependent expression of BDNF mRNA in hippocampal neurons. *Neuroreport, 4,* 527–30.

Cotman, C. W. (1994). Report of Alzheimer's Disease Working Group A. *Neurobiology of Aging, 15,* S17–S22.

Cotman, C. W., & Anderson, K. J. (1988). Synaptic plasticity and functional stabilization in the hippocampal formation: possible role in Alzheimer's disease. *Advances in Neurology, 47,* 313–35.

Cotman, C. W., Gomez-Pinilla, F., & Kahle, J. S. (1994). Neural Plasticity and Regeneration. In G. J. Siegel, B. W. Agranoff, R. W. Albers, & P. B. Molinoff (Eds.), *Basic Neurochemistry: Molecular, Cellular, and Medical Aspects* (pp. 607–626). New York: Raven Press.

Crumrine, R. C., Thomas, A. L., & Morgan, P. F. (1994). Attenuation of p53 expression protects against focal ischemic damage in transgenic mice. *Journal of Cerebral Blood Flow Metabolism, 14,* 887–91.

Cummings, B. J., Yee, G. J., & Cotman, C. W. (1992). bFGF promotes the survival of entorhinal layer II neurons after perforant path axotomy. *Brain Research, 591,* 271–6.

de la Torre, J. C., Fortin, T., Park, G. A., Butler, K. S., Kozlowski, P., Pappas, B. A., de, S. H., Saunders, J. K., & Richard, M. T. (1992). Chronic cerebrovascular insufficiency induces dementia-like deficits in aged rats. *Brain Research, 582,* 186–95.

Diamond, M. C., Johnson, R. E., Protti, A. M., Ott, C., & Kajisa, L. (1985). Plasticity in the 904-day-old male rat cerebral cortex. *Experimental Neurology, 87,* 309–17.

Diamond, M. C., Greer, E. R., York, A., Lewis, D., Barton, T., & Lin, J. (1987). Rat cortical morphology following crowded-enriched living conditions. *Experimental Neurology, 96,* 241–7.

DiStefano, P. S., Friedman, B., Radziejewski, C., Alexander, C., Boland, P., Schick, C. M., Lindsay, R. M., & Wiegand, S. J. (1992). The neurotrophins BDNF, NT-3, and NGF display distinct patterns of retrograde axonal transport in peripheral and central neurons. *Neuron, 8,* 983–93.

Dustman, R. E., Emmerson, R. Y., Ruhling, R. O., Shearer, D. E., Steinhaus, L. A., Johnson, S. C., Bonekat, H. W., & Shigeoka, J. W. (1990). Age and fitness effects on EEG, ERPs, visual sensitivity, and cognition. *Neurobiology of Aging, 11,* 193–200.

Emmerson, R. Y., Dustman, R. E., Shearer, D. E., & Turner, C. W. (1989). P3 latency and symbol digit performance correlations in aging. *Experiments in Aging Research, 15,* 151–9.

Ernfors, P., Wetmore, C., Olson, L., & Persson, H. (1990). Identification of cells in rat brain and peripheral tissues expressing mRNA for members of the nerve growth factor family. *Neuron, 5,* 511–26.

Escorihuela, R. M., Tobena, A., & Fernandez, T. A. (1994). Environmental enrichment reverses the detrimental action of early inconsistent stimulation and increases the beneficial effects of postnatal handling on shuttlebox learning in adult rats. *Behavioral Brain Research, 61,* 169–73.

Falkenberg, T., Mohammed, A. K., Henriksson, B., Persson, H., Winblad, B., & Lindefors, N. (1992). Increased expression of brain-derived neurotrophic factor mRNA in rat hippocampus is associated with improved spatial memory and enriched environment. *Neuroscience Letters, 138,* 153–6.

Fischer, W., Wictorin, K., Bjorklund, A., Williams, L. R., Varon, S., & Gage, F. H. (1987). Amelioration of cholinergic neuron atrophy and spatial memory impairment in aged rats by nerve growth factor. *Nature, 329,* 65–8.

Fischer, W., Bjorklund, A., Chen, K., & Gage, F. H. (1991). NGF improves spatial memory in aged rodents as a function of age. *Journal of Neuroscience, 11,* 1889–906.

Fisher, K. N., Turner, R. A., Pineault, G., Kleim, J., & Saari, M. J. (1991). The postweaning housing environment determines expression of learning deficit associated with neonatal monosodium glutamate (M.S.G.). *Neurotoxicology and Teratology, 13,* 507–13.

Floyd, R. A., & Carney, J. M. (1992). Free radical damage to protein and DNA: mechanisms involved and relevant observations on brain undergoing oxidative stress. *Annals of Neurology,* S22–7.

Follesa, P., & Mocchetti, I. (1993). Regulation of basic fibroblast growth factor and nerve growth factor mRNA by beta-adrenergic receptor activation and adrenal steroids in rat central nervous system. *Molecular Pharmacology, 43,* 132–8.

Follesa, P., Gale, K., & Mocchetti, I. (1994). Regional and temporal pattern of expression of nerve growth factor and basic fibroblast growth factor mRNA in rat brain following electroconvulsive shock. *Experimental Neurology, 127,* 37–44.

Fordyce, D. E., & Farrar, R. P. (1991a). Enhancement of spatial learning in F344 rats by physical activity and related learning-associated alterations in hippocampal and cortical cholinergic functioning. *Behavioral Brain Research, 46,* 123–33.

Fordyce, D. E., & Farrar, R. P. (1991b). Physical activity effects on hippocampal and parietal cortical cholinergic function and spatial learning in F344 rats. *Behavior and Brain Research, 43,* 115–23.

Fordyce, D. E., Starnes, J. W., & Farrar, R. P. (1991). Compensation of the age-related decline in hippocampal muscarinic receptor density through daily exercise or underfeeding. *Journal of Gerontology, 46,* B245–8.

Forloni, G., Chiesa, R., Smiroldo, S., Verga, L., Salmona, M., Tagliavini, F., & Angeretti, N. (1993). Apoptosis mediated neurotoxicity induced by chronic application of beta amyloid fragment 25–35. *Neuroreport, 4,* 523–6.

Gall, C. M., & Isackson, P. J. (1989). Limbic seizures increase neuronal production of messenger RNA for nerve growth factor. *Science, 245,* 758–61.

Gall, C., Murray, K., & Isackson, P. J. (1991). Kainic acid-induced seizures stimulate increased expression of nerve growth factor mRNA in rat hippocampus. *Brain Research: Molecular Brain Research, 9,* 113–23.

Gall, C. M., Berschauer, R., & Isackson, P. J. (1994). Seizures increase basic fibroblast growth factor mRNA in adult rat forebrain neurons and glia. *Brain Research: Molecular Brain Research, 21*, 190–205.

Ghosh, A., Carnahan, J., & Greenberg, M. (1994). Requirement for BDNF in activity-dependent survival of cortical neurons. *Science, 263*, 1618–1623.

Gilliam, P. E., Spirduso, W. W., Martin, T. P., Walters, T. J., Wilcox, R. E., & Farrar, R. P. (1984). The effects of exercise training on [³H]-spiperone binding in rat striatum. *Pharmacology, Biochemistry and Behavior, 20*, 863–7.

Gleser, J., & Mendelberg, H. (1990). Exercise and sport in mental health: a review of the literature. *Psychiatry and Related Sciences, 27*, 99–112.

Goldstein, S., & Reivich, M. (1991). Cerebral blood flow and metabolism in aging and dementia. *Clinical Neuropharmacology* S34–44.

Gomez-Pinilla, F., Cotman, C. W., & Nieto-Sampedro, M. (1989). NGF receptor immunoreactivity in aged rat brain. *Brain Research, 479*, 255–262.

Greenough, W. T., & Volkmar, F. (1973). Pattern of dendritic branching in occipital cortex of rats reared in complex environments. *Experimental Neurology, 40*, 491–504.

Greenough, W. T., Hwang, H. M. F., & Gorman, C. (1985). Evidence for active synapse formation or altered postsynaptic metabolism in visual cortex of rats reared in complex environments. *Proceedings of the National Academy of Sciences of the United States of America, 82*, 4549–4552.

Hannigan, J. H., Berman, R. F., & Zajac, C. S. (1993). Environmental enrichment and the behavioral effects of prenatal exposure to alcohol in rats. *Neurotoxicology and Teratology, 15*, 261–6.

Hefti, F., & Will, B. (1987). Nerve growth factor is a neurotrophic factor for forebrain cholinergic neurons; implications for Alzheimer's disease. *Journal of Neural Transmitters, Supplement, 24*, 309–15.

Hill, R. D., Storandt, M., & Malley, M. (1993). The impact of long-term exercise training on psychological function in older adults. *Journal of Gerontology, 48*, P12–7.

Isaacs, K. R., Anderson, B. J., Alcantara, A. A., Black, J. E., & Greenough, W. T. (1992). Exercise and the brain: angiogenesis in the adult rat cerebellum after vigorous physical activity and motor skill learning [published erratum appears in *J. Cereb. Blood Flow Metab.* (1992) *12*(3), 533]. *Journal of Cerebral Blood Flow Metabolism, 12*, 110–9.

Isackson, P. J., Huntsman, M. M., Murray, K. D., & Gall, C. M. (1991). BDNF mRNA expression is increased in adult rat forebrain after limbic seizures: temporal patterns of induction distinct from NGF. *Neuron, 6*, 937–48.

Jackson, G. R., Apffel, L., Werrbach, P. K., & Perez, P. J. (1990). Role of nerve growth factor in oxidant-antioxidant balance and neuronal injury. I. Stimulation of hydrogen peroxide resistance. *Journal of Neuroscience Research, 25*, 360–8.

Jacobs, B., Schall, M., & Scheibel, A. B. (1993). A quantitative dendritic analysis of Wernicke's area in humans. II. Gender, hemisperic, and environmental factors. *Journal of Comparative Neurology, 327*, 97–111.

Kawamura, J., Meyer, J. S., Terayama, Y., & Weathers, S. (1991). Cerebral hypoperfusion correlates with mild and parenchymal loss with severe multi-infarct dementia. *Journal of Neurological Science, 102*, 32–8.

Kokaia, Z., Gido, G., Ringstedt, T., Bengzon, J., Kokaia, M., Siesjo, B. K., Persson, H., & Lindvall, O. (1993). Rapid increase of BDNF mRNA levels in cortical neurons following spreading depression: regulation by glutamatergic mechanisms independent of seizure activity. *Brain Research: Molecular Brain Research, 19*, 277–86.

Kondo, S., Yin, D., Aoki, T., Takahashi, J. A., Morimura, T., & Takeuchi, J. (1994). bcl-2 gene prevents apoptosis of basic fibroblast growth factor-deprived murine aortic endothelial cells. *Experiments in Cell Research, 213*, 428–32.

Labbe, E. E., Welsh, M. C., & Delaney, D. (1988). Effects of consistent aerobic exercise on the psychological functioning of women. *Perception and Motor Skills, 67*, 919–25.

Lapchak, P. A., Araujo, D. M., & Hefti, F. (1993). Cholinergic regulation of hippocampal brain-derived neurotrophic factor mRNA expression: evidence from lesion and chronic cholinergic drug treatment studies. *Neuroscience, 52*, 575–85.

Larkfors, L., Ebendal, T., Whittemore, S. R., Persson, H., Hoffer, B., & Olson, L. (1987). Decreased level of nerve growth factor (NGF) and its messenger RNA in the aged rat brain. *Brain Research, 427,* 55–60.

Larkfors, L., Ebendal, T., Whittemore, S. R., Persson, H., Hoffer, B., & Olson, L. (1988). Developmental appearance of nerve growth factor in the rat brain: significant deficits in the aged forebrain. *Progress in Brain Research, 78,* 27–31.

Lichtman, S., & Poser, E. G. (1983). The effects of exercise on mood and cognitive functioning. *Journal of Psychosomatic Research, 27,* 43–52.

Linnik, M. D., Zobrist, R. H., & Hatfield, M. D. (1993). Evidence supporting a role for programmed cell death in focal cerebral ischemia in rats. *Stroke, 24,* 2002–9.

Lupinacci, N. S., Rakli, R. E., Jones, C. J., & Ross, D. (1993). Age and physical activity effects on reaction time and digit symbol substitution performance in cognitively active adults. *Research Quarterly: Exercise and Sport, 64,* 144–50.

MacRae, P. G., Spirduso, W. W., Walters, T. J., Farrar, R. P., & Wilcox, R. E. (1987). Endurance training effects on striatal D2 dopamine receptor binding and striatal dopamine metabolites in presenescent older rats. *Psychopharmacology (Berlin), 92,* 236–40.

Madden, D. J., Blumenthal, J. A., Allen, P. A., & Emery, C. F. (1989). Improving aerobic capacity in healthy older adults does not necessarily lead to improved cognitive performance. *Psychology of Aging, 4,* 307–20.

Markowska, A. L., Koliatsos, V. E., Breckler, S. J., Price, D. L., & Olton, D. S. (1994). Human nerve growth factor improves spatial memory in aged but not in young rats. *Journal of Neuroscience, 14,* 4815–24.

Mattson, M. P. (1994). Mechanism of neuronal degeneration and preventative approaches: quickening the pace of AD research. *Neurobiology of Aging, 15,* S121–S125.

Mattson, M. P., Murrain, M., Guthrie, P. B., & Kater, S. B. (1989). Fibroblast growth factor and glutamate: opposing roles in the generation and degeneration of hippocampal neuroarchitecture. *Journal of Neuroscience, 9,* 3728–40.

Mattson, M. P., Rydel, R. E., Lieberburg, I., &

Smith, S. V. (1993). Altered calcium signaling and neuronal injury: stroke and Alzheimer's disease as examples. *Annals of the New York Academy of Science, 679,* 1–21.

Mocchetti, I., & Isackson, P. (1994). Induction of NGF and bFGF by glucocorticoids in brain. *Proceedings of the 25th ASN Meeting, 62* (Suppl.), S13.

Mohammed, A. K., Winblad, B., Ebendal, T., & Larkfors, L. (1990). Environmental influence on behaviour and nerve growth factor in the brain. *Brain Research, 528,* 62–72.

Mohammed, A. H., Henriksson, B. G., Soderstrom, S., Ebendal, T., Olsson, T., & Seckl, J. R. (1993). Environmental influences on the central nervous system and their implications for the aging rat. *Behavior and Brain Research, 57,* 183–91.

Molloy, D. W., Richardson, L. D., & Crilly, R. G. (1988). The effects of a three-month exercise programme on neuropsychological function in elderly institutionalized women: a randomized controlled trial. *Age and Ageing, 17,* 303–10.

Morse, J. K., Wiegand, S. J., Anderson, K., You, Y., Cai, N., Carnahan, J., Miller, J., DiStefano, P. S., Altar, C. A., Lindsay, R. M., *et al.,* (1993). Brain-derived neurotrophic factor (BDNF) prevents the degeneration of medial septal cholinergic neurons following fimbria transection. *Journal of Neuroscience, 13,* 4146–56.

Murtha, S., Pappas, B. A., & Raman, S. (1990). Neonatal and adult forebrain norepinephrine depletion and the behavioral and cortical thickening effects of enriched/impoverished environment. *Behavior and Brain Research, 39,* 249–61.

Neeper, S. A., Gómez-Pinilla, F., Choi, J., & Cotman, C. W. (1995). Exercise and brain neurotrophins. *Nature, 373,* 109.

Nilsson, L., Mohammed, A. K., Henriksson, B. G., Folkesson, R., Winblad, B., & Bergstrom, L. (1993). Environmental influence on somatostatin levels and gene expression in the rat brain. *Brain Research, 628,* 93–8.

Nishizuka, M., Katoh, S. R., Eto, K., Arai, Y., Iizuka, R., & Kato, K. (1991). Age- and sexrelated differences in the nerve growth factor distribution in the rat brain. *Brain Research Bulletin, 27,* 685–8.

Nistico, G., Ciriolo, M. R., Fiskin, K., Iannone,

M., De, M. A., & Rotilio, G. (1992). NGF restores decrease in catalase activity and increases superoxide dismutase and glutathione peroxidase activity in the brain of aged rats. *Free Radical Biology and Medicine*, 12, 177–81.

Nonomura, T., & Hatanaka, H. (1992). Neurotrophic effect of brain-derived neurotrophic factor on basal forebrain cholinergic neurons in culture from postnatal rats. *Neuroscience Research (New York)*, 14, 226–33.

Okazawa, H., Murata, M., Watanabe, M., Kamei, M., & Kanazawa, I. (1992). Dopaminergic stimulation up-regulates the in vivo expression of brain-derived neurotrophic factor (BDNF) in the striatum. *FEBS Letters*, 313, 138–42.

Oliver, C. N., Starke, R. P., Stadtman, E. R., Liu, G. J., Carney, J. M., & Floyd, R. A. (1990). Oxidative damage to brain proteins, loss of glutamine synthetase activity, and production of free radicals during ischemia/reperfusion-induced injury to gerbil brain. *Proceedings of the National Academy of Sciences of the United States of America*, 87, 5144–7.

Oppenheim, R. W., Yin, Q. W., Prevette, D., & Yan, Q. (1992). Brain-derived neurotrophic factor rescues developing avian motoneurons from cell death. *Nature*, 360, 755–7.

Park, G. A., Pappas, B. A., Murtha, S. M., & Ally, A. (1992). Enriched environment primes forebrain choline acetyltransferase activity to respond to learning experience. *Neuroscience Letters*, 143, 259–62.

Pechan, P., Cizkova, D., Murgacova, M., & Malatova, Z. (1991). Effect of nerve growth factor on lesioned PC12 cells. *Cell Biology International Reports*, 15, 527–35.

Phillips, H. S., Hains, J. M., Laramee, G. R., Rosenthal, A., & Winslow, J. W. (1990). Widespread expression of BDNF but not NT3 by target areas of basal forebrain cholinergic neurons. *Science*, 250, 290–4.

Puumala, M., Anderson, R. E., & Meyer, F. B. (1990). Intraventricular infusion of HBGF-2 promotes cerebral angiogenesis in Wistar rat. *Brain Research*, 534, 283–6.

Rich, K. M. (1992). Neuronal death after trophic factor deprivation. *Journal of Neurotrauma*, S61–9.

Richter, C. (1993). Pro-oxidants and mitochondrial Ca^{2+}: their relationship to apoptosis and oncogenesis. *FEBS Letters*, 325, 104–7.

Riva, M. A., Gale, K., & Mocchetti, I. (1992). Basic fibroblast growth factor mRNA increases in specific brain regions following convulsive seizures. *Brain Research: Molecular Brain Research*, 15, 311–8.

Rogers, R. L., Meyer, J. S., & Mortel, K. F. (1990). After reaching retirement age physical activity sustains cerebral perfusion and cognition. *Journal of the American Geriatric Society*, 38, 123–8.

Rose, F. D., Al, K. K., Davey, M. J., & Attree, E. A. (1993). Environmental enrichment following brain damage: an aid to recovery or compensation? *Behavior and Brain Research*, 56, 93–100.

Ryan, C. L., & Pappas, B. A. (1990). Prenatal exposure to antiadrenergic antihypertensive drugs: effects on neurobehavioral development and the behavioral consequences of enriched rearing. *Neurotoxicology and Teratology*, 12, 359–66.

Sampath, D., Jackson, G. R., Werrbach, P. K., & Perez, P. J. (1994). Effects of nerve growth factor on glutathione peroxidase and catalase in PC12 cells. *Journal of Neurochemistry*, 62, 2476–9.

Sauer, H., Fischer, W., Nikkhah, G., Wiegand, S. J., Brundin, P., Lindsay, R. M., & Bjorklund, A. (1993). Brain-derived neurotrophic factor enhances function rather than survival of intrastriatal dopamine cell-rich grafts. *Brain Research*, 626, 37–44.

Schroll, M., Steen, B., Berg, S., Heikkinen, E., & Viidik, A. (1993). NORA—Nordic research on ageing. Functional capacity of 75-year-old men and women in three Nordic localities. *Danish Medical Bulletin*, 40, 618–24.

Schrott, L. M., Denenberg, V. H., Sherman, G. F., Waters, N. S., Rosen, G. D., & Galaburda, A. M. (1992). Environmental enrichment, neocortical ectopias, and behavior in the autoimmune NZB mouse. *Brain Research: Developments in Brain Research*, 67, 85–93.

Scott, S. A., Liang, S., Weingartner, J. A., & Crutcher, K. A. (1994). Increased NGF-like activity in young but not aged rat hippocampus after septal lesions. *Neurobiology of Aging*, 15, 337–46.

Sherman, K. A., & Friedman, E. (1990). Pre- and post-synaptic cholinergic dysfunction in aged rodent brain regions: new findings and an interpretive review. *International Journal of Developments in Neuroscience, 8,* 689–708.

Simons, C. W., & Birkimer, J. C. (1988). An exploration of factors predicting the effects of aerobic conditioning on mood state. *Journal of Psychosomatic Research, 32,* 63–75.

Smith, C. D., Carney, J. M., Starke, R. P., Oliver, C. N., Stadtman, E. R., Floyd, R. A., & Markesbery, W. R. (1991). Excess brain protein oxidation and enzyme dysfunction in normal aging and in Alzheimer disease. *Proceedings of the National Academy of Sciences of the United States of America, 88,* 10540–3.

Spina, M. B., Squinto, S. P., Miller, J., Lindsay, R. M., & Hyman, C. (1992). Brain-derived neurotrophic factor protects dopamine neurons against 6-hydroxydopamine and *N*-methyl-4-phenylpyridinium ion toxicity: involvement of the glutathione system [see comments]. *Journal of Neurochemistry, 59,* 99–106.

Valliant, P. M., & Asu, M. E. (1985). Exercise and its effects on cognition and physiology in older adults. *Perception and Motor Skills,* 1031–8.

Van Der Wal, E. A., Gomez-Pinilla, F., & Cotman, C. W. (1994). Seizure-associated induction of basic fibroblast growth factor and its receptor in the rat brain. *Neuroscience, 60,* 311–323.

Volkmar, F. R., & Greenough, W. T. (1972). Rearing complexity affects branching of dendrites in the visual cortex of the rat. *Science, 176,* 1145–7.

Widmer, H. R., Knusel, B., & Hefti, F. (1993). BDNF protection of basal forebrain cholinergic neurons after axotomy: complete protection of p75NGFR-positive cells. *Neuroreport, 4,* 363–6.

Wyllie, A. H., Kerr, J. F., & Currie, A. R. (1980). Cell death: the significance of apoptosis. *International Reviews in Cytology, 68,* 251–306.

Yakovlev, A. G., De, B. M., Fabrazzo, M., Brooker, G., Costa, E., & Mocchetti, I. (1990). Regulation of nerve growth factor receptor mRNA content by dexamethasone: in vitro and in vivo studies. *Neuroscience Letters, 116,* 216–20.

Young, R. J. (1979). The effect of regular exercise on cognitive functioning and personality. *British Journal of Sports Medicine, 13,* 110–7.

Zafra, F., Hengerer, B., Leibrock, J., Thoenen, H., & Lindholm, D. (1990). Activity dependent regulation of BDNF and NGF mRNAs in the rat hippocampus is mediated by non-NMDA glutamate receptors. *EMBO Journal, 9,* 3545–50.

Zafra, F., Castren, E., Thoenen, H., & Lindholm, D. (1991). Interplay between glutamate and gamma-aminobutyric acid transmitter systems in the physiological regulation of brain-derived neurotrophic factor and nerve growth factor synthesis in hippocampal neurons. *Proceedings of the National Academy of Sciences of the United States of America, 88,* 10037–41.

Zafra, F., Lindholm, D., Castren, E., Hartikka, J., & Thoenen, H. (1992). Regulation of brain-derived neurotrophic factor and nerve growth factor mRNA in primary cultures of hippocampal neurons and astrocytes. *Journal of Neuroscience, 12,* 4793–9.

Fourteen

Changes in Gene Expression during Brain Aging: A Survey

Steven A. Johnson and Caleb E. Finch

I. Introduction

Advancing age is the greatest risk factor for development of the three human neurodegenerative diseases: Alzheimer's (AD), Parkinson's (PD), and Huntington's diseases (HD), of which AD is by far the most common. With the exception of HD, these diseases do not have juvenile forms. HD can be manifested in young adults, but its onset is more typically between 30 and 50 years (Farrer, 1993; Farrer *et al.*, 1993; Finch, 1990). In contrast, PD and AD are very rare in young adults, but show exponential accelerations after age 50 (Bird, 1994; Katzman & Kawas, 1994; Marttila & Rinne, 1981). Unlike HD, there is no indication of a "safe" age at which the risk of PD or AD decreases or disappears.

Exactly how aging becomes the major risk factor for HD, PD, and AD is largely mysterious. This survey of changes in gene expression in the brain during aging is based on the premise that general age-related changes in gene expression in the brain will provide clues as to why familial as well as sporadic neurological diseases of aging increase exponentially. In the past, changes in brain-specific gene expression during "normal" aging have received less

attention than studies of specific diseases. It seems plausible to us that putative age-related changes in gene expression could initiate and promote the course of HD, PD, and AD. Thus, we may seek the initial "erosion" of the foundation upon which homeostasis and resistance to disease is built. Clearly, if we wish to understand the mechanisms underlying age-related brain disease, as well as brain physiology during senescence, we also need to study the brain during "normal" aging.

Before discussing changes in brain-specific gene expression during aging, we outline the gross anatomical and cellular changes that generally occur in the aging brain. We cannot yet assign cause or effect to most changes, such as neuron atrophy, astrocyte and microglia hypertrophy, dendritic regression, and synaptic loss. Each may cause, or be the result of, overall changes in the expression of specific genes.

A. Brain Cell Morphological Changes during Aging

The classic view that large numbers of neurons are lost during normal aging in nondemented individuals (Brody, 1955)

Handbook of the Biology of Aging, Fourth Edition
Copyright © 1996 Academic Press, Inc. All rights of reproduction in any form reserved.

has not been supported by modern studies (Terry, DeTeresa, & Hansen, 1987). Most researchers would now agree that there is little generalized neuron loss with age in the mammalian brain (Coleman & Flood, 1987). However, there are regions of particular vulnerability, such as the hippocampal CA4 field and subiculum (West, 1993).

Instead of neuron loss, neuron atrophy (or hypertrophy) is a common modern finding that may explain the earlier view of substantial cell loss [reviewed by Finch (1993)]. In general, neurons are defined by their larger size compared to glial cells. Thus, when small or medium-sized neurons atrophy, they may be counted as glia; similarly, atrophied large neurons, such as pyramidal neurons, will be counted as small or medium-sized neurons, accounting for earlier views that large neurons were preferentially lost during aging (see Fig. 1). Such issues still invoke controversy and depend to a certain degree on the investigator's ability to discriminate small neurons from glia. Indeed, a study using modern stereological methods claims no global neocortical neuron loss in AD (Regeur, Jensen, Pakkenberg, Evans, & Pakkenberg, 1994). While this result is based on well-accepted stereological principles, the major limitation, stated by the authors themselves, is the "distinction of neurons from glial cells. . . ." Several of the commentaries published with that article point out that global cortical neuron loss may be less important in AD than significant loss in specialized regions, such as the nucleus basalis, locus coeruleus, or hippocampus. The same may be true for aging, as West (1993) has found significant hippocampal neuron loss, but only in the subiculum and the hilus of the dentate gyrus (field CA4), which West speculates are "potential morphological correlates of senescent decline in relational memory" in elderly humans.

Glial cells also change prominently during normal aging. It has long been known that astrocytes hypertrophy during aging, as judged by conventional histological procedures. The morphological changes resemble those of reactive astrocytes found in the brain after injury or acute neurotoxicity (Hansen, Armstrong, & Terry, 1987; Landfield, Rose, Sandles, Wohlstadter, & Lynch, 1977; Vaughn & Peters, 1974). Widespread views hold that there are increased numbers of hypertrophied astrocytes (defined by morphological change and increased GFAP immunoreactivity) with aging. Importantly, the total number of astrocytes (defined by other glial markers, such as S-100β) does not appear to increase (Gordon & Morgan, 1991), which implies that the activation of astrocytes is more important than proliferation during senescence.

Microglia also become increasingly reactive or activated with age (Perry, Matyszak, & Fearn, 1993). Microglia are largely bone marrow-derived cells that may resemble macrophages in morphology and physiology when activated (Perry & Lawson, 1992). Activated microglia/macrophages are intimately associated with amyloid plaques in AD (Itagaki, McGeer, Akiyama, Zhu, & Selkoe, 1989; Styren, Civin, & Rogers, 1990), as are hypertrophic astrocytes (Itagaki *et al.*, 1989). Microglia have the potential for many inflammatory activities, including phagocytosis and the production of reactive oxygen species (Klegeris & McGeer, 1994), which in large amounts can be quite toxic. Thus, they are receiving much attention with respect to the pathological roles of local inflammation during brain disease. By analogy, increased microglial activation may indicate that subtle, but ongoing inflammatory processes are also at work in the aging brain.

B. Dendritic Atrophy and Synapse Loss

The dendritic arbor tends to atrophy during normal aging in many brain regions. While there is species and region

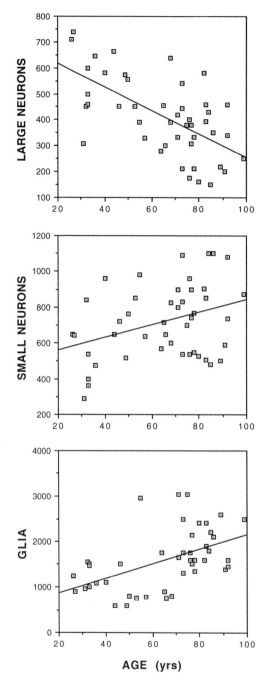

variability, a common finding among several mammals is an increase in dendritic extent during late maturation/early senescence, followed by a larger decrease during later senescence (Coleman & Flood, 1987). Other data showed regression of the dendritic arbor of human hippocampal pyramidal neurons that correlated with neuron soma shrinkage in field CA1c, but not elsewhere (Hanks & Flood, 1991).

Presynaptic terminal density decreases in the normal aged human brain. Masliah et al. (1993) showed a strong negative correlation between frontal cortex synapse density and age ($r = -0.708$, $n = 25$, $p = 0.0001$) (see Fig. 2). There was a 20% loss of synapse density in 13 individuals over 60 years of age (mean age = 76.4 ± 2.6 years) compared with 12 individuals under age 60 (mean age = 39.5 ± 3.6 years). Furthermore, these results were not adjusted for an age-related cortical atrophy of about 15% (Terry et al., 1987), which would result in an even greater loss of synapses. This work confirms earlier studies (Bertoni-Freddari et al., 1989; Gibson, 1983), but also shows that synapse loss does not correlate with diffuse amyloid density, which is determined by immunostaining with antibodies to the Alzheimer amyloid Aβ peptide. An important exception was the finding of further reduced synaptic density in the local area around the few mature plaques found in the aged brains. Hypertrophic astrocytes and activated microglia characteristically surround or invest the mature plaque, and activated microglia are phagocytes that have been reported to "strip" synapses during injury responses (Blinzinger & Kreutzberg, 1968; Streit, Graeber,

Figure 1. The number of large neurons decreases while small neurons and glia increase with aging in human neocortex. Brains from 46 nondemented individuals were included in this study. Neocortical cells in fixed, cresyl violet-stained sections (20 μm thick) were counted with a Quantimet 20 image analysis system. Counts are for a 600-μm wide strip over the full cortical thickness (pia to white matter) in midfrontal cortex. Large neuron (>90 μm²) numbers (top panel) show a strong negative correlation ($r = -0.628$) with aging in the midfrontal cortex (shown) and the superior temporal and inferioral parietal cortices. Small neurons (middle panel) and glia (<40 μm²; bottom panel) increase with aging ($r = 0.33$ and 0.51, respectively). Reprinted with permission of the authors and publisher from Annals of Neurology, 21, 530–539, copyright 1987.

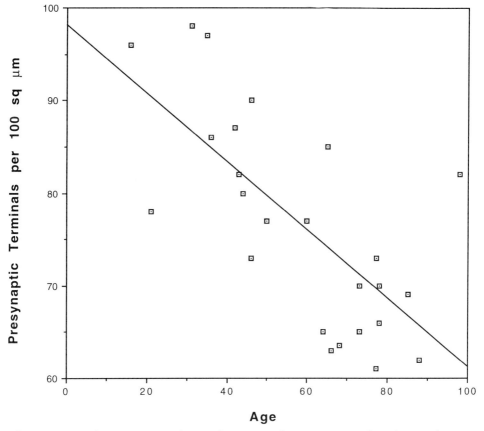

Figure 2. Frontal cortex synapse density decreases with aging. Superior frontal cortex from 25 nondemented individuals 16–98 years old was sectioned (40 μm) and immunostained with anti-synaptophysin antibody. Digitization with a laser confocal microscope allowed the quantitation of synapse density. The number of presynaptic terminals showed a strong negative linear relation ($r = -0.708$) with age. Reprinted with permission of the authors and publisher from *Neurology*, 43, 192–197, copyright 1993.

& Kreutzberg, 1988). While the mechanism for synapse loss during aging and AD is not clear, investigation into the potential role of microglia in this mechanism may prove fruitful.

C. Cerebrovascular Changes during Aging

Vascular changes are evident in the senescent mammalian brain. In a review of this literature, Mooradian (1988) discusses age-related thickening of the vascular basement membrane, loss of capillary endothelial cells, elongation of remaining endothelial cells, and fewer endothelial cell mitochondria (only in rat) in humans, monkeys, and rodents. Histochemically, the cerebral vasculature of all mammals showed increased periodic acid–Schiff reactions for hyalinization (Sobin, Bernick, & Ballard, 1992), which may indicate the presence of glycated or oxidized proteins. There is also an age-related decrease in choline and glucose transport across the blood–brain barrier (BBB), but there is no good evidence for profound age changes in the permeability of the BBB to water-soluble substances or higher molecular weight proteins. Neither [14C]sucrose nor horseradish peroxidase showed increased transit across the aged compared to young

BBB. However, if stressed, e.g., during amphetamine-induced hypertension, the senescent BBB becomes more permeable (Edvinsson, MacKenzie, & McCulloch, 1993), which suggests potential neurological consequences in the hypertensive elderly. There are controversial reports of increased concentrations of circulating brain-reactive antibodies in aging rodents, monkeys, and humans (Felsenfeld & Wolf, 1972; Miller & Blumenthal, 1978); the mechanism is unclear but may not require a defective BBB, since there is evidence that lymphocytes may cross the normal BBB at very low rates that, however, may increase in AD (Rogers, Luber-Narod, Styren, & Civin, 1988; Styren et al., 1990). Thus, most evidence concludes that barrier function is basically intact, while the carrier or transport function of the BBB is somewhat compromised during aging. However, it is still questionable whether any of these changes compromise brain function or engender disease.

Clearly, many of the phenomena we know to be associated with AD, such as reduced brain weight, vascular pathology, cortical atrophy, neuronal atrophy, astrocyte hypertrophy, microglial activation, dendritic atrophy, and synapse loss, are all found during mammalian brain aging, but are greatly accentuated during disease. Furthermore, the anatomical distribution of many of these changes in the aging human brain generally approximates that in the AD brain (Arriagada, Marzloff, & Hyman, 1992). By inference, we hypothesize that aging provides the substrate or precursor for disease. Thus, studies of the molecular changes that accompany/underlie these morphological events of aging may help us understand and perhaps prevent disease.

D. Previous Reviews

This survey is not intended to be a comprehensive review of all aspects of mRNA changes during aging, AD, or other brain diseases. Excellent chapters in previous editions of this Handbook reviewed changes in RNA and protein metabolism with age (Reff, 1985) and changes in gene expression with aging in all cell types of diverse species (Danner & Holbrook, 1990). Similarly, Van Remmen et al. (1995) provide a detailed synopsis of changes in senescence-related gene expression in all tissues, with an emphasis on liver. The present chapter focuses specifically on brain gene expression during aging in mammals.

Gene expression encompasses information transfer from DNA to the functioning protein or catalytic RNA and may be controlled at several strategic points, including transcription, nuclear RNA splicing, mRNA translation, mRNA stability, and RNA editing. Earlier work has addressed several of these processes or control points with respect to aging, leading to general conclusions: (1) RNA synthesis and degradation both decline with age in most tissues, including brain [reviewed in Danner and Holbrook (1990)]. (2) Protein synthesis and degradation also decline with age in most tissues [reviewed by Reff (1985) and updated by Danner and Holbrook (1990)]. (3) The accuracy of information transfer, based on proteins synthesized in young vs old tissues, appears unchanged (Danner & Holbrook, 1990). (4) At least for rat brain, there is no change across the life span (3–32 months) in the mass of polysomal poly(A)mRNA or in the number of different mRNAs that are present in the polysomal poly(A)RNA population. These measurements are based on the nucleotide sequence complexity of polysomal mRNA from whole brain (Colman, Kaplan, Osterburg, & Finch, 1980). The technique of RNA-driven hybridization to single-copy DNA would not resolve changes of less than 10%. Thus, these general conclusions do not rule out major changes in specific mRNAs or proteins, which may play important roles in aging processes.

II. Age-Related Increases of Brain DNA Mutations: New Evidence for Somatic Mutational Theories of Aging

Somatic mutation theories of aging hypothesize that aging is due to an increasing mutational load in somatic cell DNA over time, ultimately resulting in cellular dysfunction [Szilard, 1959; reviewed in Finch (1990)]. For the brain, where neurons are postmitotic and are not replaced if lost, somatic mutation buildup during aging could be more important than in other tissues. This theory has begun to accumulate direct experimental support. We discuss data from studies using brain DNA. The reader is also directed to Chapter 10 in this Handbook for a more in-depth review, as well as to reviews on oxidants and degenerative diseases of aging (Ames *et al.*, 1993), oxidative damage of mitochondrial DNA during aging (Shigenaga *et al.*, 1994), and the hypothesis that defects in DNA repair could be involved in the etiology of AD (Boerrigter, Wei, & Vijg, 1992).

A. Brain DNA Modification

By using human brain nuclear DNA, Randerath and colleagues (Randerath *et al.*, 1993) used a sensitive labeling assay to show a 20-fold increase in "I-spots" over the human life span. I-spots, which are bulky, covalently modified nucleotides that may be expected to affect the fidelity of RNA transcription, were not found in neonatal brain DNA and dramatically increased after the age of 60, although with considerable individual variations that could reflect environmental factors. These modified nucleotides, of which there are several variants, also increased with age in rat brain nuclear DNA. The physiological effects of I-spot accumulation are unknown.

B. Brain DNA Mutation

Evidence that somatic DNA mutations occur in the brain and may increase with age comes from elegant studies on vasopressin gene expression in the Brattleburo rat brain. The homozygous *di/di* Brattleburo rat suffers from severe diabetes insipidus due to a lack of vasopressin (VP), an antidiuretic hormone produced in the hypothalamus. A single base pair deletion in the second exon of the VP gene causes a frameshift mutation (Schmale & Richter, 1984). This mutation blocks intracellular processing and transport and, thus, prevents proper expression and secretion by hypothalamic neurons (Schmale, Borowiak, Holtgreve-Grez, & Richter, 1989). While the neonatal brain has no VP immunopositive hypothalamic neurons, the number of solitary VP immunopositive magnocellular neurons increases progressively from birth onward at the rate of one neuron per week (van Leeuwen, Evans, Meloen, & Sonnemans, 1994). The increase is remarkably linear with age irrespective of gender until about 80 weeks when, in females, the number of solitary VP neurons levels off and may decline at 120 weeks (van Leeuwen *et al.*, 1994) (see Fig. 3). The mechanism causing the decline in old females is unknown, but may be due to the presence of adenohypophyseal tumors (in 11/13 rats) that would exert pressure on and possibly cause cell loss in the hypothalamus.

Solitary VP neurons are heterozygous, expressing both mutant, unprocessed VP precursor and the VP, neurophysin, and glycoprotein products from essentially normal VP processing. New evidence, based on the sequencing of Brattleburo hypothalamic cDNA clones, shows that this age-related "reversion" of the mutant phenotype is primarily due to a 2-base-pair GA deletion, which restores the VP coding sequence reading frame downstream of the deletion (Evans, van der Kleij, Sonnemans, Burbach, & van Leeuwen, 1994).

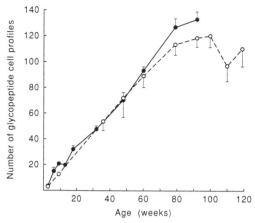

Figure 3. Total number of vasopressin glycopeptide-immunoreactive cell bodies in the hypothalamus of male (solid circle) and female (open circle) homozygous Brattleburo rats at various ages. Note that the linear increase in number declines after 79 weeks of life. Fifty-micrometer vibratome sections were immunostained with vasopressin-associated glycopeptide antiserum. Solitary glycopeptide-immunopositive hypothalamic neurons were counted and increased linearly with age. Reprinted with permission of the authors and publisher from *Brain Research, 635,* 328–330, copyright 1994.

Furthermore, this work shows that the same GA deletion occurs in the VP gene from *wild-type* rats as well. While the mechanism responsible for the GA deletion is unknown, the mutation frequency of the VP gene (10^{-6}/base pair) is several orders of magnitude higher than the overall somatic cell DNA mutation rate (10^{-9}/base pair) and raises the new issue of enhanced genomic instability in neurons vs other somatic cells (Evans *et al.*, 1994).

Accumulating evidence suggests that there is also an increasing mutational load during aging in mitochondrial DNA, which many believe is more likely to have physiological consequences than accumulating somatic nuclear DNA mutations. Mitochondria may be overly sensitive to DNA mutations because of a small genome [only 17 kilobases (kb) in human mitochondria], a paucity of DNA repair functions compared to nuclear DNA, and an environment where reactive oxygen species, such as superoxide and H_2O_2, are byproducts of normal mitochondrial physiology [reviewed in Arnheim and Cortopassi (1992); Luft, 1994]. Oxidative damage to liver mitochondrial DNA is an order of magnitude higher than that in nuclear DNA. Aging results in a further increase in the level of modified mitochondrial DNA bases. In general, all forms of mitochondrial DNA damage that have been examined have been found to accumulate with age (Wallace, 1994).

Besides oxidative damage, brain mitochondrial DNA *deletions* also increase during aging. By using a sensitive polymerase chain reaction (PCR) method, Cortopassi, Arnheim, and colleagues found an age-related *1000-fold* increase in the level of mitochondrial DNAs with a specific 5-kb deletion in select regions of the human brain and in the myocardium. The increase is greatest in tissues with particularly high oxygen consumption (Cortopassi & Arnheim, 1990). This particular deletion (MT 4977) is associated with neuromuscular disease, e.g., Kearnes–Sayre syndrome, and thus could be expected to have deleterious effects on mitochondria in aged human brain. Brain region analyses further showed regional variability, where the highest levels of deletion correlated with high dopamine metabolism and the likely production of oxygen radicals by monoamine oxidase during dopamine breakdown (Soong, Hinton, Cortopassi, & Arnheim, 1992). These authors speculate, in agreement with others (Luft, 1994; Wallace, 1994), that oxidative damage may be a major cause of somatic DNA mutation (whether mitochondrial or nuclear). Cell-type localization of mitochondrial DNA deletions remains an important question, especially with respect to potential roles in age-related neurodegenerative diseases such as AD and PD.

Some evidence suggests that free radical-induced DNA damage may lead directly to neurotoxicity. NMDA receptor activation produces large quantities of the free radical nitric oxide (NO), which mediates neuronal killing (Dawson, Dawson, Bartley, Uhl, & Snyder, 1993) and damages DNA (Wink *et al.*, 1991). Zhang *et al.* (1994) found that NO-damaged DNA greatly induced poly(ADP) ribosylation (PARS) activity in rat brain nuclear extracts and rapidly depleted energy stores (NAD and ATP are consumed during the ADP ribose transfer), which also occurs during neurotoxicity. Inhibitors that block either PARS or NO production by NO synthase prevent NMDA-induced neurotoxicity. Little is known about levels of NO during brain aging.

III. Aging Changes of CNS Disease-Associated Genes

A. Glial Fibrillary Acidic Protein: A Marker of Astrocytosis

Glial fibrillary acidic protein (GFAP), an astrocyte-specific intermediate filament protein, is now recognized as a biomarker of mammalian brain aging because an increase in GFAP has been found in all species examined and is independent of specific pathological changes in the brain or elsewhere in the individual. It is well-known that astrocytes hypertrophy, with an increase in size and fibrous appearance, during aging (Bjorklund, Eriksdotter-Nilsson, Dahl, Rose, & Olson, 1985; Hansen *et al.*, 1987; Vaughn & Peters, 1974) or in response to injury (Mathewson & Berry, 1985) or disease (Beach, Walker, & McGeer, 1989). Astrocyte hypertrophy is accompanied by an accumulation of intermediate filaments, which principally contain GFAP. Despite a large increase in the number of hypertrophied astrocytes after injury (Mathewson & Berry, 1985) or during aging (Hansen *et al.*, 1987; Lindsey, Landfield, & Lynch, 1979), most studies conclude that the total number of astrocytes does not change in either rat (Diamond, Johnson, & Gold, 1977; Gordon &

Morgan, 1991; Landfield, Braun, Pitler, Lindsey, & Lynch, 1981) or human brains (Hansen *et al.*, 1987) during aging. Astrocytes can respond very rapidly to changes in local (or distant!) brain environment, e.g., anesthetization of the cochlear nerve to suppress electrical activity rapidly activates astrocytes that are in contact with distal parts of these axons (Canady & Rubel, 1992). We have seen dramatically increased GFAP immunostaining, the common marker for hypertrophy or activation, less than an hour after acute trauma (S. Johnson, unpublished). Moreover, hypertrophy, as defined by increased radioimmunoassay (RIA)-detectable GFAP protein, may persist for weeks or months after neurotoxin administration (O'Callaghan & Miller, 1988), and during senescence, moderate activation seems to persist indefinitely, suggesting permanent changes in brain homeostasis.

Changes in GFAP mRNA during brain senescence have been documented in mice (Goss, Finch, & Morgan, 1991) and in rats and humans (Nichols, Day, Laping, Johnson, & Finch, 1993). In aging mouse brain, both Northern blot and solution titration hybridization methods showed increased GFAP mRNA in cortex, hippocampus, and cerebellum. Glutamine synthetase (GS), another astrocyte-specific mRNA, did not change in any region, demonstrating the specificity of the GFAP response with age. These data parallel increases in GFAP protein, without concomitant increases in several other proteins, in tissue extracts from six different, aged mouse brain regions, including cortex, hippocampus, and cerebellum (O'Callaghan & Miller, 1991). In this study, the oldest age was 18 months (as compared to 3, 5, and 11 months, where no change was seen), which is too young for true senescence in this mouse strain [C57BL/6J mice have lived for 4.8 years when maintained on mild diet restriction (Harrison & Archer, 1987)], yet significant increases were seen. This suggests that, at least for this strain, GFAP increases may begin during late maturation. On the other hand, these early changes may be related to hormonal phenomena occurring at this developmental stage in female mice, rather than senescence.

In aging male F344 rats, GFAP mRNA in the hippocampus increased between 6 (mature adult) and 24 months (Nichols *et al.*, 1993). Some regional variability was noticed: larger changes were found in the striatum (4-fold) than the hippocampus (2-fold) (see Fig. 4). Most of the change occurred between 15 and 24 months, which suggests that the GFAP mRNA increase is predominantly related to senescence rather than late maturational changes. Again, independent studies of GFAP protein, measured by RIA, show significant increases in six different regions of the senescent (24 months) vs mature (6 months) rat brain (O'Callaghan & Miller, 1991).

Hormonal changes during aging may contribute to changes in GFAP. Corticosterone (CORT) has been shown to be a negative regulator of GFAP transcription (Laping, Nichols, Day, Johnson, & Finch,

1994b) and mRNA prevalence (Nichols, Osterburg, Masters, Millar, & Finch, 1990). However, circulating a.m. CORT levels did not change with aging in Nichols *et al.* (1993), perhaps because of careful attention to reduce stress during housing and sacrifice. On the other hand, serum testosterone levels decreased linearly with age and were correlated with increased GFAP in this study. It is known that castration of male rats enhances GFAP mRNA in the brain (Day *et al.*, 1990). However, in one study of aging human brain that showed increased GFAP (Nichols *et al.*, 1993) there were no gender differences in GFAP mRNA levels. Thus, it is unclear what role testosterone or other gonadal steroids, such as estrogen or progesterone, may play in senescence-related increases in GFAP mRNA. This important question clearly deserves further attention, especially in light of new evidence suggesting that estrogen replacement therapy may reduce the incidence of AD in postmenopausal women (Henderson, Paganini-Hill, Emanuel, Dunn, & Buckwalter, 1994).

That GFAP mRNA also increases in

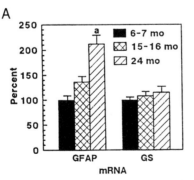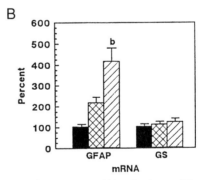

Figure 4. GFAP mRNA increases with age in rat hippocampus (A) and striatum (B). Northern blots of total hippocampal or striatal RNA were hybridized with ^{32}P-labeled antisense rat GFAP or glutamine synthetase (GS) cRNA probes, washed at high stringency, and used to expose X-ray film. Signals were quantified by computerized video densitometry. Data (mean + SE) are plotted as percent of the 6-month group. The study included 14–17 rats for each age group: (a) $p < 0.0001$ vs 6–7-month group and $p < 0.001$ vs 15–16-month group; (b) $p < 0.0001$ vs 6–7-month group and $p < 0.01$ vs 15–16-month group. GS was not significantly different at any age in hippocampus or striatum.

senescent human brain demonstrates the robust nature of GFAP as a general biomarker of mammalian brain aging. Evidence from our laboratory shows a 4-fold increase in GFAP mRNA in nonneurologically diseased brains of elderly (60–79 years, $n = 25$) vs middle-aged humans (25–59 years, $n = 22$) (Nichols *et al.*, 1993) (Fig. 5). A control mRNA for mitochondrial cytochrome oxidase I was also quantified by RNA blot hybridization and did not change with age. Interestingly, non-AD neuropathology in approximately half of the middle-aged individuals (principally due to alcoholism) did not alter GFAP mRNA. Conversely, neuropathology in the elderly group that was distinct from AD was associated with an increased GFAP mRNA level above that in the healthy elderly (Nichols *et al.*, 1993). This suggests that aging per se may be an underlying prerequisite for a generalized age-related GFAP increase, which can be resolved from injury- or neurodegeneration-induced GFAP mRNA responses, as seen earlier for humans.

Studies of aged vs aged/lesioned mice support this concept (Goss & Morgan, 1995). After receiving the fimbria/fornix lesion, aging mice showed a much exaggerated response that developed more slowly (delayed superinduction). It was hypothesized that the age-related increase was different from or secondary to the injury-related response. Another study of GFAP responses to neurodegenerative lesion during aging is partly supportive of this conclusion. In a series of 6-, 15-, and 24-month-old rats lesioned by stereotaxic placement of the neurotoxin 6-hydroxydopamine in the substantia nigra, there was a 2.5-fold greater increase in the GFAP immunocytochemical signal in the substantia nigra of rats aged 24 vs 6 months (Holcomb, Gordon, Schreier, & Morgan, 1994). However, the surprising result was that there was no detectable increase of GFAP immunoreactivity with aging in the substantia nigra of the unlesioned, control rats. Nevertheless, the lesion-induced

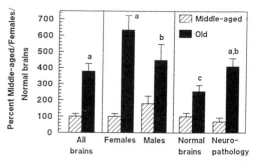

Figure 5. GFAP mRNA prevalence is increased in old vs middle-aged human brain. Northern blots containing total RNA from hippocampus and frontal and temporal cortices were hybridized to ^{32}P-labeled human GFAP cRNA; X-ray film signals were quantified by computerized video densitometry. Mean + SE is presented as a percentage of the middle-aged value: (a) $p < 0.0001$ vs middle age by t-test or ANOVA; (b) $p < 0.01$ vs middle age or vs old normal by ANOVA; (c) $p < 0.05$ vs middle age by ANOVA.

GFAP response again was increased during aging and could be differentiated from a baseline aging response, which, in the latter case of rat substantia nigra, was not seen for unknown reasons.

Different temporal responses in GFAP to injury or aging may represent fundamentally different levels of control of GFAP gene transcription or translation. To address such issues, studies have used nuclear run-on transcription analyses to measure the transcription of GFAP and other genes. In this analysis, nuclei are isolated from the brain region of choice after experimental manipulation, or from animals of various ages, and incubated with radiolabeled ribonucleotide precursors. The synthesis of preinitiated nuclear RNA transcripts is completed, but no new transcripts are initiated, and the result is a radiolabeled pool of nuclear RNA that is representative of the transcriptional status of each gene in the tissue examined. This run-on transcript pool is then analyzed by slot-blot hybridization, and the signal reflects the relative rate of transcription of the gene in question. When GFAP transcription is examined by nuclear run-on after brain injury, a clear increase is seen

(Laping *et al.*, 1994a), showing that the typical lesion-induced increases in GFAP mRNA prevalence are transcriptional in nature. Conversely, GFAP transcription is inhibited by glucocorticoids (Laping *et al.*, 1994b), again showing that the negative glucorticoid regulation of GFAP mRNA prevalence occurs at the transcriptional level. However, run-on analysis of rat brain GFAP transcription during aging shows no significant changes (Laping *et al.*, 1994c), suggesting that the robust age-related increases in mammalian brain GFAP mRNA and protein may be due to posttranscriptional events, such as increased GFAP mRNA stability.

This study also failed to detect any senescence-related changes in the methylation status of 19 CpG sites in the GFAP gene (5′ promoter and exon 1) between 5- vs 30-month-old F344 rats or between 5- vs 35-month-old F344 × Brown Norway F1 hybrid rats (Laping *et al.*, submitted). Many of these CpG sites in the GFAP promoter region were evaluated because their methylation status changed during early brain development, when GFAP expression increases during astrocytosis (Teter *et al.*, in preparation). Decreased DNA methylation has been associated with increased gene expression during embryogenesis and cell differentiation (Brandeis, Ariel, & Cedar, 1993). Other reports show age-related demethylation of whole brain nuclear DNA (e.g., Mays-Hoopes, 1989).

New studies have shown that GFAP mRNA prevalence is significantly reduced in the hypothalamus (Nichols, Finch, & Nelson, 1995) or hippocampus (Major, Kesslak, Cotman, Finch, & Day, 1994) of diet-restricted vs *ad libitum*-fed rats of equivalent age. In the hypothalamus, diet restriction slowed the age-related increase of GFAP mRNA, such that levels in 33-month-old rats were the same as those of *ad libitum*-fed 24-month-old rats. Glutamine synthetase, another astrocyte mRNA, was not affected by caloric restriction. Similarly, in several regions of rat hippocampus, lifelong caloric restriction reduced astrocytic GFAP mRNA prevalence, as determined by *in situ* hybridization, but did not affect the prevalence of clusterin mRNA, another astrocyte marker. Since dietary restriction is known to increase life span and delay the appearance of many age-related markers, including disease, these data further support the hypothesis that GFAP up-regulation is a biomarker of brain aging.

A key question is what do GFAP up-regulation and astrocyte hypertrophy represent with respect to the processes of brain aging? When a manipulation such as dietary restriction reduces the age-related GFAP increase, does it indicate that the aging processes that normally cause GFAP to increase in the brain have been slowed? Increased GFAP expression during brain injury and neurodegeneration, in response to adrenal and gonadal steroids or to various cytokines and growth factors like transforming growth factor β or IL-1 [reviewed in Laping *et al.* (1994d)], shows that astrocytes respond to many physiological stimuli or homeostatic perturbations in the brain. Additional studies show the regulation of GFAP by extracellular potassium, in response to neuronal blockade by tetrodotoxin (Canady & Rubel, 1992), or after seizure activity (Steward, Torre, Tomasulo, & Lothman, 1991). Furthermore, GFAP responses may occur in astrocytes far removed from the site of injury, suggesting that astrocytes monitor and respond to changes in neuronal activity (Steward *et al.*, 1991). Thus, while age-related astrocyte hypertrophy with increased GFAP may be due to the minimal neurodegeneration known to occur in senescent mammalian brain (Terry *et al.*, 1987; West, 1993), it may also represent a response to a number of other subtle perturbations in brain inflammatory status, neuronal activity, peripheral hormone status, etc. We can only speculate that a reduction in the normal age-related GFAP increase, by a manipulation such as diet restriction, may represent a reduction in positive stimuli, such as neurodegeneration or inflammation.

B. Amyloid Precursor Protein

The amyloid precursor protein (APP) has received an enormous amount of attention because a small portion of this protein, the 42-amino acid (aa) Aβ peptide, is the dominant constituent of the extracellular senile plaques and cerebrovascular amyloid deposits that, along with intracellular neurofibrillary tangles, are the hallmarks used in the diagnosis of AD. The mature senile plaque typically contains amyloid (plus other minor protein components) surrounded by a neuritic component, composed of dystrophic neurites, and activated astrocytes and microglia/macrophages. Aβ peptide is also present in so-called diffuse deposits that are generally only detected with anti-Aβ antibodies. Diffuse deposits lack a neuritic component or glial cell investment and are not considered pathologic, but they may represent a precursor form of the mature, fibrillar neuritic plaque. Both diffuse and mature amyloid deposits are found in increasing numbers in the human brain during normal aging (Davies et al., 1988; Delaere, He, Fayet, Duyckaerts, & Hauw, 1993; Ogomori, Kitamoto, Tateishi, Sato, & Tashima, 1988). Diffuse and, occasionally, mature amyloid plaques are also found in aged, long-lived mammals, such as rhesus monkey and dog (Gearing, Rebeck, Hyman, Tigges, & Mirra, 1994; Russell et al., 1992; Wisniewski, Ghetti, & Terry, 1973), but never in short-lived mammals such as rats or mice. This could be a consequence of the different life spans of these mammals, where a certain minimum time is required for detectable amyloid deposition. However, sequencing of the Aβ region of the APP from these species shows that the long-lived mammals all have the same amino acid sequence, whereas the Aβ sequence of rats (Shivers et al., 1988)

and mice (Yamada et al., 1987) differs from that of humans in 3 of 42 aa. Changing these three amino acids in human Aβ to those of the rat peptide decreases the propensity of the altered peptide to aggregate (Dyrks, Dyrks, Masters, & Beyreuther, 1993). Furthermore, there has been success in developing an animal model of brain amyloidosis. Transgenic mice that overexpress mutant human APP (Val 717 Phe) develop amyloid deposits within 8–9 months of age (Games et al., 1995). This success should help to reveal the mechanism of Aβ deposition in either diffuse or mature fibrillar form, which remains a critical area of study in AD research. Nevertheless, the fact that most normal individuals over 60 years of age have numerous diffuse Aβ deposits in their brains (Davies et al., 1988; Ogomori et al., 1988) only underscores the concept that changes that occur during normal aging may provide the initial components necessary for disease progression.

The isolation and amino acid sequencing of the Aβ peptide (Glenner & Wong, 1984) allowed the cloning and sequencing of the APP mRNA (Kang & Muller, 1989). Not long thereafter, several groups independently found that three differentially spliced mRNAs could be spliced from the single-copy APP gene (Kitaguchi, Takahashi, Tokushima, Shiojiri, & Ito, 1988; Ponte et al., 1988; Tanzi et al., 1988). We now know that there are at least six different APP gene transcripts that result from differential splicing of three of the 19 exons that make up the APP gene. There are three predominant forms in brain cells, coding for APP proteins of 695, 751, and 770 aa; the latter two contain the so-called Kunitz-like protease inhibitor domain (KPI), which has trypsin or chymotrypsin inhibitory activity (Kitaguchi et al., 1988).

There is little evidence for much change, increase or decrease, in the prevalence of total brain APP mRNA during aging or AD. However, studies that selectively examined each differentially spliced

APP transcript found changes in the splicing ratio both during aging and in AD. The predominant transcript in human fetal brain is APP-695, varying from 70 to 90% of the total APP transcript in two different studies (Konig et al., 1991; Koo et al., 1990). In aged human brain the situation is reversed: APP-751/APP-770 are the predominant transcripts, representing 50–90% of the total APP transcript (Konig et al., 1991; Koo et al., 1990; Tanaka et al., 1992a). These changes in the splicing ratio may be considered to be aging phenomena since young or middle-aged individuals (20–50 years) have intermediate APP splicing ratios. Furthermore, these same studies each independently show a gradual increase in the KPI-APP/APP-695 ratio with age in individuals over 60 years.

Several studies also showed increased KPI-APP/APP-695 ratios in AD compared to age-matched non-AD brain (Johnson, Rogers, & Finch, 1989; Tanaka et al., 1989), including an in situ hybridization study showing increased cellular KPI-APP/APP-695 in AD hippocampus that correlated with neuritic plaque density (Johnson, McNeill, Cordell, & Finch, 1990). Other studies, however, have not replicated an increased APP splicing ratio in AD brain (Konig et al., 1991; Koo et al., 1990). Tanaka et al. (1992b) present a careful analysis of this issue, concluding that the KPI-APP/APP-695 ratio increases at approximately the same rate in both non-AD and AD patients, but that AD patients have a higher KPI/695 ratio, equivalent to that of non-AD individuals who are on average 20 years or more older. It is not clear whether there is a connection between increased KPI-APP and age-associated deposition of Aβ peptide in non-AD (or AD) brain. Nevertheless, this represents one of the few known examples of age-related changes in differential mRNA splicing in brain. The mechanism responsible for this is not known, but it could hypothetically be due to the age-related loss of a splicing factor that protects the splice site adjacent to the KPI exon.

Only a few studies have determined changes in APP protein and subfragments during brain aging (Nordstedt et al., 1991; Rumble, Retallak, Montgomery, Beyreuther, & Masters, 1989). Nordstedt et al. (1991) found no clear change in the total APP protein between a set of very young (mean age = 4.9 ± 5.9 years) and elderly individuals (78 ± 7 years), which agreed with the earlier results of Rumble et al. (1989). However, Nordstedt et al. (1991) found a 2–3-fold increase in the 133-kDa holoprotein (equivalent to KPI-APP) and, interestingly, in a 19-kDa subfragment that would be expected to be amyloidogenic. Since they found no further increase in these APP species in AD brain, they caution that the increases are "not sufficient for generation of amyloid deposits seen in AD."

C. Microtubule-Associated Tau. The Paired Helical Filament Protein

Abnormal phosphorylation of the microtubule-associated protein tau appears to underlie the formation of the paired helical filaments (PHF) that make up the neurofibrillary tangle (NFT), the other hallmark pathology used to confirm a diagnosis of AD (Goedert, Spillantini, & Crowther, 1991; Lee & Trojanowski, 1992). Abnormal phosphorylation of tau has been shown to destabilize microtubules (Bramblett et al., 1993), as well as to promote the polymerization of tau into fibrillar structures that resemble PHF (Drewes et al., 1992). NFT, like senile plaques, are present in the normal senescent brain, but to a much lesser degree than in AD, and are not found in the brains of normal individuals less than 50 years old. Antibodies to PHF-tau, the hyperphosphorylated version found in AD NFT, paint a similar picture: no signals with the young human brain (except fetal brain), occasional signals in the cognitively normal senescent brain, especially in the entorhinal cortex, and widespread signals in the AD brain (Vermersch, Frigard, David, Fallet-Bianco, & Delacourte, 1992). By using the abnormal phosphorylation-specific tau antibody AT8, Braak *et al.* (1994) found AT8-positive neurons in senescent brain from sheep and goats, but not dogs or cats. They detected two classes: one with apparently normal cell bodies and processes, and another neuron class with intensely stained distal dendritic swellings, a situation similar to that found in AD.

There are six isoforms of tau, each resulting from differential splicing of a single tau gene (Kosik, Orecchio, Bakalis, & Neve, 1989). Tau gene splicing is developmentally regulated. Only one tau isoform is found in fetal brain, but all six are present in an adult brain (Goedert, Spillantini, Potier, Ulrich, & Crowther, 1989b; Kosik *et al.*, 1989). While tau has been under intense scrutiny, there is a frustrating lack of information on changes in tau expression during normal brain aging. Two studies actually determined specific tau mRNA levels in 37 aging brains (50–101 years) by the sensitive nuclease protection assay, but only reported the data as a comparison to APP mRNA isoforms (Oyama, Shimada, Oyama, Titani, & Ihara, 1992) or to plaque and NFT counts (Oyama, Shimada, Oyama, Titani, & Ihara, 1993). While there was no correlation between any tau or APP isoform and NFT or plaque density (Oyama *et al.*, 1993), this group showed an interesting coregulation of total APP mRNA and total tau mRNA prevalence among the 37 individuals ($r^2 = 0.78$). Thus, while levels of each varied substantially between individuals, their levels were tightly coupled among all individuals. Furthermore, the three-repeat, fetal tau isoform was coregulated with APP-695 ($r^2 = 0.74$), as were the four-repeat, adult tau subclass mRNA and APP-KPI mRNA levels ($r^2 = 0.65$) (Oyama *et al.*, 1992). Anoth-

er limited study of seven normal individuals aged 23–79 years examined tau mRNA subclasses that are either present or absent during brain development, but found no obvious change with age (Goedert, Spillantini, Jakes, Rutherford, & Crowther, 1989a). Nevertheless, there is still insufficient data to address changes in tau isoforms that might occur during aging. However, the current hypothesis that abnormal phosphorylation of tau at sites that recapitulate a developmental or fetal phosphorylation pattern during AD (Bramblett *et al.*, 1993; Goedert *et al.*, 1993), coupled with the lack of change in tau mRNA isoform prevalence between AD and an age-matched control (Goedert *et al.*, 1989a), suggests that age-related changes in tau gene expression may not be involved in predisposition to AD.

IV. Neuroendocrine Aging and Gene Expression

Because of the fundamental role of the hypothalamus and the limbic system in physiological regulation, any changes in gene expression that occur in these brain regions are of great interest. The best-defined changes are described in the female rodent hypothalamus, which is strongly implicated in the impairments of fertility cycles that happen in rodents during middle age, in which exposure to ovarian estrogens appears to induce physiological dysfunction (Finch, Felicio, Mobbs, & Nelson, 1984; Chapter 12 in this Handbook). The neuronal systems that are primary targets of aging or estradiol (E2) in the rodent brain are not known. In rodents, hypothalamic changes become prominent during the loss of fertility by 10–18 months, e.g., the preovulatory gonadotrophin surge becomes smaller in still-cycling rats and mice, and smaller surges are induced by treatments with E2 that induce preovulatory-like surges.

Nonetheless, after menopause, women also show altered hypothalamic regulation of gonadotrophins, e.g., slower pulse frequencies and less inhibition by clomiphine, an estrogen antagonist (Rossmanith, Reichelt, & Scherbaum, 1994). These species differences in the pattern of aging are more quantitative than qualitative, since similar impairments eventually occur.

There are several examples of altered response to E2 in the hypothalamus during aging. The occupancy of nuclear receptor complexes by E2 shows substantial declines: a loss of about 35% by middle age, which is chiefly due to a faster dissociation of the E2–receptor complex (Bergman, Karelus, Felicio, & Nelson, 1991). Consistent with this impairment of the transacting E2–receptor, the normal activity of E2 in suppressing POMC mRNA is decreased during aging in the female mouse hypothalamus (Karelus & Nelson, 1992).

There is no loss of the neurons that contain the neuropeptide GnRH (gonadotrophin hormone-releasing hormone) in the hypothalamus during the loss of estrous cycles in aging mice (Hoffman & Finch, 1986). The GnRH neurons contain the pacemakers that drive the preovulatory surge of gonadotrophins and are among the most vital of all neurons in the brain for reproductive success. Impairments of GnRH neurons include the regulation of c-fos and Jun by E2; these immediate early gene responses of GnRH neurons during proestrus in young rats occur in about 50% fewer GnRH neurons by middle age (Lloyd, Hoffman, & Wise, 1994). The mechanisms of aging on GnRH neurons could be indirect and might be mediated by astrocytic changes. For example, the increase in GFAP that occurs in female mice, even if ovariectomized when young (Kohama et al., 1995), could impair astrocyte interactions with neurons. Other hypothalamic astrocytic markers in the arcuate nucleus show a marked hyperactivity during aging that is reduced by ovariec-

tomy of mice when young (Schipper et al., 1981) and prematurely induced by chronic elevations of E2 (Brawer, Beaudet, Desjardins, & Schipper, 1993).

A subject that should develop well in the future is the relation of hippocampal aging to corticosteroids (also see Chapter 12 of this Handbook). The data on changes of the mRNAs that encode the two types of corticosteroid receptors indicate that there is a loss of mRNA during aging for the type II (low affinity) receptor in the rat hippocampus, with little loss elsewhere in the brain (van Eekelen, Rots, Sutanto, Oitzl, & de Kloet, 1991). The effects of aging on receptor protein levels are more controversial. A consensus view is that the loss in the number of receptors during aging is more prominent than changes in their affinity for corticosteroids (Landfield & Eldridge, 1994; Sapolsky, 1992, pp. 63–69).

V. Inflammation during Brain Aging and Disease

There is a growing body of evidence in support of the hypothesis that inflammation plays a pathological role during AD and other degenerative brain diseases. Inflammation has a pathological role in the periphery, e.g., in glomerulonephritis (kidney) or rheumatoid arthritis (joints), as well as in the brain during multiple sclerosis. A number of "acute phase proteins," which are serum proteins synthesized by the liver or circulating lymphocytes in response to proinflammatory stimuli [e.g., interleukin-6 (IL-6)], are found in senile plaques during aging and AD. Examples include the protease inhibitors α_2-macroglobulin (Strauss et al., 1992), α_1-antitrypsin (Gollin, Kalaria, Eikelenboom, Rozemuller, & Perry, 1992), and α_1-antichymotrypsin (Abraham, Selkoe, & Potter, 1988), potent cytokines such as TGF-β1 and IL-6 (Strauss et al., 1992), classical complement cascade proteins C1q, C3, and C4

(Eikelenboom, Hack, Rozemuller, & Stam, 1989), complement inhibitors C4-binding protein (Kalaria & Kroon, 1992) and clusterin (McGeer, Kawamata, & Walker, 1992), and the invariant amyloid-associated protein serum amyloid protein (Kalaria, 1992). The rapid up-regulation of these and other proteins during the acute phase response is driven primarily by IL-6, which is produced by circulating monocytes. That these acute phase serum proteins are found in the brain has prompted several groups to look for evidence of synthesis in the brain, which secondarily addresses the question of BBB damage and serum extravasation during disease. Surprisingly, mRNAs for nearly all of the above-mentioned plaque-associated (serum) proteins have been found in the brain by RNA gel blot analysis, and many have been localized to specific brain cell types by *in situ* hybridization.

Astrocytes contain mRNAs encoding α_1-antichymotrypsin (Koo, Abraham, Potter, Cork, & Price, 1991), IL-1 (Griffin *et al.*, 1989), and clusterin (Day *et al.*, 1990). Microglia, the resident brain macrophages, contain mRNAs for TGF-β (Morgan, Nichols, Pasinetti, & Finch, 1993), IL-6, IL-1 (Yao, Keri, Taffs, & Colton, 1992), and complement components C1q and C4 (Johnson, Lampert-Etchells, Pasinetti, Rozovsky, & Finch, 1992; Pasinetti *et al.*, 1992), and neurons contain C4 mRNA (Johnson *et al.*, 1992). These data strongly suggest that the brain has the capability to mount an inflammatory response. Moreover, the up-regulation of many of these molecules during AD (compared to age-matched non-AD cases), coupled with the localization of cognate proteins to plaques and NFT-bearing neurons, indicates that there is a chronic inflammatory condition in the AD brain. In addition, case-control twin studies (Breitner *et al.*, 1994) and preliminary clinical studies (Rogers *et al.*, 1993) are beginning to suggest that the use of antiinflammatory drugs may be effective in slowing the progression of AD.

Whether brain inflammation occurs during normal aging or, more importantly, whether inflammation has a pathological role during brain aging is less clear. As discussed earlier in this chapter, both astrocytes and microglia become increasingly activated during aging, but not necessarily to the levels they would in response to acute brain injury or during chronic disease, such as AD. Nevertheless, increased glial activation suggests inflammation, since microglia and astrocytes are generally considered the immune/inflammatory cells of the brain. Microglial activation is often determined by increased expression of class II histocompatability antigens, such as HLA-DR in humans, which is necessary for phagocytosis. In culture, activated microglia secrete complement components (Haga, Ikeda, Sato, & Ishii, 1993), proinflammatory cytokines (IL-1, IL-6, TNF-α) (Frei *et al.*, 1989; Sawada, Kondo, Suzumura, & Marunouchi, 1989; Yao *et al.*, 1992), proteases and protease inhibitors, and reactive oxygen compounds (Colton & Gilbert, 1987), all of which can be detrimental to normal cell function.

There is limited evidence for age-related increases in the expression of immune/inflammatory genes during aging in the brain. α_1-Antichymotrypsin (ACT), a typical acute phase serum protein produced in the liver, is also a common senile plaque component whose mRNA is found in astrocytes (Abraham, Shirahama, & Potter, 1990). ACT mRNA is difficult to detect in fetal or young adult human or monkey brains, but is easily detected in aged human or monkey brains and is quite prevalent in AD brains (Koo *et al.*, 1991). Interestingly, there is 2-fold increase in ACT in the cerebrospinal fluid (CSF) of aged vs young individuals, but no additional increase in AD CSF (Delamarche, Berger, Gallard, & Pouplard-Barthelaix, 1991). In addition, preliminary evidence indicates slight age-related increases in mRNAs for clusterin (Apo J), apolipoprotein E, and complement component C1q (B chain) in rat brain (Pasinetti *et al.*, unpublished). Clusterin and Apo E are serum proteins whose mRNAs are found in astrocytes; C1q is an acute phase protein that is the initiation complex of the potentially cytotoxic complement cascade. C1q is typically produced in circulating monocytes, but its mRNA is found in microglia (Johnson *et al.*, 1992; Pasinetti *et al.*, 1992) and is up-regulated during AD (Johnson *et al.*, 1992). These limited data are generally consistent with microglial and astrocyte activation in senescent brain. Thus, while much additional evidence is needed, existing information suggests that there may be low-level inflammation in the aging brain. As stated earlier, important goals of future research should be to determine whether inflammation has a pathological role during brain aging and whether the use of antiinflammatory drugs would be beneficial.

VI. Other Genes Examined in the Aging Brain

The accompanying table (Table I) presents a list of genes whose mRNA prevalence has been examined in aged compared to mature adult brain since 1990. Of the 37 different genes in the list, 20 show decreases, 14 show no change or have contradictory results in different studies, and only 3 show consistent increases. The latter 3 are found in astrocytes, and their increase may be tied to age-related astrocyte hypertrophy discussed in section I.A. It is important to note, however, that another astrocyte mRNA, glutamine synthetase, is not increased with aging. Neuronal mRNAs include both nonchangers and those that decrease, but interpretation of this is difficult since different methods, such as Northern blot or *in situ* hybridization measure global tissue prevalence vs cellular prevalence, respectively. Furthermore, decreased prevalence of a neuronal mRNA in a neuronal population that has

atrophied may simply reflect a reduced need of the cognate protein by smaller cells, instead of an underlying cause of cell atrophy during aging. Clearly, many additional carefully designed studies that take these and other issues into account are needed before it will be possible to show cause and effect at the level of gene expression during brain aging.

References

Abraham, C. R., Selkoe, D. J., & Potter, H. (1988). Immunochemical identification of the serine protease inhibitor alpha 1-antichymotrypsin in the brain amyloid deposits of Alzheimer's disease. *Cell, 52* (4), 487–501.

Abraham, C. R., Shirahama, T., & Potter, H. (1990). Alpha1-antichymotrypsin is associated solely with amyloid deposits containing the β-protein. Amyloid and cell localization of alpha1-antichymotrypsin. *Neurobiology of Aging, 11*, 123–129.

Ames, B., Shigenaga, M. K., & Hagen, T. M. (1993). Oxidants, antioxidants, and the degenerative diseases of aging. *Proceedings of the National Academy of Sciences of the United States of America, 90*, 7915–7922.

Ammendola, R., Mesuraca, M., Russo, T., & Cimino, F. (1992). Sp1 DNA binding efficiency is highly reduced in nuclear extracts from aged rat tissues. *Journal of Biological Chemistry, 267* (25), 17944–17948.

Arnheim, N., & Cortopassi, G. (1992). Deleterious mitochondrial DNA mutations accumulate in aging human tissues. *Mutation Research, 275*, 157–167.

Arriagada, P. V., Marzloff, K., & Hyman, B. T. (1992). Distribution of Alzheimer-type pathological changes in nondemented elderly individuals matches the pattern in Alzheimer's disease. *Neurology, 42*, 1681–1688.

Bacci, B., Petrelli, L., Dal Toso, R., & Nunzi, M. G. (1992). Age-associated alteration in the expression of synapsin I mRNA in the rat central nervous system. *Annals of the New York Academy of Science, 663*, 463–465.

Beach, T. G., Walker, R., & McGeer, E. G. (1989). Patterns of gliosis in Alzheimer's disease and aging cerebrum. *Glia, 2*, 420–436.

Bergman, M. D., Karelus, K., Felicio, L. S., & Nelson, J. F. (1991). Age-related alterations in

Table I

Articles on Gene Expression in Senescent Mammalian Brain[a]

Gene[b]	Species	Region[c]	Method[d]	Change: aged vs adult[e]	Reference
α-actin	Rat	Brain	NB	No change	Slagboom et al. (1990)
Adenosine A2 R	Rat	Striatum	ISH	30% decrease	Schiffmann and Vanderhaeghen (1993)
APP-KPI/APP-695	Human	Cortex/gray	RP	Increase	Tanaka et al. (1993)
APP-KPI/APP-695	Human	Cortex	RP	1.5× increase	Tanaka et al. (1992a,b)
APP-KPI/APP-695	Human	Cortex	RP	2× increase	Koo et al. (1990)
APP-KPI/APP-695	Monkey	Cortex	RP	No change	Koo et al. (1990)
BDNF	Rat	Hippocampus	NB, ISH	No change	Lapchak et al. (1993)
β-Endorphin	Mouse	Hypothalamus	ICC	35% fewer neurons	Miller et al. (1991)
C-fos	Rat	ctx, cbl	NB	50% decrease	Kitraki et al. (1993)
CRF	Rat	pvn	NB	Decrease	Cizza et al. (1994)
cytochrome oxidase	Rat	ctx, cbl	NRO	Decrease	Gadaleta et al. (1990)
D2 dopamine R	Rat	Striatum	NB	Decrease	Mesco et al. (1991)
D2 dopamine R	Rat	Striatum	NRO	50% lower transcription	Mesco et al. (1993)
D2 dopamine R	Rat	Various	RT-PCR	Decrease	Della Vedova et al. (1992)
D2 dopamine R	Rat	Striatum	NB	No change	Sakata et al. (1992)
EIF-2α	Rat	Brain	Slot blot	No change	Kimball et al. (1992)
Elongation factor 1α	Rat	Brain	NB	No change	Lee et al. (1992)
Ferritin heavy chain	Rat	Brain	NB	50% decrease	Ammendola et al. (1992)
Fibronectin	Rat	Brain	RP	Decreased splicing of elIIa	Pagani et al. (1991)
Fx (actin sequestering)	Rat	Hippocampus	NB	Decrease	Gomez-Marquez et al. (1993)
GFAP	Mouse	ctx, cbl, hip, str	NB, RP	2× increase	Goss et al. (1991)
GFAP	Human	Cortex	NB	3.5× increase	Nichols et al. (1993)
GFAP	Rat	hip, str	NB	2×, 4× increase	Nichols et al. (1993)
GFAP	Rat	Hippocampus	NB	2× increase	Wagner et al. (1993)
Glucocorticoid R	Rat	Hippocampus	NB	Decrease	Peiffer et al. (1991)
Glucocorticoid R	Rat	hip CA4, CA3, DG	ISH	40% decrease	van Eekelen et al. (1992)
Glucocorticoid R	Rat	Hippocampus	NB	No change	Cizza et al. (1994)
GLUT1	Rat	Brain	NB	No change	Oka et al. (1992)
Glutathione peroxidase	Rat	Brain	NB	Linear increase (1–100 weeks)	Rao et al. (1990)
Glutathione peroxidase	Mouse	Brain	NB	Decrease (after heat stress)	de Hann et al. (1992)
HSP-70	Rat	Hippocampus	ISH	Decrease (after heat stress)	Pardue et al. (1992)
HSP-70	Rat	Brain	NB	Decrease (after heat stress)	Blake et al. (1991)

(continued)

Table I (*Continued*)

Gene[b]	Species	Region[c]	Method[d]	Change: aged vs adult[e]	Reference
IGF-I	Rat	Brain	NB	Decrease	Park and Beutow (1991)
IGF-II	Rat	Various	NB	50% decrease	Kitraki et al. (1993)
IGF-II	Rat	Brain	NB	No change	Park and Buetow (1991)
M2 ACh R	Rat	Brain	NB	Decrease	Wang et al. (1992)
M1, M3, M4, ACh R	Rat	Various	ISH	No change	Blake et al. (1991)
Mineralicorticoid R	Rat	Hippocampus	ISH	No change	van Eekelen et al. (1992)
Mineralicorticoid R	Rat	Hippocampus	NB	No change	Cizza et al. (1994)
NCAM	Rat	Brain	NB	No change	Linnemann et al. (1993)
POMC	Rat	ant. pit.	NB	25% loss/cell; 40% less cells	Heroux et al. (1991)
POMC	ovx rat	Arcuate	ISH	Lack of E2-induced suppression	Lloyd et al. (1991)
POMC	Rat	Arcuate	ISH	Lack of E2-induced suppression	Weiland et al. (1992)
POMC	Rat	Hypothalamus	RP	Lack of E2-induced suppression	Karelus et al. (1992)
POMC	Rat	Hypothalamus	NB	Decrease	Cizza et al. (1994)
Prepro Substance P	Rat	Brain stem	ISH	Decrease	Johnson et al. (1993)
Prepro TRH	Rat	Brain stem	ISH	Decrease	Johnson et al. (1993)
Prolactin	Rat	Pituitary	NB	No change	Stewart et al. (1992)
S-100β	Rat	Hippocampus	NB	1.5 × increase	Wagner et al. (1993)
SNAP-25	Rat	Hippocampus	ISH	No change	Lapchak et al. (1993)
Somatostatin	Rat	ctx, str	NB	50% decrease	Florio et al. (1991)
Somatostatin	Rat	Hypothalamus	ISH	Decrease	Martinoli et al. (1991)
Superoxide dismutase	Rat	Brain	NB	Decrease	Rao et al. (1990)
SOD; catalase	Rat	Brain	NB	40% decrease	Semsei et al. (1991)
Synapsin I	Rat	Hippocampus	NB	Decrease	Bacci et al. (1992)
Tyrosine hydroxylase	Human	Substantia nigra	NB, ISH	No change	Nagatsu (1991)
TRK B	Rat	Hippocampus	ISH	Decrease	Lapchak et al. (1993)
Vasopressin	Rat	BNST	ISH	Decrease	Dobie et al. (1991)
Vasopressin	Rat	BNST	ISH	TEST reverses age decrease	Dobie et al. (1992)
Vasopressin	Rat	Hypothalamus	NB	Increase	Cizza et al. (1994)

[a]Includes articles published in 1990 or later.

[b]R in many gene catagories stands for receptor. APP-KPI, Kunitz inhibitor containing amyloid precursor protein; BDNF, brain-derived neurotrophic factor; EIF-2α, eukaryotic initiation factor 2 alpha; GFAP, glial fibrillary acidic protein; GLUT1, glucose transporter protein 1; HSP-70, heat shock protein 70; IGF-I, insulin-like growth factor 1; IGF-II, insulin-like growth factor 2; M1–M4 ACh R, muscarinic acetylcholine receptor subunits; NCAM, neural cell adhesion molecule; POMC, pro-opiomelanocortin; TRH, thyrotropin-releasing hormone; SNAP-25, synaptosomal-associated protein (25,000 MW); SOD, superoxide dismutase; TRK B, tyrosine receptor kinase B (BDNF receptor).

[c]ant. pit, anterior pituitary; CA3, hippocampal field Cornu Ammonis 3; CA4, field CA4; DG, dentate gyrus; cbl, cerebellum; ctx, cortex; hip, hippocampus; pvn, paraventricular nucleus of the hypothalamus; str, striatum.

[d]ICC, immunocytochemistry; ISH, *in situ* hybridization; NB, Northern blot hybridization; RP, ribonuclease protection/solution titration; NRO, nuclear run-on transcription assay; RT-PCR, reverse transcriptase/polymerase chain reaction.

[e]All specificied changes are statistically significant.

estrogen receptor dynamics are independent of cycling status in middle-aged C57BL/6J mice. *Journal of Steroid Biochemistry and Molecular Biology, 38*, 127–133.

Bertoni-Freddari, C., Fattoretti, P., Casoli, T., Masera, F., Meier-Ruge, W., & Ulrich, J. (1989). Computer-assisted morphometry of synaptic plasticity during aging and dementia. *Pathology Research Practices, 185*, 799–802.

Bird, T. D. (1994). Clinical Genetics of Familial Alzheimer Disease. In R. K. R. D. Terry & K. L. Bick (Eds.), *Alzheimer Disease.* New York: Raven Press, Ltd.

Bjorklund, H., Eriksdotter-Nilsson, M., Dahl, D., Rose, G., & Olson, L. (1985). Image analysis of GFA-positive astrocytes from adolescence to senescence. *Experiments in Brain Research, 58*, 163–170.

Blake, M. J., Fargnoli, J., Gershon, D., & Holbrook, N. J. (1991). Concomitant decline in heat-induced hyperthermia and HSP70 mRNA expression in aged rats. *American Journal of Physiology, 260* (4, Part 2), R663–667.

Blinzinger, K., & Kreutzberg, G. W. (1968). Displacement of synaptic terminals from regenerating motoneurons by microglial cells. *Zeitschrift fuer Zellforschung, 85*, 145–157.

Boerrigter, M. E. T. I., Wei, J. Y., & Vijg, J. (1992). DNA repair and Alzheimer's disease. *Journal of Gerontology: Biological Science, 47*, B177–B184.

Braak, H., Braak, E., & Strothjohann, M. (1994). Abnormally phosphorylated tau protein related to the formation of neurofibrillary tangles and neuropil threads in the cerebral cortex of sheep and goat. *Neuroscience Letters, 171*, 1–4.

Bramblett, G. T., Goedert, M., Jakes, R., Merrick, S. E., Trojanowski, J. Q., & Lee, V. M.-Y. (1993). Abnormal Tau phosphorylation at Ser396 in Alzheimer's disease recapitulates development and contributes to reduced microtubule binding. *Neuron, 10*, 1089–1099.

Brandeis, M., Ariel, M., & Cedar, H. (1993). Dynamics of DNA methylation during development. *BioEssays, 15*, 709–713.

Brawer, J. R., Beaudet, A., Desjardins, G. C., & Schipper, H. M. (1993). Pathologic effect of estradiol on the hypothalamus. *Biology of Reproduction, 49*, 647–652.

Breitner, J. C. S., Gau, B. A., Welsh, K. A., Plass-

man, B. L., McDonald, W. M., Helms, M. J., & Anthony, J. C. (1994). Inverse association of anti-inflammatory treatments and Alzheimer's disease. *Neurology, 44*, 227–232.

Brody, H. (1955). Organization of the cerebral cortex. III. A study of aging in the human cerebral cortex. *Journal of Comparative Neurology, 102*, 511–556.

Canady, K. S., & Rubel, E. W. (1992). Rapid and reversible astrocytic reaction to afferent blockade in chick cochlear nucleus. *Neuroscience, 13*, 769–779.

Cizza, G., Calogero, A. E., Brady, L. S., Bagdy, G., Bergamini, E., Blackman, M. R., Chrousos, G. P., & Gold, P. W. (1994). Male Fischer 344/N rats show a progressive central impairment of the hypothalamic-pituitary-adrenal axis with advancing age. *Endocrinology, 134* (4), 1611–1620.

Coleman, P. D., & Flood, D. G. (1987). Neuron numbers and dendritic extent in normal aging and Alzheimer's disease. *Neurobiology of Aging, 8*, 521–545.

Colman, P. C., Kaplan, B. B., Osterburg, H. H., & Finch, C. E. (1980). Brain poly(A)RNA during aging: Stability of yield and sequence complexity in two rat strains. *Journal of Neurochemistry, 34*, 335–345.

Colton, C., & Gilbert, D. (1987). Production of superoxide anion by a CNS macrophage, the microglia. *FEBS Letters, 223*, 284–288.

Cortopassi, G., & Arnheim, N. (1990). Detection of a specific mitochondrial deletion in tissues of older individuals. *Nucleic Acids Research, 18*, 6927–6933.

Danner, D. B., & Holbrook, N. J. (1990). Alterations in Gene Expression with Aging. In *Handbook of the Biology of Aging* (3rd ed.). New York: Academic Press.

Davies, L., Wolska, B., Hilbich, C., Multhaup, G., Martins, K., Simms, G., Beyreuther, K., & Masters, C. L. (1988). A4 amyloid deposition and the diagnosis of Alzheimer's disease: Prevalence in aged brains determined by immunochemistry compared with conventional neuropathologic techniques. *Neurology, 38*, 1688–1693.

Dawson, V. L., Dawson, T. M., Bartley, D. A., Uhl, G. R., & Snyder, S. H. (1993). Mechanisms of nitric oxide-mediated neurotoxicity in primary brain cultures. *Journal of Neuroscience, 13* (6), 2651–2661.

Day, J. R., Laping, N. J., McNeill, T. H.,

Schreiber, S. S., Pasinetti, G. M., & Finch, C. E. (1990). Castration enhances expression of GFAP and SGP-2 in the intact and lesion-altered hippocampus of the adult male rat. *Molecular Endocrinology, 4,* 1995–2002.

de Haan, J. B., Newman, J. D., & Kola, I. (1992). Cu/Zn superoxide dismutase mRNA and enzyme activity, and susceptibility to lipid peroxidation, increases with aging in murine brains. *Brain Research: Molecular Brain Research, 13* (3), 179–187.

Delaere, P., He, Y., Fayet, G., Duyckaerts, C., & Hauw, J. J. (1993). Beta A4 deposits are constant in the brain of the oldest old: an immunocytochemical study of 20 French centenarians. *Neurobiology of Aging, 14* (2), 191–194.

Delamarche, C., Berger, F., Gallard, L., & Pouplard-Barthelaix, A. (1991). Aging and Alzheimer's disease: Protease inhibitors in cerebrospinal fluid. *Neurobiology of Aging, 12,* 71–74.

Della Vedova, F., Fumagalli, F., Sacchetti, G., Racagni, G., & Brunello, N. (1992). Age-related variations in relative abundance of alternative spliced D2 receptor mRNAs in brain areas of two rat strains. *Brain Research: Molecular Brain Research, 12* (4), 357–359.

Diamond, M. C., Johnson, R. E., & Gold, M. W. (1977). Changes in neuron number and size and glial number in the young adult and aging rat medial occipital cortex. *Behavioral Biology, 20,* 409–418.

Dobie, D. J., Miller, M. A., Urban, J. H., Raskind, M. A., & Dorsa, D. M. (1991). Age-related decline of vasopressin mRNA in the bed nucleus of the stria terminalis. *Neurobiology of Aging, 12* (5), 419–423.

Dobie, D. J., Miller, M. A., Raskind, M. A., & Dorsa, D. M. (1992). Testosterone reverses a senescent decline in extrahypothalamic vasopressin mRNA. *Brain Research, 583* (1–2), 247–252.

Drewes, G., Lichtenberg-Kraag, B., Doring, F., Mandelkow, E.-M., Biernat, J., Goris, J., Doree, M., & Mandelkow, E. (1992). Mitogen activated protein (MAP) kinase transforms tau protein into an Alzheimer-like state. *EMBO Journal, 11,* 2131–2138.

Dyrks, T., Dyrks, E., Masters, C. L., & Beyreuther, K. (1993). Amyloidogenicity of rodent and human βA4 sequences. *FEBS Letters, 324,* 231–236.

Edvinsson, L., MacKenzie, E. T., & McCulloch, J. (1993). In *Cerebral Blood Flow and Metabolism.* New York: Raven Press.

Eikelenboom, P., Hack, C. E., Rozemuller, J. M., & Stam, F. C. (1989). Complement activation in amyloid plaques in Alzheimer's dementia. *Virchows Archives B: Cell Pathology, 56* (4), 259–262.

Evans, D. A. P., van der Kleij, A. A. M., Sonnemans, M. A. F., Burbach, J. P. H., & van Leeuwen, F. W. (1994). Frameshift mutations at two hotspots in vasopressin transcripts in post-mitotic neurons. *Proceedings of the National Academy of Sciences of the United States of America, 91,* 6059–6063.

Farrer, L. A. (1993). Neurogenetics of Aging. In J. E. K. M. L. Albert (Ed.), *Clinical Neurology of Aging* (2nd ed.). New York: Oxford University Press.

Farrer, L. A., Cupples, L. A., Wiater, P., Conneally, P. M., Gusella, J. F., & Myers, R. H. (1993). The normal Huntington Disease (HD) allele, or a closely linked gene, influences age at onset of HD. *American Journal of Human Genetics, 53,* 125–130.

Felsenfeld, O., & Wolf, R. H. (1972). Relationship of age and serum immunoglobulins to autoantibodies against brain constituents in primates. I. A study in apparently healthy men, *Macaca mulatta* and *Erythrocebus patas. Journal of Medical Primatology, 1,* 287–296.

Finch, C. E. (1990). In *Longevity, Senescence, and the Genome.* Chicago: The University of Chicago Press.

Finch, C. E. (1993). Neuron atrophy during aging: programmed or sporadic? *Trends in Neurosciences, 16* (3), 104–110.

Finch, C. E., Felicio, L. S., Mobbs, C. V., & Nelson, J. F. (1984). Ovarian and steroidal influences on neuroendocrine aging processes in female rodents. *Endocrine Reviews, 5,* 467–497.

Florio, T., Ventra, C., Postiglione, A., & Schettini, G. (1991). Age-related alterations of somatostatin gene expression in different rat brain areas. *Brain Research, 557* (1–2), 64–68.

Frei, K., Malipiero, U., Leist, T., Sinkernagel, R., Schwab, D. F., & Fontana, A. (1989). On the source and function of interleukin-6 produced in the central nervous system in viral disease. *European Journal of Immunology, 19,* 689–694.

Gadaleta, M. N., Petruzzella, V., Renis, M., Fracasso, F., & Cantatore, P. (1990). Reduced transcription of mitochondrial DNA in the senescent rat; tissue dependence and effect of L-carnitine. *European Journal of Biochemistry, 187,* 501–506.

Games, D., et al. (1995). Alzheimer-type neuropathology in transgenic mice overexpressing V717F β-amyloid precursor protein. *Nature, 373,* 523–527.

Gearing, M., Rebeck, G. W., Hyman, B. T., Tigges, J., & Mirra, S. S. (1994). Neuropathology and apolipoprotein E profile of aged chimpanzees: Implications for Alzheimer disease. *Proceedings of the National Academy of Sciences of the United States of America, 91,* 9382–9386.

Gibson, P. H. (1983). EM study of the number of cortical synapses in the brains of ageing people and people with Alzheimer-type dementia. *Acta Neuropathologica (Berlin), 62,* 127–133.

Glenner, G. G., & Wong, C. W. (1984). Initial report of the purification and characterization of a novel cerebrovascular amyloid protein. *Biochemical and Biophysical Research Communications, 120,* 885–890.

Goedert, M., Spillantini, M. G., Jakes, R., Rutherford, D., & Crowther, R. A. (1989a). Multiple isoforms of human microtubule-associated protein tau: Sequences and localization in neurofibrillary tangles of Alzheimer's disease. *Neuron, 3,* 519–526.

Goedert, M., Spillantini, M. G., Potier, M. C., Ulrich, J., & Crowther, R. A. (1989b). Cloning and sequencing of the cDNA encoding an isoform of microtubule-associated protein tau containing four tandem repeats: differential expression of tau protein mRNAs in human brain. *EMBO Journal, 8,* 393–399.

Goedert, M., Spillantini, M. G., & Crowther, R. (1991). Tau protein and neurofibrillary degeneration. *Brain Pathology, 1,* 279–286.

Goedert, M., Jakes, R., Crowther, R. A., Six, J., Lubke, U., Vandermeeren, M., Cras, P., Trojanowski, J. Q., & Lee, V. M.-Y. (1993). The abnormal phosphorylation of tau protein at Ser-202 in Alzheimer disease recapitulates phosphorylation during development. *Proceedings of the National Academy of Sciences of the United States of America, 90,* 5066–5070.

Gollin, P. A., Kalaria, R. N., Eikelenboom, P., Rozemuller, A., & Perry, G. (1992). a1-antitrypsin and a1-antichymotrypsin are in the lesions of Alzheimer's disease. *Neuroreport, 3,* 201–203.

Gomez-Marquez, J., Pedrares, J. I., Otero, A., & Anadon, R. (1993). Prominent expression of the actin-sequestering peptide Fx gene in the hippocampal region of rat brain. *Neuroscience Letters, 152* (1–2), 41–44.

Gordon, M. N., & Morgan, D. G. (1991). Increased GFAP expression in the aging brain does not result from increased astrocyte density. *Society for Neuroscience, Abstracts, 17,* 53 (No. 26.4).

Goss, J. R., & Morgan, D. G. (1995). Enhanced glial fibrillary acidic protein RNA response to fornix transection in aged mice. *Journal of Neurochemistry, 64,* 1351–1360.

Goss, J. R., Finch, C. E., & Morgan, D. G. (1991). Age-related changes in glial fibrillary acidic protein mRNA in the mouse brain. *Neurobiology of Aging, 12* (2), 165–170.

Griffin, W. S. T., Stanley, L. C., Ling, C., White, L., MacLeod, V., Perrot, L. J., White, C. L., III, & Araoz, C. (1989). Brain interleukin 1 and S-100 immunoreactivity are elevated in Down syndrome and Alzheimer's disease. *Proceedings of the National Academy of Sciences of the United States of America, 86,* 7611–7615.

Haga, S., Ikeda, K., Sato, M., & Ishii, T. (1993). Synthetic Alzheimer amyloid beta/A4 peptides enhance production of complement C3 component by cultured microglial cells. *Brain Research, 601* (1–2), 88–94.

Hanks, S. D., & Flood, D. G. (1991). Region-specific stability of dendritic extent in normal human aging and regression in Alzheimer's disease. I. CA1 of hippocampus. *Brain Research, 540* (1–2), 63–82.

Hansen, L. A., Armstrong, D. M., & Terry, R. D. (1987). An immunohistochemical quantification of fibrous astrocytes in the aging human cerebral cortex. *Neurobiology of Aging, 8,* 1–6.

Harrison, D. E., & Archer, J. R. (1987). Genetic differences in effects of food restriction on aging in mice. *Journal of Nutrition, 117,* 376–382.

Henderson, V. W., Paganini-Hill, A., Emanuel, C. K., Dunn, M. E., & Buckwalter, J. G. (1994). Estrogen replacement therapy in older women. Comparisons between Alzheimer's disease cases and nondemented control subjects. *Archives of Neurology, 51* (9), 896–900.

Heroux, J. A., Grigoriadis, D. E., & De Souza, E. B. (1991). Age-related decreases in corticotropin-releasing factor (CRF) receptors in rat brain and anterior pituitary gland. *Brain Research, 542* (1), 155–158.

Hoffman, G. E., & Finch, C. E. (1986). LHRH neurons in the female C57BL/6J mouse brain during reproductive aging: No loss up to middle-age. *Neurobiology of Aging, 7*, 45–48.

Holcomb, L. A., Gordon, M. N., Schreier, W. A., & Morgan, D. G. (1994). Enhanced glial response to nigrostriatal lesion in aged rats. *Society for Neuroscience, Abstracts, 20*, 48 (No. 28.9).

Itagaki, S., McGeer, P. L., Akiyama, H., Zhu, S., & Selkoe, D. (1989). Relationship of microglia and astrocytes to amyloid deposits of Alzheimer disease. *Journal of Neuroimmunology, 24*, 173–182.

Johnson, H., Ulfhake, B., Dagerlind, A., Bennett, G. W., Fone, K. C., & Hokfelt, T. (1993). The serotoninergic bulbospinal system and brainstem-spinal cord content of serotonin-, TRH-, and substance P-like immunoreactivity in the aged rat with special reference to the spinal cord motor nucleus. *Synapse, 15* (1), 63–89.

Johnson, S. A., Rogers, J., & Finch, C. E. (1989). APP-695 transcript prevalence is selectively reduced during Alzheimer's disease in cortex and hippocampus but not in cerebellum. *Neurobiology of Aging, 10* (3), 267–272.

Johnson, S. A., McNeill, T., Cordell, B., & Finch, C. E. (1990). Relation of Neuronal APP-751/APP-695 mRNA Ratio and Neuritic Plaque Density in Alzheimer's Disease. *Science, 248*, 854–857.

Johnson, S. A., Lampert-Etchells, M., Pasinetti, G. M., Rozovsky, I., & Finch, C. E. (1992). Complement mRNA in the mammalian brain: responses to Alzheimer's disease and experimental brain lesioning. *Neurobiology of Aging, 13* (6), 641–648.

Kalaria, R. N. (1992). Serum amyloid P and related molecules associated with the acute phase response in Alzheimer's disease. *Research in Immunology, 143* (6), 637–641.

Kalaria, R. N., & Kroon, S. N. (1992). Complement inhibitor C4-binding protein in amyloid deposits containing serum amyloid P in Alzheimer's disease. *Biochemical and Biophysical Research Communications, 186* (1), 461–466.

Kang, J., & Muller, H. B. (1989). The sequence of the two extra exons in rat preA4. *Nucleic Acids Research, 17* (5).

Karelus, K., & Nelson, J. F. (1992). Aging impairs estrogenic suppression of hypothalamic proopiomelanocortin messenger ribonucleic acid in the mouse. *Neuroendocrinology, 55* (6), 627–633.

Katzman, R., & Kawas, C. (1994). The Epidemiology of Dementia and Alzheimer Disease. In R. K. R. D. Terry & K. L. Bick (Eds.), *Alzheimer Disease*. New York: Raven Press, Ltd.

Kimball, S. R., Vary, T. C., & Jefferson, L. S. (1992). Age-dependent decrease in the amount of eukaryotic initiation factor 2 in various rat tissues. *Biochemistry Journal, 286* (Part 1), 263–268.

Kitaguchi, N., Takahashi, Y., Tokushima, Y., Shiojiri, S., & Ito, H. (1988). Novel precursor of Alzheimer's disease amyloid protein shows protease inhibitory activity. *Nature, 331* (6156), 530–532.

Kitraki, E., Bozas, E., Philippidis, H., & Stylianopoulou, F. (1993). Aging-related changes in IGF-II and c-fos gene expression in the rat brain. *International Journal of Developments in Neuroscience, 11* (1), 1–9.

Klegeris, A., & McGeer, P. L. (1994). Rat brain microglia and peritoneal macrophages show similar responses to respiratory burst stimulants. *Journal of Neuroimmunology, 53*, 83–90.

Kohama, S. G., Goss, J. R., Finch, C. E., & McNeill, T. H. (1995). Increases of glial fibrillary acidic protein in the aging female mouse brain. *Neurobiology of Aging, 16*, 59–67.

Konig, G., Salbaum, J. M., Wiestler, O., Lang, W., Schmitt, H. P., Masters, C. L., & Beyreuther, K. (1991). Alternative splicing of the βA4 amyloid gene of Alzheimer's disease in cortex of control and Alzheimer's disease patients. *Molecular Brain Research, 9*, 159–262.

Koo, E. H., Sisodia, S. S., Cork, L. C., Unterbeck, A., Bayney, R. M., & Price, D. L. (1990). Differential expression of amyloid precursor protein mRNAs in cases of Alzheimer's disease and in aged nonhuman primates. *Neuron, 4* (1), 97–104.

Koo, E. H., Abraham, C. R., Potter, H., Cork, L. C., & Price, D. L. (1991). Developmental Expression of alpha1-Antichymotrypsin in Brain May Be Related to Astrogliosis. *Neurobiology of Aging, 12*, 495–501.

Kosik, K. S., Orecchio, L. D., Bakalis, S., & Neve, R. L. (1989). Developmentally regulated expression of specific tau sequences. *Neuron, 2,* 1389–1397.

Landfield, P. W., & Eldridge, J. C. (1994). Evolving aspects of the glucocorticoid hypothesis of brain aging: Hormonal modulation of neuronal calcium homeostasis. *Neurobiology of Aging, 15* (4), 579–588.

Landfield, P. W., Rose, G., Sandles, L., Wohlstadter, T. C., & Lynch, G. (1977). Patterns of astroglial hypertrophy and neuronal degeneration in the hippocampus of aged memory-deficient rats. *Journal of Gerontology, 32,* 3–12.

Landfield, P. W., Braun, L. D., Pitler, T. A., Lindsey, J. D., & Lynch, G. (1981). Hippocampal aging in rats: a morphometric study of multiple variables in semithin sections. *Neurobiology of Aging, 2,* 265–275.

Lapchak, P. A., Araujo, D. M., Beck, K. D., Finch, C. E., Johnson, S. A., & Hefti, F. (1993). BDNF and trkB mRNA expression in the hippocampal formation of aging rats. *Neurobiology of Aging, 14* (2), 121–126.

Laping, N. J., Morgan, T. E., Nichols, N. R., Rozovsky, I., Young-Chan, C. S., Zarow, C., & Finch, C. E. (1994a). Transforming growth factor β-1 induces neuronal and astrocyte genes: Tubulin alpha-1, glial fibrillary acidic protein, and clusterin. *Neuroscience, 58,* 563–572.

Laping, N. J., Nichols, N. R., Day, J. R., Johnson, S. A., & Finch, C. E. (1994b). Transcriptional control of hippocampal glial fibrillary acidic protein and glutamine synthetase in vivo: opposite responses to corticosterone. *Endocrinology, 135,* 1928–1933.

Laping, N. J., Teter, B., Anderson, C., O'Callaghan, J. P., Johnson, S. A., & Finch, C. E. (1994c). Age-related increases in glial fibrillary acidic protein are not associated with proportionate changes in transcription rates or DNA methylation in the cerebral cortex and hippocampus of male rats. *Journal of Neuroscience Research, 39,* 710–717.

Laping, N. J., Teter, B., Nichols, N. R., Rosovsky, I., & Finch, C. E. (1994d). Glial fibrillary acidic protein: regulation by hormones, cytokines, and growth factors. *Brain Pathology, 4,* 259–274.

Lee, S., Francoeur, A. M., Liu, S., & Wang, E. (1992). Tissue-specific expression in mammalian brain, heart, and muscle of S1, a member of the elongation factor-1 alpha gene family. *Journal of Biological Chemistry, 267* (33), 24064–24068.

Lee, V. M.-Y., & Trojanowski, J. Q. (1992). The disordered neuronal cytoskeleton in Alzheimer's disease. *Current Opinions in Neurobiology, 2,* 653–656.

Lindsey, J. D., Landfield, P. W., & Lynch, G. (1979). Early onset and topographical distribution of hypertrophied astrocytes in hippocampus of aging rats: a quantitative study. *Journal of Gerontology, 34,* 661–671.

Linnemann, D., Gaardsvoll, H., Olsen, M., & Bock, E. (1993). Expression of NCAM mRNA and polypeptides in aging rat brain. *International Journal of Developments in Neuroscience, 11* (1), 71–81.

Lloyd, J. M., Scarbrough, K., Weiland, N. G., & Wise, P. M. (1991). Age-related changes in proopiomelanocortin (POMC) gene expression in the periarcuate region of ovariectomized rats. *Endocrinology, 129* (4), 1896–1902.

Lloyd, J., Hoffman, G., & Wise, P. (1994). Decline in immediate early gene expression in GnRH-neurons during proestrus regularly cycling, middle-aged rats. *Endocrinology, 134,* 1800–1805.

Luft, R. (1994). The development of mitochondrial medicine. *Proceedings of the National Academy of Sciences of the United States of America, 91,* 8731–8738.

Major, D. E., Kesslak, J. P., Cotman, C. W., Finch, C. E., & Day, D. R. (1994). Life-long dietary restriction attenuates age-related increases in glial fibrillary acidic protein (GFAP) mRNA in the rat hippocampus. Paper presented at the Society for Neuroscience, Miami.

Martinoli, M. G., Ouellet, J., Rheaume, E., & Pelletier, G. (1991). Growth hormone and somatostatin gene expression in adult and aging rats as measured by quantitative in situ hybridization. *Neuroendocrinology, 54,* 607–615.

Marttila, R. J., & Rinne, U. K. (1981). Epidemiology of Parkinson's disease—an overview. *Journal of Neural Transmitters, 51,* 135–148.

Masliah, E., Mallory, M., Hansen, L., DeTeresa, R., & Terry, R. D. (1993). Quantitative synaptic alterations in the human neocortex during aging. *Neurology, 43,* 192–197.

Mathewson, A. J., & Berry, M. (1985).

Observations on the astrocyte response to a cerebral stab wound in adult rats. *Brain Research, 327,* 61–69.

Mays-Hoopes, L. L. (1989). Age-related changes in DNA methylation: Do they represent continued developmental changes? *International Reviews in Cytology, 114,* 181–220.

McGeer, P. L., Kawamata, T., & Walker, D. G. (1992). Distribution of clusterin in Alzheimer brain tissue. *Brain Research, 579* (2), 337–341.

Mesco, E. R., Joseph, J. A., Blake, M. J., & Roth, G. S. (1991). Loss of D2 receptors during aging is partially due to decreased levels of mRNA. *Brain Research, 545* (1–2), 355–357.

Mesco, E. R., Carlson, S. G., Joseph, J. A., & Roth, G. S. (1993). Decreased striatal D2 dopamine receptor mRNA synthesis during aging. *Brain Research: Molecular Brain Research, 17* (1–2), 160–162.

Miller, D. T., & Blumenthal, H. T. (1978). Neuron-thymic lymphocyte binding by serum IgG of 90- and 500-day-old female Wistar albino rats. *Journal of Gerontology, 33,* 329–336.

Miller, M. M., Joshi, D., Billiar, R. B., & Nelson, J. F. (1991). Loss during aging of beta-endorphinergic neurons in the hypothalamus of female C57BL/6J mice. *Neurobiology of Aging, 12* (3), 239–244.

Mooradian, A. D. (1988). Effect of aging on the blood-brain barrier. *Neurobiology of Aging, 9,* 31–39.

Morgan, T. E., Nichols, N. R., Pasinetti, G. M., & Finch, C. E. (1993). TGF-β1 mRNA increases in macrophage/microglial cells of the hippocampus in response to deafferentation and kainic acid-induced neurodegeneration. *Experimental Neurology, 120,* 291–301.

Nagatsu, T. (1991). Genes for human catecholamine-synthesizing enzymes. *Neuroscience Research, 12* (2), 315–345.

Nichols, N. R., Osterburg, H. H., Masters, J. N., Millar, S. L., & Finch, C. E. (1990). Messenger RNA for glial fibrillary acidic protein is decreased in rat brain following acute and chronic corticosterone treatment. *Molecular Brain Research, 7,* 1–7.

Nichols, N. R., Day, J. R., Laping, N. J., Johnson, S. A., & Finch, C. E. (1993). GFAP mRNA increases with age in rat and human brain. *Neurobiology of Aging, 14* (5), 421–429.

Nichols, N. R., Finch, C. E., & Nelson, J. F. (1995). Effect of food restriction on the age-related increases of glial fibrillary acidic protein and glutamine synthetase mRNAs in the hypothalamus of male F344 rats. *Neurobiology of Aging, 16,* 105–110.

Nordstedt, C., Gandy, S. E., Alafuzoff, I., Caporaso, G. L., Iverfeldt, K., Grebb, J. A., Winblad, B., & Greengard, P. (1991). Alzheimer β/A4 amyloid precursor protein in human brain: Aging-associated increases in holoprotein and in a proteolytic fragment. *Proceedings of the National Academy of Sciences of the United States of America, 88,* 8910–8914.

O'Callaghan, J. P., & Miller, D. B. (1988). Acute exposure of the neonatal rat to triethyltin results in persistent changes in neurotypic and gliotypic proteins. *Journal of Pharmacology and Experimental Therapeutics, 244,* 368–378.

O'Callaghan, J. P., & Miller, D. B. (1991). The concentration of glial fibrillary acidic protein increases with age in the mouse and rat brain. *Neurobiology of Aging, 12,* 171–174.

Ogomori, K., Kitamoto, T., Tateishi, J., Sato, Y., & Tashima, T. (1988). Aging and cerebral amyloid: Early detection of amyloid in the human brain using biochemical extraction and immunostain. *Journal of Gerontology, 43,* B157–B162.

Oka, Y., Asano, T., Tsukuda, K., Katagiri, H., Ishihara, H., Inukai, K., & Yazaki, Y. (1992). Expression of glucose transporter isoforms with aging. *Gerontology, 38,* 3–9.

Oyama, F., Shimada, H., Oyama, R., Titani, K., & Ihara, Y. (1992). A novel correlation between the levels of beta-amyloid protein precursor and tau transcripts in the aged human brain. *Journal of Neurochemistry, 59* (3), 1117–1125.

Oyama, F., Shimada, H., Oyama, R., Titani, K., & Ihara, Y. (1993). Beta-amyloid protein precursor and tau mRNA levels versus beta-amyloid plaque and neurofibrillary tangles in the aged human brain. *Journal of Neurochemistry, 60* (5), 1658–1664.

Pagani, F., Zagato, L., Vergani, C., Casari, G., Sidoli, A., & Baralle, F. E. (1991). Tissue-specific splicing pattern of fibronectin messenger RNA precursor during development and aging in rat. *Journal of Cell Biology, 113* (5), 1223–1229.

Pardue, S., Groshan, K., Raese, J. D., & Morrison-Bogorad, M. (1992). Hsp70 mRNA induction is reduced in neurons of aged rat hippocampus after thermal stress. *Neurobiology of Aging, 13* (6), 661–672.

Park, G. H., & Buetow, D. E. (1991). Genes for insulin-like growth factors I and II are expressed in senescent rat tissues. *Gerontology, 37* (6), 310–316.

Pasinetti, G., Johnson, S., Rozovsky, I., Lampert-Etchells, M., Morgan, D., Gordon, M., Morgan, T., Willoughby, D., & Finch, C. (1992). Complement C1qB and C4 mRNA Responses to Lesioning in Rat Brain. *Experimental Neurology, 118,* 117–125.

Peiffer, A., Barden, N., & Meaney, M. J. (1991). Age-related changes in glucocorticoid receptor binding and mRNA levels in rat brain and pituitary. *Neurobiology of Aging, 12* (5), 475–479.

Perry, V. H., & Lawson, L. J. (1992). Macrophages in the central nervous system. In C. E. L. a. J. O. D. McGee (Ed.), *The Macrophage* (pp. 391–414). Oxford: Oxford University Press.

Perry, V. H., Matyszak, M. K., & Fearn, S. (1993). Altered antigen expression of microglia in the aged rodent CNS. *Glia, 7,* 60–67.

Ponte, P., Gonzalez, D. P., Schilling, J., Miller, J., Hsu, D., Greenberg, B., Davis, K., Wallace, W., Lieberburg, I., & Fuller, F. (1988). A new A4 amyloid mRNA contains a domain homologous to serine proteinase inhibitors. *Nature, 331* (6156), 525–527.

Randerath, K., Putman, K. L., Osterburg, H. H., Johnson, S. A., Morgan, D. G., & Finch, C. E. (1993). Age-dependent increases of DNA adducts (I-compounds) in human and rat brain DNA. *Mutation Research, 295,* 11–18.

Rao, G., Xia, E., & Richardson, A. (1990). Effect of age on the expression of antioxidant enzymes in male Fischer 344 rats. *Mechanisms of Ageing and Development, 53,* 49–60.

Reff, M. E. (1985). RNA and Protein Metabolism. In C. E. Finch & E. L. Schneider (Eds.), *Handbook of the Biology of Aging* (2nd ed., pp. 1025). New York: Van Nostrand Reinhold Co.

Regeur, L., Jensen, G. B., Pakkenberg, H., Evans, S. M., & Pakkenberg, B. (1994). No global neocortical nerve cell loss in brains from patients with senile dementia of the Alzheimer's type. *Neurobiology of Aging, 15* (3), 347–352.

Rogers, J., Luber-Narod, J., Styren, S. D., & Civin, W. H. (1988). Expression of immune system-associated antigens by cells of the human central nervous system: Relationship to the pathology of Alzheimer disease. *Neurobiology of Aging, 9* (4), 339–349.

Rogers, J., Kirby, L. C., Hempleman, S. R., Berry, D. L., McGeer, P. L., Kasniak, A. W., Zalinski, J., Cofield, M., Mansukhani, M. H. S. A., Willson, P., & Kogan, F. (1993). Clinical trial of indomethacin in Alzheimer's disease. *Neurology, 43,* 1609–1611.

Rossmanith, W., Reichelt, C., & Scherbaum, W. (1994). Neuroendocrinology of aging in humans: Attenuated sensitivity to sex steroid feedback in elderly postmenopausal women. *Neuroendocrinology, 59,* 355–362.

Rumble, B., Retallak, R., Montgomery, P., Beyreuther, K., & Masters, C. L. (1989). Amyloid A4 protein and its precursor in Down's syndrome and Alzheimer's disease. *New England Journal of Medicine, 320,* 1446–1452.

Russell, M. J., White, R., Patel, E., Markesbery, W. R., Watson, C. R., & Geddes, J. W. (1992). Familial influence on plaque formation in the beagle brain. *NeuroReport, 3,* 1093–1096.

Sakata, M., Farooqui, S. M., & Prasad, C. (1992). Post-transcriptional regulation of loss of rat striatal D2 dopamine receptor during aging. *Brain Research, 575* (2), 309–314.

Sapolsky, R. M. (1992). *Stress, the Aging Brain, and the Mechanisms of Neuron Death.* MIT Press.

Sawada, M., Kondo, N., Suzumura, A., & Marunouchi, T. (1989). Production of tumor necrosis factor-alpha by microglia and astrocytes in culture. *Brain Research, 491,* 394–397.

Schiffmann, S. N., & Vanderhaeghen, J. J. (1993). Age-related loss of mRNA encoding adenosine A2 receptor in the rat striatum. *Neuroscience Letters, 158* (2), 121–124.

Schipper, H., Brawer, J. R., Nelson, J. F., Felicio, L. S., & Finch, C. E. (1981). The role of gonads in the histologic aging of the hypothalamic arcuate nucleus. *Biology of Reproduction, 25,* 413–419.

Schmale, H., & Richter, D. (1984). Single base deletion in the vasopressin gene is the cause of diabetes insipidus in Brattleburo rats. *Nature, 308,* 705–709.

Schmale, H., Borowiak, B., Holtgreve-Grez, H., & Richter, D. (1989). Impact of altered protein structures on the intracellular traffic of a mutated vasopressin precursor from Brattleburo rats. *European Journal of Biochemistry, 182*, 621–627.

Semsei, I., Rao, G., & Richardson, A. (1991). Expression of superoxide dismutase and catalase in rat brain as a function of age. *Mechanisms of Ageing and Development, 58* (1), 13–19.

Shigenaga, M. K., Hagen, T. M., & Ames, B. N. (1994). Oxidative damage and mitochondrial decay in aging. *Proceedings of the National Academy of Sciences of the United States of America, 91*, 10771–10778.

Shivers, B. D., Hilbich, C., Multhaup, G., Salbaum, M., Beyreuther, K., & Seeburg, P. H. (1988). Alzheimer's disease amyloidogenic glycoprotein: expression pattern in rat brain suggests a role in cell contact. *EMBO Journal, 7* (5), 1365–1370.

Slagboom, P. E., De Leeuw, W. J., & Vijg, J. (1990). Messenger RNA levels and methylation patterns of GAPDH and β-actin genes in rat liver, spleen and brain in relation to aging. *Mechanisms of Ageing and Development, 53*, 243–257.

Sobin, S. S., Bernick, S., & Ballard, K. W. (1992). Histochemical characterization of the aging microvasculature in the human and other mammalian and non-mammalian vertebrates by periodic acid-Schiff reaction. *Mechanisms of Ageing and Development, 63*, 183–192.

Soong, N. W., Hinton, D. R., Cortopassi, G., & Arnheim, N. (1992). Mosaicism for a specific somatic mitochondrial DNA mutation in adult human brain. *Nature Genetics, 2* (4), 318–323.

Steward, O., Torre, F. R., Tomasulo, R., & Lothman, E. (1991). Neuronal activity up-regulates astroglial gene expression. *Proceedings of the National Academy of Sciences of the United States of America, 88*, 6819–6823.

Stewart, D. A., Blackman, M. R., Kowatch, M. A., Danner, D. B., & Roth, G. S. (1992). Discordant effects of aging on prolactin and luteinizing hormone-β messenger ribonucleic acid levels in the female rat. *Endocrinology, 126*, 773–778.

Strauss, S., Bauer, J., Ganter, U., Jonas, U., Ber-

ger, M., & Volk, B. (1992). Detection of Interleukin-6 and a2-macroglobulin immunoreactivity in cortex and hippocampus of Alzheimer's disease patients. *Laboratory Investigations, 66* (2), 223–230.

Streit, W. J., Graeber, M. B., & Kreutzberg, G. W. (1988). Functional Plasticity of Microglia: A review. *Glia, 1*, 301–307.

Styren, S. D., Civin, W. H., & Rogers, J. (1990). Molecular, cellular, and pathologic characterization of HLA-DR immunoreactivity in normal elderly and Alzheimer's disease brain. *Experimental Neurology, 110*, 93–104.

Szilard, L. (1959). On the nature of the aging process. *Proceedings of the National Academy of Sciences of the United States of America, 45*, 30–45.

Tanaka, S., Shiojiri, S., Takahashi, Y., Kitaguchi, N., Ito, H., Kameyama, M., Kimura, J., Nakamura, S., & Ueda, K. (1989). Tissue-specific expression of three types of beta-protein precursor mRNA: enhancement of protease inhibitor-harboring types in Alzheimer's disease brain. *Biochemical Biophysical Research Communications, 165* (3), 1406–1414.

Tanaka, S., Liu, L., Kimura, J., Shiojiri, S., Takahashi, Y., Kitaguchi, N., Nakamura, S., & Ueda, K. (1992a). Age-related changes in the proportion of amyloid precursor protein mRNAs in Alzheimer's disease and other neurological disorders. *Brain Research: Molecular Brain Research, 15* (3–4), 303–310.

Tanaka, S., Liu, L., Kimura, J., Shiojiri, S., Takahashi, Y., Kitagushi, N., Makamura, S., & Ueda, K. (1992b). Age-related changes in the proportion of amyloid precursor protein mRNAs in Alzheimer's disease and other neurological disorders. *Molecular Brain Research, 15*, 303–310.

Tanaka, S., Nakamura, S., Kimura, J., & Ueda, K. (1993). Age-related change in the proportion of amyloid precursor protein mRNAs in the gray matter of cerebral cortex. *Neuroscience Letters, 163*, 19–21.

Tanzi, R. E., McClatchey, A. I., Lamperti, E. D., Villa, K. L., Gusella, J. F., & Neve, R. L. (1988). Protease inhibitor domain encoded by an amyloid protein precursor mRNA associated with Alzheimer's disease. *Nature, 331* (6156), 528–530.

Terry, R. D., DeTeresa, R., & Hansen, L. A.

(1987). Neocortical cell counts in normal human adult aging. *Annals of Neurology, 21,* 530–539.

van Eekelen, J. A., Rots, N. Y., Sutanto, W., Oitzl, M. S., & de Kloet, E. R. (1991). Brain corticosteroid receptor gene expression and neuroendocrine dynamics during aging. *Journal of Steroid Biochemistry and Molecular Biology, 40* (4–6), 679–683.

van Leeuwen, F. W., Evans, D. A., Meloen, R., & Sonnemans, M. A. (1994). Differential neurophysin immunoreactivities in solitary magnocellular neurons of the homozygous Brattleboro rat indicate an altered neurophysin moiety. *Brain Research, 635* (1–2), 328–330.

Van Remmen, H., Ward, W., Sabia, R. V., & Richardson, A. (1995). Effect of Age on Gene Expression and Protein Degradation. In E. Maser (Ed.), *Handbook of Physiology Volume on Aging.* Oxford: Oxford University Press.

Vaughn, D. W., & Peters, A. (1974). Neuroglial cells in the cerebral cortex of rats from young adulthood to old age: An electron microscope study. *Journal of Neurocytology, 3,* 405–429.

Vermersch, P., Frigard, B., David, J. P., Fallet-Blanco, C., & Delacourte, A. (1992). Presence of abnormally phosphorylated Tau proteins in the entorhinal cortex of aged non-demented subjects. *Neuroscience Letters, 144,* 143–146.

Wagner, A. P., Reck, G., & Platt, D. (1993). Evidence that V+ fibronectin, GFAP and S100 beta mRNAs are increased in the hippocampus of aged rats. *Experimental Gerontology, 28* (2), 135–143.

Wallace, D. C. (1994). Mitochrondrial DNA sequence variation in human evolution and disease. *Proceedings of the National Academy of Sciences of the United States of America, 91,* 8739–8746.

Wang, S. Z., Zhu, S. Z., Joseph, J. A., & el-Fakahany, E. E. (1992). Comparison of the level of mRNA encoding m1 and m2 muscarinic receptors in brains of young and aged rats. *Neuroscience Letters, 145* (2), 149–152.

Weiland, N. G., Scarbrough, K., & Wise, P. M. (1992) Aging abolishes the estradiol-induced suppression and diurnal rhythm of pro-opiomelanocortin gene expression in the arcuate nucleus. *Endocrinology, 131* (6), 2959–2964.

West, M. J. (1993). Regionally specific loss of neurons in the aging human hippocampus. *Neurobiology of Aging, 14,* 287–293.

Wink, D. A., Kasprzak, K. S., Maragos, C. M., Elespuru, R. K., Misra, M., Dunams, T. M., Cebula, T. A., Koch, W. H., Andrews, A. W., Allen, J. S., *et al.* (1991). DNA deaminating ability and genotoxicity of nitric oxide and its progenitors. *Science, 254* (5034), 1001–1003.

Wisniewski, H. M., Ghetti, B., & Terry, R. D. (1973). Neuritic (senile) plaques and filamentous changes in aged Rhesus monkeys. *Journal of Neuropathology Experiments in Neurology, 32* (4), 566–584.

Yamada, T., Sasaki, H., Furuya, H., Miyata, T., Goto, I., & Sakaki, Y. (1987). Complementary DNA for the mouse homolog of the human amyloid beta protein precursor. *Biochemical and Biophysical Research Communications, 149,* 665–671.

Yao, J., Keri, J., Taffs, R., & Colton, C. (1992). Characterization of interleukin-1 production by microglia in culture. *Brain Research, 591,* 88–93.

Zhang, J., Dawson, V. L., Dawson, T. M., & Snyder, S. H. (1994). Nitric oxide activation of poly(ADP-ribose) synthetase in neurotoxicity. *Science, 263,* 687–689.

Part Five

Physiology, Endocrinology, and Nutrition

Edited by John W. Rowe and Edward L. Schneider

Fifteen

Exercise Physiology and Aging

Andrew P. Goldberg, Donald R. Dengel, and James M. Hagberg

I. Introduction

Aging in healthy, sedentary people is accompanied by a decline in cardiovascular and endocrine metabolic functions. Physical inactivity and immobility also result in numerous undesirable physiological consequences, including declines in cardiovascular fitness and lean body mass and the development of obesity. These changes contribute to the progressive decline in cardiovascular and endocrine metabolic functions with aging, increasing susceptibility for the development of noninsulin-dependent diabetes (NIDDM), hyperlipidemia, and hypertension, conditions that accelerate the development of atherosclerotic cardiovascular disease (CVD). Evaluation of the role of physical inactivity in the decline in physiological function with aging and the potential for regular physical exercise to maintain functional capacity and reduce risk factors for CVD is an important area of gerontologic research.

Aging and physical inactivity often coexist due to changes in lifestyle or the development of diseases that limit function to cause disability. Examination of the independent effects of primary biological aging on organ function is confounded by limitations inherent to the systematic examination of the effects of age, lifestyle, and disease on the functional capacity of the aging human. Careful attention to experimental design in the conduct of gerontologic research enhances the ability to distinguish the physiological changes associated with primary aging from the effects of lifestyle habits and chronic diseases, conditions considered secondary aging processes (Rowe & Kahn, 1987). Results of research studies that compare individuals of varying age, i.e., cross-sectional studies, are unable to discern the effects of nutrition, exercise, and coexistent diseases on changes in functional capacity with aging. However, when physiological function is examined over a lifetime in the same individual, i.e., a longitudinal study design, mechanisms for the progression of functional declines with aging can be ascertained by documentation of the effects of disease and changes in diet, exercise, smoking, and other habits on physiological function. Indeed, it may be possible to evaluate the pathophysiological effects of primary aging in a longitudinal study of healthy, older people carefully screened at entry for

Handbook of the Biology of Aging, Fourth Edition
Copyright © 1996 Academic Press, Inc. All rights of reproduction in any form reserved.

diseases and functional disabilities. Laboratory animals kept free of disease also might be suitable models to examine the effects of physical activity and diet on age-related functional declines. Insight into the processes by which aging affects function and the potential for exercise to maximize health and prevent morbidity would permit the development of guidelines for the prevention of disease and the promotion of health in older persons.

The deterioration in physiological function that occurs in healthy, physically active older individuals with prudent lifestyles is, by definition, "normal aging." Regularly performed vigorous exercise prevents abnormalities that are the result of being sedentary; even short periods of physical inactivity worsen cardiovascular performance, muscle structure and function, and glucose and lipid metabolism (Coyle *et al.*, 1984; Saltin *et al.*, 1968). The profiles of these physiological changes parallel many of the changes often attributed to aging. Regularly performed activity induces adaptations that compensate for some of the functional declines associated with aging, primarily because the habits of physically active older people may have prevented the development of the endocrine metabolic and cardiovascular risk factors that accelerate CVD and its complications (Bjorntorp, 1993; Blair *et al.*, 1989; Bouchard, Despres, & Tremblay, 1993; Kissebah & Krakower, 1994; Lakatta, 1993; Manson *et al.*, 1992; Paffenbarger *et al.*, 1993; Sandvik *et al.*, 1993). This would suggest that the development of NIDDM, hypertension, or hyperlipidemia in some older individuals is not the result of aging or disease, but is related to the effects of sedentariness and imprudent dietary habits. An understanding of the effects of regular exercise training on the physiological factors that influence the declines in cardiovascular and endocrine metabolic functions with aging may improve the health and functional well-being of the elderly.

This chapter reviews the interactions between physical conditioning status and the physiological changes that often accompany aging. Some aspects of the effects of obesity on these processes are reviewed, but a more thorough discussion is found elsewhere (Bjorntorp, 1993; Bouchard *et al.*, 1993; Kissebah & Krakower, 1994). Evidence will be presented that demonstrates that regular physical exercise training can prevent or reverse many of the physiological declines in cardiovascular and endocrine metabolic functions that occur with aging to increase risk for CVD. This suggests that the implementation of exercise training on a regular basis early or even later in life may help prevent the development of risk factors for CVD and prove to be a realistic strategy to maintain the functional status, health, and independence of older people.

II. Principles of Exercise Physiology

A. Maximal Aerobic Capacity and Aging

Maximal oxygen uptake (V_{O_2max}) is the primary measure of maximal cardiovascular function in older as well as younger individuals. It is defined as the highest rate of oxygen consumption attained during exercise of progressively increasing intensity that requires the use of a large proportion of the total skeletal muscle mass. V_{O_2max} is a function of both maximal cardiac output and maximal arteriovenous oxygen difference $[(A - V)_{O_2}]$, and in healthy people it is generally not believed to be limited by pulmonary function, blood flow, or oxygen uptake by skeletal muscle. Central cardiac and peripheral muscle structure and function are the primary physiological factors limiting V_{O_2max} in healthy older people because they affect the ability of the heart to pump (stroke volume × heart rate) and the ability of muscle to take up and utilize oxygen

(Table I). At submaximal work rates the cardiac output and blood pressure (BP) of trained and untrained individuals are generally similar. However, because trained individuals have larger diastolic left ventricular (LV) volumes and increased stroke volumes (SV) than untrained individuals of the same age, they can achieve a higher maximal cardiac output (Q_{max}), despite similar maximal heart rates (HR_{max}) (Lakatta, 1993). As the intensity of the exercise stimulus increases, cardiac output rises and there is vasoconstriction in the vessels of visceral organs and the skin to redistribute blood flow so that the maximal supply of oxygen is provided to the myocardium and exercising muscle. As $V_{O_2 max}$ is approached during a progressive exercise test, HR, SV, Q, and the $(A - V)_{O_2}$ difference peak and then plateau. $V_{O_2 max}$ is highly reproducible during treadmill exercise using a multistage protocol, provided >50% of muscle mass is exercised (Tonino & Driscoll, 1988).

Older endurance-trained athletes have $V_{O_2 max}$ values nearly twice those of sedentary age-matched peers and nearly comparable to that of an average 20-year-old sedentary individual (Heath, Hagberg, Ehsani, & Holloszy, 1981) (Fig. 1). An age-related decline in $V_{O_2 max}$ is reported in numerous longitudinal and cross-sectional studies of sedentary and physically active subjects. This decline may be exaggerated in longitudinal studies when $V_{O_2 max}$ is expressed in ml kg^{-1} min^{-1}, because of the gain in body weight that occurs in sedentary

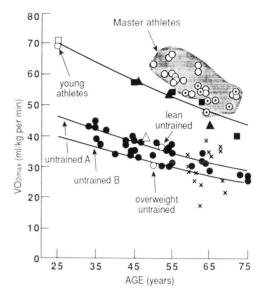

Figure 1. $V_{O_2 max}$ is depicted as a function of age as measured in males of varying ages, cardiovascular fitness, and body composition. Points are average $V_{O_2 max}$ levels for groups of men of different ages from reports in the literature for younger and older athletes and lean and overweight untrained men (Heath *et al.*, 1981; Lakatta, 1993). Symbols as in Lakatta (1993): Champion young athletes, ○ and □; exchampion athletes, △; cross-country runners, ▲; runners, ■; groups of men from nine studies, ● and ×; and master athletes, ○ and ⊙.

people; conversely, the decrease in $V_{O_2 max}$ may be attenuated when adjusted per kilogram of lean body mass because of the decline in lean body mass with aging. Thus, we believe it is most appropriate to express $V_{O_2 max}$ in liters minute^{-1} in longitudinal studies where aerobic fitness and body composition are likely to change. The

Table I
Factors Affecting $V_{O_2 max}$ with Aging

Cardiovascular	Peripheral tissues
1. Myocardial contractility	1. Muscle mass/structure
2. Venous capacitance/vascular resistance	2. Blood flow to tissues
3. Coronary blood flow	3. Muscle capillary density
4. Valvular function	4. Oxygen transport/tissue extraction
5. Myocardial mass	5. Blood volume
6. β-Adrenergic (SNS) responses/maximal heart rate	6. Pulmonary function

aforementioned caveats also should be considered in the interpretation of V_{O_2max} levels from cross-sectional studies (Toth, Goran, Ades, Howard, & Poehlman, 1993). The decline in V_{O_2max} with aging can have a multifactorial etiology, beginning around age 25–30 years and progressing over time due to declines in both central and peripheral functions, the primary factors limiting V_{O_2max} (Table I). Depending on an individual's level of physical activity, V_{O_2max} can vary by as much as 100%. The development of disease, especially CVD, dramatically lowers V_{O_2max}, but exercise rehabilitation and endurance training will improve V_{O_2max} in individuals with CVD (Hiatt, Regensteiner, & Wolfel, 1993).

Cross-sectional data estimate that the relative rate of decline in V_{O_2max} is 8% per decade in males and 10% per decade in females (Toth, Gardner, Ades, & Poehlman, 1994). Although a number of these studies showed that older athletes experienced the same, and in some cases a greater, decline in V_{O_2max} with age than their sedentary peers (Grimby & Saltin, 1966; Pollock, Miller, & Wilmore, 1974), they did not consider the physiological effects of the reduction in training observed in longitudinal studies of older athletes (Pollock, Foster, Knapp, Rod, & Schmidt, 1987; Robinson, Dill, Robinson, Tzankoff, & Wagner, 1976; Rogers, Hagberg, Martin, Ehsani, & Holloszy, 1990a). Most of the cross-sectional studies also did not screen the older subjects for occult disease. Participants in the Baltimore Longitudinal Study on Aging (BLSA) undergo careful evaluations of cardiovascular health prior to evaluation. Results from the BLSA suggest that in healthy older people changes in peripheral skeletal muscle, circulatory factors, and disease contribute to the decline in V_{O_2max} with advancing age more than changes in central cardiac function (Fleg & Lakatta, 1988; Fleg et al., 1993; Rodeheffer et al., 1984). After the decline in V_{O_2max} with aging is attenuated by con-

trolling differences in fat free and fat mass (Fleg & Lakatta, 1988), further adjustment for leisure time physical activity suggests that physical inactivity also contributes to the decline in V_{O_2max} with aging (Toth et al., 1994). Thus, over the human life span, the maintenance of muscle mass, prevention of obesity, and performance of regular physical activity may lessen the magnitude of the decline in V_{O_2max} with aging (Lakatta, Goldberg, Fleg, Fortney, & Drinkwater, 1988).

A number of longitudinal studies performed in sedentary individuals also show that V_{O_2max} declines with aging at a rate of 10–13% per decade in males and 7–11% per decade in females. In general, V_{O_2max} declines at an average rate of 5–9% per decade in older athletes when physical activity levels are maintained and body composition does not change (Pollock et al., 1974, 1987; Robinson et al., 1976; Rogers, Hagberg, et al., 1990a). In studies that compared the cardiovascular performance of young and older endurance athletes matched on the basis of their training, the difference in V_{O_2max} between the young and older athletes was 5% per decade, a rate approximately 50% less than that reported in relatively unscreened sedentary populations (Hagberg et al., 1985; Heath et al., 1981). In longitudinal studies, V_{O_2max} did not decrease in 60-year-old athletes who maintained a relatively constant training program over the preceding decade; however, in comparably healthy athletes whose training decreased over the same period, V_{O_2max} fell by 12.5% (Pollock et al., 1987). In a later study (Rogers, Hagberg, et al., 1990a), endurance-trained older athletes decreased their V_{O_2max} over an 8-year follow-up by 5.5% per decade, which is half that of a sedentary control population. The limited information comparing cardiovascular function in healthy older and younger athletes matched on the basis of their training regimens and screened carefully for disease suggests that the hemodynamic determinants of V_{O_2max}, other than maximal heart rate, change very little with age in the absence of disease.

Thus, cross-sectional and longitudinal studies examining the age-related decline in $V_{O_2 max}$ generally indicate that it is influenced by the extent of regular physical conditioning, body composition, and disease. A reversal of the decline in $V_{O_2 max}$ with aging by 50 or even 25% would have considerable health benefits, since a reduction in physical activity and $V_{O_2 max}$ is associated with a greater risk of morbidity and mortality, primarily because of their relationship to risk for CVD (Blair et al., 1989; Manson et al., 1992; Paffenbarger et al., 1993; Sandvik et al., 1993). The level of $V_{O_2 max}$ is also an important determinant of endocrine metabolic function, total daily energy requirements, and nutritional status of older individuals, as well as an independent predictor of the decline in resting metabolic rate and lean tissue mass with aging (Gardner & Poehlman, 1993; Goran & Poehlman, 1992; Poehlman et al., 1993; Poehlman, McAuliffe, Van Houten, & Danforth, 1990). The progressive deterioration in the structure and function of connective tissue, joints, muscle, vascular capacity, and myocardial contractility with aging substantially affects the ability of the older individual to maintain a high level of physical activity necessary to prevent a decline in $V_{O_2 max}$ (Fries et al., 1994). Disability is inevitable when $V_{O_2 max}$ decreases to a level where the energy cost of social and recreational activities and activities of daily living approaches an older person's maximal capacity to produce energy by oxidative processes. Thus, the ability to prevent, reverse, or delay the decline in $V_{O_2 max}$ with aging has important implications for sustaining the health and well-being of older people.

B. Cardiovascular Function and Aging

Aging is associated with a decrease in β-adrenergic stimulation of myocardial contractility, an increase in arterial stiffness and total peripheral vascular resistance, a rise in systolic BP, moderate hypertrophy of the LV, a prolongation of myocardial contraction, and a reduction in HR_{max} (Lakatta, 1993). Aging may be responsible for much of this decline in cardiac function; however, the impairment in LV function is greatly exaggerated even in healthy sedentary compared to highly conditioned older individuals. This suggests that a significant component of the decline in cardiovascular function with aging is due to the physical inactivity associated with aging. Cross-sectional comparisons among young and older sedentary and athletic individuals show that older athletes have a pattern of LV filling more similar to younger subjects than their sedentary peers, with enhanced early diastolic filling and stroke volume and a greater rise in cardiac index in response to exercise (Fleg et al., 1994; Ogawa et al., 1992; Rivera et al., 1989; Seals et al., 1994). The finding of the same oxygen pulse during maximal exercise in young and older athletes suggested that the decrease in $V_{O_2 max}$ with aging in older athletes may be due only to the decrease in HR_{max} (Seals et al., 1994). In a cross-sectional report, the higher peak V_{O_2} achieved during exhaustive cycle exercise in older master athletes compared to sedentary peers was related to a higher peak $(A - V)_{O_2}$ difference, with only a modest rise in SV and other central circulatory factors during maximal exercise (Fleg et al., 1994). In studies using the acetylene rebreathing method to measure Q_{max}, the higher $V_{O_2 max}$ in older athletes than in sedentary peers was associated with a higher $(A - V)_{O_2}$ difference maximum and Q_{max} (Ogawa et al., 1992; Rivera et al., 1989); nevertheless, SV_{max} and HR_{max} during exercise were approximately 15% lower in the older than the younger athletes. It is possible that a decline in exercise habits as the athletes aged, the development of occult CVD, or primary aging prevented compensatory cardiovascular changes, such as an augmentation of LV end diastolic volume to prevent the reduction in SV_{max} and Q_{max} in older athletes. Examination of the effects of aerobic exercise training on cardiovascular function in healthy, sedentary older subjects might determine the extent to which some of the declines in cardiovascular function with aging are reversible.

C. Exercise Training and Cardiovascular Function

Healthy older men and women up to age 80 years can adapt to endurance exercise training with an increase in V_{O_2max} that, on a relative basis, is comparable in magnitude to that seen with training younger individuals (Ehsani, Ogawa, Miller, Spina, & Jilka, 1991; Spina, Ogawa, Kohrt, et al., 1993; Stratton, Levy, Cereueira, Schwartz, & Abrass, 1994). If the training intensity, duration, and frequency are sufficient, exercise training can result in substantial improvements in physical performance as well as in hemodynamic and endocrine metabolic functions in the elderly. Left ventricular function, indexed as the rise in the LV ejection fraction from rest to peak exercise, increased less in older men than in young healthy men before exercise, but after aerobic training the increase in ejection fraction from rest to peak exercise was similar in older and younger men (Ehsani et al., 1991). Exercise training in the elderly increased cardiac index at peak exercise in both young and older subjects by increasing the SV index. The increase in SVI was related to the increase in end diastolic volume index and peak ejection fraction, with comparable declines in end SV index in both younger and older men at peak exercise. The increase in systolic BP and decrease in diastolic BP at peak exercise after training were associated with an increased ejection fraction (Ehsani et al., 1991; Stratton et al., 1994). These findings are consistent with an augmentation of

cardiac inotropy after exercise training in older men comparable to that observed in younger men. Thus, despite aging-related changes in cardiovascular function, exercise training can produce adaptations in central cardiac function in healthy older men that are similar to those in younger men. However, older women do not appear to undergo a similar increase in central cardiac function, i.e., Q_{max} or SV_{max}, despite an increase in V_{O_2max} (Spina, Ogawa, Kohrt, et al., 1993a), a difference postulated to be related to estrogen deficiency associated with menopause.

An enhancement in skeletal muscle's ability to extract oxygen also contributes to the rise in V_{O_2max} with exercise training in older individuals. High-intensity training increased V_{O_2max} by about 20% in 60–70-year-old subjects, primarily due to an increase in the estimated $(A - V)_{O_2}$ difference maximum, with little increase in the estimated Q_{max}. In a longitudinal 12-month intensive exercise training study, there was a 15% increase in SV and peak V_{O_2} during treadmill exercise and a 7% increase in the $(A - V)_{O_2}$ difference maximum in older men (Spina, Ogawa, Kohrt, et al., 1993a). In the same study, women increased V_{O_2max} by raising the $(A - V)_{O_2}$ difference maximum achieved during exhaustive exercise, but there was no increase in SV_{max} or HR_{max} (Spina, Ogawa, Miller, Kohrt, & Ehsani, 1993b). In contrast to these findings, low-intensity exercise does not enhance cardiac performance in older individuals (Schocken, Blumenthal, Port, Hindle, & Coleman, 1983). This suggests that the intensity, duration, and frequency of exercise must be substantial for the older individual to increase central cardiovascular function.

D. Exercise and Muscle Structure and Function in the Elderly

Numerous studies confirm a decline in muscle mass with aging. The loss of muscle accounts for much of the decline in basal metabolic rate, muscle strength, and physical activity levels seen in the elderly. Skeletal muscle oxidative enzymes, capillary density, and type II muscle fiber area are also lower in sedentary older men and women than in young, untrained people (Coggan *et al.*, 1992a; Meredith *et al.*, 1989). This reduces the capacity of muscle for aerobic metabolism, and the decrease in mitochondrial enzyme activities limits fatty acid oxidation, glucose and lipid metabolism, and glycogen storage (Holloszy & Coyle, 1984). This decreases oxygen uptake by muscle during exhaustive exercise and contributes to the decline in V_{O_2max} in sedentary older people by reducing the $(A - V)_{O_2}$ difference maximum (Ogawa *et al.*, 1992; Makrides, Heigenhauser, & Jones, 1990).

Skeletal muscle undergoes major structural and functional adaptations in response to physical inactivity, just as it does in response to disease, nutritional status, and obesity, and these effects must be considered when examining the independent effects of aging on muscle structure and function. Gastrocnemius muscle biopsies from endurance-trained athletes in their 60's had capillary densities and mitochondrial enzyme levels similar to those of young athletes and did not show the reduction in type II muscle area seen in sedentary older people (Coggan *et al.*, 1990). Exercise training studies demonstrated increases in mitochondrial enzyme activity, the conversion of type II-B muscle fibers to type II-A fibers, capillary density, and the increased ability of muscles to extract oxygen from the blood during exercise in older subjects (Coggan *et al.*, 1992b; Meredith *et al.*, 1989). This increase was greater on a relative basis than that seen in younger individuals due to the lower initial levels of these indices of muscular function in the elderly prior to training. These skeletal muscle adaptations contribute to the rise in V_{O_2max} in the elderly with training, as these skeletal muscle enzyme adaptations and the in-

crease in blood flow to muscle with exercise training raise the V_{O_2max} in the elderly by increasing the $(A - V)_{O_2}$ difference maximum (Makrides *et al.*, 1990).

Aging-related reductions in muscle mass are a direct cause of declines in muscle strength with aging. This reduction in muscle strength is a major cause of disability in the elderly, as strength and power are major components of gait, balance, and the ability to walk (Bassey *et al.*, 1992). Although resistance or strength training does not increase V_{O_2max}, the muscle hypertrophy and increased strength, changes in body composition, and hormonal and nervous system adaptations have a substantial impact on the daily activities of living and functional independence of the elderly. In frail elderly people living in a nursing home, a high-intensity progressive resistance training program of 8 weeks duration increased strength on the average of 174% with a mean increase in muscle cross-sectional area of 15% (Fiatarone *et al.*, 1990). These increases in muscle size and strength were associated with clinically significant improvements in gait speed, balance, and functional independence. Strength training could also have substantial benefits for protection from injury in the elderly, as falling is strongly related to hip weakness, poor balance, and postural sway. Exercise training rehabilitation instituted after hospitalization due to disease, acute illness, or surgery could prevent disability and institutionalization in the elderly by enhancing muscle function (Felsenthal, Garrison, & Steinberg, 1994).

Although both aerobic and resistance (strength) training are recommended to improve muscular function in the elderly, only resistance training can reverse or delay the decline in muscle mass and strength with aging. Increased strength and mass in the elderly can be an important step in maintaining daily functional activities of independence in older persons where "disuse" atrophy has limited their daily activities. Thus, a substantial proportion of the decline in muscle mass, structure, and function in the elderly is due to disuse, physical inactivity, and disease; the incorporation of aerobic and resistance exercise training into the lifestyle of older individuals can have a considerable impact on the functional capacity and independence, as well as cardiovascular and endocrine metabolic functions, of sedentary, older adults.

E. Summary

A substantial proportion of the decline in cardiovascular function and V_{O_2max} seen with aging in healthy, sedentary older individuals is due to physical inactivity and deconditioning. The decline in cardiovascular and muscle function with aging can be improved by endurance and resistance (strength) exercise training. The physiological adaptations that occur in older individuals in response to this training are, in relative terms (percent of initial), comparable to those of younger subjects and partially explain differences in function derived from cross-sectional comparisons of function across the age span. Physiological improvements with endurance training are mediated by adaptations in central cardiac and peripheral muscular functions and are, to a large extent, related to the intensity of the exercise and the initial conditioning level of the participant.

Resistance exercise training increases muscle mass and strength, with little improvement in V_{O_2max}, while the converse is seen with aerobic exercise training in healthy, deconditioned elderly people. However, improvements in muscle strength in frail, elderly people can enhance their functional capacity and independence in daily activities such as stair climbing, household chores, and even walking. Longitudinal studies that examine the effects of exercise training and detraining on cardiac and musculoskeletal functions with-

in and between older subjects can elucidate the effects of aging, exercise, body composition, and disease on the maximal functional capacity of the aging cardiovascular and muscular systems. This is because these kinds of studies examine interindividual differences in the effects of physical activity habits and other "secondary aging processes" on cardiovascular and muscular structure–function relationships. This information would permit the design and institution of appropriately prescribed exercise training programs to prevent declines in functional capacity and risk factors for disease with aging.

III. Influence of Exercise on Specific Physiological Systems in the Elderly

A. Physical Activity and Glucose Homeostasis

Aging is associated with a deterioration in glucose metabolism, increasing the susceptibility of older people to develop diabetes mellitus. Diabetes is consistently among the 10 most common diseases in the elderly population, accounting for greater than 10% of outpatient doctor visits plus an additional 3 million visits to hospital emergency rooms. Older diabetics are hospitalized 2.5 times more frequently and have an average length of stay 2–3 days longer than nondiabetic patients. Furthermore, other acute and chronic conditions such as atherosclerotic disease, claudication, microvascular disease involving the eye, kidney, and nervous systems, and increased infections are associated with diabetes. The cost of hospital care is approximately 56% greater for the diabetic than the nondiabetic patient, and the total cost of medical care for diabetes in 1991 was estimated at greater than $40 billion per year in the United States (Helms, 1992). Thus, prevention and/or reduction in the severity and economic impact of diabetes in the elderly population would have important health implications.

Age is one of the strongest risk factors for the development of glucose intolerance and diabetes. Major abnormalities in glucose homeostasis occur in the elderly due to physical inactivity and the development of abdominal obesity. These conditions are potentially modifiable by changes in physical activity and nutritional habits, while family history, aging, race, and genetics, which are also important risk factors for diabetes, are not modifiable. Abnormalities in glucose homeostasis often occur in the elderly without the characteristic clinical complications of diabetes mellitus, suggesting that in some older individuals glucose intolerance does not have pathophysiological consequences and may be modifiable through changes in lifestyle.

The development of insulin resistance and glucose intolerance in older men up to the age of 80 years are related primarily to the development of abdominal obesity and physical deconditioning, not aging per se (Bierman, 1992; Coon, Bleecker, Drinkwater, Meyers, & Goldberg, 1989; Coon, Rogus, Drinkwater, Muller, & Goldberg, 1992). When older and younger men are matched for regional fat distribution, percent body fat, and V_{O_2max}, insulin sensitivity is comparable in young and older subjects over a wide range of insulin levels. Thus, there is good evidence that insulin resistance is the primary pathophysiological mechanism by which impaired glucose tolerance and NIDDM develop in the elderly population (Bierman, 1992; DeFranzo & Ferrannini, 1991; Fink, Kolterman, & Olefsky, 1984; Reaven, 1988). Yet diabetes is a syndrome and involves complementary metabolic defects in muscle, the endocrine pancreas, and the liver that contribute to the decline in glucose homeostasis with aging. These abnormalities reduce insulin-mediated glucose utilization, decrease insulin secretion required

for glucose regulation, and cause the liver to overproduce glucose in the fasted state to worsen hyperglycemia. The decline in glucose tolerance in older persons is related to peripheral tissue and hepatic resistance to the action of insulin at low and high doses, as well as an impairment in insulin secretion (Coon et al., 1992; Fink et al., 1984; Kahn et al., 1990). These mechanisms are worsened by physical inactivity and the development of abdominal adiposity, increasing sympathetic nervous system activity (SNS) and the delivery of free fatty acids to the liver to increase insulin resistance, impair peripheral insulin-mediated glucose utilization, and cause hyperinsulinemia (Kissebah & Krakower, 1994). Exercise increases glucose utilization by peripheral tissues, i.e., by muscle, the largest organ responsible for glucose utilization, while exercise combined with weight loss also decreases total and abdominal fat stores. The mechanisms responsible for these improvements in glucose metabolism with exercise and weight loss involve increases in GLUT-4, glycogen synthase, capillary density, and blood flow to muscle, as well as enhanced pancreatic β-cell function (Elahi et al., 1984; Hughes et al., 1993; Kahn et al., 1990; Kirwan, Kohrt, Wojta, Bourey, & Holloszy, 1993; Pratley, Hagberg, Rogus, & Goldberg, 1995; Seals, Hagberg, et al., 1984b; Tonino, 1989). Although studies in middle-aged patients suggest that there are modest improvements in glucose tolerance and insulin sensitivity when aerobic exercise training is combined with weight loss (Bogardus et al., 1984; Holloszy, Schultz, Kusnierkiewicz, Hagberg, & Ehsani, 1986), there are no prospective studies which examine the effect of endurance exercise training and weight loss on glucose homeostasis in older patients with impaired glucose tolerance or NIDDM. Considering the potential for considerable health benefits at low expense, it would seem prudent to conduct such an intervention study in elderly diabetics.

Glucose metabolism, measured by the glucose clamp, improved by 13–36% after 3–6 months of aerobic exercise training (Kirwan *et al.*, 1993; Tonino, 1989), a level comparable to the 24% improvement in insulin sensitivity observed after 16 weeks of whole body resistance exercise training (Miller *et al.*, 1994). Intensive aerobic exercise for 12 weeks in healthy glucose-intolerant older men and women was associated with a 9% increase in V_{O_2max}, but only a small improvement in glucose tolerance (Hughes *et al.*, 1993). There was an 11% increase in insulin-mediated glucose disposal, a 24% increase in muscle glycogen, and a 60% increase in GLUT-4 levels. The diabetics who improved the most had the lowest percent of body fat and greatest muscle capillary density, but there was no relationship between the increases in GLUT-4 concentration with glucose disposal rates or glucose tolerance. The improvement in glucose metabolism with aerobic exercise training correlated better with the reduction in body fat in upper body sites (Kirwan *et al.*, 1993) (Fig. 2) than the increase in V_{O_2max}, suggesting that the improvement in glucose metabolism with aerobic exercise training is related to the changes in abdominal obesity and muscle adaptations to exercise training. These mechanisms may also contribute to the improvements in glucose metabolism and insulin sensitivity associated with resistance exercise training.

Insulin sensitivity is greater in well-trained younger and older athletes than in their sedentary peers (Pratley *et al.*, 1995; Seals, Hagberg, *et al.*, 1984b). These improvements dissipate after 7–10 days without exercise, partially due to reductions in insulin receptor binding affinity and nonoxidative glucose disposal (Heath *et al.*, 1983; Rogers, King, Hagberg, Ehsani, & Holloszy, 1990b). Endurance exercise-trained older individuals also have less body fat than sedentary people, especially in abdominal sites, and this increase in insulin sensitivity in older sedentary people

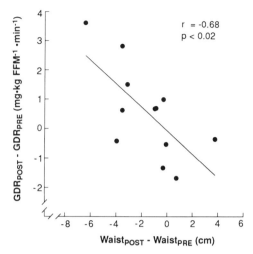

Figure 2. Training-induced changes in the glucose disposal rate (GDR) during a hyperglycemic clamp as a function of changes in waist circumference after exercise training in 12 older men and women. From Kirwan *et al.*, *J. Gerontol.* **48** (1993). Copyright © The Gerontological Society of America.

and master athletes correlated independently with their regional distribution of body fat, not their physical conditioning status (Kohrt *et al.*, 1993; Pratley *et al.*, 1995). Thus, it is not only the increase in V_{O_2max} but also the adaptations in body composition that result from exercise training that mediate improvements in glucose metabolism in elderly people.

Thus, one should consider interventions that alter body composition as well as aerobic capacity in the prevention and treatment of the insulin resistance, glucose intolerance, and NIDDM associated with aging. With the expected increase in the number of Americans aged 60 years and older from 31 million in 1990 to 60 million by the year 2025, there could be an increase in the prevalence of diabetes from 4% in the 45–55-year-old group to 9% in the 65–74-year-old group, with an additional 10% of subjects in the older age group having undiagnosed, asymptomatic diabetes. The prevalence of diabetes in the elderly obese subject is even higher, at nearly 27%. Considering the rapid increase in the prevalence of obesity in older men and women (Kuczmarski, Flegal, Campbell, & Johnson, 1994), examination of the benefits of aerobic exercise and weight loss to glucose metabolism in obese, insulin-resistant older individuals with impaired glucose tolerance and NIDDM would have important health and socioeconomic implications.

B. Physical Activity and Lipoprotein Metabolism

Aging is associated with the rise in plasma total and LDL cholesterol levels from the third to the sixth decade, followed by a decline thereafter (Hazzard, 1994). Triglyceride levels rise across the age span, and ratios of HDL-C to total cholesterol and LDL-C fall by some 20–30% during the same period before reaching a plateau. The concentration of HDL-C increases slightly across the age span in both men and women due to an increase in the HDL-2 subfraction, with no change in HDL-3 (Ettinger, Verdery, Wahl, & Fried, 1994). The prevalence of low HDL-C and high LDL-C levels in older persons with chronic vascular diseases indicates that dyslipidemia is important in the pathogenesis of atherosclerosis in the elderly (Ettinger et al., 1992, 1994; Zimetbaum et al., 1992). This suggests that the increase in HDL with age is due to the increase in HDL-2, and that individuals who undergo healthy, normal aging without the development of CVD are likely to have very high HDL and low LDL-C levels because of their protective effect against the development of coronary heart disease (Ettinger et al., 1992; Seals, Allen, et al., 1984a). Plasma lipoprotein lipid levels in the elderly also are influenced by physiological alterations in body composition, hormone levels, diet, and physical activity habits, factors which also affect atherogenesis and the risk for cardiovascular complications. Thus, there is a great deal of heterogeneity in the lipoprotein lipids of older people, especially those with chronic diseases, but more impor-

tantly among healthy older people living in different environments where exercise and dietary habits may have a substantial influence on risk for CVD.

In cross-sectional as well as longitudinal studies in young, middle-aged, and older individuals, higher levels of physical activity are associated with a less atherogenic lipoprotein profile. A number of cross-sectional studies show that older athletes have higher HDL-C and lower triglyceride and LDL-C levels than their sedentary peers (Seals, Allen, et al., 1984a) and lipoprotein lipid profiles comparable to those of younger athletes (Fig. 3a,b). In these studies, the older trained group was consistently leaner and had less central body fat than their sedentary peers. In a population of healthy obese older men (Meyers et al., 1991), there was an inverse relationship between central adiposity, as defined by the waist-to-hip ratio, and V_{O_2max}; furthermore, plasma triglyceride and HDL levels correlated more strongly with central adiposity than V_{O_2max}. In another study of healthy older men, HDL-C concentrations were more closely related to aerobic fitness, body composition, and fat distribution than to age, and HDL-C was higher and total cholesterol, LDL-C, and the total cholesterol to HDL-C ratio were lower in trained older men, even after correcting for central adiposity (Williams, Krauss, Vranizan, & Wood, 1990).

In several longitudinal studies where exercise training raised HDL-C and reduced plasma triglyceride and LDL-C concentrations, there were also concomitant, substantial reductions in body weight (Despres et al., 1991; Schwartz, 1988), making it difficult to distinguish the metabolic effects of exercise from those of weight loss. Direct measurement of visceral fat by computerized tomography distinguished changes in V_{O_2max} and body fat from those of central adipose tissue, providing evidence that increases in HDL with exercise may be more closely related to the decrease in visceral (intraabdominal) fat than

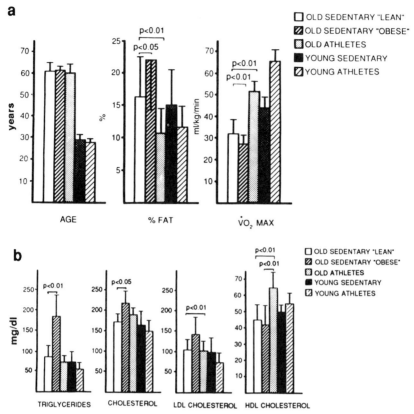

Figure 3. (a) Healthy, active, lean, untrained, older men (older sedentary "lean," $n =$ 10) and young athletes (young athletes, $n = 8$) were matched as closely as possible to healthy, highly conditioned master athletes (older athletes, $n = 15$) for age and percent body fat to determine the effects of regular physical conditioning on lipoprotein metabolism. An active, obese group of older untrained men (older sedentary "obese," $n = 15$) and a group of young sedentary men ("young sedentary" men, $n = 10$) determined the effects of obesity and reduced V_{O_2max} metabolic function. The ages of the older men were comparable, but percent fat was higher in the older sedentary lean men than in the older athletes ($P < 0.01$); the obese men had a higher percent body fat than all the other groups. The percent body fat of the young and older athletes and the young sedentary men did not differ significantly, but was lower than that of the sedentary groups of older men. V_{O_2max} differed significantly among the older sedentary groups and the older and young athletes and young sedentary subjects. V_{O_2max} was not different in the young and older athletes. (b) Plasma triglyceride and total and low-density lipoprotein cholesterol (LDL-C) levels were significantly higher in the older sedentary obese group than in the other groups ($P < 0.01$). Plasma high-density lipoprotein cholesterol (HDL-C) levels were lowest in the older sedentary lean and obese men ($P <$ 0.01 versus older athletes; $P < 0.05$ versus young athletes), but did not differ significantly between the young and older athletes or the young sedentary and older sedentary lean men.

total body fat or the increase in V_{O_2max} (Schwartz, 1988). In these studies, aerobic exercise appeared to directly affect Apo A-I and HDL-2 levels, while the changes in body composition during exercise training accounted for the rise in HDL-C (Despres et al., 1991; Herbert et al., 1984; Schwartz, 1988). This suggests that exercise may affect the HDL reverse cholesterol transport system to raise both HDL and Apo A-I levels proportionately, while weight loss reduces the catabolism of HDL-2 by hepatic lipase and increases the clearance of triglyceride-rich lipoproteins by lipoprotein lipase to raise the absolute concentration of HDL-C without changing its particle size or Apo A-I composition. It is not known whether exercise training affects LDL and Apo-B metabolism independently, but when other health and lifestyle modifications in diet and body composition occur during intensive aerobic training, there are also reductions in total and LDL cholesterol concentrations.

Changes in body composition with aging contribute substantially to the dyslipidemia in the elderly, as central obesity and physical deconditioning have complementary affects on triglyceride, cholesterol, and HDL metabolism. Adult weight gain in an upper body or central pattern has more significant adverse effects on lipoprotein metabolism than does the development of obesity in the lower body (Kissebah & Krakower, 1994; Despres & Marette, 1994; Krauss & Kesaniemi, 1994). The adverse metabolic effect of upper body weight gain are particularly significant in women after menopause, when the risk of premature atherosclerosis and diabetes mellitus is greatly enhanced with increasing fat deposition within the abdominal cavity (Dennis & Goldberg, 1993). This type of upper body weight gain is also associated with multiple lipoprotein abnormalities, characterized by increased small, dense, Apo B-enriched LDL particles, elevated plasma triglycerides levels, and reduced HDL-C levels (Dennis & Goldberg, 1993; Despres, Allard, Tremblay, Talbot, & Bouchard, 1985; Despres & Marette, 1994; Krauss & Kesaniemi, 1994). This lipoprotein disorder is termed atherogenic LDL pattern B and is the most prevalent dyslipidemia in the elderly, evident in 30–35% of older men and 15–25% of postmenopausal women (Krauss & Kesaniemi,

1994). Population studies suggest that the atherogenic LDL pattern B is inherited as either an autosomal dominant or codominant trait, but its increased expression with aging seems to be related to the male gender and the development of abdominal obesity and physical deconditioning. Metabolic conditions also associated with the insulin resistance syndrome, such as glucose intolerance and NIDDM, are also prevalent in patients with the LDL-B phenotype (Reaven, Chen, Jeppesen, Maheux, & Krauss, 1993). This suggests that this dyslipidemia may be worsened by insulin resistance, as hyperinsulinemia increases triglyceride production rates and the formation of dense LDL particles as well as accelerates the catabolism of HDL-C by hepatic lipase (Despres & Marette, 1994; Katzel et al., 1992; Krauss & Kesaniemi, 1994). Individuals with the LDL-B phenotype not only have central obesity but also tend to be more sedentary, suggesting that there is an interaction between lifestyle habits and a genetic predisposition to the development of these metabolic risk factors for CVD in the elderly.

The presence of coexistent medical diseases, medications, dietary habits, and cigarette smoking, as well as genetic factors, also has a substantial effect on lipoprotein metabolism and should be considered in the evaluation of the effects of exercise on lipoprotein lipids. Diets high in cholesterol and saturated fat increase total and LDL-C levels and raise triglyceride levels, while diets high in carbohydrates lower plasma HDL and LDL cholesterol levels. Diseases such as diabetes, renal disease, hypothyroidism, and liver disease cause hyperlipidemia and lower HDL-C levels, as do the medications thiazide diuretics, beta blockers, and corticosteroids. The assessment of the independent effects of primary aging on lipoprotein metabolism requires the isolation of the effects of aging from these factors. Careful medical evaluation can exclude patients with disease, medications, and cigarette smoking habits from the study, and diet can be controlled. A number of studies attempted to limit changes in body composition with exercise training; however, such an effect may only be able to be accomplished with low-intensity training and careful attention to diet. There are minimal changes in lipoprotein lipid concentrations with low-intensity training, and it is only when the exercise stimulus is increased substantially that there are reductions in plasma triglyceride and cholesterol levels and an increase in HDL-C level. However, high-intensity exercise is usually accompanied by weight loss, particularly in the abdominal region, thereby confounding the interpretation of the direct effects of aerobic exercise training on plasma lipoprotein lipids. This reenforces the fact that both physical fitness and body composition are important determinants of lipoprotein lipids in older people.

C. Physical Exercise and Hypertension

Hypertension afflicts nearly 50 million Americans, including 13% of all Caucasian and 35% of African Americans, predisposing them to premature death and disability from cardiovascular disease. Hypertension is particularly prevalent in the elderly and is present in greater than 50% of some subsets of older Americans (Schoenberger, 1986). There are numerous medications to lower BP, but they are more effective in reducing BP in younger individuals with marked hypertension than in the elderly, where mild-to-moderate elevations in blood pressure are most prevalent (Joint National Committee, 1993; Kuller, Hulley, Cohen, & Meaton, 1986). Furthermore, many antihypertensive medications have substantial side effects in older patients who are susceptible to postural hypertension, drug interactions because of the coexistent use of other medications, and changes in mental status and depression. Nonpharmacological means for controlling blood pressure would be more effective than medications for the aforementioned reasons and because of the higher prevalence of obesity, dietary indiscretion, and sedentary lifestyles in the elderly. Therefore, the introduction of nonpharmacological measures such as weight loss (Stevens et al., 1993), sodium restriction (Ferrara, deSimone, Pisanisi, & Mancini, 1984), and regular physical activity (Fagard & Tipton, 1994) may be more beneficial as a first step in the treatment of mild essential hypertension in the elderly than the use of pharmacological therapy.

A number of studies show that athletes have lower blood pressure levels than individuals who do not engage in regular exercise. The lack of regular strenuous exercise was an independent risk for the development of hypertension among Harvard male alumni who were followed for 6–10 years from ages 16 to 50 after entering college (Paffenbarger, Leung, Jung, & Hyde, 1991). Similar evidence of a direct relationship between physical inactivity and blood pressure is reported from the Cooper Clinic in Dallas (Blair, Goodyear, Gibbons, & Cooper, 1984) and in males from Tecumseh, MI (Montoye, Metzner, & Keller, 1972). Numerous studies examining the effects of exercise in individuals with hypertension demonstrate that mild-to-moderate intensity exercise training lowers systolic and diastolic BP on the average by roughly 10 mm Hg (Fagard & Tipton, 1994). Nine months of endurance exercise training at a low intensity of 50% of heart rate reserve (HRR) elicited an 18-mm Hg reduction in systolic BP and a 12-mm Hg decrease in diastolic BP in 60–69-year-old subjects with moderate hypertension, in contrast to the finding of only an 8-mm Hg drop in systolic and diastolic BP attained with a higher intensity (70% of HRR) exercise training program (Hagberg, Montain, Martin, & Ehsani, 1989). In another study, regular physical activity reduced BP to comparable degrees in 70–79-year-old men and women with moderate hypertension subjected to low-to-moderate intensity training (Cononie *et al.*, 1991). Earlier studies, although less well-controlled, also report greater BP reductions in older hypertensive subjects with low-intensity exercise training.

Improvements in BP associated with exercise training can be seen independent of weight loss (Cade, Patterson, & Hood-Lewis, 1984). However, the addition of weight loss to exercise training dramatically lowers BP in older, obese, sedentary men with multiple risk factors for CVD (Dengel, Pratley, Hagberg, & Goldberg, 1994). In addition to the benefits seen with aerobic exercise training, there are a few reports demonstrating that circuit weight training (Keleman, Effron, & Valente, 1990) lowers BP in middle-aged individuals. A 10-week program of circuit weight training involving multiple muscle groups increased aerobic fitness and decreased systolic and diastolic BP of sufficient magnitude to reduce the need for BP-lowering medications and also normalized the BP of hypertensive individuals on a placebo. Although there are a number of studies demonstrating improvements in BP in the elderly, few distinguish the effects of changes in body composition and diet on the beneficial BP lowering effects of exercise training. Carefully controlled studies in which diet, body composition, and other lifestyle habits are modified and/or controlled before exercise training intervention will be necessary to elucidate the mechanisms by which aerobic exercise training lowers BP in the elderly.

Cardiovascular morbidity and mortality rise as blood pressure increases, and small changes in systolic and diastolic BP with age can have profound health implications in the elderly. Physical conditioning status, body composition, and dietary factors correlate well with blood pressure. Changes in these variables occur with aging, and in a population of healthy Caucasian men and women, where the relationship between mean arterial BP and age was strong in women and men, the increase in arterial pressure with aging in men was primarily related to an increase in body fatness, whereas in women the distribution of fat was the primary factor (Gardner & Poehlman, 1995). Thus, appropriate dietary and exercise practices may exert complementary effects to reduce the prevalence of hypertension in the elderly.

IV. Conclusions and Recommendations

The American population, and those in most developed countries, is aging at a rapid rate. The projection is that within 25 years the American population will have 50%, or 17 million, more people over age 65. At present, persons 65 and over represent 1 of every 8 Americans; however, by the year 2020 this will increase to 1 of every 6 and by 2040 to 1 of every 4–5 Americans. Thus, there will be many more older people in the United States, and they will represent an ever-increasing percentage of the total population.

Cardiovascular diseases are the major cause of morbidity and mortality in older individuals; therefore, maximizing the cardiovascular health and function of older individuals is a major health care priority. Functional independence and the ability to perform activities of daily life are also critical factors affecting the health status and the quality of life of older persons. The 65 and older portion of the population is responsible for a majority of the nation's health care expenditures; hence, preventive or rehabilitative strategies that reduce morbidity and mortality have the potential to be very beneficial in improving quality of life and reducing economic costs of health care in the elderly.

Numerous studies clearly indicate that many of the functional and structural deteriorations previously attributed to primary aging are, in fact, affected substantially by lifestyle habits that reduce cardiovascular fitness and muscle mass and increase total and central obesity. There is now substantial clinical and experimental evidence that regular physical activity programs are feasible and effective in improving health and function in nearly all elderly individuals. These results indicate that both aerobic and resistance exercises should be included in these training programs to maximize cardiovascular fitness and musculoskeletal function. The aerobic components of these programs will improve cardiovascular function and reduce risk factors for CVD, while resistance training primarily benefits skeletal muscle mass and strength. Collectively, such programs will optimize future health and well-being and minimize the risk of falling and loss of functional independence in older people. Thus, regular physical activity has potential as a preventive and rehabilitative strategy to impact morbidity, mortality, and quality of life in the elderly; this could markedly alter the health care expenditures required by this burgeoning portion of the American population.

A. Exercise Training Program

The higher prevalence of asymptomatic as well as symptomatic CVD and other chronic diseases such as hypertension, diabetes, arthritis, and coronary artery and renal disease necessitates that an exercise program be individualized on the basis of health status and the older person's goals. The most important recommendation is that, prior to beginning exercise training, older persons have a comprehensive health evaluation, including an exercise treadmill test with ECG monitoring (American College of Sports Medicine, 1991). The contraindications for exercise in the elderly are well-reviewed in the textbook of the American College of Sports Medicine (1991) and briefly outlined in Table II. After initiation of training, the cardiopulmonary, central nervous, and musculoskeletal systems should be

monitored for symptoms that are warning signs of excessive effort (Table III). The guidelines provided (herein) for aerobic and resistance exercise training are intended for healthy older sedentary persons and should be modified in intensity, duration, and frequency on the basis of the health and functional limitations of the patient population (Felsenthal *et al.*, 1994).

1. Aerobic Exercise Training

The actual workout should consist of (1) a warm-up, (2) the conditioning period, and (3) a cool-down. The warm-up prepares the body for the upcoming workout and is a precaution against unnecessary injuries and muscle soreness. A proper warm-up stretches the muscles and tendons in preparation for more forceful contractions. The conditioning period is the main workout and should involve activities that are continuous and rhythmic, such as walking, swimming, and bicycling. Recreational activities such as golf or tennis are usually not continuous or rhythmic and do not promote the development of cardiovascular fitness. The main conditioning period should incorporate the basic principles of intensity, duration, and frequency. The cool-down following the conditioning period should allow the body to return toward its resting level. Walking and light stretching to avoid cramping are the most common means of diminishing the cardiovascular and muscular side effects of aerobic exercise.

The most important factor in developing an aerobic exercise program is the intensity of the exercise. To improve cardiorespiratory fitness, the HR during exercise should be raised by approximately 60% of the HRR, or the difference between the maximal and resting HR ($HR_{max} - HR_{rest}$). The training or target rate (THR) is calculated by multiplying the difference between the maximal and resting rates by 0.60 and adding the result to the resting

Table II
Contraindications to Exercise in the Elderly

1. Unstable angina
2. Resting systolic blood pressure >200 or diastolic pressure >100 mm Hg
3. Hypertension with exercise: systolic pressure >250 or diastolic >120 mm Hg
4. Moderate-to-severe aortic stenosis
5. Acute systemic illness, active infectious disease, or fever
6. Uncontrolled atrial or ventricular dysrhythmias, third-degree heart block, resting ST segment depression (greater than 3 mm)
7. Uncontrolled symptomatic congestive heart failure
8. Active pericarditis, myocarditis, or endocarditis
9. Thrombophlebitis or recent embolism
10. Active or uncontrolled hyperthyroidism, adrenal insufficiency, gout, or diabetes
11. Orthopedic problems that would prohibit exercise
12. Severe anemia
13. Adverse environmental conditions (high temperature and relative humidity, significant air pollution)
14. Cerebral dysfunction (vertigo, gait disturbance, multiple falls)

heart rate. For the older adult, an intensity between 60 and 75% of HRR is both safe and effective for developing cardiovascular fitness. To determine whether an individual is exercising at the prescribed intensity, have the person count his/her pulse immediately after exercise, since the HR falls rapidly after the cessation of exercise, and multiply by 6. There are a number of devices on the market that monitor HR during exercise that might prove easier for some older people than actually trying to count their pulse. The next component of the aerobic exercise program involves determining the duration of the exercise session. For the beginner or deconditioned older individual, it is unwise to start out exercising continuously for longer than

Table III
Criteria for Termination of Exercise Training

1. Fatigue
2. Angina, new onset; cardiac arrhythmias, PVCs
3. Ataxia, light-headedness, confusion, pallor, cyanosis, nausea and vomiting, prolonged dyspnea, insomnia
4. Inappropriate cardiovascular responses (bradycardia, hypo- or hypertension, claudication, PVCs, or prolonged tachycardia after exercise)
5. Orthopedic problems aggravated by exercise

10–15 min. The sedentary beginner initially should start a gradual program with 5–10 min exercise bouts interspersed with 3–5 min rest periods for 2 weeks. An additional 5 min could be added every 2 weeks until 20–30 min of continuous exercise is reached. We recommend that sessions be at least 30 min of exercise. As the individual becomes more aerobically fit, more time can be added, but aerobic exercise sessions greater than 45 min in length offer few additional health benefits. The final component of the program is the frequency of aerobic exercise. Cardiorespiratory fitness can be adequately achieved by exercising 3–4 times per week. More than 4 workouts per week provide very little additional improvement; however, the chance for injury does increase with additional workouts.

Thus, an aerobic exercise program for a healthy, sedentary older person should be progressive, with gradual increases in intensity and duration every 2 weeks. The goal is to reach an exercise intensity of at least 70% of HRR for 30–45 min, 3–4 times per week; however, the appropriateness of the exercise prescription may need to be modified on the basis of subjective and objective (cardiovascular) responses and precautions to avoid injury.

2. Resistance Exercise Training

A resistance training program to increase muscular strength and/or muscular endurance should include warm-up and cool-down periods of conditioning exercises that involve stretching each muscle group involved in the resistance training routine. The equipment and facilities available to the participant for resistance training, such as Nautilus or Universal weight machines and barbells, should be considered and the program individualized to meet the subject's needs and functional goals.

A resistance training program with the goal to develop both muscular strength and endurance should focus on four components: (a) the number of contractions per bout (repetitions); (b) the number of bouts (sets); (c) the quantity of weight lifted (load); and (d) the rest period between sets and exercise sessions. There should be a gradual progression in all phases of resistance training individualized to meet the needs and accomplishments of the older patient, with appropriate safety features to avoid injury. General training guidelines and proper techniques should be taught, including stretching of the muscle groups involved in training at the onset and after the session, avoidance of breath holding during heavy lifting, selection of the load based on results of strength testing, conservative progression in the number of repetitions and sets, length of rest intervals, and limiting the frequency of training sessions to 3 times/week.

An initial load that allows 6 or less repetitions is most effective for the development of muscular strength, while loads that allow 20 or more repetitions are designed to develop of muscular endurance. A work load that permits between 8 and 15 repetitions is effective for the development of both muscular endurance and strength and also results in fewer cases of injury and muscle soreness. The selection

of a load should be based on the individual being able to perform 8 repetitions, with the last 2 repetitions requiring a concentrated effort. The individual should strive to lift the weight as many times as possible; however, it is important to stress proper lifting form and technique. In the beginning stages, training should be directed initially at large muscle groups involved in everyday activities, including arms, shoulders, legs, hips, and spine muscles. The number of sets used in a workout is directly related to training results. In programs for older individuals, a maximum of three sets is recommended. The subject should be taught the proper lifting form and technique by performing the first few (2–3) training sessions without any weight or load. During the next 2–3 weeks, older individuals should only use 1–2 sets and continue to focus on proper lifting technique. Another set can be added after 2–3 weeks, and after another 2 weeks the third set finally can be added. If the individual is sore the day after the training session, a more conservative approach should be used for adding additional weight or sets. The length of the rest period allowed between sets is usually 1–3 min, but is determined by the goals of the training program and the subject's adaptations. If the goal of the program is to increase muscular strength, then relatively long rest periods (2–3 min) are used. When the goal is to increase muscular endurance, then rest periods are 1 min or less.

Resistance training programs usually are conducted 3 times per week, with at least 1 day between workouts. In addition to the rest allowed between sets, it is important to consider the order of exercises. Following an arm exercise with a leg exercise is helpful for older individuals beginning resistance training programs because it allows for some recovery of the arm muscles while the leg muscles are being exercised. Some individuals involved in resistance training like to do all arm exercises on one day and all leg exercises on another; the drawback to this approach is that the program is now 6 days instead of 3 days. Most older individuals like to train only 3 times per week, thereby allowing freedom to benefit from their newly acquired fitness level by participating in recreational activities.

Thus, some of the declines in cardiovascular and muscular function with aging can be reversed or prevented by aerobic and resistance exercise training. The adaptations that occur in response to training are usually related to the initial exercise capacity of the older participant, because exercise training improves functional declines that are related to being sedentary. Hence, functional improvements in response to exercise training can be large in older persons and, in relative terms (percent of basal), comparable to that in younger subjects. This may partially explain the exaggerated functional declines attributed to aging that are derived from cross-sectional studies. This suggests that the health consequences of secondary aging processes related to cardiovascular morbidity and mortality and musculoskeletal disability in the elderly are potentially modifiable through exercise training. Increased cardiovascular function, reduced risk factors for CVD, and increased muscle mass and strength through regular exercise can be realistic goals for older persons.

Acknowledgments

This work was supported by a Geriatric Leadership Academic Award (1KO7AG00609), Dept. of Veterans Affairs Geriatric Research, Education and Clinical Center (GRECC), Claude D. Pepper Older Americans Independence Center (P60AG12583), NIA training grant (5T32AG00291), and a grant-in-aid from the Maryland Affiliate of the American Heart Association. The authors are grateful to Mrs. Loretta Hetmanski and Mrs. Helen Spencer for typing this chapter.

References

American College of Sports Medicine. (1991). *Guidelines for Exercise Testing and Prescription* (4th ed.). Philadelphia: Lea & Febiger.

Bassey, E. J., Fiatarone, M. A., O'Neil, E. F., Kelly, M., Evans, W. J., & Lipsitz, L. A. (1992). Leg extensor power and functional performance in very old men and women. *Clinical Science, 82,* 321–327.

Bierman, E. L. (1992). George Lyman Duff Memorial Lecture. Atherogenesis in diabetes. *Arteriosclerosis and Thrombosis, 12,* 647–656.

Bjorntorp, P. (1993). Visceral obesity: A "civilization syndrome." *Obesity Research, 1,* 206–222.

Blair, S. N., Goodyear, N. N., Gibbons, L. W., & Cooper, K. H. (1984). Physical fitness and the incidence of hypertension in healthy, normotensive men and women. *Journal of the American Medical Association, 252,* 487–490.

Blair, S. N., Kohl, H. W., III, Paffenbarger, R. S., Jr., Clark, D. G., Cooper, K. H., & Gibbons, L. W. (1989). Physical fitness cause mortality. A prospective study of healthy men and women. *Journal of the American Medical Association, 262,* 2395–2401.

Bogardus, C., Ravussin, E., Robbins, D. C., Wolfe, R. R., Horton, E. S., & Sims, E. A. H. (1984). Effects of physical training and diet therapy on carbohydrate metabolism in patients with glucose intolerance and non-insulin dependent diabetes mellitus. *Diabetes, 33,* 311–318.

Bouchard, C., Despres, J.-P., & Tremblay, A. (1993). Exercise and obesity. *Obesity Research, 1,* 133–147.

Cade, M., Patterson, J., & Hood-Lewis, D. (1984). Effect of aerobic exercise training on patients with systemic arterial hypertension. *American Journal of Medicine, 77,* 785–790.

Coggan, A. R., Spina, R. J., Rogers, M. A., King, D. S., Brown, M., Nemeth, P. M., & Holloszy, J. O. (1990). Histochemical and enzymatic characteristics of skeletal muscle in master athletes. *Journal of Applied Physiology, 68,* 1896–1901.

Coggan, A. R., Spina R. J., King, D. S., Rogers, M. A., Brown, M., Nemeth, P. M., & Holloszy, J. O. (1992a). Histochemical and enzymatic comparison of the gastrocnemius muscle of young and elderly men and women. *Journal of Gerontological Biology Science, 46B,* 71–76.

Coggan, A. R., Spina, R. J., King, D. S., Rogers, M. A., Brown, M., Nemeth, P. M., & Holloszy, J. O. (1992b). Skeletal muscle adaptations to endurance training in 60- to 70-yr-old men and women. *Journal of Applied Physiology, 72,* 1780–1786.

Cononie, C. C., Graves, J. E., Pollack, M. L., Phillips, M. I., Sumners, C., & Hagberg, J. M. (1991). Effects of exercise training on blood pressure in 70–79 year old men and women. *Medicine Science Sports Exercise, 23,* 505–511.

Coon, P. J., Bleecker, E. R., Drinkwater, D. T., Meyers, D. A., & Goldberg, A. P. (1989). Effects of body composition and exercise capacity on glucose tolerance, insulin and lipoprotein lipids in healthy older men: A cross-sectional and longitudinal intervention study. *Metabolism, 38,* 1201–1209.

Coon, P. J., Rogus, E. M., Drinkwater, D., Muller, D. C., & Goldberg, A. P. (1992). Role of body fat distribution in the decline in insulin sensitivity and glucose tolerance with age. *Journal of Clinical Endocrinology and Metabolism, 75,* 1125–1132.

Coyle, E. F., Martin, W. H., III, Sinacore, D. R., Joyner, M. J., Hagberg, J. M., & Holloszy, J. O. (1984). Time course of loss of adaptations after stopping prolonged intense endurance training. *Journal of Applied Physiology, 57,* 1857–1864.

DeFronzo, R. A., & Ferrannini, E. (1991). Insulin resistance: A multifaceted syndrome responsible for NIDDM, obesity, hypertension, dyslipidemia, and atherosclerotic cardiovascular disease. *Diabetes Care, 14,* 173–194.

Dengel, D. R., Pratley, R. E., Hagberg, J. M., & Goldberg, A. P. (1994). Aerobic exercise and weight loss ameliorate coronary artery disease risk factors associated with the insulin resistance syndrome. *Clinical Research, 42* (2), 216A.

Dennis, K. E., & Goldberg, A. P. (1993). Differential effects of body fatness and body fat distribution on risk factors for cardiovascular disease in women: Impact of weight loss. *Arteriosclerosis and Thrombosis, 13,* 1487–1494.

Despres, J. P., & Marette, A. (1994). Relation of components of insulin resistance syndrome to coronary disease risk. *Current Opinion in Lipidology, 5,* 274–289.

Despres, J. P., Allard, C., Tremblay, A., Talbot, J., & Bouchard, C. (1985). Evidence for a regional component of body fatness in the association with serum lipids in men and women. *Metabolism, 34,* 967–973.

Despres, J. P., Pouliot, M. C., Moorjarri, S., Nadeau, A., Tremblay, M., Lupien, P. J., Thereault, G., & Bouchard, C. (1991). Loss of abdominal fat and the metabolic response to exercise training in obese women. *American Journal of Physiology, 261,* 159–167.

Ehsani, A. A., Ogawa, T., Miller, T. R., Spina, R. J., & Jilka, S. M. (1991). Exercise training improves left ventricular systolic function in older men. *Circulation, 83,* 96–103.

Elahi, D., Andersen, D. K., Muller, D. C., Tobin, J. D., Brown, J. C., & Andres, R. (1984). The enteric enhancement of glucose-stimulated insulin release: The role of GIP in aging, obesity, and non-insulin-dependent diabetes mellitus. *Diabetes, 33,* 950–957.

Ettinger, W. H., Wahl, P. W., Kuller, L. H., Bush, T. L., Tracy, R. P., Manolio, T. A., Bouhani, N. O., Wong, N. D., & O'Leary, D. H. (1992). Lipoprotein lipids in older people: Results from the Cardiovascular Health Study. The CHS Collaborative Research group. *Circulation, 86,* 858–869.

Ettinger, W. H., Verdery, R. B., Wahl, P. W., & Fried, L. P. (1994). High density lipoprotein cholesterol subfractions in older people. *Journal of Gerontology, 49,* M116–M122.

Fagard, R. H., & Tipton, C. M. (1994). Physical activity fitness and hypertension. In C. Bouchard, R. J. Shephard, & T. Stephens (Eds.), *Physical Activity, Fitness and Health* (pp. 633–655). Illinois: Human Kinetics.

Felsenthal, G., Garrison, S. J., & Steinberg, F. U. (Eds.) (1994). *Rehabilitation of the Aging Patient.* Baltimore: Williams and Wilkins.

Ferrara, L. A., deSimone, G., Pasanisi, F., & Mancini, M. (1984). Left ventricular mass reduction during salt depletion in arterial hypertension. *Hypertension, 6,* 755–759.

Fiatarone, M. A., Marks, E. C., Ryan, N. D., Meredith, C. N., Lipsitz, L. A., & Evans, W. J. (1990). High-intensity strength training in nonagenarians: Effects on skeletal muscle. *Journal of the American Medical Association, 263,* 3029–3034.

Fink, R. I., Kolterman, O. G., & Olefsky, J. M.

(1984). The physiological significance of the glucose intolerance of aging. *Journal of Gerontology, 39,* 273–278.

Fleg, J. L., & Lakatta, E. G. (1988). Role of muscle loss in the age-associated reduction in VO2max. *Journal of Applied Physiology, 65,* 1147–1151.

Fleg, J. L., Schulman, S. P., Gerstenblith, G., Becker, L. C., O'Connor, F. C., & Lakatta, E. G. (1993). Additive effects of age and silent myocardial ischemia on the left ventricular response to upright cycle exercise. *Journal of Applied Physiology, 75,* 499–504.

Fleg, J. L., Schulman, S. P., O'Connor, F. C., Gerstenblith, G., Becker, L. C., Fortney, S., Goldberg, A. P., & Lakatta, E. G. (1994). Cardiovascular responses to exhaustive upright cycle exercise in highly trained older men. *Journal of Applied Physiology, 77,* 1500–1506.

Fries, J. F., Singh, G., Morfeld, D., Hubert, H. B., Lane, N. E., & Brown, B. W., Jr. (1994). Running and the development of disability with age. *Annals of Internal Medicine, 121,* 502–509.

Gardner, A. W., & Poehlman, E. T. (1993). Physical activity is a significant predictor of body density in women. *American Journal of Clinical Nutrition, 57,* 8–14.

Gardner, A. W., & Poehlman, E. T. (1995). Predictors of the age related increase in blood pressure in men and women. *Journal of Gerontology, 50,* M1–M6.

Goran, M. I., & Poehlman, E. T. (1992). Total energy expenditure and energy requirements in healthy elderly persons. *Metabolism, 41,* 744–753.

Grimby, G., & Saltin, B. (1966). Physiological analysis of middle-aged and old athletes. *ACTA Medica Scandinavica, 179,* 513–526.

Hagberg, J. M., Allen, W. K., Seals, D. R., Hurley, B. F., Ehsani, A. A., & Holloszy, J. O. (1985). A hemodynamic comparison of young and older endurance athletes during exercise. *Journal of Applied Physiology, 58,* 2041–2046.

Hagberg, J. M., Montain, S. J., Martin, W. H., & Ehsani, A. A. (1989). Effect of exercise training on 60–69 year old persons with essential hypertension. *American Journal of Cardiology, 64,* 348–353.

Hazzard, W. R. (1994). Dyslipoproteinemia. In W. R. Hazzard, E. L. Bierman, J. P. Blass, W. H.

Ettinger, & J. B. Halter (Eds.), *Principles of Geriatric Medicine and Gerontology* (3rd ed., Chapter 73, pp. 855–866). New York: McGraw-Hill, Inc.

Heath, G. W., Hagberg, J. M., Ehsani, A. A., & Holloszy, J. O. (1981). A physiological comparison of young and older endurance athletes. *Journal of Applied Physiology, 51,* 634–640.

Heath, G. W., Gavin, J. R., III, Hinderliter, J. M., Hagberg, J. M., Bloomfield, S. A., & Holloszy, J. O. (1983). Effects of exercise and lack of exercise on glucose tolerance and insulin sensitivity. *Journal of Applied Physiology, 55,* 512–517.

Helms, R. B. (1992). Implications of population growth on prevalence of diabetes: a look at the future. *Diabetes Care, 15* (Suppl. 1), 6–9.

Herbert, P. N., Bernier, D. N., Cullinane, E. M., Edelstein, L., Kantor, M. A., & Thompson, P. D. (1984). High density lipoprotein metabolism in runners and sedentary men. *Journal of the American Medical Association, 252,* 1034–1037.

Hiatt, W. R., Regensteiner, J. G., & Wolfel, E. E. (1993). Special populations in cardiovascular rehabilitation. Peripheral arterial disease, noninsulin dependent diabetes mellitus, and heart failure. *Cardiology Clinics, 11,* 309–321.

Holloszy, J. L., & Coyle, E. F. (1984). Adaptations of skeletal muscle to endurance exercise and their metabolic consequences. *Journal of Applied Physiology, 56,* 831–838.

Holloszy, J. O., Schultz, J., Kusnierkiewicz, J., Hagberg, J. M., & Ehsani, A. A. (1986). Effects of exercise on glucose tolerance and insulin resistance. *ACTA Medica Scandinavica, Suppl. 711,* 55–65.

Hughes, V. A., Fiatarone, M. A., Fielding, R. A., Kahn, B. B., Ferrara, C. M., Shepherd, P., Fisher, E. C., Wolfe, R. R., Elahi, D., & Evans, W. J. (1993). Exercise increases muscle GLUT-4 levels and insulin action in subjects with impaired glucose tolerance. *American Journal of Physiology, 264,* E855–E862.

Joint National Committee on Detection, Evaluation, and Treatment of High Blood Pressure, Fifth Report (JNC-5). (1993). *Archives of Internal Medicine, 153,* 154–183.

Kahn, S. E., Larson, V. G., Beard, J. C., Cain, K. C., Fellingham, G. W., Schwartz, R. S., Veith, R. C., Stratton, J. R., Cerqueira, M. D.,

& Abrass, I. B. (1990). Effect of exercise on insulin action, glucose tolerance, and insulin secretion in aging. *American Journal of Physiology, 258,* E937–E943.

Katzel, L. I., Coon, P. J., Busby, M. J., Gottlieb, S. O., Krauss, R. M., & Goldberg, A. P. (1992). Reduced HDL$_2$ cholesterol subspecies and elevated postheparin hepatic lipase activity in older men with abdominal obesity and symptomatic myocardial ischemia. *Arteriosclerosis and Thrombosis, 12,* 814–823.

Keleman, A., Effron, M., & Valente, S. (1990). Effect of exercise training combined with antihypertensive drug therapy. *Journal of the American Medical Association, 263,* 2766–2771.

Kirwan, J. P., Kohrt, W. M., Wojta, D. M., Bourey, R. E., & Holloszy, J. O. (1993). Endurance exercise training reduces glucose-stimulated insulin levels in 60-to-70-year old men and women. *Journal of Gerontology, 48,* M84–M90.

Kissebah, A. H., & Krakower, G. R. (1994). Regional adiposity and morbidity. *Physiological Reviews, 74,* 761–811.

Kohrt, W. M., Kirwan, J. P., Staten, M. A., Bourey, R. E., King, D. S., & Holloszy, J. O. (1993). Insulin resistance in aging is related to abdominal obesity. *Diabetes, 42,* 273–281.

Krauss, R. M., & Kesaniemi, Y. A. (1994). Cardiovascular disease and hyperlipidemia. *Current Opinions in Lipidology, 5,* 249–251.

Kuczmarski, R. J., Flegal, K. M., Campbell, S. M., & Johnson, C. L. (1994). Increasing prevalence of overweight among US adults. The National Health and Nutrition Examination Surveys, 1960–1991. *Journal of the American Medical Association, 272,* 205–211.

Kuller, L. H., Hulley, S. D., Cohen, J. D., & Meaton, J. (1986). Unexpected effects of treating hypertension in men with ECG abnormalities: a critical analysis. *Circulation, 73,* 114–123.

Lakatta, E. G. (1993). Cardiovascular regulatory mechanisms in advanced age. *Physiological Reviews, 73,* 413–467.

Lakatta, E. G., Goldberg, A. P., Fleg, J. L., Fortney, F. M., & Drinkwater, D. T. (1988). Reduced cardiovascular and metabolic reserves in older persons: Disuse, disease, or aging? In R. Chernoff & D. A. Lipschitz (Eds.), *Health Promotion and Disease Prevention in the El-* *derly: Vol. 35, Aging Series* (pp. 75–88). New York: Raven Press.

Makrides, L., Heigenhauser, G. J., & Jones, N. L. (1990). High intensity endurance training in 20 to 30 and 60 to 70 year old healthy men. *Journal of Applied Physiology, 69,* 1792–1798.

Manson, J. E., Nathan, D. M., Krolewski, A. S., Stampfer, M. J., Willett, W. C., & Hennekens, C. H. (1992). A prospective study of exercise and incidence of diabetes among U.S. male physicians. *Journal of the American Medical Association, 268,* 63–67.

Meredith, C., Frontera, W., Fisher, E., Hughes, V., Herland, J., Edwards, J., & Evans, W. (1989). Peripheral effects of endurance training in young and old subjects. *Journal of Applied Physiology, 66,* 2844–2849.

Meyers, D. A., Goldberg, A. P., Bleecker, M. L., Coon, P. J., Drinkwater, D. T., & Bleecker, E. R. (1991). Relationship of obesity and physical fitness to cardiopulmonary and metabolic function in healthy older men. *Journal of Gerontology, 46,* M57–M65.

Miller, J., Pratley, R. E., Goldberg, A. P., Gordon, P., Rubin, M., Treuth, M. S., Ryan, A. S., & Hurley, B. F. (1994). Strength training increases insulin action in healthy 50 to 65 year old men. *Journal of Applied Physiology, 77,* 1122–1127.

Montoye, E. H., Metzner, H., & Keller, J. (1972). Habitual physical activity and blood pressure. *Medicine Science Sports Exercise, 4,* 175–181.

Ogawa, T., Spina, R. J., Martin, W. H., III, Kohrt, W. M., Schechtman, K. B., Holloszy, J. O., & Ehsani, A. A. (1992). Effects of aging, sex, and physical training on cardiovascular responses to exercise. *Circulation, 86,* 494–503.

Paffenbarger, R. S., Jr., Leung, R. W., Jung, D. L., & Hyde, R. T. (1991). Physical activity and hypertension. An epidemiological view. *Annual Review of Medicine, 23,* 319–327.

Paffenbarger, R. S., Jr., Hyde, R. T., Wing, A. L., Lee, I. M., Jung, D. L., & Kampert, J. B. (1993). The association of changes in physical activity level and other lifestyle characteristics with mortality among men. *New England Journal of Medicine, 328,* 538–545.

Poehlman, E. T., McAuliffe, T. L., Van Houten, D. R., & Danforth, E., Jr. (1990). Influence of age and endurance training on metabolic rate and hormones in healthy men. *American Journal of Physiology, 259,* E66–E72.

Poehlman, E. T., Goran, M. I., Gardner, A. W., Ades, P. A., Arciero, P. J., Katzman-Rooks, S. M., Montgomery, S. M., Toth, M. J., & Sutherland, P. T. (1993). Determinants of decline in resting metabolic rate in aging females. *American Journal of Physiology, 264,* E450–E455.

Pollock, M. L., Foster, C., Knapp, D., Rod, J. L., & Schmidt, D. H. (1987). Effect of age and training on aerobic capacity and body composition of master althletes. *Journal of Applied Physiology, 62,* 725–731.

Pollock, M. L., Miller, H. S., & Wilmore, J. (1974). Physiological characteristics of champion American track athletes 40 to 75 years of age. *Journal of Gerontology, 29,* 645–649.

Pratley, R. E., Hagberg, J. M., Rogus, E. M., & Goldberg, A. P. (1995). Enhanced insulin sensitivity and waist-to-hip ratio in master athletes. *American Journal of Physiology, 268* (Endocrinol. Metab 31), E484–E490.

Reaven, G. M. (1988). Banting lecture 1988. Role of insulin resistance in human disease. *Diabetes, 37,* 1595–1607.

Reaven, G. M., Chen, Y. D. I., Jeppesen, J., Maheux, P., & Krauss, R. M. (1993). Insulin resistance and hyperinsulinemia in individuals with small dense low density lipoprotein particles. *Journal of Clinical Investigation, 92,* 141–146.

Rivera, A. M., Pells, A. E., III, Sady, S. P., Sady, M. A., Cullinane, E. M., & Thompson, P. D. (1989). Physiological factors associated with the lower maximal oxygen consumption of master runners. *Journal of Applied Physiology, 66,* 949–954.

Robinson, S., Dill, D. B., Robinson, R. D., Tzankoff, S. P., & Wagner, J. A. (1976). Physiological aging of champion runners. *Journal of Applied Physiology, 41,* 46–51.

Rodeheffer, R. J., Gerstenblith, G., Becker, L. C., Fleg, J. L., Weisfeldt, M. L., & Lakatta, E. G. (1984). Exercise cardiac output is maintained with advancing age in healthy human subjects: cardiac dilatation and increased stroke volume compensate for diminished heart rate. *Circulation, 69,* 203–213.

Rogers, M. A., Hagberg, J. M., Martin, W. H., III, Ehsani, A. A., & Holloszy, J. O. (1990a). De-cline in VO$_2$max with aging in master athletes and sedentary men. *Journal of Applied Physiology, 68,* 2195–2199.

Rogers, M. A., King, D. S., Hagberg, J. M., Ehsani, A. A., & Holloszy, J. O. (1990b). Effect of 10 days of physical inactivity on glucose tolerance in master athletes. *Journal of Applied Physiology, 68,* 1833–1837.

Rowe, J. W., & Kahn, R. L. (1987). Human aging: usual and successful. *Science, 237,* 143–149.

Saltin, B., Blomqvist, G., Mitchell, J. H., Johnson, R. L., Jr., Widenthal, K., & Chapman, C. B. (1968). Response to exercise after bed rest and after training. *Circulation, 38* (5, Suppl. VII), 1–78.

Sandvik, L., Erikssen, J., Thaulow, E., Erikssen, G., Mundal, R., & Rodahl, K. (1993). Physical fitness as a predictor of mortality among healthy middle-aged Norwegian men. *New England Journal of Medicine, 328,* 533–537.

Schocken, D. D., Blumenthal, J. A., Port, S., Hindle, P., & Coleman, R. E. (1983). Physical conditioning in left ventricular performance in the elderly: Assessment by radionuclide angiocardiography. *American Journal of Cardiology, 52,* 359–364.

Schoenberger, J. A. (1986). Epidemiology of systolic and diastolic systemic blood pressure elevation in the elderly. *American Journal of Cardiology, 57,* 45C–51C.

Schwartz, R. S. (1988). Effects of exercise training on high-density lipoproteins and apolipoprotein A-I in old and young men. *Metabolism, 37,* 1128–1133.

Seals, D. R., Allen, W. K., Hurley, B. F., Dalsky, G. P., Ehsani, A. A., & Hagberg, J. M. (1984a). Elevated high density lipoprotein cholesterol levels in older endurance athletes. *American Journal of Cardiology, 54,* 390–393.

Seals, D. R., Hagberg, J. M., Allen, W. K., Hurley, B. F., Dalsky, G. P., Ehsani, A. A., & Holloszy, J. O. (1984b). Glucose tolerance in young and older athletes and sedentary men. *Journal of Applied Physiology, 56,* 1521–1525.

Seals, D. R., Hagberg, J. M., Spina, R. J., Rogers, M. A., Schechtman, K. B., & Ehsani, A. A. (1994). Enhanced left ventricular performance in endurance trained older men. *Circulation, 89,* 198–205.

Spina, R. J., Ogawa, T., Kohrt, W. M., Martin,

W. H., III, Holloszy, J. O., & Ehsani, A. A. (1993a). Differences in cardiovascular adaptations to endurance exercise training between older men and women. *Journal of Applied Physiology, 75,* 849–855.

Spina, R. J., Ogawa, T., Miller, T. R., Kohrt, W. M., & Ehsani, A. A. (1993b). Effect of exercise training on left ventricular performance in older women free of cardiopulmonary disease. *American Journal of Cardiology, 71,* 99–104.

Stevens, V. J., Corrigan, S. A., Obarzanek, E., *et al.* (1993). Weight loss intervention in phase I of the trials of hypertension prevention. *Archives of Internal Medicine, 153,* 849–858.

Stratton, J. R., Levy, W. C., Cereueira, M. D., Schwartz, R. S., & Abrass, I. B. (1994). Cardiovascular responses to exercise: Effects of aging and exercise training in healthy men. *Circulation, 89,* 1648–1655.

Tonino, R. P. (1989). Effect of physical training on the insulin resistance of aging. *American Journal of Physiology, 256,* E352–E356.

Tonino, R. P., & Driscoll, P. A. (1988). Reliability of maximal and submaximal parameters of treadmill testing for the measurement of physical training in older persons. *Journal of Gerontology, 43,* 101–104.

Toth, M. J., Goran, M. I., Ades, P. A., Howard, D. B., & Poehlman, E. T. (1993). An examination of data normalization procedures for expressing peak VO$_2$ data. *Journal of Applied Physiology, 75,* 2288–2292.

Toth, M. J., Gardner, A. W., Ades, P. A., & Poehlman, E. T. (1994). Contribution of body composition and physical activity to age-related decline in peak VO$_2$ in men and women. *Journal of Applied Physiology, 77,* 647–652.

Williams, P. T., Krauss, R. M., Vranizan, K. M., & Wood, P. B. (1990). Changes in lipoprotein subfractions during diet-induced and exercise induced weight loss in moderately overweight men. *Circulation, 81,* 1293–1304.

Zimetbaum, P., Frishman, W. H., Ooi, W. L., Derman, M. P., Aronson, M., Gidez, L. I., & Eder, H. A. (1992). Plasma lipids and lipoproteins and the incidence of cardiovascular disease in the very elderly. The Bronx Aging Study. *Arteriosclerosis and Thrombosis, 12,* 416–423.

Sixteen

Aging and the Immune Response

Richard A. Miller

I. Introduction

The immune system provides a particularly attractive arena for gerontological
investigation. Unlike most other organ
systems, the immune system largely consists of naturally motile cells, and for this
reason physiologically relevant intercellular responses can often be modeled in
short-term *in vitro* culture conditions and
in "host" animals that have received mixtures of cells from different sources, including donors of varying ages. The substantial (and rapidly growing) appreciation
of the molecular and cellular details of immune regulation in young humans and rodents furnishes the gerontologist with
reagents and ideas needed to probe immunosenescent change, while the role of the
immune system in defenses against infectious and neoplastic diseases renders these
investigations highly germane to geriatric
medicine.

This chapter will summarize the status
of our understanding of the mechanisms
and implications of immune senescence,
with emphasis on work that has been carried out in the 5 years since the last edition
of this Handbook. Much of the work done
prior to 1990 has been reviewed in earlier

editions of this series (Hausman & Weksler, 1985; Miller, 1990), and reviews by
other authors also offer useful perspectives (Murasko & Goonewardene, 1990;
Thoman & Weigle, 1989).

II. Cellular Interactions in the Immune Response

The immune system generates highly specific effector cells and molecules that provide defenses against microbial agents and
may also participate in antineoplastic responses. There are three broad classes of
specific immune reactions, which often
occur simultaneously in response to an antigenic stimulus. In the humoral immune
response, B lymphocytes produce antigen-
specific antibody molecules that can bind
to microbes and microbial products and
then activate a variety of defensive responses mediated by complement proteins and phagocytic cells. Second, the cytotoxic T-cell response involves the generation of effector T cells that can recognize
and lyse abnormal or infected target cells.
Third, in the delayed-type hypersensitivity response, antigen-specific T cells
initiate a defensive reaction by attracting

Handbook of the Biology of Aging, Fourth Edition
Copyright © 1996 Academic Press, Inc. All rights of reproduction in any form reserved.

tracting other cell types, including macrophages, to the site of an infectious agent or other antigenic stimulus.

Although each of these three reactions involves a distinct effector mechanism, in most cases they are initiated and controlled through a common process; the activation of helper T cells. Extracellular antigens (for example, bacterial toxins) are ingested by specialized antigen-processing cells (APCs), digested into peptide fragments, and then exposed on the APC surface in a form that is strongly stimulatory for the helper T cell. These helper T cells in turn perform several activities: (1) activation of B cells to initiate the humoral response; (2) production of the soluble cytokine interleukin-2 (IL-2) to promote the growth of cytotoxic T cells; and (3) initiation of the delayed-type hypersensitivity response by the secretion of other cytokines that attract and activate effector macrophages. Each of the relevant cell types can be identified and purified on the basis of characteristic patterns of cell surface molecules, including immunoglobulin (Ig) on B cells, CD4 on the cytokine-producing helper T cells, and CD8 on the T cells able to generate potent cytotoxic effectors. The principal challenge for the immunogerontologist is to elucidate the ways in which aging alters these interactions among T cells, B cells, and APCs so as to diminish the effectiveness of protective immune reactions.

III. T Lymphocyte Function: Production of and Response to Cytokines

Early work [reviewed in Hausman and Weksler (1985) and Miller (1990; 1991a] established that most tests of T-cell function—including in vivo assays of DTH and in vitro tests for growth in response to T-cell mitogens and foreign cells—showed consistent and quantitatively impressive declines in aging hu-

mans and rodents. The central focus of modern work on T-cell function has been to clarify the ways in which changes in these end points depend upon alterations in the production and response to cytokines, which are soluble proteins secreted by immunologically active cells that modulate the activities of other cells in the interacting immune network. Unlike antibodies, cytokines themselves are not specific for any given antigen, but their production is often stimulated by the recognition of a specific antigen by T cells. The first of the T-cell cytokines to be investigated thoroughly was IL-2, which serves as a potent growth factor for T and B lymphocytes. Since the proportion of T and B cells that are specific for any single antigen is very small (typically 10^{-5}), IL-2-driven clonal expansion is a critically important early step in the development of adequate numbers of effector lymphocytes for protective immunity. Once good assays for IL-2 were developed, many laboratories were able to demonstrate consistent age-related declines in IL-2 production by T cells from old humans and mice (Gillis et al., 1981; Thoman & Weigle, 1981; Miller & Stutman, 1981; Nagel et al., 1988; Hertogh-Huijbregts et al., 1990; Huang et al., 1992). Production of IL-2 mRNA also declines with age in humans and mice (Nagel et al., 1988; Fong & Makinodan, 1989). Both in situ hybridization analysis of mRNA (Fong & Makinodan, 1989) and limiting dilution tests for IL-2 secretion (Miller, 1984) have suggested that the decline represents a diminution of the number of T cells that are able to generate IL-2 after stimulation, rather than a uniform decline in IL-2 production by all T cells. Studies of IL-2 and IL-2 mRNA production by rats have demonstrated age-related declines in some laboratories (Wu et al., 1986; Odio et al., 1987; Davila & Kelley, 1988), but not in others (Holbrook et al., 1989; Goya et al., 1991) with a greater effect of age in male than in female rats (Davila & Kelley, 1988) and in mixed lymphocyte cultures than in mitogen-stimulated cultures (Gilman et al., 1982). Immobilized antibody to the CD3 chains of the T-cell receptor generates a very strong stimulus for IL-2 production that bypasses the requirement for APC/T-cell interaction; this stimulus produces equally high amounts of IL-2 and IL-2 mRNA from young and old mouse T cells (Hobbs et al., 1991).

Defects in the production of IL-2 could plausibly account for much of the age-related decline in T-cell function, and indeed in certain cases, the addition of exogenous IL-2 to cultures containing T cells from old donors can greatly increase responsiveness (Thoman & Weigle, 1982; Chang et al., 1982; Bruley-Rosset & Payelle, 1987; Beckman et al., 1990). High doses of IL-2 injected along with antigen can also restore the generation of cytotoxic T cells in live mice (Thoman & Weigle, 1985). In most circumstances, however, IL-2 supplementation has only a partial or negligible ability to repair age-associated immunodeficiencies (Gillis et al., 1981; Gilman et al., 1982; Nordin & Collins, 1983; Miller, 1984; Gottesman et al., 1985; Negoro et al., 1986). Two distinct defects seem to be involved in this loss of IL-2 responsiveness: defects in IL-2 receptor (IL-2R) expression and alterations in signal transduction through the IL-2R complex. IL-2R is a three-chain, signal-transducing complex that is not present on T cells in their typical resting state, but that can be induced (in T cells from young individuals) after contact with an activating agent. Induction of the 25-kDa IL-2Rα chain by mitogenic agents has been reported to decline in aged mice (Vie & Miller, 1986; Ernst et al., 1989) and humans (Negoro et al., 1986; Orson et al., 1989). The proportion of resting T cells that, after activation, can express high-affinity IL-2R (which requires the expression of both the α-chain and the 75-kDa β-chain) also declines with age (Negoro et al., 1986; Proust et al., 1988; Froelich et al., 1988; Nagel et

al., 1989; Hara et al., 1988; Schwab et al., 1990), as does the proportion of T cells that can proliferate when activated and then further cultured with IL-2 (Nordin & Collins, 1983; Miller, 1984; Proust et al., 1988). In addition to defects in the expression of IL-2R, three groups have noted a decline in proliferative responses to IL-2, even in purified IL-2R-expressing blasts (Negoro et al., 1986; Nagel et al., 1989; Thoman, 1991). The potential role of the third component of the IL-2R complex, the signal-transducing γ-chain (Kondo et al., 1993), has yet to be examined in aging subjects, but it is worth noting that conditions that induce full expression of the α- and β-chains in T cells from old humans do not always induce the formation of high-affinity IL-2R complexes (Schwab et al., 1990). It seems very likely that defects in the production of IL-2 and in the response to IL-2 contribute to the age-related declines in the strength and speed of protective immune responses.

A study in which elderly subjects were tested for immune responsiveness twice over a 2- to 4-week interval has shown that the degree of impairment may vary markedly over time for a given aged individual (Brill et al., 1987). Another analysis (Huang et al., 1992) showed that influenza vaccination could lead to a transient decline in the ability of T cells from old humans to generate IL-2 in mitogen-stimulated in vitro cultures; this decline was detectable 15 days but not 30 days after vaccination. In tests performed prior to vaccination, a fraction (31%) of elderly subjects were found to have high serum levels of IL-2 and depressed ability to produce IL-2 in vitro; members of this subgroup were found to be poor responders to the vaccine. The authors suggested that recent exposure to an immunogen, in the form of a vaccine or transient infection, may render the elderly person temporarily hyporesponsive for IL-2-dependent immune reactions. More detailed longitudinal analyses will be required to test the implications of this interesting idea.

The demonstration (Mosmann *et al.*, 1986) that long-term mouse helper T-cell clones fall into two subsets with distinct patterns of cytokine production has had a strong influence on studies of aging and cytokine production. Helper T-cell clones of the T_H1 type produce IL-2 as well as interferon-γ (IFN-γ), which has potent pleiotropic effects on immune reactions in addition to its antiviral properties. Clones of the T_H2 type do not produce IL-2 or IFN-γ, but instead produce IL-4 and IL-5, which are cytokines that play important roles in the stimulation of antibody production by B cells. The demonstration that IL-2 production declines with aging has prompted the speculation that aging might lead to defects of other cytokines of the T_H1 series and corresponding increases in the generation of T_H2 cytokines such as IL-4 and IL-5. The evidence for this question is only partially consistent. Several groups have found, as predicted, an age-related increase in IL-4 production by stimulated mouse T cells (Ernst *et al.*, 1990; Kubo & Cinader, 1990; Nagelkerken *et al.*, 1991; Daynes & Araneo, 1992; Cillari *et al.*, 1992); generation of IL-4 mRNA is also reported to increase with age (Hobbs *et al.*, 1993). In contrast, the production of IL-4 by human T cells was found to decrease with age (al-Rayes *et al.*, 1992), as does the production of IL-4 in cultures of mouse T cells supplemented with IL-2, a potent activator of IL-4 production (Li & Miller, 1993). The number of IL-4-secreting T cells produced in mitogen-activated cultures of mouse spleen or lymph node also falls dramatically with age (Green-Johnson *et al.*, 1991), although in this report the numbers of mice tested were too small to preclude chance effects. Two reports have also shown an age-associated increase in T-cell IL-5 production (Daynes & Araneo, 1992; Hobbs *et al.*, 1993), consistent with the idea of an increase in cells predisposed to T_H2 cytokine secretion.

A shift from T_H1 to T_H2 patterns of CD4 T-cell differentiation would be expected to produce a decline in IFN-γ production to parallel the loss of IL-2, but the data for this question are inconsistent. In studies of mice, three groups have reported the predicted decrease in IFN-γ generation (Green-Johnson *et al.*, 1991; Cillari *et al.*, 1992; Bloom & Horvath, 1994), but four others have shown an increase in IFN-γ synthesis (Saxena *et al.*, 1988; Kirschmann & Murasko, 1992; Daynes & Araneo, 1992; Hobbs *et al.*, 1993). Stimulated human T cells from aged donors have been reported to produce higher (Chopra *et al.*, 1989), lower (Abb *et al.*, 1984; Gauchat *et al.*, 1988; al-Rayes *et al.*, 1992), or unchanged (Rytel *et al.*, 1986) levels of IFN-γ. Interpretation of these data in the context of the T_H1/T_H2 dichotomy is complicated by variations in culture conditions, stimulus used, and species and cell type (human blood versus mouse spleen and lymph node). The production of IFN-γ by CD8 T cells may also contribute to disparities among these reports.

A macrophage-dependent cytokine IL-10 has been discovered to promote the production of T_H2 cytokines at the expense of the T_H1 set. Generation of IL-10 seems to increase with age in mice (Hobbs *et al.*, 1994) and could contribute to a decline in IL-2 and increases in IL-4 and IL-5 production in the aged.

The hematopoietic growth factor IL-3 is produced equally well by both T_H1 and T_H2 cells (Mosmann *et al.*, 1986). Thus, a shift with age from T_H1 to T_H2 cells would not, by itself, be expected to alter IL-3 production. Five groups, however, have reported an age-related decline in IL-3 production (Li *et al.*, 1988; Chang *et al.*, 1988; Koyama *et al.*, 1990; Daynes & Araneo, 1992; Flurkey *et al.*, 1992b). This result suggests that shifts in patterns of cytokine production may be superimposed on a general decline in CD3 cell responsiveness. Three other groups, however, have reported higher levels of IL-3 secretion or IL-3 mRNA production by T cells from aged donors (Iwashima *et al.*, 1987; Kubo & Cinader, 1990; Hobbs *et al.*, 1993). One of these reports (Hobbs *et al.*, 1993) used a signal, immobilized anti-CD3 antibody, that overcomes the age-associated defect in IL-2 production, while another (Kubo & Cinader, 1990) used extremely short culture intervals (18–24 hr) that might indicate IL-3 production by previously activated effectors, rather than the induction of new IL-3-secreting cells from resting lymphocytes.

On balance, the evidence is most consistent with an increase with age in the production of T$_H$2 cytokines IL-4 and IL-5, with a parallel loss in IL-2 production and an uncertain effect on IFN-γ. The decline in IL-3 production seen in most studies suggests that an overall decline in T-cell responsiveness may be superimposed on any shifts in subsets with differing propensities for cytokine production. There is, however, considerable interlaboratory variability in the degree and even the direction of the age-related change for many of the cytokines studied. It seems likely that variations in stimuli, cell density, and APC influences may, in certain combinations, favor T cells from young donors, but in other conditions favor T cells from older individuals. Indeed, one group has reported an age-dependent shift in T cells from a population that preferentially responds to macrophage-presented antigens to another that prefers antigens presented by B lymphocytes (Hayakawa & Hardy, 1989). Further advances in this field will require careful dissection of the age sensitivity of variations in specific forms of costimuli and intercellular signals.

IV. T-Cell Subsets

The question of whether aging might lead to an alteration in the relative proportions of the CD4 (helper) and CD8 (cytotoxic) subsets has stimulated the publication of over 15 reports, which have been tabulated elsewhere (Miller, 1991a, 1994) and which

taken together suggest that changes in the relative or absolute numbers of CD4 and CD8 T cells, while sometimes demonstrable in individual strains of mice or human populations, are small and inconsistent. Reports of increases, decreases, or stability in the CD4/CD8 ratio are about equally distributed in this set of publications, and there is little reason to suspect that the numerical changes seen have biological significance.

Studies using approaches that further subdivide the CD4 and CD8 populations have been much more provocative. Both the CD4 and CD8 subsets contain a mixture of naive T cells, which are thought to have emigrated from the thymus to the periphery but not yet encountered an activating antigen, and memory T cells, the progeny of naive cells that have undergone one or perhaps several rounds of antigen- and cytokine-driven proliferation. In both mice and humans, naive and memory T cells can be distinguished from one another on the basis of differences in cell surface glycoprotein markers. Naive and memory T cells differ not just in their surface markers but also in their requirements for stimulation and their ability to produce different batteries of cytokines (Akbar *et al.*, 1991).

Numerous laboratories have now reported that aging in mice, rats, and humans leads to increases in the proportion of T cells expressing the memory cell phenotype and declines in the proportion of naive T cells (De Paoli *et al.*, 1988; Serra *et al.*, 1988; Walker *et al.*, 1990; Lerner *et al.*, 1989; Ernst *et al.*, 1990; Pilarski *et al.*, 1991; Grossmann *et al.*, 1991; Utsuyama *et al.*, 1992; Gabriel *et al.*, 1993; Tielen *et al.*, 1993). This transition affects both the CD4 and CD8 pools and also affects T cells in the blood, lymph nodes, and spleen; in mice the shift leads to 2- to 3-fold increases in the proportion of memory cells and 2- to 3-fold declines in the proportion of naive T cells (Lerner *et al.*, 1989). There is some controversy among immunologists as to whether the markers used to delineate the memory cell pool also detect cells that have been recently activated, and whether cells of the memory phenotype retain that phenotype indefinitely, but the majority of the memory cells that accumulate in aged subjects seem to be resting lymphocytes in size, DNA profile, lack of activation markers (Kendig et al., 1991; Utsuyama et al., 1992), and requirement for further stimulation for cell cycle entry. Since the size (Nakahama et al., 1990) and productivity (Scollary et al., 1980) of the thymus gland decline with age, and since removal of the thymus in adult life leads to a rapid decline in the number and proportion of naive T cells in the periphery (Budd et al., 1987), the age-associated shift from naive to memory T cells is explicable in developmental terms, although the extent to which thymic involution is the root cause of this shift has not been carefully evaluated.

There are several lines of evidence suggesting that the shift from naive to memory T cells contributes to immunodeficiency in old age. Aging leads to a decline in the proportion of T cells that can make IL-2 or IL-3 after exposure to Con A (a mitogenic plant lectin) or staphylococcal enterotoxin B (SEB) and to a decline in the proportion of cells that can respond to Con A plus IL-2 by proliferation or by generation of cytotoxic effectors (Lerner et al., 1989; Flurkey et al., 1992b). In each of these cases, naive T cells (from young or old mice) respond much more frequently than memory T cells, so that the age effect can largely be attributed to the increase with age in the less responsive memory cell pool. Since IL-4 is thought to be largely a memory cell product (Akbar et al., 1991), the increase with age in IL-4 production can also plausibly be attributed to the shift in subsets (Ernst et al., 1990; Nagelkerken et al., 1991), although it should be noted that the question of whether memory T cells from old mice are actually responsible for IL-4 production has not been studied carefully. The one published comparison of IL-4 production by purified memory T cells from young and old mice suggests that aging may impair memory cell IL-4 production under certain culture conditions (Li & Miller, 1993) and thus is not consistent with the suggestion that higher IL-4 production in aging reflects memory cell accumulation. The increase with age in IL-10 production also seems to reflect a shift to memory cell predominance, in that memory T cells from mice of any age produce much more IL-10 than naive cells (Hobbs et al., 1994). In summary, it seems likely that the loss with age of the naive T-cell populations within the CD4 and CD8 subsets may diminish responses to polyclonal mitogens by impairing both IL-2 production and IL-2 responsiveness. The extent to which this transition might also impair responses to novel cognate antigens (for example, newly arising strains of influenza virus or tumor neoantigens), and might contribute to altered patterns of lymphokine production, will require further investigation.

New data suggest that the naive and memory T-cell subsets can be further subdivided into smaller, functionally distinct subsets whose relative distribution is age-sensitive. A small fraction of T cells in young mice and a much larger fraction of T cells from old mice exhibit high levels of cell surface P-glycoprotein, the ATP-dependent translocator that mediates multiple-drug resistance in tumor cells (Juranka et al., 1989). P-glycoprotein-expressing T cells increase with age in the naive and memory cell pools in both the CD4 and CD8 lineages (Witkowski & Miller, 1993). Within the CD4 memory pool, only cells with low levels of P-glycoprotein are able to respond to stimulatory antibodies and IL-2 by proliferation and IL-4 secretion (Witkowski et al., 1994), and the shift to cells with high levels of P-glycoprotein thus accounts for some, though not all, of the decline with age in IL-2 responsiveness.

Other shifts among T-cell subsets have

been reported, although not yet fully evaluated for functional significance. There is, for example, a 3-fold increase with age in human peripheral blood T cells that express the 3G5 ganglioside (Rabinowe et al., 1987). T cells expressing the γδ form of the T-cell receptor have been variously inferred to increase (Matsuzaki et al., 1988) or to decrease (O'Leary et al., 1988) with aging, in each case on equivocal data. T cells expressing relatively low levels of the αβ form of the T-cell receptor have been reported to be prominent in the liver of mice and to increase with age, escaping in small numbers into the peripheral immune system of the oldest animals examined (Ohteki et al., 1992). CD4 T cells expressing the surface marker 3G11 are also reported to increase with age (Hayakawa & Hardy, 1988) and to be specialized for the recognition of antigens presented by B lymphocytes and for the production of IL-2 (Hayakawa & Hardy, 1989). Within the CD8 pool, aging leads to an increase in cells expressing surface markers characteristic of memory cells and an increase in the production of high levels of IFN-γ, a characteristic product of CD8 memory T cells (Ernst et al., 1993). The CD8 memory pool can be further subdivided using antibodies to other surface markers (3G11 and MEL-14), and it seems possible that further work on these CD8 memory subsets may provide additional insights into the cellular basis for immune changes in the cytotoxic T-cell response.

V. Activation Defects in T Cells from Old Donors

The demonstration that many T cells in old mice fail to respond to stimuli that would ordinarily activate T cells from young donors has prompted analysis of the biochemical basis for this unresponsiveness. The conversion of resting T cells to actively proliferating blasts and then to differentiated effector cells is a complex, sequential process involving (a) increases in cellular calcium levels, changes in second messengers, and protein kinase-mediated phosphorylations in the first few minutes of activation, followed by (b) activation of specific genes including protooncogenes c-fos and c-myc within the first 60 min and (c) activation of other sets of genes, including those for IL-2 and components of the IL-2 receptor within the first 6 hr. Later events lead to DNA synthesis, cell division, and the generation of clones of effector lymphocytes. T cells from old mice (and perhaps also old humans) show defects at several stages of this process, although it is not yet clear whether all of the defects in later events can be attributed simply to defects at earlier stages.

One of the earliest detectable events in T-cell activation is the increase in level of intracellular free calcium ion concentration, $[Ca]_i$, from its resting level of 100 to 300–1000 nM; increases in $[Ca]_i$ can be seen within 30 s of T-cell exposure to an activating stimulus. T cells from old mice exhibit defects in calcium signal generation when triggered by Con A or antibody to the CD3 components of the T-cell receptor (Miller et al., 1987; Proust et al., 1987; Grossmann et al., 1991; Saini & Sei, 1993). Both CD4 and CD8 cells are affected in at least four strains of mice (Philosophe & Miller, 1990; Grossmann et al., 1990, 1991), although spleen and blood cells seem to be more age-sensitive in this regard than lymph node cells (Grossmann et al., 1991). Three groups have also reported an age-dependent impairment of calcium signal generation in human peripheral blood T cells (Gupta, 1989; Whisler et al., 1991; al-Rayes et al., 1992), although a fourth group noted only a small (though statistically convincing) age effect (Grossmann et al., 1989), and two others (Lustyik & O'Leary, 1989; Naylor et al., 1992) found no effect of age on calcium signals.

The biochemical basis for this defect is unclear. One group has reported (Proust et *al.*, 1987) that T cells from old mice exhibit an increased level of [Ca]$_i$ in the resting, unactivated state and that old and young T cells produce similar [Ca]$_i$ levels after activation, but most laboratories found no increases in [Ca]$_i$ of resting T cells from older subjects (Miller *et al.*, 1987; Gupta, 1989; Grossmann *et al.*, 1989, 1991; Whisler *et al.*, 1991; Naylor *et al.*, 1992). Poor calcium signal induction could reflect a defect in the production of the secondary messenger inositol trisphosphate (IP3), which is responsible for the release of intracellular Ca^{2+} stores early in activation, and indeed some (Proust *et al.*, 1987; Kawanishi, 1993), but not all (Lerner *et al.*, 1988; Whisler *et al.*, 1991), laboratories have noted a loss in IP3 production by aged T cells. Sustained increases in [Ca]$_i$ depend not so much on IP3-mediated release of stored Ca^{2+} as on the influx of Ca^{2+} from extracellular sources (Gelfand *et al.*, 1988), and mitogen-stimulated Ca^{2+} influx does indeed decline with age in mice (Lerner *et all.*, 1988), although the process by which influx is linked to receptor-mediated signals is still unclear. T cells from old mice are resistant to changes in [Ca]$_i$ even when these are induced by ionomycin, which bypasses receptor-mediated signal transduction steps (Miller *et al.*, 1989; Philosophe & Miller, 1990); such a defect suggests that poor calcium signal generation in old T cells might result from overactivity of the ATP-dependent plasma membrane calcium pump that regulates [Ca]$_i$ in the 100–1000 nM range (Carafoli, 1987). Although two groups have noted ionomycin resistance in T cells from aged mice (Miller *et al.*, 1989; Negoro & Hara, 1992), studies of rats (Franklin *et al.*, 1990) and humans (Whisler *et al.*, 1991) have shown no such effect of age. The basis for this disparity is unclear, although it may be pertinent to note that calcium ionophores are mitogenic (in the absence of phorbol ester costimuli) in rats and humans but not in mice. Indeed, the mitogenic effects

of calcium ionophores are more apparent in aged than in young rats (Franklin *et al.*, 1990).

The combination of a phorbol ester (typically phorbol myristic acetate or PMA) plus a calcium ionophore is strongly mitogenic for T cells, causing activation at intracellular sites and thus bypassing the earliest steps in the signal transduction cascade. Several groups thus have tried to determine whether the defect(s) in signal transduction in T cells from old donors lie upstream or downstream from the PMA- and calcium-sensitive steps by measuring PMA/ionophore-stimulated proliferation or lymphokine production. Most reports indicate that PMA and a calcium ionophore induce higher levels of function in old T cells than do receptor-dependent signals (Miller, 1986; Thoman & Weigle, 1988; Hertogh-Huijbregts *et al.*, 1990; Nagelkerken *et al.*, 1991; Negoro & Hara, 1992; Naylor *et al.*, 1992) and that the differences between young and old mice or humans are less dramatic (though often still apparent) when these receptor-bypassing stimuli are used. In T cells from old humans, lectin-induced activation of the DNA-binding factor AP-1 is usually poor, but in many cases can be repaired by the addition of PMA to the culture medium (Whisler *et al.*, 1993). The ability of PMA and calcium ionophore to produce only a partial correction of the age-associated activation defect suggests that T cells from aged individuals may exhibit defects at several stages of the activation cascade, including some that precede the generation of calcium signals and the diacylglycerols mimicked by PMA.

Several classes of protein kinases are known to participate in T-cell activation in a set of linked reactions that are still only partly worked out (Mustelin & Burn, 1993). These include tyrosine-specific protein kinases (TPKs) of the *src* family, including *lck* and *fyn*, that are thought to mediate some of the very early steps in

T-cell receptor-mediated activation. TPK-mediated phosphorylation induced by Con A, anti-CD3, and anti-TCR antibodies is lower in T cells from old than from young mice (Shi & Miller, 1992), and both CD4 and CD8 cells are affected (Shi & Miller, 1993). Most of the protein phosphorylation in the cell is mediated by serine- and threonine-specific kinases, including protein kinase C, and T cells from old mice show dramatic alterations in the patterns of phosphorylated substrates induced by Con A or by anti-CD3 antibody (Patel & Miller, 1992). Each of 16 phosphoproteins (PPNs) whose phosphorylation was vigorously induced by anti-CD3 in young T cells was essentially unresponsive in 2-year-old mice, with intermediate levels of response seen for each PPN at intermediate ages, with measurable effects seen in mice as young as 10–12 months. Anti-CD3 did, however, induce in old T cells the phosphorylation of a set of three PPNs that were unreactive in T cells from young animals. Some of the PPNs were characteristically reactive only in CD4 cells and others only in CD8 cells, but both classes were equally susceptible to the age effect. This abnormal pattern of PPN phosphorylation can be attributed in part to defects in responses to intracellular calcium, since levels of calcium ionophore that were able to alter $[Ca]_i$ in both young and old T cells led to the phosphorylation of a set of 10 PPNs only in T cells from young donors (Patel & Miller, 1992). The pattern of PPN responses to the PK-C activator PMA was more complex: of 12 PPNs that were phosphorylated in PMA-activated young T cells, 10 were entirely unresponsive and the other 2 were fully responsive in T cells from old mice, and in addition the old T cells phosphorylated a set of three PPNs not PMA-reactive in young T cells. This pattern is not consistent with models in which PK-C is entirely absent, nor with models in which PK-C signals are entirely normal, but may reflect alterations in the distribution of PK-C, PK-C substrates, or protein phosphatases that remove PO_4 from PK-C-phosphorylated PPNs. PK-C activation involves its translocation from cytoplasm to plasma membrane, a process reported to be impaired in T cells from old mice (Proust et al., 1987; Kawanishi, 1993). Further studies of age-related changes in specific kinases and specific substrates known to be involved in T-cell activation seem likely to be informative and are long overdue.

Some, though not all, of these biochemical abnormalities can be linked to the replacement of naive by memory T cells in aging mice. Thus, memory T cells—in young or old mice—are intrinsically more resistant than naive T cells to the development of high $[Ca]_i$ (Philosophe & Miller, 1990; Miller et al., 1991; Rajasekar & Augustin, 1994), and their relative predominance in the aged immune system largely accounts for the average decline in calcium signal generation (Miller, 1991c). Since only those cells that generate early, strong calcium signals are likely to produce IL-2 and respond to IL-2 in lectin-stimulated T-cell cultures (Philosophe & Miller, 1989; Miller et al., 1991), the calcium resistance of mouse memory T cells also accounts for much of the loss with age in IL-2-dependent proliferative responses induced by lectins. Some of the defects in TPK-dependent phosphorylation also reflect underlying variations in the patterns of naive and memory T cells (Shi & Miller, 1993), although the functional implications will remain uncertain until more is known about the detailed biochemistry of subset-specific kinase pathways. Some protein kinase reactions, including some initiated by PMA or by calcium ionophores, are altered in both naive and memory T cells (Patel & Miller, 1992) and thus cannot be attributed to memory T-cell accumulation.

The details of the steps by which kinase

function and calcium signal generation lead to the activation of new gene transcription are gradually being pieced together (Pelech & Sanghera, 1992; Northrup et al., 1994). Reports of age-related changes in early gene activation are scanty and for the most part merely descriptive. Production of c-myc mRNA by Con A-stimulated mouse T cells (Buckler et al., 1988) and PHA-stimulated human T cells (Gamble et al., 1990) is reported to diminish with age; induction of c-myc protein synthesis also declines with age in humans (Pieri et al., 1992). The decline reflects a loss in the proportion of responding T cells, rather than a uniform abnormality affecting all cells to an equal degree (Gamble et al., 1990; Pieri et al., 1992); whether the nonresponsive cells are indeed those that fail to generate calcium signals (Miller et al., 1987) and fail to go on to IL-2 production and IL-2R generation (Miller, 1984; Nagel et al., 1989) has not yet been examined, nor has the hypothesis that the unresponsive cells are in the memory subset. Induction by PHA of mRNA for c-fos and junB in human T cells does not seem to be affected by age (Song et al., 1992), although induction of c-jun does show a slight (33%), significant decline. The transcription factor AP-1, which is composed of a mixture of fos-related and jun-related proteins, is not stimulated as well by PHA in T cells of old compared to young human donors (Whisler et al., 1993). It seems likely that defects in gene activation and the intranuclear appearance of transcription factors may result from upstream alterations in protein kinase activation and formation of second messengers, but little evidence is available to test this notion.

In summary, immune models linking early aspects of signal transduction, slightly later activation of protooncogenes and then cytokine mRNAs, and ultimate generation of clones of effector cells in age-sensitive T-cell subsets have received just enough attention to hint at the potential power of this approach for the elucidation of the mechanism of immunosenescence and perhaps also general principles of cellular gerontology, but remain woefully underexploited.

VI. T-Lymphocyte Development

Most discussions of T-cell production and the effects of aging focus on thymic involution: the decline with age in thymus size, cellularity, and production of thymic emigrants bound for the peripheral immune system (Scollay et al., 1980; Nakahama et al., 1990). The ability of the thymus to support the development of bone marrow-derived prothymocytes into mature peripheral T cells has been reported to diminish severely between the third and twelfth months of life in mice (Hirokawa et al., 1976), although another report surprisingly found little difference between thymus glands from 1- and 24-month-old mice in a very similar assay system (Utsuyama et al., 1991). The number of cells that arrive in the periphery from the thymus is, however, much too low to account for peripheral turnover, and essentially nothing is known about the effects of aging on the very substantial self-renewal process in the peripheral immune system (Miller & Stutman, 1984; Rocha, 1987). Thymectomy in young adult life does rapidly lead to the exhaustion of naive cells and the predominance of cells with the memory phenotype (Budd et al., 1987); this subset shift, though even more pronounced than in normal aged mice, leads to abnormalities of immune responsiveness that in many ways do not resemble those seen in old mice or humans (Miller, 1965; Kappler et al., 1974; Simpson & Cantor, 1975). Thymic transplantation into aging mice leads to the restoration of immune responsiveness only if accompanied by host irradiation and coadministration of bone marrow cells as a source of prothymocytes (Hirokawa et al.,

1976); functional restoration is transient, although repeated restorations can be accomplished by successive rounds of irradiation and transplantation (Hirokawa & Utsuyama, 1984). The hypothesis that thymic involution is central to T-lymphocyte immunosenescence deserves strengthening by critical tests or replacement by new ideas that give attention to postthymic aspects of T-cell development.

The question of whether aging diminishes the function of prothymocytes, bone marrow-derived cells that enter the thymus gland to develop into mature T cells, has been addressed in a variety of ways. Quantitative assays for prothymocyte number have shown no effect of age (Kadish & Basch, 1976) in their principal source, the bone marrow, although their number does decline in the spleens of aging mice (Basch, 1990). Functional assessment by culture of bone marrow cells on thymic epithelial (stromal) organ cultures has shown that the prothymocytes from aged mice are fully competent to undergo intrathymic maturation, although they are somewhat less vigorous in this assay than the marrow cells from young donors (Eren et al., 1988). Adoptive transfer experiments, in which marrow cells from young or old donors are injected into a host mouse along with a neonatal thymus gland, do not show any differences between the prothymocyte pools of young and old animals (Harrison et al., 1978; Gozes et al., 1982) when the immune competence of peripheral T cells is assessed within a few months of the transplantation procedure. T-cell immune systems reconstituted from old bone marrow may, however, show a relatively rapid decline in function compared to those derived from the marrow of young donors (Gozes et al., 1982; Averill & Wolf, 1985; Hirokawa et al., 1986), although this matter is in dispute (Harrison et al., 1978). Competitive assays using mixtures of bone marrow from young and old donors suggest that pluripotent hematopoietic stem cells do

not become less frequent with age, although there may be an age-dependent increase in the proportion of slightly less primitive stem cells with a substantial, but not indefinite, capacity for self-renewal (Harrison et al., 1989). The issue of whether these subtle shifts in prothymocyte and stem cell populations have functional consequences for peripheral immune function is still unresolved.

The repertoire of T-cell receptor specificities is determined by a mixture of intrathymic selection processes, both positive and negative, and potentially by postthymic processes that could lead to clonal depletion, anergy, or expansion. Studies of T-cell reactivity have provided some evidence for possible alterations in old mice (Schwab et al., 1992; Russo et al., 1993), but are complicated by technical concerns about in vitro clonal selection, absence of expected allogeneic effects in negative controls, and evidence for multicellular suppressive interactions. The first truly compelling suggestion of altered TCR repertoire formation has come from two studies of TCR V gene utilization in mice (Callahan et al., 1993) and in humans (Posnett et al., 1994). An earlier publication (Gonzalez-Quintial & Theofilopoulos, 1992) had measured mRNA transcript levels for 18 different $V\beta$ genes in pools of thymic and splenic cells from mice of various ages and found no evidence of age-dependent change. When $V\beta$ utilization was tested in individual aging mice, however, there was an impressive degree of idiosyncrasy in V gene usage within the CD8 populations of individual mice, with some mice showing unexpectedly high levels of T cells with $V\beta3$, others with expanded $V\beta7$ expression, and so forth. Almost every mouse tested over the age of 14 months showed some such abnormality in the CD8 subset of peripheral T cells. Similarly, the peripheral blood CD8 T-cell populations of most elderly humans were found to exhibit abnormally high proportions expressing one or another $V\beta$ chain

(Posnett *et al.*, 1994); this report, alas, did not include young adult controls and thus provides no information as to whether the unexpected Vβ distributions are a phenomenon restricted to the elderly. In neither species was there any corresponding abnormality of Vβ expression within the CD4 pool. There are also suggestions in both publications of interindividual differences in Vα heterogeneity in the CD8 subset, although the data on this point are still skimpy. There is some, still weak, evidence to suggest that the expansion is monoclonal or oligoclonal, e.g., involving cells derived from a very small number of original cells, although it is unlikely that these monoclonal events are a prelude to frank T-lymphoid neoplasia, which is quite rare in humans. Much more work is needed to determine the developmental origin, molecular basis, and functional implications of this phenomenon.

VII. B-Cell Function

There is ample evidence for an age-related decline in humoral immunity, characterized not only by a decline in the amount of antibody produced but also by dispro-

portionate losses in the ability to make IgG and IgA antibodies and antibodies with high affinities for their complementary antigens. Since the production of high-affinity antibodies of the IgG and IgA classes is particularly dependent on T-cell helper function, it has seemed reasonable that much of the senescent decline in humoral immunity might reflect alterations in helper T-cell function rather than an intrinsic change in B-cell function. Indeed, the major technical challenge facing students of aged B cells is to devise experimental situations in which T-cell help is either irrelevant or provided in excess. Under such conditions, defects in B-cell function—measured by antibody production or B-cell proliferation—are seen about half of the time. Table I summarizes many of these reports. It is noteworthy that none of the reports suggests an age-related increase in proliferation or antibody production, despite claims for increases with age in the production of the B-cell-stimulatory molecules IL-4 and IL-5.

Diminished B-cell function could reflect changes in the number of B cells, their distribution into functionally distinct subsets, the proportion of B cells that

Table I
Age-Associated Changes in B-Lymphocyte Function

Assay method/stimulus	Species	Result	Citation(s)
Proliferation/LPS	Mouse	Decline	Abraham *et al.* (1977)
Proliferation/LPS	Mouse	No change	Snow (1987)
Proliferation/anti-Ig	Mouse	Decline	Scribner *et al.* (1978)
Proliferation/anti-Ig	Human	No change	Weiner *et al.* (1978)
Proliferation/anti-Ig	Rat	No change	Gilman *et al.* (1982)
Proliferation/T cells + Fc	Mouse	Decline	Morgan *et al.* (1981)
Proliferation/staphylococcus	Human	Decline	Hara *et al.* (1987)
Ig/LPS	Mouse	No change	Snow (1987)
Ig/T cells + Fc	Mouse	Decline	Morgan *et al.* (1981)
Ig/T cells + antigen	Mouse	No change	Snow (1987)
Ig/T cells + antigen	Mouse	Decline	Callard and Basten (1978)
Ig/pokeweed mitogen	Human	Decline	Ceuppens and Goodwin (1982)
Ig/pokeweed mitogen	Human	No change	Kishimoto *et al.* (1978)
Ig/various mitogens	Human	Decline	Wrabatz *et al.* (1982)
Ig/tetanus toxoid	Human	Decline	Kishimoto *et al.* (1982)

respond to stimuli, or the ability of B cells to respond to antigen and/or T-cell helper signals. B-cell number seems to remain steady in mouse spleen for many (Kay et al., 1979; Patel, 1981; Subbarao et al., 1990), but not all (Flurkey et al., 1992a) strains. The data on human peripheral blood B-cell number are in conflict, with one group finding no evidence for any effect of age (Utsuyama et al., 1992) and a second (Paganelli et al., 1992) reporting a 4-fold decline in adult life. By using CD19 as a marker, a third group has reported a significant decline (about 2-fold) in peripheral blood B-cell number in men, but not in women (Chrest et al., 1993), and cautioned against reliance on studies that compare groups of young volunteers (often balanced in gender distribution or biased toward males) with groups of aged volunteers that may include largely women.

Discrimination of three B-cell subsets based upon relative levels of surface IgM and IgD revealed no systematic age-dependent trend except for a tendency of aged mice to have unusually high or low numbers of one or another of the subsets (Subbarao et al., 1990). B-cell activation usually leads to an increase in expression of the Ia antigens encoded within the major histocompatibility complex. The average level of B-cell Ia expression does not change with age (Subbarao et al., 1990; Seth et al., 1990), although there is again increased variation among elderly humans above and below the mean levels seen in young controls (Subbarao et al., 1990). Resting B cells do not express CD23 antigen, and the proportion of resting (CD23$^-$) B cells is decreased with age in men but increased in older women (Chrest et al., 1993).

The subset of B cells that expresses CD5 is of particular interest in that CD5$^+$ B cells are thought to play a major role in autoantibody production and to be prone to clonal expansion and malignant transformation. These cells are rare in spleen and lymph node, but are found in high pro-portions in the peritoneal cavity. The number and proportion of peritoneal CD5$^+$ B cells increase with aging in female, but not in male mice (Weksler et al., 1990; Gottesman et al., 1993; Linton & Klinman, 1993); these cells do not become significantly more frequent in the lymph nodes of aging mice (Linton & Klinman, 1993). A subset of B cells that expresses low levels of the J11D antigen is primarily responsible for the production of memory B cells after encounters with novel antigens, but this subset, too, is unaltered in frequency or function in aged mice (Linton, 1993). Thus, in summary, although shifts in T-cell subsets are intimately involved in age-related alterations of immune function, age-dependent changes in B-cell subsets seem unlikely to be critically involved in immunosenescence (Linton & Klinman, 1993).

Poor T-cell function in aged subjects often reflects a decline in the proportion of T cells that participate in the response; similar analyses of B cells have produced partially conflicting reports, with most data suggesting that the fraction of responding B cells declines slightly, but significantly with age. By using limit dilution approaches in liquid culture, one group (Andersson et al., 1977) documented a 95% decline in the proportion of mature B cells that could respond to the polyclonal activator lipopolysaccharide (LPS), while a second group found no effect of aging on this measure (Hooijkaas et al., 1983), and a third found only a 2-fold decline (Ravichandran et al., 1994). An assay system based upon B-cell growth on filter paper led to an estimate of a 2- to 3-fold decline in the frequency of LPS-responsive B cells (Schulze et al., 1992), while a splenic focus system in which B-cell colonies develop in an adoptive host suggested that the frequency of B cells responsive to several haptenic groups declined by about 2-fold in old mice (Zharhary & Klinman, 1983), although responses to some antigens, including influenza virus, were found not to decline with age in this system (Zharhary & Klinman, 1984).

Stimulation of resting B lymphocytes involves a complex series of interactions that allow helper T cells to recognize processed antigenic peptides on the B-cell surface and then to deliver contact-dependent signals to the B cell through the latter's CD40 molecules. T cells also provide cytokines, including IL-2, IL-4, and IL-5, that promote different components of B-cell clonal expansion, maturation into antibody-secreting plasma cells, and somatic mutation to generate higher affinity antibodies. Production of high-affinity, non-IgM antibodies is particularly T-cell-dependent in young individuals and particularly impaired by the aging process. T cells from old mice and humans are known to be defective in providing helper signals to B cells (Krogsrud & Perkins, 1977; Callard & Basten, 1978; Liu et al., 1982), but it is not yet clear whether the missing signals include contact-dependent interactions, cytokines, or both. One group (Thoman et al., 1988) has reported that B cells from old mice are less responsive than young B cells to IL-4 in tests of proliferation and antibody production, although a second group (al-Rayes et al., 1992) found no evidence for altered IL-4 responsiveness in B cells from old human donors. IL-5 responsiveness is reported not to be altered by aging in mice (Thoman, 1993). Experiments in which B cells from young or old individuals are stimulated by activated T cells or by graded doses of the CD40 ligand derived from T cells would be very informative in sorting out the basis for impaired T-cell help, but data of this kind are not yet available.

Naive B cells express, on their surface, an antibody of the IgD type, which is not secreted but appears to be involved in binding antigen and delivering signals that determine whether the B cell will be activated or tolerized. T cells can be stimulated, by IgD or other agents, to produce surface receptors for IgD, and this response

declines with age in mice and humans (Coico et al., 1987; Wei et al., 1993). Although the role of this T-cell IgD receptor in the promotion of T/B interactions is unclear, it is intriguing to note that those elderly humans who show a deficiency in IgDR induction are also the least likely to respond strongly to influenza vaccination (Wei et al., 1992).

VIII. Antibody Levels and Specificity

The apparently simple question of whether levels of serum immunoglobulins increase with age is, surprisingly, still unsettled. An early study of human Ig levels (Lyngbye & Kroll, 1971) found less than a 10% change in IgG and IgA levels between a group aged 20–39 years and another aged 60–95; IgM levels declined 10% over this age range. Another study (French & Harrison, 1984) produced similarly undramatic results, documenting a small decline in IgG1 levels and no change in other IgG antibody isotypes. Two other groups (Haaijman et al., 1977; Paganelli et al., 1992), however, have reported a 40% increase in IgG and striking 3- to 5-fold increases in IgA levels in aging humans; increases were reported in IgG1, IgG2a, and IgG2b subclasses (Paganelli et al., 1992). The situation in mice is equally confusing. Two groups have reported dramatic increases in serum IgM and in all four subclasses of IgG (Goidl et al., 1988; Daynes et al., 1993); the latter group documents, for example, a 5-fold increase in serum IgM, a 6-fold increase in IgA, and a 60% to 4-fold increase in each of the IgG subclasses in C3H mice. In contrast, a third group (Haaijman et al., 1977) sees no change in IgA, IgM, IgG2a, or IgG3 between the ages of 9 and 24 months, a 2-fold increase in IgG2b, and a 3-fold increase in IgG1 levels in CBA mice. Last, a report of Ig levels in C3H and C57BL/6 mice found no evidence for age-related increases in the levels of IgM, IgA, or any IgG subclass, except for an increase in IgG2a in the C3H strain (Albright *et al.*, 1990). Although interstrain variations could, in principle, account for some of the discrepancies among laboratories, other major discrepancies remain in the mouse and human data for which there is no obvious explanation.

There is a consistent increase in both mice and humans in the appearance of autoreactive serum immunoglobulins that recognize homologous proteins, cells, and organelles (Goodwin *et al.*, 1982; Rodriguez *et al.*, 1982; Moulias *et al.*, 1984; Sawin *et al.*, 1985; Hayashi *et al.*, 1989; Fields *et al.*, 1989; Klinman, 1992; Daynes *et al.*, 1993). Although the appearance of high-titered self-reactive antibodies is a prominent feature in autoimmune inflammatory diseases in humans and in mouse models, it is not at all clear whether the low-titered autoantibodies routinely demonstrable in as many as 80% of healthy elderly people and animals have any pathological significance; the age distribution for incidence of these autoantibodies clearly differs from that of the common human autoimmune diseases, which usually afflict victims in their 30's. It is, however, noteworthy that calorie restriction regimens that retard age-related physiological and pathological changes, including signs of immune aging (Miller, 1991b), are also effective at delaying the onset of disease in strains of mice that are prone to develop diseases that closely resemble human lupus erythematosis (Kubo *et al.*, 1987), and it seems plausible that both asymptomatic and symptomatic autoimmunity may in part be coupled to similar age-sensitive changes in immune regulation. Studies of the effects of aging on animal models of cellular autoimmune diseases have been limited and conflicting, with reports of increased (Ben-Nun *et al.*, 1980), decreased (Tomer *et al.*, 1991), or unchanged (Romball & Weigle, 1987) severity of symptoms in aged subjects.

B cells assemble their immunoglobulin genes from germ line-encoded fragments, thus generating a very diverse group of antibody specificities from a much smaller amount of genetic material. Each antibody molecule contains amino acids encoded by gene fragments of the V, D, and J families, and several laboratories have carried out studies to determine whether the contribution of different V, D, and J genes to antibody repertoire varies with age. One group (Schulze *et al.*, 1992) examined over 10^5 B-cell clones from young and old mice of two strains (BALB/c and C57BL/6) and noted no significant differences with age in the use of eight families of heavy chain V genes and eight families of light chain V genes. (The one exception was overuse by aged BALB/c mice of the V_H S107 V gene, which is discussed in more detail in the following.) A second group, using a different method for clonal expansion, found no evidence for changes in the use of three V_H gene families (J558, S107, and 7183) in aging BALB/c mice (Ravichandran *et al.*, 1994). A third group, however, reached very different conclusions (Viale *et al.*, 1994). In the C57BL/6 strain, they noted a significant increase in the expression of V_H genes of the J558 family and declines in the expression of each of the other 10 V_H families examined. In BALB/c mice, they found idiosyncratic patterns, with three individual aged BALB/c mice overexpressing either J558, Q52, or J606 V_H genes. None of the three aged BALB/c mice that they studied showed overuse of the S107 V_H family. This pattern of idiosyncratic expansion in V_H-bearing B cells is reminiscent of the patterns of CD8 T-cell Vβ genes noted earlier in aging mice (Callahan *et al.*, 1993) and humans (Posnett *et al.*, 1994). It is not clear why these latter two reports (Ravichandran *et al.*, 1994; Viale *et al.*, 1994) are so dramatically at odds: both used high-efficiency cloning methods that produce testable B-cell colonies from 1 in every 5–20 B cells. It should be noted that even these methods fail to stimulate the majority of resting B cells, and it thus is possible that they produce a biased picture of the available B-cell repertoire.

Although most antigens stimulate a very large number of B-cell clones, there are several that elicit a highly restricted pattern of antibody production. Among the most useful of these "idiotypically restricted" antigens is the phosphorylcholine (PC) molecule, which represents the key antigen present on the pneumococcus. Nearly all of the antibody to PC generated by young BALB/c mice uses a single V_H gene, S107, as well as a single set of D and J gene fragments. Two groups have shown that the pattern of anti-PC antibodies produced by aged mice is dramatically different from that of young mice in several respects. The frequency of B cells that can respond to PC increases by 2-fold with age in BALB/c mice, in contrast to the decline in the proportion of reactive cells seen in responses to other haptens (Zharhary & Klinman, 1986). A similar increase in frequency is also seen in the B-cell precursor pools that do not yet express surface Ig, showing that the bias toward anti-PC antibody does not depend upon interaction with the antigen itself; indeed, PC-specific pro-B cells are 7-fold more common in the bone marrow of 2-year-old mice than in 2–4 month-old animals. Analysis of the usage of different V_H families revealed, remarkably, that although essentially all of the anti-PC antibodies produced in young mice used the S107 V_H gene, 31% of the anti-PC-specific pro-B cells in aged BALB/c mice used other V_H genes for their anti-PC antibodies (Riley et al., 1989). Among pro-B cells that were able to generate clones of PC-specific B cells, the frequency of S107$^+$ cells increased with age by a factor of 6, while the proportion of S107$^-$ cells increased by at least 18-fold. There is no convincing explanation for the age-dependent increase in either class of anti-PC B cells. Work in a second laboratory showed that B cells from mice of several strains showed an age-dependent ability to respond to PC by the use of both heavy and light chain V

genes, which are rarely if ever used for this purpose in young mice (Nicoletti et al., 1991). These findings, if extended to humans, might have clinical implications, in that the anti-PC antibodies generated by aged BALB/c mice were found to be less potent than the antibodies of young mice at protecting from lethal pneumococcal infections (Nicoletti et al., 1993). Further work on the PC system may shed important light on the way in which aging alters gene expression in (and possibly outside of) the immune system, although it is as yet unclear whether similar phenomena affect responses to other, more typical, antigens.

Analysis of age-related changes in use of the D and J gene fragments has been extremely limited, but the limited data that exist are nonetheless provocative. A single study (Bangs et al., 1991), using a single young adult mouse and a single older (15 month) mouse, has demonstrated a variety of potentially important changes. The frequency with which individual D and J fragments were incorporated into the working antibody genes of mature B cells was found to differ with age, and the amount of D region DNA that remained in the sequence after the completion of the gene-splicing process also increased with age. In addition, these authors noted that, although specific gene sequences were very rarely isolated more than once in their set of 53 sequenced clones from the young mouse, 17 of the 61 different sequences seen in the old mouse were duplicated at least once, with some sequences seen as many as 10 or 11 times. To the extent that the genes sequenced are representative of the B-cell repertoire in this mouse (and, perhaps, other mice), it appears that the repertoire of antibody sequences in the aged mouse, while still highly diverse, nonetheless contains a moderate number of greatly expanded B-cell clones, each of which substantially contributes to the pool of available antibody specificities. The cellular basis and functional implications of this finding, if confirmed in other animals and other species, will merit vigorous exploration.

IX. B-Cell Development

B cells are continually produced from adult bone marrow through a series of progressively more differentiated precursors. There are several lines of evidence that B-cell production by the marrow of aged mice is impaired. Transplant studies have shown (Francus et al., 1986) a decline with aging in the ability of bone marrow to repopulate the B-cell pool of adoptive hosts. Functional tests for in vitro growth and differentiation of marrow also revealed defects in aged mice, and the marrow of aged mice was found to have smaller numbers of cells with the surface phenotype characteristic of B-cell precursors (Zharhary, 1988). A third study (Riley et al., 1991) showed an age-dependent decline in both immature and relatively mature B-cell precursors, with the latter type being particularly scarce in aged marrow. The functional implications of these observations are, however, uncertain.

A variety of approaches have suggested that some of the age-dependent changes in B-cell responses are likely to result from developmental processes controlled by T cells. The 2-fold decline in the fraction of B cells that can generate antibody in the presence of antigen and T-cell help is corrected by allowing the B cells to develop from their precursors in an environment that does not contain T cells from old mice (Zharhary, 1986). B cells from old mice produce elevated levels of "antiidiotype" antibodies, which react to immunoglobulins on the surface of other B cells and tend to suppress B-cell responses; production of these antiidiotypic antibodies is also dependent on the presence of T cells from old mice during B-cell development (Kim et al., 1985; Tsuda et al., 1988). There is also some evidence that T cells from old

mice can suppress B-cell function by recognition of their Ig molecules, in that T cells from old mice seem to block B-cell responses in adoptive hosts only if T and B cells come from mice with the same Ig genes (Klinman, 1981). It is, however, far from certain whether these Ig-based regulatory interactions play an important role in immunosenescence.

X. Antigen-Presenting Cells

There are a variety of cells throughout the immune system that can ingest antigens, process them, and present them to T cells in an activating form. The details vary depending on the antigen-presenting cell (APC) and the form of the antigen. B cells, for example, are highly efficient at presenting antigens to which their surface Ig is complementary, while macrophages are specialized for presenting particulate antigens (e.g., whole bacteria), and follicular dendritic cells are particularly good at the presentation of antigens that appear in antigen/antibody complexes.

The classical method for examining the effects of aging on APCs has been to construct cultures in which the T cells come from donors of one age and the APCs come from donors of a different age. A sample of such work is listed in Table II; most of the studies suggest that aging has no detectable effect on APC function, or at least that altered APC function cannot account for age-related changes in T-cell function in cultures containing T and APC from old donors. There is a need for additional studies that make full use of our growing appreciation of the subtleties of antigen processing, including detailed analyses of the specific cleavage, intracellular traffic, and eventual surface appearance of well-defined peptides derived from endogenous and exogenous antigens. Studies that allow for the differences between B cells, macrophages, and dendritic cells in stimulating specific classes of T cells will also be

Table II
Assays for Accessory Cell Function in Mixed T/APC Cultures

Stimulus	Species	Age effect	Citation
Con A	Mouse	No change	Grinblat et al. (1983)
Con A	Mouse	Decline	Chang et al. (1982)
Various lectins	Mouse	No change	Bruley-Rosset and Vergnon (1984)
Various lectins	Human	No change	Antel et al. (1980)
Fc fragments	Mouse	No change	Morgan et al. (1981)
Protein antigens	Mouse	No change	Perkins et al. (1982)
Alloantigens	Mouse	No change	Gottesman et al. (1985)
Influenza	Mouse	Decline	Effros and Walford (1984)

needed to produce a convincing account of the potential effects of age on T-cell/APC interactions.

APC function in skin is largely assumed by the pool of Langerhans dendritic cells, whose number per unit area of skin declines modestly with age (Gilchrest et al., 1982; Choi & Sauder, 1987; Belsito et al., 1987; Sprecher et al., 1990). In vitro tests have suggested that the decline in Langerhans cell number may lead to functional impairment (Sprecher et al., 1990), although tests for contact sensitivity in intact skin argue instead that age-dependent changes in skin T-cell responses are not likely to be attributable to the Langerhans cell loss (Belsito et al., 1987).

There is, however, mounting evidence for an age-dependent decline in the function of the lymph node follicular dendritic cell (FDC), which is thought to play a critical role in the formation of memory B cells and high-affinity antibodies in the lymph node germinal centers. In old mice, antigen brought to the lymph nodes seems to remain at the outskirts of the node rather than becoming associated with the FDC in the germinal centers (Holmes et al., 1984). The ability of the FDC to generate highly immunogenic vesicles coated with antigen (in the form of complexes with antibody) also is impaired by age in mice (Szakal et al., 1988; Burton et al., 1991). Although more work is needed to assess the implications of these findings, it seems plausible that changes in FDC function may contribute to senescent decline in T-cell-dependent humoral immune responses.

XI. Monokine Production and Response

APCs, and particularly macrophages, can have a strong positive or negative influence on immune responses by the production of cytokines and other soluble, antigen-nonspecific mediators that modulate the responses of other cell types, including T cells. Early work in this area focused on IL-1, a macrophage product with potent effects on T- and B-cell function. Table III lists seven such studies. The first four used bioassay methods now known not to discriminate well between the effects of IL-1α, IL-1β, and IL-6, a distinct macrophage product with overlapping biological functions. The most comprehensive of these reports (Chen et al., 1993) illustrates well the interpretive difficulties, in that aging led to an increase in the production of IL-1 in cells stimulated by candida, a decrease in responses to staphylococci, and no change in responses to intact Escherichia coli. Perhaps more to the point, several reports show that addition of IL-1 to in vitro cultures fails to correct age-related declines in T-cell responses (Bruley-Rosset & Vergnon, 1984; Negoro et al., 1986), suggesting that defects in IL-1 production, if they exist at all, are unlikely

Table III
Reports of Interleukin-1 Production in Aging

Citation	Species	Effect	Comment
Bruley-Rosset and Vergnon (1984)	Mice	Decline	Bioassay
Hiramoto et al. (1986)	Mice	Decline	Bioassay
Jones et al. (1984)	Humans	No change	Bioassay
Kauffman (1986)	Rats	No change	Bioassay
Goldberg et al. (1991)	Humans	No change	ELISA (IL-1β)
Putnam and Peterson (1991)	Humans	No change	ELISA
Chen et al. (1993)	Mice	Varied	See text

to play a major role in cell-mediated immunosenescence.

There are several reports (Wei et al., 1992; Daynes et al., 1993) of age-related increases in the plasma level of IL-6, which is produced by many cell types, including macrophages, and has a wide range of effects on immune function. Stimulation of murine inflammatory macrophages in vitro by heat-killed Escherichia coli, Staphylococcus aureus, or Candida albicans resulted in higher IL-6 production by cells from older animals (Chen et al., 1993). In one report, spleen and lymph node cells from old mice are reported to produce IL-6 in culture without added stimulus (Daynes et al., 1993), but in a second case there was no increase with age in spontaneous IL-6 production by human peripheral blood cells (Fagiolo et al., 1993). IL-6 production in endotoxin-treated rats increases greatly in old age (Foster et al., 1992). In contrast, one group, however, has reported a decline in IL-6 production by mouse macrophages (Effros et al., 1991).

There are also reports of age effects on the production of a third macrophage cytokine, tumor necrosis factor (TNFα). TNF production seems to increase in endotoxin-treated rats (Foster et al., 1992), but seems to decrease in cultures of macrophages from old mice (Effros et al., 1991). The production of TNF and other cytokines may be very sensitive to details of stimulus, timing, and cell preparation: in studies of mouse inflammatory macrophages, aging leads to an increase in TNF production in cultures stimulated by C. albicans, a decrease in S. aureus-stimulated cultures, and either an increase or no change (depending on stimulator dose) in response to intact E. coli.

The results of most of these studies are all of only limited relevance to the question of age-dependent changes in IL-1, IL-6, and TNF production during the course of immune responses in intact animals or humans, since the procedures involve tests of cells from inflammatory exudates (used to generate sufficient quantities of cells for convenient assay) and optimal doses of highly potent stimuli, including bacterial endotoxin and phorbol esters. Further progress is likely to require subtler designs that pay closer attention to multicellular feedback controls and cytokine circuits. The growing availability of gene-knockout mice in which particular pathways are rendered inoperable undoubtedly will assist in this effort.

Some attention has also been paid to the possible involvement of macrophage prostaglandin (PG) production in the regulation of immune function of the elderly. In an early study, PG synthesis inhibitors were found to restore much of the ability of T cells from older humans to proliferate in response to mitogens (Goodwin & Messner, 1979), and follow-up work suggested that T cells from older people were relatively more sensitive to PG-mediated inhibition than T cells from young donors

(Delfraissy *et al.*, 1982). Diets rich in vitamin E, which diminishes macrophage PG synthesis, have also been reported to improve *in vitro* mouse T-cell responsiveness (Meydani *et al.*, 1986). Other laboratories, however, find no effects of PG inhibitors on the T cells of aged humans (Sohnle *et al.*, 1980), and it is clear that T-cell-proliferative defects, at least in the CD8 subset, can still be seen in cultures in which macrophages have been replaced by costimulatory (anti-CD28) antibodies (Grossmann *et al.*, 1989).

XII. Natural Cytotoxicity

Natural killer (NK) cells are present as a minority population in blood and spleen and are able to recognize a wide range of tumor cells and virus-infected targets. Unlike the T and B cells, NK cells do not express a clonally specific antigen receptor, and their method of distinguishing tumor from nontransformed cells is still unclear. Responses of T and B cells to novel antigens require several weeks to reach maximal effectiveness, but NK cells do not require priming of this kind and thus are thought to provide a first line of defense. Most studies of human peripheral blood (see Table IV) show no effect of age on NK cell function or a small increase. In contrast, studies of mouse spleen and lymph nodes (also listed in Table IV) show clear

evidence of an age-dependent decrease. Mouse blood, tested in only a single report (Lanza & Djeu, 1982), resembles human blood in showing decline with age in NK function. Thus, it seems plausible that aging humans may well exhibit a decline in NK cell activity in their internal organs (like that documented for mouse), which is not adequately evaluated by tests of blood NK function. Such a hypothetical decline could, in principle, contribute to the increased vulnerability of aged humans to neoplastic disease. There are reports that NK cell function can be increased in aged mice by treatments with IL-2 (Kawakami & Bloom, 1987; Ho *et al.*, 1990) or IFN-γ (Weindruch *et al.*, 1983; Blair *et al.*, 1987), and it is possible that antitumor defenses might be augmented by therapeutic strategies involving this pathway. Another report, however, points to some potential complications, showing that while IFN-γ could increase IL-2 stimulation of NK cell growth in cultures of young mice, it paradoxically inhibited these NK responses in cultures from older animals (Kawakami & Bloom, 1988).

XIII. Rejuvenation of Immune Function

A major motivation for immunogerontological research is the hope that an understanding of the basis for immune fail-

Table IV
Effects of Age on NK Function in Mice and Humans

Species/sample	Effect of age	Citation(s)
Human blood	No change	Pross and Baines (1982); Thompson *et al.* (1984); Murasko *et al.* (1986); Bender *et al.* (1986a)
Human blood	Increase	Krishnaraj and Blandford (1988)
Human blood	Decline	Tsang *et al.* (1985); Mysliwska *et al.* (1992)
Mouse spleen or lymph node	Decline	Weindruch *et al.* (1983); Albright and Albright (1983); Saxena *et al.* (1984); Blair *et al.* (1987); Kawakami and Bloom (1987); Ho *et al.* (1990)
Mouse blood	No change	Lanza and Djeu (1982)

ure in old age could suggest therapeutic approaches to preserve or restore protective immunity. Many approaches have met with sporadic success, although none has yet been established as practical, safe, and efficacious in humans. Caloric restriction, which retards most of the physiological and pathological effects of aging in rodents (Masoro, 1988), also delays the majority of those age-related changes in immunity that have been examined (Weindruch & Walford, 1988; Miller, 1991b). Although caloric restriction has not yet been shown to work in primates, and is in any case impractical as a human intervention, further understanding of its physiological basis is likely to suggest new methods for the prevention of age-related immune defects. Transplantation of bone marrow and thymic tissue into old hosts also permits the redeployment of an immune system that functions much like that of a young animal (Hirokawa et al., 1982). Other work suggests that transplanted thymic epithelial cells may also have a significant functional effect (Haar et al., 1989); this approach deserves more careful attention.

The idea that thymic involution might contribute to immunosenescence has prompted a series of studies of the effects of soluble substances isolated from the thymus gland and of synthetic peptide analogues, and this line of work has continued despite the general skepticism of many immunologists that the thymus indeed produces bioactive hormones. Isolated studies have reported some success with this approach in humans, mice, and monkeys (Meroni et al., 1987; Frasca et al., 1987; Ershler et al., 1988); more systematic studies, which included a wide range of doses of several preparations with numerous explicit end points, have been much less encouraging (Hiramoto et al., 1986; Ghanta et al., 1991). The most dramatic reports are nonetheless impressive. In one such study, for example, a single injection of a synthetic octapeptide into old mice

was found to lead to a 6-fold increase in IL-2 production and a 4-fold increase in T-cell help in in vitro assays (Goso et al., 1992). In a second study, injections of a synthetic pentapeptide increased IL-2 and IFN-γ production and dramatically improved the resistance of the old mice to Leishmania infection (Cillari et al., 1992). It will be of great interest to determine whether these provocative reports can be confirmed by other laboratories.

A similar degree of cautious optimism applies to the reports that immune function in aged mice can be largely overcome by either chronic or indeed single-dose exposure to dehydroepiandrosterone (DHEA) or its orally administered sulfate derivative, DHEA-S (Daynes & Araneo, 1992; Daynes et al., 1993; Araneo et al., 1993). Administration of DHEA is said to increase the production of IL-2, IL-3, and other cytokines, diminish the production of IL-4 and IL-5, diminish plasma levels of IL-6, diminish serum levels of autoantibodies and acute phase reactants, and improve both primary antibody responses and the generation of immune memory as tested in secondary responses. Although interest in the possible therapeutic value of DHEA was sparked by the observation that its level in serum progressively declined with age in humans and correlated with disease risk (Barrett-Conner et al., 1986), its levels in mice of any age are very low, and thus its effects when administered to mice probably do not reflect the simple restoration of an age-sensitive endocrinological pathway. Reproduction of these dramatic findings in another laboratory will justify detailed further exploration of the molecular and cellular bases of the DHEA effect and exploration of its possible role in the prevention or treatment of human disease.

An early report of thymic atrophy and severe immune deficiency in growth hormone (GH)-deficient mutant mice (Fabris et al., 1972) has since been shown to represent merely a temporary delay attributable to the stress associated with weaning (Cross *et al.*, 1992), but several laboratories have nonetheless tested the idea that administration of GH might repair immune defects in aged rodents. GH-secreting pituitary tumors were found to increase thymic size and cellularity in old rats, but had a very modest effect on peripheral immune function (Kelley *et al.*, 1986). Tests of purified GH injections in aged mice also led to the rejuvenation of thymic anatomy, but there was no improvement in splenic helper or killer T-cell function (McCormick *et al.*, 1991). Implantation of pituitary gland fragments into old mice led to very small increases in antibody responses, which remained 90% lower than those of young animals (Cross *et al.*, 1990). One study (Khansari & Gustad, 1991) did report statistically significant increases in responses to a mitogen in aged mice given a 13-week course of GH injections; in this study, GH dramatically increased survival compared to injection controls. Nearly all of the control mice, however, died prior to 21 months of age, suggesting that the GH effect may have served to mitigate the immunosuppressive effects of some endemic infection in this colony. Interestingly, removal of the pituitary is also reported to improve immune function in rats and mice (Scott *et al.*, 1979; Harrison *et al.*, 1982). Thus, the weight of evidence does not suggest that GH is a promising candidate for immune rejuvenation.

It is worth noting that the most useful human intervention reported has involved the simplest approach: a 12-month course of multivitamin supplementation was found to lead to improvements in IL-2 production, NK function, and antibody responses, as well as to a statistically significant and clinically impressive (2-fold) decline in infectious illness (Chandra, 1992). This report suggests that correctable micronutrient deficiencies might underlie some of the age-related declines in human immune function and resistance to infection.

XIV. Aging, Infection, and Immunity

Several model systems have been used to test the idea that diminished immune function late in life might contribute to the increased vulnerability of the elderly to infectious illness. Infection late in life is more likely to lead to hospitalization and death, and recrudescence of latent infections (e.g., by tuberculosis or herpes zoster) in the elderly could, in principle, reflect diminished immune defenses, although there are many factors besides changes in specific immunity that may also render the elderly more susceptible to serious infectious disease. The strongest evidence for an involvement of immunosenescence in this process comes from animal models in which cells can be transferred from young donors to old recipients: T cells have, in this way, been shown to protect aged hosts from polio virus (Bentley & Morris, 1982), Listeria infection (Patel, 1981), and tuberculosis (Orme, 1987), and in *in vitro* cultures they have been shown to support improved responses to hepatitis viral antigens in B cells from elderly individuals who were hyporesponsive to hepatitis vaccination (Cook *et al.*, 1987).

Two model systems—influenza virus and tuberculosis—have been used to explore more deeply the possible mechanisms for age-related increases in disease severity. Intranasal infection of elderly mice with influenza virus led to a prolonged period of viral shedding and to impaired cytotoxic T-cell function compared to younger controls (Bender *et al.*, 1991). Heterotypic immunity, i.e., the ability of antigenically distinct virus to confer partial immunity to the challenge virus, was found to develop in young, but not in old, mice and was again correlated with delayed cytotoxic T-cell development (Bender & Small, 1993). Cytotoxic T-cell responses to influenza are also diminished by aging in humans (Powers, 1993). Studies of the rate at which vaccine-induced immunity declines have suggested that memory cells induced by an encounter with influenza may be relatively short-lived in the elderly (McElhaney et al., 1992). The possible role of virus-specific helper T-cell function in these antiviral responses has not yet been explored.

In the tuberculosis system, Orme (1987) has shown that aged mice are much less resistant than young animals to mycobacterial proliferation and that this vulnerability is accompanied (and presumably caused) by a diminished ability to generate effector T cells. Furthermore, mice infected with TB at 3 months of age were shown (Orme, 1988) to develop recrudescence of the disease at a median age of 24 months, in a model of the typical human presentation; analysis of these aged mice showed a decline in their ability to express antimicrobial immunity that was dependent at least partly on CD4 memory T cells. The CD4 T cells that do develop in infected animals appear after a delayed interval and may express low levels of the surface markers required for localization in areas of inflammation (Orme et al., 1993). This model seems worthy of more detailed exploration, particularly in terms of T-cell memory development and endurance, although it should also be noted that a second laboratory has failed to replicate the central observation of an age-dependent increase in susceptibility to mycobacterial infection (North, 1993).

XV. Immune Status and Late-Life Illness

Although it seems entirely plausible that diminished immune function might lead to increased risks of infection and perhaps cancer in the elderly, a causal connection has been difficult to establish. Humans live too long to reliably exclude preexisting disease as a cause of immune decline in studies of economical length, while short-lived rodents are too small to permit repeated sampling of immune tissues at early ages without specially designed microassay methods. Several groups have tested the hypothesis that aged people with immune defects are more likely to become ill than those with more vigorous levels of immune protection. Two laboratories (Roberts-Thomson et al., 1974; Murasko et al., 1988) have reported significant associations between anergy and subsequent mortality, but did not convincingly exclude either age or preexisting illness as potential confounders. The most nearly convincing report (Wayne et al., 1990) found an association between skin test anergy and subsequent mortality after the adjustment of subject age in a group of 273 initially healthy people: the relative risk (1.89; 95% confidence interval 0.94–3.79) fell just below conventionally accepted criteria for statistical significance. Low peripheral blood lymphocyte counts also predict subsequent mortality, after correction for age, in demonstrably healthy middle-aged and older humans (Bender et al., 1986b); it would be useful to know whether these low lymphocyte counts reflected corresponding declines in any specific T- or B-cell subset or were accompanied by evidence of impaired functional immunity.

Studies of mice also provide suggestive, but not compelling, support for a connection between immune senescence and susceptibility to late-life disease. In one study, low levels of CD8 T cells correlated with low life expectancy in two strains of mice (Boersma et al., 1985) at remarkably early ages, i.e., well before the animals were likely to be suffering from any detectable illness. It is troubling, however, that this group of mice exhibited a severe, life-long decline in CD8 cell number that has not been noted in most other studies of aging mice, and thus it remains to be seen whether these provocative observations can be reproduced elsewhere. A second approach involved the construction of a segregating back-cross between strains of mice selectively bred for high or low early-life immune function (Covelli et al., 1989). The back-cross mice showed, as expected, a wide range in immune function, as tested by the induction of antierythrocyte antibodies at 2–3 months of age. Genetic analysis showed that variation among the animals was controlled by as few as 3–9 loci. In this population, those mice that had high levels of immune function when they were young were also likely to have a long life span and a low age-adjusted incidence of disease, including neoplasia. This study provides the best evidence that levels of immune function influence late-life illness and survival, but is somewhat weakened by the relatively short life spans of even the longest lived animals and the likelihood of endemic infection in this conventional colony. Data on late-life immunity also are not available but would be helpful. A third study (Miller et al., 1994) has also used genetically heterogeneous mice to show that T-cell subset distribution can predict life span: those mice found at 6 months of age to have high levels of T cells characteristic of aged mice (i.e., memory CD4 and CD8 cells) were significantly more likely to die prior to the 18th month of life. The value of this study is limited by short follow-up and relatively small numbers of animals tested. Taken together, however, the three reports lend support to the idea that individual differences in protective immunity may lead to variations in susceptibility to neoplasia and perhaps other late-life diseases.

XVI. Conclusion

We now have the beginnings of a cellular model for the immunodeficiency of old age, in which shifts in T-cell subsets, perhaps in synergy with changes in certain APCs and changes in B-cell specificity, lead to alterations in cell-mediated and humoral aspects of protective immune reactions to pathogens. Although some progress has been made, most of the key questions remain in areas of cellular physiology, molecular genetics, and pathology of late-life illnesses. The immune system continues both to offer an accessible route to the exploration of how aging alters intracellular reactivity and intercellular communication and to provide useful insights into the developmental biology of the immune system in healthy young adults.

Acknowledgments

Much of the work from the author's laboratory has been supported by Grants AG08808, AG09801 and AG03978.

References

Abb, J., Abb, H., & Deinhardt, F. (1984). Age-related decline of human interferon alpha and interferon gamma production. Blut, 48, 285–289.

Abraham, C., Tal, Y., & Gershon, H. (1977). Reduced in vitro response to concanavalin A and lipopolysaccharide in senescent mice: a function of reduced number of responding cells. European Journal of Immunology, 7, 301–304.

Akbar, A. N., Salmon, M., & Janossy, G. (1991). The synergy between naive and memory T cells during activation. Immunology Today, 12, 184–188.

al-Rayes, H., Pachas, W., Mirza, N., Ahern, D. J., Geha, R. S., & Vercelli, D. (1992). IgE regulation and lymphokine patterns in aging humans. Journal of Allergy and Clinical Immunology, 90, 630–636.

Albright, J. W., & Albright, J. F. (1983). Age-associated impairment of murine natural killer activity. Proceedings of the National Academy of Sciences of the United States of America, 80, 6371–6375.

Albright, J. W., Holmes, K. L., & Albright, J. F. (1990). Fluctuations in subsets of splenocytes and isotypes of Ig in young adult and aged mice resulting from *Trypanosoma musculi* infections. *Journal of Immunology, 144,* 3970–3979.

Andersson, J., Coutinho, A., & Melchers, F. (1977). Frequencies of mitogen-reactive B cells in the mouse. I. Distribution in different lymphoid organs from different inbred strains of mice at different ages. *Journal of Experimental Medicine, 145,* 1511–1530.

Antel, J. P., Oger, J. F. D. E., Richman, D. P., Huo, H. H., & Arnason, B. G. W. (1980). Reduced T-lymphocyte cell reactivity as a function of human aging. *Cellular Immunology, 54,* 184–192.

Araneo, B. A., Woods, M. L., & Daynes, R. A. (1993). Reversal of the immunosenescent phenotype by dehyrdoepiandrosterone: hormone treatment provides an adjuvant effect on the immunization of aged mice with recombinant hepatitis B surface antigen. *Journal of Infectious Diseases, 167,* 830–840.

Averill, L. E., & Wolf, N. S. (1985). The decline in murine splenic PHA and LPS responsiveness with age is primarily due to an intrinsic mechanism. *Journal of Immunology, 134,* 3859–3863.

Bangs, L. A., Sanz, I. E., & Teale, J. M. (1991). Comparison of D, J_H, and junctional diversity in the fetal, adult, and aged B cell repertoires. *Journal of Immunology, 146,* 1996–2004.

Barrett-Conner, E., Khaw, K.-T., & Yen, S. S. C. (1986). A prospective study of dehydroepiandrosterone sulfate, mortality, and cardiovascular disease. *New England Journal of Medicine, 315,* 1519–1524.

Basch, R. S. (1990). Thymic repopulation after irradiation in aged mice. *Aging: Immunology and Infectious Disease, 2,* 229–235.

Beckman, I., Dimopoulos, K., Xu, X. N., Bradley, J., Henschke, P., & Ahern, M. (1990). T cell activation in the elderly: evidence for specific deficiencies in T cell/accessory cell interactions. *Mechanisms of Ageing and Development, 51,* 265–276.

Belsito, D. V., Derarkissian, R. M., Thorbecke, G. J., & Baer, R. L. (1987). Reversal by lymphokines of the age-related hyporesponsiveness to contact sensitization and reduced Ia expression on langerhans cells. *Archives of Dermatological Research, 279,* S76–S80.

Ben-Nun, A., Ron, Y., & Cohen, I. R. (1980).

Spontaneous remission of autoimmune encephalomyelitis is inhibited by splenectomy, thymectomy or ageing. *Nature, 288,* 389–390.

Bender, B. S., & Small, P. A., Jr. (1993). Heterotypic immune mice lose protection against influenza virus infection with senescence. *Journal of Infectious Disease, 168,* 873–880.

Bender, B. S., Chrest, F. J., & Adler, W. H. (1986a). Phenotypic expression of natural killer cell associated membrane antigens and cytolytic function of peripheral blood cells from different aged humans. *Journal of Clinical and Laboratory Immunology, 21,* 31–36.

Bender, B. S., Nagel, J. E., Adler, W. H., & Andres, R. (1986b). Absolute peripheral blood lymphocyte count and subsequent mortality of elderly men. The Baltimore Longitudinal Study of Aging. *Journal of the American Geriatric Society, 34,* 649–654.

Bender, B. S., Johnson, M. P., & Small, P. A. (1991). Influenza in senescent mice: impaired cytotoxic T-lymphocyte activity is correlated with prolonged infection. *Immunology, 72,* 514–519.

Bentley, D. M., & Morris, R. E. (1982). T cell subsets required for protection against age-dependent polioencephalomyelitis of C58 mice. *Journal of Immunology, 128,* 530–534.

Blair, P. B., Staskawicz, M. O., & Sam, J. S. (1987). Suppression of natural killer cell activity in young and old mice. *Mechanisms of Ageing and Development, 40,* 57–70.

Bloom, E. T., & Horvath, J. A. (1994). Cellular and molecular mechanisms of the IL-12-induced increase in allospecific murine cytolytic T cell activity. Implications for the age-related decline in CTL. *Journal of Immunology, 152,* 4242–4254.

Boersma, W. J. A., Steinmeier, F. A., & Haaijman, J. J. (1985). Age-related changes in the relative numbers of Thy-1 and Lyt-2-bearing peripheral blood lymphocytes in mice: a longitudinal approach. *Cellular Immunology, 93,* 417–430.

Brill, S., Kukulansky, T., Tal, E., Abel, L., Polgin, Y., Dassa, C., & Globerson, A. (1987). Individual changes in T lymphocyte parameters of old human subjects. *Mechanisms of Ageing and Development, 40,* 71–79.

Bruley-Rosset, M., & Vergnon, I. (1984). Interleukin-1 synthesis and activity in aged mice.

Mechanisms of Ageing and Development, 24, 247–264.

Bruley-Rosset, M., & Payelle, B. (1987). Deficient tumor-specific immunity in old mice: in vivo mediation by suppressor cells, and correction of the defect by interleukin 2 supplementation in vitro but not in vivo. *European Journal of Immunology, 17*, 307–312.

Buckler, A., Vie, H., Sonenshein, G., & Miller, R. A. (1988). Defective T lymphocytes in old mice: diminished production of mature c-myc mRNA after mitogen exposure not attributable to alterations in transcription or RNA stability. *Journal of Immunology, 140*, 2442–2446.

Budd, R. C., Cerottini, J. C., Horvath, C., Bron, C., Pedrazzini, T., Howe, R. C., & MacDonald, H. R. (1987). Distinction of virgin and memory T lymphocytes. Stable acquisition of the Pgp-1 glycoprotein concomitant with antigenic stimulation. *Journal of Immunology, 138*, 3120–3129.

Burton, G. F., Kosco, M. H., Szakal, A. K., & Tew, J. G. (1991). Iccosomes and the secondary antibody response. *Immunology, 73*, 271–276.

Callahan, J. E., Kappler, J. W., & Marrack, P. (1993). Unexpected expansions of CD8-bearing cells in old mice. *Journal of Immunology, 151*, 6657–6669.

Callard, R. E., & Basten, A. (1978). Immune function in aged mice. IV. Loss of T cell and B cell function in thymus-dependent antibody responses. *European Journal of Immunology, 8*, 552–558.

Carafoli, E. (1987). Intracellular calcium homeostasis. *Annual Review of Biochemistry, 56*, 395–433.

Ceuppens, J. L., & Goodwin, J. S. (1982). Regulation of immunoglobulin production in pokeweed mitogen-stimulated cultures of lymphocytes from young and old adults. *Journal of Immunology, 128*, 2429–2434.

Chandra, R. K. (1992). Effect of vitamin and trace-element supplementation on immune responses and infection in elderly subjects. *Lancet, 340*, 1124–1127.

Chang, M., Makinodan, T., Peterson, W. J., & Strehler, B. L. (1982). Role of T cells and adherent cells in age-related decline in murine interleukin 2 production. *Journal of Immunology, 129*, 2426–2430.

Chang, M. P., Utsuyama, M., Hirokawa, K., & Makinodan, T. (1988). Decline in the production of interleukin-3 with age in mice. *Cellular Immunology, 115*, 1–12.

Chen, Y., Ramsey, M. A., & Bradley, S. F. (1993). Differential monokine production by macrophages from aged mice stimulated with various microorganisms. *Aging: Immunology and Infectious Diseases, 4*, 155–167.

Choi, K. L., & Sauder, D. N. (1987). Epidermal Langerhans cell density and contact sensitivity in young and aged BALB/c mice. *Mechanisms of Ageing and Development, 39*, 69–79.

Chopra, R. K., Holbrook, N. J., Powers, D. C., McCoy, M. T., Adler, W. H., & Nagel, J. E. (1989). Interleukin 2, interleukin 2 receptor, and interferon-gamma synthesis and mRNA expression in phorbol myristate acetate and calcium ionophore A23187-stimulated T cells from elderly humans. *Clinical Immunology and Immunopathology, 3*, 297–308.

Chrest, F. J., Pyle, R. S., Schoonmaker, M. M., Nagel, J. E., & Adler, W. H. (1993). Age and gender differences in human CD19+ and CD19+/CD23+ peripheral blood B lymphocytes. *Aging: Immunology and Infectious Diseases, 4*, 231–244.

Cillari, E., Milano, S., Dieli, M., Arcoleo, F., Perego, R., Leoni, F., Gromo, G., Severn, A., & Liew, F. Y. (1992). Thymopentin reduces the susceptibility of aged mice to cutaneous leishmaniasis by modulating CD4 T cell subsets. *Immunology, 76*, 362–366.

Coico, R. F., Gottesman, S. R. S., & Thorbecke, G. J. (1987). Physiology of IgD. VIII. Age-related decline in the capacity to generate T cells with receptors for IgD and partial reversal of the defect with IL-2. *Journal of Immunology, 138*, 2776–2781.

Cook, J. M., Gualde, N., Hessel, L., Mounier, M., Michel, J. P., Denis, F., & Ratinaud, M. H. (1987). Alterations in the human immune response to the hepatitis B vaccine among the elderly. *Cellular Immunology, 109*, 89–96.

Covelli, V., Mouton, D., Di Majo, V., Bouthillier, Y., Bangrazi, C., Mevel, J. C., Rebessi, S., Doria, G., & Biozzi, G. (1989). Inheritance of immune responsiveness, life span, and disease incidence in interline crosses of mice selected for high or low multispecific antibody production. *Journal of Immunology, 142*, 1224–1234.

Cross, R. J., Campbell, J. L., Markesbery, W. R., & Roszman, T. L. (1990). Transplantation of pituitary grafts fail to restore immune function and to reconstitute the thymus glands of aged mice. *Mechanisms of Ageing and Development, 56,* 11–22.

Cross, R. J., Bryson, J. S., & Roszman, T. L. (1992). Immunologic disparity in the hypopituitary dwarf mouse. *Journal of Immunology, 148,* 1347–1352.

Davila, D. R., & Kelley, K. W. (1988). Sex differences in lectin-induced interleukin-2 synthesis in aging rats. *Mechanisms of Ageing and Development, 44,* 231–240.

Daynes, R. A., & Araneo, B. A. (1992). Prevention and reversal of some age-associated changes in immunologic responses by supplemental dehydroepiandrosterone sulfate therapy. *Aging: Immunology and Infectious Disease, 3,* 135–154.

Daynes, R. A., Araneo, B. A., Ershler, W. B., Maloney, C., Li, G.-Z., & Ryu, S.-Y. (1993). Altered regulation of interleukin-6 production with normal aging: possible linkage to the age-associated decline in dehydroepiandrosterone (DHEA) and its sulfated derivative. *Journal of Immunology, 150,* 5219–5230.

De Paoli, P., Battistin, S., & Santini, G. F. (1988). Age-related changes in human lymphocyte subsets: progressive reduction of the CD4 CD45R (suppressor inducer) population. *Clinical Immunology and Immunopathology, 48,* 290–296.

Delfraissy, J. F., Gelanaud, P., Wallon, C., Balavoine, J. F., & Dormont, J. (1982). Abolished in vitro antibody response in elderly: exclusive involvement of prostaglandin-induced T suppressor cells. *Clinical Immunology and Immunopathology, 24,* 377–385.

Effros, R. B., & Walford, R. L. (1984). The effect of age on the antigen-presenting mechanism in limiting dilution precursor cell frequency analysis. *Cellular Immunology, 88,* 531–539.

Effros, R. B., Svoboda, K., & Walford, R. L. (1991). Influence of age and caloric restriction on macrophage IL-6 and TNF production. *Lymphokine Cytokine Research, 10,* 347–351.

Eren, R., Zharhary, D., Abel, L., & Globerson, A. (1988). Age-related changes in the capacity of bone marrow cells to differentiate in thymic organ cultures. *Cellular Immunology, 112,* 449–455.

Ernst, D. N., Weigle, W. O., McQuitty, D. N., Rothermel, A. L., & Hobbs, M. H. (1989). Stimulation of murine T cell subsets with anti-CD3 antibody. Age-related defects in the expression of early activation molecules. *Journal of Immunology, 142,* 1413–1421.

Ernst, D. N., Hobbs, M. V., Torbett, B. E., Glasebrook, A. L., Rehse, M. A., Bottomly, K., Hayakawa, K., Hardy, R. R., & Weigle, W. O. (1990). Differences in the expression profiles of CD45RB, Pgp-1, and 3G11 membrane antigens and in the patterns of lymphokine secretion by splenic CD4¹ T cells from young and aged mice. *Journal of Immunology, 145,* 1295–1302.

Ernst, D. N., Weigle, W. O., Noonan, D. J., McQuitty, D. N., & Hobbs, M. V. (1993). The age-associated increase in IFN-gamma synthesis by mouse CD8+ T cells correlates with shifts in the frequencies of cell subsets defined by membrane CD44, CD45RB, 3G11, and MEL-14 expression. *Journal of Immunology, 151,* 575–587.

Ershler, W. B., Coe, C. L., Laughlin, N., Klopp, R. G., Gravenstein, S., Roecker, E. B., & Schultz, K. T. (1988). Aging and immunity in non-human primates. II. Lymphocyte response in thymosin treated middle-aged monkeys. *Journal of Gerontology, 43,* B142–B146.

Fabris, N., Pierpaoli, W., & Sorkin, E. (1972). Lymphocytes, hormones and ageing. *Nature, 240,* 557–559.

Fagiolo, U., Cossarizza, A., Scala, E., Fanales-Belasio, E., Ortolani, C., Cozzi, E., Monti, D., Franceschi, C., & Paganelli, R. (1993). Increased cytokine production in mononuclear cells of healthy elderly people. *European Journal of Immunology, 23,* 2375–2378.

Fields, R. A., Toubbeh, H., Searles, R. P., & Bankhurst, A. D. (1989). The prevalence of anticardiolipin antibodies in a healthy elderly population and its association with antinuclear antibodies. *Journal of Rheumatology, 16,* 623–625.

Flurkey, K., Miller, R. A., & Harrison, D. E. (1992a). Cellular determinants of age-related decrements in the T-cell mitogen response of B6CBAF1 mice. *Journal of Gerontology: Biological Science, 47,* B115–B120.

Flurkey, K., Stadecker, M., & Miller, R. A. (1992b). Memory T lymphocyte hyporesponsiveness to non-cognate stimuli: a key factor in age-related immunodeficiency. *European Journal of Immunology, 22,* 931–935.

Fong, T. C., & Makinodan, T. (1989). In situ

hybridization analysis of the age-associated decline in IL-2 mRNA expressing murine T cells. *Cellular Immunology, 118,* 199–207.

Foster, K. D., Conn, C. A., & Kluger, M. J. (1992). Fever, tumor necrosis factor, and interleukin-6 in young, mature, and aged Fischer 344 rats. *American Journal of Physiology, 262,* R211–R215.

Francus, T., Chen, Y. W., Staiano-Coico, L., & Hefton, J. M. (1986). Effect of age on the capacity of the bone marrow and the spleen cells to generate B lymphocytes. *Journal of Immunology, 137,* 2411–2417.

Franklin, R. A., Arkins, S., & Kelley, K. W. (1990). The proliferative response of rat T cells to calcium ionophores increases with age. *Cellular Immunology, 130,* 416–428.

Frasca, D., Adorini, L., & Doria, G. (1987). Enhanced frequency of mitogen-responsive T cell precursors in old mice injected with thymosin alpha-1. *European Journal of Immunology, 17,* 727–730.

French, M. A. H., & Harrison, G. (1984). Serum IgG subclass concentrations in healthy adults: a study using monoclonal antisera. *Clinical and Experimental Immunology, 56,* 473–475.

Froelich, C. J., Burkett, J. S., Guiffaut, S., Kingsland, R., & Brauner, D. (1988). Phytohemagglutinin induced proliferation by aged lymphocytes: reduced expression of high affinity interleukin-2 receptors and interleukin-2 secretion. *Life Science, 43,* 1583–1590.

Gabriel, H., Schmitt, B., & Kindermann, W. (1993). Age-related increase of CD45RO+ lymphocytes in physically active adults. *European Journal of Immunology, 23,* 2704–2706.

Gamble, D. A., Schwab, R., Weksler, M. E., & Szabo, P. (1990). Decreased steady state c-myc mRNA in activated T cell cultures from old humans is caused by a smaller proportion of T cells that transcribe the c-myc gene. *Journal of Immunology, 144,* 3569–3573.

Gauchat, J. F., DeWeck, A. L., & Stadler, B. M. (1988). Decreased cytokine mRNA levels in the elderly. *Aging: Immunology and Infectious Disease, 1,* 191–204.

Gelfand, E. W., Cheung, R. T., Mills, G. B., & Grinstein, S. (1988). Uptake of extracellular Ca^{2+} and not recruitment from internal stores is essential for T lymphocyte prolifera-

tion. *European Journal of Immunology, 18,* 917–922.

Ghanta, V. K., Hiramoto, N. S., Soong, S. J., & Hiramoto, R. N. (1991). Survey of thymic hormone effects on physical and immunological parameters in C57BL/6NNia mice of different ages. *Annals of the New York Academy of Science, 621,* 239–255.

Gilchrest, B. A., Murphy, G. F., & Soter, N. A. (1982). Effect of chronologic aging and ultraviolet irradiation on Langerhans cells in human epidermis. *Journal of Investigative Dermatology, 79,* 85–88.

Gillis, S., Kozak, R., Durante, M., & Weksler, M. E. (1981). Immunological studies of aging. Decreased production of and response to T cell growth factor by lymphocytes from aged humans. *Journal of Clinical Investigation, 67,* 937–942.

Gilman, S. C., Rosenberg, J. S., & Feldman, J. D. (1982). T lymphocytes of young and aged rats. II. Functional defects and the role of Interleukin-2. *Journal of Immunology, 128,* 644–650.

Goidl, E. A., Stashak, P. W., McEvoy, S. J. M., & Hiernaux, J. R. (1988). Age-related changes in serum immunoglobulin isotypes and isotype sub-class levels among standard long-lived and autoimmune and immunodeficient strains of mice. *Aging: Immunology and Infectious Disease, 1,* 227–236.

Goldberg, T. H., Baker, D. G., & Schumacher, H. R. (1991). Interleukin-1 and the immunobiology of aging. *Aging: Immunology and Infectious Disease, 3,* 81–89.

Gonzalez-Quintial, R., & Theofilopoulos, A. N. (1992). V beta gene repertoires in aging mice. *Journal of Immunology, 149,* 230–236.

Goodwin, J. S., & Messner, R. P. (1979). Sensitivity of lymphocytes to prostaglandin E2 increases in subjects over age 70. *Journal of Clinical Investigation, 64,* 434–439.

Goodwin, J. S., Searles, R. P., & Tung, K. S. K. (1982). Immunological responses of a healthy elderly population. *Clinical Experiments in Immunology, 48,* 403–410.

Goso, C., Frasca, D., & Doria, G. (1992). Effect of synthetic thymic humoral factor (THF-gamma 2) on T cell activities in immunodeficient ageing mice. *Clinical Experiments in Immunology, 87,* 346–351.

Gottesman, S. R. S., Walford, R. L., & Thorbecke, G. J. (1985). Proliferative and cytotoxic immune functions in aging mice. III. Exogenous interleukin-2 rich supernatant only partially restores alloreactivity in vitro. *Mechanisms of Ageing and Development*, *31*, 103–113.

Gottesman, S. R. S., Edington, J., Tsiagbe, V. K., & Thorbecke, G. J. (1993). Influence of cytokines and the effect of aging on colony formation by B-cell subsets. *Aging: Immunology and Infectious Diseases*, *4*, 197–211.

Goya, R. G., Brooks, K., & Meites, J. (1991). A comparison between hormone levels and T lymphocyte function in young and old rats. *Mechanisms of Ageing and Development*, *61*, 275–285.

Gozes, Y., Umiel, T., & Trainin, N. (1982). Selective decline in differentiating capacity of immunohemopoietic stem cells with aging. *Mechanisms of Ageing and Development*, *18*, 251–259.

Green-Johnson, J. M., Haq, J. A., & Szewczuk, M. R. (1991). Effects of aging on the production of cytoplasmic interleukin-4 and 5, and interferon-γ by mucosal and systemic lymphocytes after activation with phytohemagglutinin. *Aging: Immunology and Infectious Disease*, *3*, 43–57.

Grinblat, J., Schauenstein, K., Saltz, E., Trainin, N., & Globerson, A. (1983). Regulatory effects of thymus humoral factor on T cell growth factor in aging mice. *Mechanisms of Ageing and Development*, *22*, 209–218.

Grossmann, A., Ledbetter, J. A., & Rabinovitch, P. S. (1989). Reduced proliferation in T lymphocytes in aged humans is predominantly in the CD8+ subset, and is unrelated to defects in transmembrane signaling which are predominantly in the CD4+ subset. *Experimental Cell Research*, *180*, 367–382.

Grossmann, A., Ledbetter, J. A., & Rabinovitch, P. S. (1990). Aging-related deficiency in intracellular calcium response to anti-CD3 or concanavalin A in murine T-cell subsets. *Journal of Gerontology: Biological Sciences*, *45*, B81–B86.

Grossmann, A., Maggio-Price, L., Jinneman, J. C., & Rabinovitch, P. S. (1991). Influence of aging on intracellular free calcium and proliferation of mouse T-cell subsets from various lymphoid organs. *Cellular Immunology*, *135*, 118–131.

Gupta, S. (1989). Membrane signal transduction in T cells in aging humans. *Annals of the New York Academy of Science*, *568*, 277–282.

Haaijman, J. J., van den Berg, P., & Brinkhof, J. (1977). Immunoglobulin class and subclass levels in the serum of CBA mice throughout life. *Immunology*, *32*, 923–927.

Haar, J. L., Taubenberger, J. K., Doane, L., & Kenyon, N. (1989). Enhanced in vitro bone marrow cell migration and T-lymphocyte responses in aged mice given subcutaneous thymic epithelial cell grafts. *Mechanisms of Ageing and Development*, *47*, 207–219.

Hara, H., Negoro, S., Miyata, S., Saiki, O., Yoshizaki, K., Tanaka, T., Igarashi, T., & Kishimoto, S. (1987). Age-associated changes in proliferative and differentiative response of human B cells and production of T cell-derived factors regulating B cell functions. *Mechanisms of Ageing and Development*, *38*, 245–258.

Hara, H., Tanaka, T., Negoro, S., Deguchi, Y., Nishio, S., Saiki, O., & Kishimoto, S. (1988). Age-related changes of expression of IL-2 receptor subunits and kinetics of IL-2 internalization in T cells after mitogenic stimulation. *Mechanisms of Ageing and Development*, *45*, 167–175.

Harrison, D. E., Astle, C. M., & Delaittre, J. A. (1978). Loss of proliferative capacity in immunohemopoietic stem cells caused by serial transplantation rather than aging. *Journal of Experimental Medicine*, *147*, 1526–1531.

Harrison, D. E., Archer, J. R., & Astle, C. M. (1982). The effect of hypophysectomy on thymic aging in mice. *Journal of Immunology*, *129*, 2673–2677.

Harrison, D. E., Astle, C. M., & Stone, M. (1989). Numbers and functions of transplantable primitive immunohematopoietic stem cells. Effects of age. *Journal of Immunology*, *142*, 3833–3840.

Hausman, P. B., & Weksler, M. E. (1985). Changes in the immune response with age. In C. E. Finch & E. L. Schneider (Eds.), *Handbook of the Biology of Aging*, (pp. 414–432). New York: Van Nostrand Reinhold Company.

Hayakawa, K., & Hardy, R. R. (1988). Murine CD4+ T cells subsets defined. *Journal of Experimental Medicine*, *168*, 1825–1838.

Hayakawa, K., & Hardy, R. R. (1989). Phenotypic and functional alteration of CD4+ T cells after antigenic stimulation. Resolution of two populations of memory T cells that both secrete Interleukin 4. *Journal of Experimental Medicine, 169,* 2245–2250.

Hayashi, Y., Utsuyama, M., Kurashima, C., & Hirokawa, K. (1989). Spontaneous development of organ-specific autoimmune lesions in aged C57BL/6 mice. *Clinical and Experimental Immunology, 78,* 120–126.

Hertogh-Huijbregts, A., Vissinga, C., Rozing, J., & Nagelkerken, L. (1990). Impairment of CD3-dependent and CD3-independent activation pathways in CD4+ and in CD8+ T cells from old CBA/RIJ mice. *Mechanisms of Ageing and Development, 53,* 141–155.

Hiramoto, R. N., Ghanta, V. K., & Soong, S. J. (1986). Effect of thymic hormones on immunity and lifespan. In E. Goidl (Ed.), *Aging and the Immune Response* (pp. 177–198). New York: Marcel Dekker, Inc.

Hirokawa, K., & Utsuyama, M. (1984). The effect of sequential multiple grafting of syngeneic newborn thymus on the immune functions and life expectancy of aging mice. *Mechanisms of Ageing and Development, 28,* 111–121.

Hirokawa, K., Albright, J. W., & Makinodan, T. (1976). Restoration of impaired immune functions in aging animals. I. Effect of syngeneic thymus and bone marrow grafts. *Clinical Immunology and Immunopathology, 5,* 371–376.

Hirokawa, K., Sato, K., & Makinodan, T. (1982). Restoration of impaired immune functions in aging animals. V. Long-term immunopotentiating effects of combined young bone marrow and newborn thymus grafts. *Clinical Immunology and Immunopathology, 22,* 297–304.

Hirokawa, K., Kubo, S., Utsuyama, M., Kurashima, C., & Sado, T. (1986). Age-related change in the potential of bone marrow cells to repopulate the thymus and splenic T cells in mice. *Cellular Immunology, 100,* 443–451.

Ho, S. P., Kramer, K. E., & Ershler, W. B. (1990). Effect of host age upon interleukin-2-mediated anti-tumor responses in a murine fibrosarcoma model. *Cancer Immunology Immunotherapy, 31,* 146–150.

Hobbs, M. V., Ernst, D. N., Torbett, B. E., Glasebrook, A. L., Rehse, M. A., McQuitty, D. N., Thoman, M. L., Bottomly, K., Rothermel, A. L., & Noonan, D. J. (1991). Cell proliferation and cytokine production by CD4+ cells from old mice. *Journal of Cellular Biochemistry, 46,* 312–320.

Hobbs, M. V., Weigle, W. O., Noonan, D. J., Torbett, B. E., McEvilly, R. J., Koch, R. J., Cardenas, G. J., & Ernst, D. N. (1993). Patterns of cytokine gene expression by CD4+ T cells from young and old mice. *Journal of Immunology, 150,* 3602–3614.

Hobbs, M. V., Weigle, W. O., & Ernst, D. N. (1994). Interleukin-10 production by splenic CD4+ cells and cell subsets from young and old mice. *Cellular Immunology, 154,* 264–272.

Holbrook, N. J., Chopra, R. K., McCoy, M. T., Nagel, J. E., Powers, D. C., Adler, W. H., & Schneider, E. L. (1989). Expression of interleukin 2 and the interleukin 2 receptor in aging rats. *Cellular Immunology, 120,* 1–9.

Holmes, K. L., Schnizlein, C. T., Perkins, E. H., & Tew, J. G. (1984). The effect of age on antigen retention in lymphoid follicles and in collagenous tissue of mice. *Mechanisms of Ageing and Development, 25,* 243–255.

Hooijkaas, H., Preesman, A. A., Van Oudenaren, A., Benner, R., & Haaijman, J. J. (1983). Frequency analysis of functional immunoglobulin C and V gene expression in murine B cells at various ages. *Journal of Immunology, 131,* 1629–1633.

Huang, Y.-P., Pechere, J.-C., Michel, M., Gauthey, L., Loreto, M., Curran, J. A., & Michel, J.-P. (1992). In vivo T cell activation, in vitro defective IL-2 secretion, and response to influenza vaccination in elderly women. *Journal of Immunology, 148,* 715–722.

Iwashima, M., Nakayama, T., Kubo, M., Asano, Y., & Tada, T. (1987). Alterations in the proliferative response of T cells from aged and chimeric mice. *International Archives of Allergy and Applied Immunology, 83,* 129–137.

Jones, P. G., Kauffman, C. A., Bergman, A. G., Hayes, C. M., Kluger, M. J., & Cannon, J. G. (1984). Fever in the elderly. Production of leukocytic pyrogen by monocytes from elderly persons. *Gerontology, 30,* 182–187.

Juranka, P. F., Zastawny, R. L., & Ling, V. (1989). P-glycoprotein: multidrug-resistance and a superfamily of membrane-associated transport proteins. *FASEB Journal, 3,* 2583–2592.

Kadish, J. L., & Basch, R. S. (1976). Hematopoietic thymocyte precursors. I. Assay and kinetics of the appearance of progeny. *Journal of Experimental Medicine, 143,* 1082–1099.

Kappler, J. W., Hunter, P. C., Jacobs, D., & Lord, E. (1974). Functional heterogeneity among the T-derived lymphocytes of the mouse. I. Analysis by adult thymectomy. *Journal of Immunology, 113,* 27–38.

Kauffman, C. A. (1986). Endogenous pyrogen/interleukin-1 production in aged rats. *Experimental Gerontology, 21,* 75–78.

Kawakami, K., & Bloom, E. T. (1987). Lymphokine-activated killer cells and aging in mice: significance for defining the precursor cell. *Mechanisms of Ageing and Development, 41,* 229–240.

Kawakami, K., & Bloom, E. T. (1988). Lymphokine-activated killer cells derived from murine bone marrow: age-associated difference in precursor cell populations demonstrated by response to interferon. *Cellular Immunology, 116,* 163–171.

Kawanishi, H. (1993). Activation of calcium (Ca)-dependent protein kinase C in aged mesenteric lymph node T and B cells. *Immunology Letters, 35,* 25–32.

Kay, M. M. B., Mendoza, J., Diven, J., Denton, T., Union, N., & Lajiness, M. (1979). Age-related changes in the immune system of mice of eight medium and long-lived strains and hybrids. I. Organ, cellular and activity changes. *Mechanisms of Ageing and Development, 11,* 295–346.

Kelley, K. W., Brief, S., Westly, H. J., Novakofski, J., Bechtel, P. J., Simon, J., & Walker, E. B. (1986). GH3 pituitary adenoma cells can reverse thymic aging in rats. *Proceedings of the National Academy of Sciences of the United States of America, 83,* 5663–5667.

Kendig, N. E., Chrest, F. J., Nagel, J. E., Chaisson, R. E., Saah, A. J., & Adler, W. H. (1991). Age-related changes in the immune function of HIV-1 seropositive adults. *Aging: Immunology and Infectious Disease, 3,* 67–80.

Khansari, D. N., & Gustad, T. (1991). Effects of long-term, low-dose growth hormone therapy on immune function and life expectancy of mice. *Mechanisms of Ageing and Development, 57,* 87–100.

Kim, Y. T., Goidl, E. A., Samarut, C., Weksler, M. E., Thorbecke, G. J., & Siskind, G. W. (1985). Bone marrow function. I. Peripheral T cells are responsible for the increased auto-antiidiotype response of older mice. *Journal of Experimental Medicine, 161,* 1237–1242.

Kirschmann, D. A., & Murasko, D. M. (1992). Splenic and inguinal lymph node T cells of aged mice respond differently to polyclonal and antigen-specific stimuli. *Cellular Immunology, 139,* 426–437.

Kishimoto, S., Tomino, S., Inomata, K., Kotegawa, S., Saito, T., Kuroki, M., Mitsuya, H., & Hisamitsu, S. (1978). Age-related changes in the subsets and functions of human T lymphocytes. *Journal of Immunology, 121,* 1773–1780.

Kishimoto, S., Tomino, S., Mitsuya, H., & Nishimura, H. (1982). Age-related decrease in frequencies of B-cell precursors and specific helper T cells involved in the IgG anti-tetanus toxoid antibody production in humans. *Clinical Immunology and Immunopathology, 25,* 1–10.

Klinman, D. M. (1992). Similarities in B cell repertoire development between autoimmune and aging normal mice. *Journal of Immunology, 148,* 1353–1358.

Klinman, N. R. (1981). Antibody-specific immunoregulation and the immunodeficiency of aging. *Journal of Experimental Medicine, 154,* 547–551.

Kondo, M., Takeshita, T., Ishii, N., Nakamura, M., Watanabe, S., Arai, K., & Sugamura, K. (1993). Sharing of the Interleukin-2 (IL-2) receptor γ chain between receptors for IL-2 and IL-4. *Science, 262,* 1874–1877.

Koyama, K., Hosokawa, T., & Aoike, A. (1990). Aging effect on the immune functions of murine gut-associated lymphoid tissues. *Developmental and Comparative Immunology, 14,* 465–473.

Krishnaraj, R., & Blandford, G. (1988). Age-associated alterations in human natural killer cells. 2. Increased frequency of selective NK subsets. *Cellular Immunology, 114,* 137–148.

Krogsrud, R. L., & Perkins, E. H. (1977). Age-related changes in T cell function. *Journal of Immunology, 118,* 1607–1611.

Kubo, C., Johnson, B. C., Gajjar, A., & Good, R. A. (1987). Crucial dietary factors in maximizing life span and longevity in autoimmune-prone mice. *Journal of Nutrition, 117,* 1129–1135.

Kubo, M., & Cinader, B. (1990). Polymorphism

of age-related changes in interleukin (IL) production: differential changes of T helper subpopulations, synthesizing IL 2, IL 3 and IL 4. *European Journal of Immunology, 20,* 1289–1296.

Lanza, E., & Djeu, J. Y. (1982). Age-independent natural killer cell activity in murine peripheral blood. In R. B. Herberman (Ed.), *NK Cells and Other Natural Effectors* (pp. 335–340). New York: Academic Press.

Lerner, A., Philosophe, B., & Miller, R. A. (1988). Defective calcium influx and preserved inositol phosphate generation in T cells from old mice. *Aging: Immunology and Infectious Disease, 1,* 149–157.

Lerner, A., Yamada, T., & Miller, R. A. (1989). PGP-1[hi] T lymphocytes accumulate with age in mice and respond poorly to Concanavalin A. *European Journal of Immunology, 19,* 977–982.

Li, D. D., Chien, Y. K., Gu, M. Z., Richardson, A., & Cheung, H. T. (1988). The age-related decline in interleukin-3 expression in mice. *Life Science, 43,* 1215–1222.

Li, S. P., & Miller, R. A. (1993). Age-associated decline in IL-4 production by murine T lymphocytes in extended culture. *Cellular Immunology, 151,* 187–195.

Linton, P.-J. (1993). The status of progenitors of memory B cells in aged mice. *Aging: Immunology and Infectious Disease, 4,* 35–46.

Linton, P.-J., & Klinman, N. R. (1993). Functionality of B-cell subsets in aged mice. *Aging: Immunology and Infectious Disease, 4,* 135–137.

Liu, J. J., Segre, M., & Segre, D. (1982). Changes in suppressor, helper, and B-cell functions in aging mice. *Cellular Immunology, 66,* 372–382.

Lustyik, G., & O'Leary, J. J. (1989). Aging and intracellular free calcium response in human T cells after stimulation by phytohemagglutinin. *Journal of Gerontology, 44,* B30–B36.

Lyngbye, J., & Kroll, J. (1971). Quantitative immunoelectrophoresis of proteins in serum from a normal population: season-, age-, and sex-related variations. *Clinical Chemistry, 17,* 495–500.

Masoro, E. J. (1988). Food restriction in rodents: an evaluation of its role in the study of aging. *Journal of Gerontology, 43,* B59–B64.

Matsuzaki, G., Yoshikai, Y., Kishihara, K., Nomoto, K., & Yokokura, T. (1988). Age-associated increase in the expression of T cell antigen receptor gamma chain genes in mice. *European Journal of Immunology, 18,* 1779–1784.

McCormick, K. R., Harr, J. L., Taubenberger, J. K., & Krieg, R. J. (1991). A murine model for regeneration of the senescent thymus using growth hormone therapy. *Aging: Immunology and Infectious Disease, 3,* 19–26.

McElhaney, J. E., Meneilly, G. S., Beattie, B. L., Helgason, C. D., Lee, S.-F., Devine, R. D. O., & Bleackley, R. C. (1992). The effect of influenza vaccination on IL2 production in healthy elderly: implications for current vaccination practices. *Journal of Gerontology: Medical Science, 47,* M3–M8.

Meroni, P. L., Barcellini, W., Frasca, D., Sguotti, C., Borghi, M. O., De Bartolo, G., Doria, G., & Zanussi, C. (1987). In vivo immunopotentiating activity of thymopentin in aging humans: increase of IL-2 production. *Clinical Immunology and Immunopathology, 42,* 151–159.

Meydani, S. N., Meydani, M., Verdon, C. P., Shapiro, A. A., Blumberg, J. B., & Hayes, K. C. (1986). Vitamin E supplementation suppresses prostaglandin E2 synthesis and enhances the immune response of aged mice. *Mechanisms of Ageing and Development, 34,* 191–201.

Miller, J. F. A. P. (1965). Effect of thymectomy in adult mice on immunological responsiveness. *Nature, 208,* 1337–1338.

Miller, R. A. (1984). Age-associated decline in precursor frequency for different T cell-mediated reactions, with preservation of helper or cytotoxic effect per precursor cell. *Journal of Immunology, 132,* 63–68.

Miller, R. A. (1986). Immunodeficiency of aging: restorative effects of phorbol ester combined with calcium ionophore. *Journal of Immunology, 137,* 805–808.

Miller, R. A. (1990). Aging and the immune response. In E. L. Schneider & J. W. Rowe (Eds.), *Handbook of the Biology of Aging* (pp. 157–180). San Diego, CA: Academic Press.

Miller, R. A. (1991a). Caloric restriction and immune function: developmental mechanisms. *Aging: Clinical and Experimental Research, 3,* 395–398.

Miller, R. A. (1991b). Aging and immune function. *International Review in Cytology, 124,* 187–216.

Miller, R. A. (1991c). Accumulation of hypo-responsive, calcium extruding memory T cells as a key feature of age-dependent immune dysfunction. *Clinical Immunology and Immunopathology, 58,* 305–317.

Miller, R. A. (1994). Aging and the Immune System. In E. Masoro (Ed.), *Handbook of Physiology: Physiology of Aging* (in press). New York: Oxford University Press.

Miller, R. A., & Stutman, O. (1981). Decline, in aging mice, of the anti-TNP cytotoxic T cell response attributable to loss of Lyt-2⁻, IL-2 producing helper cell function. *European Journal of Immunology, 11,* 751–756.

Miller, R. A., & Stutman, O. (1984). T cell repopulation from functionally restricted splenic precursors: 10,000 fold expansion documented by using limiting dilution analyses. *Journal of Immunology, 133,* 2925–2932.

Miller, R. A., Jacobson, B., Weil, G., & Simons, E. R. (1987). Diminished calcium influx in lectin-stimulated T cells from old mice. *Journal of Cellular Physiology, 132,* 337–342.

Miller, R. A., Philosophe, B., Ginis, I., Weil, G., & Jacobson, B. (1989). Defective control of cytoplasmic calcium concentration in T lymphocytes from old mice. *Journal of Cellular Physiology, 138,* 175–182.

Miller, R. A., Flurkey, K., Molloy, M., Luby, T., & Stadecker, M. J. (1991). Differential sensitivity of virgin and memory T lymphocytes to calcium ionophores suggests a bouyant density separation method and a model for memory cell hyporesponsiveness to Con A. *Journal of Immunology, 147,* 3080–3086.

Miller, R. A., Turke, P., Chrisp, C., Ruger, J., Luciano, A., Peterson, J., Chalmers, K., Gorgas, G., & VanCise, S. (1994). Age-sensitive T cell phenotypes covary in genetically heterogeneous mice and predict early death from lymphoma. *Journal of Gerontology: Biological Science, 49,* B255–B269.

Morgan, E. L., Thoman, M. L., & Weigle, W. O. (1981). The immune response in aged C57BL/6 mice. I. Assessment of lesions in the B-cell and T-cell compartments of aged mice utilizing the Fc fragment-mediated polyclonal antibody response. *Cellular Immunology, 63,* 16–27.

Mosmann, T. R., Cherwinski, H., Bond, M. W.,

Giedlin, M. A., & Coffman, R. L. (1986). Two types of murine helper T cell clone. I. Definition according to profiles of lymphokine activities and secreted proteins. *Journal of Immunology, 136,* 2348–2357.

Moulias, R., Proust, J., Wang, A., Congy, F., Marescot, M. R., Deville Chabrolle, A., Paris Hamelin, A., & Lesourd, B. (1984). Age-related increase in autoantibodies [letter]. *Lancet, 1,* 1128–1129.

Murasko, D. M., & Goonewardene, I. M. (1990). T-cell function in aging: mechanisms of decline. *Annual Review of Gerontology and Geriatrics, 10,* 71–96.

Murasko, D. M., Nelson, B. J., Silver, R., & Matour, D. (1986). Immunologic response in an elderly population with a mean age of 85. *American Journal of Medicine, 81,* 612–618.

Murasko, D. M., Weiner, P., & Kaye, D. (1988). Association of lack of mitogen-induced lymphocyte proliferation with increased mortality in the elderly. *Aging: Immunology and Infectious Disease, 1,* 1–6.

Mustelin, T., & Burn, P. (1993). Regulation of src family tyrosine kinases in lymphocytes. *Trends in Biochemical Science, 18,* 215–220.

Mysliwska, J., Mysliwski, A., Romanowski, P., Bigda, J., Sosnowska, D., & Foerster, J. (1992). Monocytes are responsible for depressed natural killer (NK) activity in both young and elderly low NK responders. *Gerontology, 38,* 41–49.

Nagel, J. E., Chopra, R. K., Chrest, F. J., McCoy, M. T., Schneider, E. L., Holbrook, N. J., & Adler, W. H. (1988). Decreased proliferation, interleukin 2 synthesis, and interleukin 2 receptor expression are accompanied by decreased mRNA expression in phytohemagglutinin-stimulated cells from elderly donors. *Journal of Clinical Investigation, 81,* 1096–1102.

Nagel, J. E., Chopra, R. K., Powers, D. C., & Adler, W. H. (1989). Effect of age on the human high affinity interleukin 2 receptor of phytohaemagglutinin stimulated peripheral blood lymphocytes. *Clinical and Experimental Immunology, 75,* 286–291.

Nagelkerken, L., Hertogh-Huijbregts, A., Dobber, R., & Drager, A. (1991). Age-related changes in lymphokine production related to a decreased number of CD45RB^{hi} CD4+ T cells. *European Journal of Immunology, 21,* 273–281.

Nakahama, M., Mohri, N., Mori, S., Shindo, G., Yokoi, Y., & Machinami, R. (1990). Immunohistochemical and histometrical studies of the human thymus with special emphasis on age-related changes in medullary epithelial and dendritic cells. *Virchows Archives B: Cell Pathology, 58,* 245–251.

Naylor, J. R., James, S. R., & Trejdosiewicz, L. K. (1992). Intracellular free Ca^{2+} fluxes and responses to phorbol ester in T lymphocytes from healthy elderly subjects. *Clinical and Experimental Immunology, 89,* 158–163.

Negoro, S., & Hara, H. (1992). The effect of taurine on the age-related decline of the immune response in mice: the restorative effect on the T cell proliferative response to costimulation with ionomycin and phorbol myristate acetate. *Advances in Experimental Medical Biology, 315,* 229–239.

Negoro, S., Hara, H., Miyata, S., Saiki, O., Tanaka, T., Yoshizaki, K., Igarashi, T., & Kishimoto, S. (1986). Mechanisms of age-related decline in antigen-specific T cell proliferative response: IL-2 receptor expression and recombinant IL-2 induced proliferative response of purified TAC-positive T cells. *Mechanisms of Ageing and Development, 36,* 223–241.

Nicoletti, C., Borghesi-Nicoletti, C., Yang, X., Schulze, D. H., & Cerny, J. (1991). Repertoire diversity of antibody response to bacterial antigens in aged mice. II. Phosphorylcholine-antibody in young and aged mice differ in both V_H/V_L gene repertoire and in specificity. *Journal of Immunology, 147,* 2750–2755.

Nicoletti, C., Yang, X., & Cerny, J. (1993). Repertoire diversity of antibody response to bacterial antigens in aged mice. III. Phosphorylcholine antibody from young and aged mice differ in structure and protective activity against infection with *Streptococcus pneumoniae. Journal of Immunology, 150,* 543–549.

Nordin, A. A., & Collins, G. D. (1983). Limiting dilution analysis of alloreactive cytotoxic precursor cells in aging mice. *Journal of Immunology, 131,* 2215–2218.

North, R. J. (1993). Minimal effect of advanced aging on susceptibility of mice to infection with *Mycobacterium tuberculosis. Journal of Infectious Disease, 168,* 1059–1062.

Northrup, J. P., Ho, S. N., Chen, L., Thomas, D. J., Timmerman, L. A., Nolan, G. P., Admon, A., & Crabtree, G. R. (1994). NF-AT components define a family of transcription factors targeted in T-cell activation. *Nature, 369,* 497–502.

Odio, M., Brodish, A., & Ricardo, M. J., Jr. (1987). Effects on immune responses by chronic stress are modulated by aging. *Brain Behavior Immunology, 1,* 204–215.

Ohteki, T., Okuyama, R., Seki, S., Abo, T., Sugiura, K., Kusumi, A., Ohmori, T., Watanabe, H., & Kumagai, K. (1992). Age-dependent increase of extrathymic T cells in the liver and their appearance in the periphery of older mice. *Journal of Immunology, 149,* 1562–1570.

O'Leary, J. J., Fox, R., Bergh, N., Rodysill, K. J., & Hallgren, H. M. (1988). Expression of the human T cell antigen receptor complex in advanced age. *Mechanisms of Ageing and Development, 45,* 239–252.

Orme, I. M. (1987). Aging and immunity to tuberculosis: increased susceptibility of old mice reflects a decreased capacity to generate mediator T lymphocytes. *Journal of Immunology, 138,* 4414–4418.

Orme, I. M. (1988). A mouse model of the recrudescence of latent tuberculosis in the elderly. *American Review of Respiratory Disease, 137,* 716–718.

Orme, I. M., Griffin, J. P., Roberts, A. D., & Ernst, D. N. (1993). Evidence for a defective accumulation of protective T cells in old mice infected with *Mycobacterium tuberculosis. Cellular Immunology, 147,* 222–229.

Orson, F. M., Saadeh, C. K., Lewis, D. E., & Nelson, D. L. (1989). Interleukin 2 receptor expression by T cells in human aging. *Cellular Immunology, 124,* 278–291.

Paganelli, R., Quinti, I., Fagiolo, U., Cossarizza, A., Ortolani, C., Guerra, E., Sansoni, P., Pucillo, L. P., Scala, E., & Cozzi, E. (1992). Changes in circulating B cells and immunoglobulin classes and subclasses in a healthy aged population. *Clinical and Experimental Immunology, 90,* 351–354.

Patel, H. R., & Miller, R. A. (1992). Age-associated changes in mitogen-induced protein phosphorylation in murine T lymphocytes. *European Journal of Immunology, 22,* 253–260.

Patel, P. J. (1981). Aging and antimicrobial immunity. Impaired production of mediator T cells as a basis for the decreased resistance of senescent mice to Listeriosis. *Journal of Experimental Medicine, 154,* 821–831.

Pelech, S. L., & Sanghera, J. S. (1992). MAP kinases: charting the regulatory pathways. *Science, 257,* 1355–1356.

Perkins, E. H., Massucci, J. M., & Glover, P. L. (1982). Antigen presentation by peritoneal macrophages from young adult and old mice. *Cellular Immunology, 70,* 1–10.

Philosophe, B., & Miller, R. A. (1989). T lymphocyte heterogeneity in old and young mice: functional defects in T cells selected for poor calcium signal generation. *European Journal of Immunology, 19,* 695–699.

Philosophe, B., & Miller, R. A. (1990). Diminished calcium signal generation in subsets of T lymphocytes that predominate in old mice. *Journal of Gerontology: Biological Science, 45,* B87–B93.

Pieri, C., Recchioni, R., Moroni, F., Marcheselli, F., & Lipponi, G. (1992). Phytohemagglutinin induced changes of membrane lipid packing, c-myc and c-myb encoded protein expression in human lymphocytes during aging. *Mechanisms of Ageing and Development, 64,* 177–187.

Pilarski, L. M., Yacyshyn, B. R., Jensen, G. S., Pruski, E., & Pabst, H. F. (1991). β1 integrin (CD29) expression on human postnatal T cell subsets defined by selective CD45 isoform expression. *Journal of Immunology, 147,* 830–837.

Posnett, D. N., Sinha, R., Kabak, S., & Russo, C. (1994). Clonal populations of T cells in normal elderly humans: the T cell equivalent to "benign monoclonal gammapathy" [published erratum appears in *J. Exp. Med.* (1994) *179*(3), 1077]. *Journal of Experimental Medicine, 179,* 609–618.

Powers, D. C. (1993). Influenza A virus-specific cytotoxic T lymphocyte activity declines with advancing age [see comments]. *Journal of the American Geriatric Society, 41,* 1–5.

Pross, H. F., & Baines, M. G. (1982). Studies of human natural killer cells. I. In vivo parameters affecting normal cytotoxic function. *International Journal of Cancer, 29,* 383–390.

Proust, J. J., Filburn, C. R., Harrison, S. A., Buchholz, M. A., & Nordin, A. A. (1987). Age-related defect in signal transduction during lectin activation of murine T lymphocytes. *Journal of Immunology, 139,* 1472–1478.

Proust, J. J., Kittur, D. S., Buchholz, M. A., & Nordin, A. A. (1988). Restricted expression of mitogen-induced high affinity IL-2 receptors in aging mice. *Journal of Immunology, 141,* 4209–4216.

Putnam, A. D., & Peterson, T. C. (1991). Effect of aging and other factors on monocyte aryl hydrocarbon hydroxylase activity. *Mechanisms of Ageing and Development, 60,* 61–74.

Rabinowe, S. L., Nayak, R. C., Krisch, K., George, K. L., & Eisenbarth, G. S. (1987). Aging in man. Linear increase of a novel T cell subset defined by antiganglioside monoclonal antibody 3G5. *Journal of Experimental Medicine, 165,* 1436–1441.

Rajasekar, R., & Augustin, A. (1994). Antigen-dependent selection of T cells that are able to efficiently regulate free cytoplasmic calcium levels. *Journal of Immunology, 153,* 1037–1045.

Ravichandran, K. S., Osborne, B. A., & Goldsby, R. A. (1994). Quantitative analysis of the B cell repertoire by limiting dilution analysis and fluorescent in situ hybridization. *Cellular Immunology, 154,* 309–327.

Riley, R. L., Kruger, M. G., & Elia, J. (1991). B cell precursors are decreased in senescent BALB/c mice, but retain normal mitotic activity in vivo and in vitro. *Clinical Immunology and Immunopathology, 59,* 301–313.

Riley, S. C., Froscher, B. G., Linton, P. J., Zharhary, D., Marcu, K., & Klinman, N. R. (1989). Altered V_h gene segment utilization in the response to phosphorylcholine of aged mice. *Journal of Immunology, 143,* 3798–3805.

Roberts-Thomson, I. C., Whittingham, S., Youngchaiyud, U., & Mackay, I. R. (1974). Ageing, immune response, and mortality. *Lancet, 2,* 368–370.

Rocha, B. B. (1987). Population kinetics of precursors of IL 2-producing peripheral T lymphocytes: evidence for short life expectancy, continuous renewal, and post-thymic expansion. *Journal of Immunology, 139,* 365–372.

Rodriguez, M. A., Ceuppens, J. L., & Goodwin, J. S. (1982). Regulation of IgM rheumatoid factor production in lymphocyte cultures from young and old subjects. *Journal of Immunology, 128,* 2422–2428.

Romball, C. G., & Weigle, W. O. (1987). The effect of aging on the induction of experimental autoimmune thyroiditis. *Journal of Immunology, 139,* 1490–1495.

Russo, C., Cherniack, E. P., Wali, A., & Weksler, M. E. (1993). Age-dependent appearance of non-major histocompatibility complex-restricted helper T cells. *Proceedings of the National Academy of Sciences of the United States of America, 90,* 11718–11722.

Rytel, M. W., Larratt, K. S., Turner, P. A., & Kalbfleisch, J. H. (1986). Interferon response to mitogens and viral antigens in elderly and young adult subjects. *Journal of Infectious Disease, 153,* 984–987.

Saini, A., & Sei, Y. (1993). Age-related impairment of early and late events of signal transduction in mouse immune cells. *Life Science, 52,* 1759–1765.

Sawin, C. T., Bigos, S. T., Land, S., & Bacharach, P. (1985). The aging thyroid. Relationship between elevated serum thyrotropin level and thyroid antibodies in elderly patients. *American Journal of Medicine, 79,* 591–595.

Saxena, R. K., Saxena, Q. B., & Adler, W. H. (1984). Interleukin-2-induced activation of natural killer activity in spleen cells from old and young mice. *Immunology, 51,* 719–726.

Saxena, R. K., Saxena, Q. B., & Adler, W. H. (1988). Lectin-induced cytotoxic activity in spleen cells from young and old mice. Age-related changes in types of effector cells, lymphokine production and response. *Immunology, 64,* 457–461.

Schulze, D. H., Mancillas, P., Kaushik, A., Bona, C., & Kelsoe, G. (1992). Mitogen-induced V_H and V_K expression is similar in young adult and aged mice. *Aging: Immunology and Infectious Disease, 3,* 127–134.

Schwab, R., Pfeffer, L. M., Szabo, P., Gamble, D., Schnurr, C. M., & Weksler, M. E. (1990). Defective expression of high affinity IL-2 receptors on activated T cells from aged humans. *International Immunology, 2,* 239–246.

Schwab, R., Russo, C., & Weksler, M. E. (1992). Altered major histocompatibility complex-restricted antigen recognition by T cells from elderly humans. *European Journal of Immunology, 22,* 2989–2993.

Scollary, R. G., Butcher, E. C., & Weissman, I. L. (1980). Thymus cell migration. Quantitative aspects of cellular traffic from thymus to the periphery in mice. *European Journal of Immunology, 10,* 210–218.

Scott, M., Bolla, R., & Denckla, W. D. (1979). Age-related changes in immune function of rats and the effect of long-term hypophysectomy. *Mechanisms of Ageing and Development, 11,* 127–136.

Scribner, D. J., Weiner, H. L., & Moorhead, J. W. (1978). Anti-immunoglobulin stimulation of murine lymphocytes. V. Age-related decline in Fc receptor-mediated immunoregulation. *Journal of Immunology, 121,* 377–382.

Serra, H. M., Krowka, J. F., Ledbetter, J. A., & Pilarski, L. M. (1988). Loss of CD45R (Lp220) represents a post-thymic T cell differentiation event. *Journal of Immunology, 140,* 1435–1441.

Seth, A., Nagarkatti, M., Nagarkatti, P. S., Subbarao, B., & Udhayakumar, V. (1990). Macrophages but not B cells from aged mice are defective in stimulating autoreactive T cells in vitro. *Mechanisms of Ageing and Development, 52,* 107–124.

Shi, J., & Miller, R. A. (1992). Tyrosine-specific protein phosphorylation in response to anti-CD3 antibody is diminished in old mice. *Journal of Gerontology: Biological Science, 47,* B147–B153.

Shi, J., & Miller, R. A. (1993). Differential tyrosine-specific protein phosphorylation in mouse T lymphocyte subsets. Effect of age. *Journal of Immunology, 151,* 730–739.

Simpson, E., & Cantor, H. (1975). Regulation of the immune response by subclasses of T lymphocytes. II. The effect of adult thymectomy upon humoral and cellular responses in mice. *European Journal of Immunology, 5,* 337–343.

Snow, E. C. (1987). An evaluation of antigen-driven expansion and differentiation of hapten-specific B lymphocytes purified from aged mice. *Journal of Immunology, 139,* 1758–1762.

Sohnle, P. G., Larson, S. E., Collins-Lech, C., & Guansing, A. R. (1980). Failure of lymphokine-producing lymphocytes from aged humans to undergo activation by recall antigens. *Journal of Immunology, 124,* 2169–2174.

Song, L., Stephens, J. M., Kittur, S., Collins, G. D., Nagel, J. E., Pekala, P. H., & Adler, W. H. (1992). Expression of c-fos, c-jun and jun B in peripheral blood lymphocytes from young and elderly adults. *Mechanisms of Ageing and Development, 65,* 149–156.

Sprecher, E., Becker, Y., Kraal, G., Hall, E., Harrison, D., & Shultz, L. D. (1990). Effect of aging on epidermal dendritic cell populations in C57BL/6J mice. *Journal of Investigative Dermatology, 94,* 247–253.

Subbarao, B., Morris, J., & Kryscio, R. J. (1990). Phenotypic and functional properties of B lymphocytes from aged mice. *Mechanisms of Ageing and Development, 51,* 223–241.

Szakal, A. K., Taylor, J. K., Smith, J. P., Kosco, M. H., Burton, G. F., & Tew, J. G. (1988). Morphometry and kinetics of antigen transport and developing antigen retaining reticulum of follicular dendritic cells in lymph nodes of aging mice. *Aging: Immunology and Infectious Disease, 1,* 7–22.

Thoman, M. L. (1991). Impaired responsiveness of IL-2 receptor-expressing T lymphocytes from aged mice. *Cellular Immunology, 135,* 410–417.

Thoman, M. L. (1993). Impact of aging on B lymphocyte responsiveness to IL-5. *Aging: Immunology and Infectious Disease, 4,* 123–134.

Thoman, M. L., & Weigle, W. O. (1981). Lymphokines and aging: Interleukin-2 production and activity in aged animals. *Journal of Immunology, 127,* 2101–2106.

Thoman, M. L., & Weigle, W. O. (1982). Cell-mediated immunity in aged mice: an underlying lesion in IL 2 synthesis. *Journal of Immunology, 128,* 2358–2361.

Thoman, M. L., & Weigle, W. O. (1985). Reconstitution of in vivo cell-mediated lympholysis responses in aged mice with Interleukin 2. *Journal of Immunology, 134,* 949–952.

Thoman, M. L., & Weigle, W. O. (1988). Partial restoration of Con A-induced proliferation, IL-2 receptor expression, and IL-2 synthesis in aged murine lymphocytes by phorbol myristate acetate and ionomycin. *Cellular Immunology, 114,* 1–11.

Thoman, M. L., & Weigle, W. O. (1989). The cellular and subcellular bases of immunosenescence. *Advances of Immunology, 46,* 221–261.

Thoman, M. L., Keogh, E. A., & Weigle, W. O. (1988). Response of aged T and B lymphocytes to IL-4. *Aging: Immunology and Infectious Disease, 1,* 245–253.

Thompson, J. S., Wekstein, D. R., Rhoades, J. L., Kirkpatrick, C., Brown, S. A., Roszman, T., Straus, R., & Tietz, N. (1984). The immune status of healthy centenarians. *Journal of the American Geriatric Society, 32,* 274–281.

Tielen, F. J., van Vliet, A. C., de Geus, B., Nagelkerken, L., & Rozing, J. (1993). Age-related changes in CD4+ T-cell subsets associated with prolonged skin graft survival in aging rats. *Transplantation Proceedings, 25,* 2872–2874.

Tomer, Y., Mendlovic, S., Kukulansky, T., Mozes, E., Shoenfeld, Y., & Globerson, A. (1991). Effects of aging on the induction of experimental systemic lupus erythematosus (SLE) in mice. *Mechanisms of Ageing and Development, 58,* 233–244.

Tsang, K. Y, Pan, J. F., Swanger, D. L., & Fudenberg, H. H. (1985). In vitro restoration of immune response in aging humans by isoprinosine. *Immunopharmacology, 7,* 199–206.

Tsuda, T., Kim, Y. T., Siskind, G. W., & Weksler, M. E. (1988). Old mice recover the ability to produce IgG and high-avidity antibody following irradiation with partial bone marrow shielding. *Proceedings of the National Academy of Sciences of the United States of America, 85,* 1169–1173.

Utsuyama, M., Kasai, M., Kurashima, C., & Hirokawa, K. (1991). Age influence on the thymic capacity to promote differentiation of T cells: induction of different composition of T cell subsets by aging thymus. *Mechanisms of Ageing and Development, 58,* 267–277.

Utsuyama, M., Hirokawa, K., Kurashima, C., Fukayama, M., Inamatsu, T., Suzuki, K., Hashimoto, W., & Sato, K. (1992). Differential age-change in the numbers of CD4+CD45RA+ and CD4+CD29+ T cell subsets in human peripheral blood. *Mechanisms of Ageing and Development, 63,* 57–68.

Viale, A. C., Chies, J. A., Huetz, F., Malenchere, E., Weksler, M., Freitas, A. A., & Coutinho, A. (1994). VH-gene family dominance in ageing mice. *Scandinavian Journal of Immunology, 39,* 184–188.

Vie, H., & Miller, R. A. (1986). Decline, with age, in the proportion of mouse T cells that express IL-2 receptors after mitogen stimulation. *Mechanisms of Ageing and Development, 33,* 313–322.

Walker, D., Gauchat, J. F., De Weck, A. L., & Stadler, B. M. (1990). Analysis of leukocyte markers in elderly individuals. *Aging: Immunology and Infectious Disease, 2,* 31–43.

Wayne, S. J., Rhyne, R. L., Garry, P. J., & Goodwin, J. S. (1990). Cell-mediated immunity as a predictor of morbidity and mortality in subjects over 60. *Journal of Gerontology: Medical Science, 45,* M45–M48.

Wei, C.-F., Wali, A., Cherniack, E. P., Saririan, K., Weksler, M. E., Russo, C., & Thorbecke, G. J. (1992). Correlation between the ability of elderly individuals to respond to influenza vaccination and the capacity of their peripheral blood lymphocytes to express receptors for IgD. *Aging: Immunology and Infectious Disease, 3,* 195–202.

Wei, C. F., Tamma, S. L., Coico, R. F., Swenson, C. D., Secord, E. A., Amin, A. R., & Thorbecke, G. J. (1993). The IgD-receptor positive human T lymphocytes II: Total absence of any IgD-receptor expression in a large percentage of healthy aged individuals. *Aging: Immunology and Infectious Disease, 4,* 169–185.

Wei, J., Xu, H., Davies, J. L., & Hemmings, G. P. (1992). Increase of plasma IL-6 concentration with age in healthy subjects. *Life Science, 51,* 1953–1956.

Weindruch, R., & Walford, R. L. (1988). *The Retardation of Aging and Disease by Dietary Restriction.* Springfield, IL: Charles C. Thomas.

Weindruch, R., Devens, B. H., Raff, H. V., & Walford, R. L. (1983). Influence of dietary restriction and aging on natural killer cell activity in mice. *Journal of Immunology, 130,* 993–996.

Weiner, H. L. Scribner, D. J., Schocket, A. L., & Moorhead, J. W. (1978). Increased proliferative response of human peripheral blood lymphocytes to anti-immunoglobulin antibodies in elderly people. *Clinical Experiments in Immunology, 9,* 356–362.

Weksler, M. E., Schwab, R., Huetz, F., Kim, Y. T., & Coutinho, A. (1990). Cellular basis for the age-associated increase in autoimmune reactions. *International Immunology, 2,* 329–335.

Whisler, R. L., Newhouse, Y. G., Donnerberg, R. L., & Tobin, C. M. (1991). Characterization of intracellular ionized calcium responsiveness and inositol phosphate production among resting and stimulated peripheral blood T cells from elderly humans. *Aging: Immunology and Infectious Disease, 3,* 27–36.

Whisler, R. L., Liu, B., Wu, L. C., & Chen, M. (1993). Reduced activation of transcriptional factor AP-1 among peripheral blood T cells from elderly humans after PHA stimulation: restorative effect of phorbol diesters. *Cellular Immunology, 152,* 96–109.

Witkowski, J. M., & Miller, R. A. (1993). Increased function of P-glycoprotein in T lymphocytes of aging mice. *Journal of Immunology, 150,* 1296–1306.

Witkowski, J. M., Li, S. P., Gorgas, G., & Miller, R. A. (1994). Extrusion of the P-glycoprotein substrate rhodamine-123 distinguishes CD4 memory T cell subsets that differ in IL-2-driven IL-4 production. *Journal of Immunology, 153,* 658–665.

Wrabatz, L. G., Antel, J. P., Oger, J. J. F., Arnason, B. G. W., Goust, J. M., & Hopper, J. E. (1982). Age-related changes in in vivo immunoglobulin secretion: comparison of responses to T-dependent and T-independent polyclonal activators. *Cellular Immunology, 74,* 398–403.

Wu, W. T., Pahlavani, M., Cheung, H. T., & Richardson, A. (1986). The effect of aging on the expression of interleukin 2 messenger ribonucleic acid. *Cellular Immunology, 100,* 224–231.

Zharhary, D. (1986). T cell involvement in the decrease of antigen-responsive B cells in aged mice. *European Journal of Immunology, 16,* 1175–1178.

Zharhary, D. (1988). Age-related changes in the capability of the bone marrow to generate B cells. *Journal of Immunology, 141,* 1863–1869.

Zharhary, D., & Klinman, N. R. (1983). Antigen responsiveness of the mature and generative B cell populations of aged mice. *Journal of Experimental Medicine, 157,* 1300–1308.

Zharhary, D., & Klinman, N. R. (1984). B cell repertoire diversity to PR8 influenza virus does not decrease with age. *Journal of Immunology, 133,* 2285–2287.

Zharhary, D., & Klinman, N. R. (1986). A selective increase in the generation of phosphorylcholine-specific B cells associated with aging. *Journal of Immunology, 136,* 368–370.

Seventeen

Status and Functional Impact of Nutrition in Older Adults

Jeffrey B. Blumberg

I. Introduction

Nutrition has been recognized as an important factor influencing the functional outcome of aging. The adherence to particular dietary patterns by older as well as younger adults can affect the terminal years of the life span. Conversely, aging is accompanied by a variety of physiological, psychological, economic, and social changes that compromise nutritional status and/or affect nutritional requirements (Munro & Danford, 1989). Nutritional status surveys of the elderly have shown a relatively low prevalence of frank nutrient deficiencies, but a marked increase in the risk of malnutrition and evidence of subclinical deficiencies with a direct impact on function (Rosenberg, 1995). Nutrition is also an important factor in the progressive changes in body composition associated with aging, such as the loss of bone and lean body mass (Cumlea & Baumgartner, 1989). Moreover, the evidence is now undisputed that diet and nutrition are directly linked to many of the chronic diseases afflicting older and elderly adults (Nutrition Policy Board, 1988; Committee on Diet and Health, 1989). Thus, nutrition now represents an important part of the solution to the demographic challenge of the growing population of older adults and to the public health policy need to compress morbidity (Schneider & Brody, 1983; Schneider & Guralnik, 1990).

Aging produces physiological changes that affect the need for several essential nutrients (Munro & Schlierf, 1992). Although most standards of nutritional requirements for older adults continue to be based upon extrapolation from the recommendations for younger adults, evidence is accumulating that indicates different dietary goals are necessary to achieve optimal health in later life (Blumberg, 1991). Some of the apparent age-related changes in body composition and physiological function that appear to influence nutrient requirements in older adults are listed in Table I. In addition, decrements in the senses of taste and smell can have a significant impact on food selection and nutrient intake. Sedentary lifestyles, drug therapies, social isolation, physical disabilities, and chronic diseases can also substantially affect food choices, interfere with shopping and cooking, and impair nutritional status.

The absence of validated age-adjusted values for anthropometric, biochemical,

Handbook of the Biology of Aging, Fourth Edition
Copyright © 1996 Academic Press, Inc. All rights of reproduction in any form reserved.

Table I
Examples of Age-Related Changes in Body Composition and Physiological Function
That Influence Nutrient Requirements

Change in body composition or physiological function	Impact on nutrient requirement
Decreased muscle mass (sarcopenia)	Decreased need for calories
Decreased bone density (osteopenia)	Increased need for calcium and vitamin D
Decreased immune function	Increased need for vitamins B_6 and E and zinc
Increased gastric pH (atrophic gastritis)	Increased need for vitamin B_{12}, folic acid, calcium, iron, and zinc
Decreased skin capacity for cholecalciferol synthesis	Increased need for vitamin D
Increased wintertime parathyroid hormone production	Increased need for vitamin D
Decreased calcium bioavailability	Increased need for calcium and vitamin D
Decreased hepatic uptake of retinol	Decreased need for vitamin A
Decreased efficiency in metabolic utilization of pyridoxal	Increased need for vitamin B_6
Increased oxidative stress status	Increased need for β-carotene, vitamin C, and vitamin E
Increased levels of homocysteine	Increased need for folate, vitamin B_6, and vitamin B_{12}

and clinical standards has always confounded an adequate nutritional assessment of elderly individuals and the older adult population. Indeed, many standards of interpretation have been based on studies of younger populations. Research approaches in nutrition have begun to focus on measures of nutrient intake and status not merely as normative means but as part of an effort to identify and predict the functional and health consequences of these assessments. Thus, while the chapter on nutrition and aging in the previous edition of this series appropriately emphasized the nutritional status of the elderly (Ausman & Russell, 1990), attention here is devoted to the impact of selected nutrients on physiological function and the risk of chronic disease.

II. Body Composition

A. Bone Density and Fractures

The major determinants of bone volume include genetics and the status of sex hormones, exercise, and calcium and vitamin D nutriture (Nelson et al., 1991; Nelson

et al., 1988). Peak bone mass is achieved at about age 23, but as much as 40% of skeletal calcium can be lost thereafter; in women, almost half of this loss occurs within 5 years after menopause. The age-related decline in the capacity to absorb calcium (Bullamore, Wilkinson, Gallagher, Nordin, & Marshall, 1970) appears to be due to a gut resistance to the action of 1,25-dihydroxyvitamin D_3, resulting from a loss of vitamin D receptors in the duodenal mucosa (Ebeling et al., 1992). A decrease in the renal production of 1,25-dihydroxyvitamin D_3 with age has also been reported (Tsai, Heath, Kumar, & Riggs, 1984). Importantly, several other situations common to older people compromise their calcium nutriture and help to explain the striking deficiency of dietary calcium among persons aged 65 years and older. For example, lactose intolerance leads to the avoidance of dairy products and increased fiber intake for laxation impairs calcium bioavailability (Knox et al., 1991), as does atrophic gastritis (Recker, 1985).

Oral tests of physiological (but not pharmacological) doses of cholecalciferol indicate that the absorption efficiency of dietary vitamin D is reduced in older adults (Barragry et al., 1978; Clemens, Zhou, Myles, Endres, & Lindsay, 1986). In addition, there is also an age-related decline in the epidermal concentration of 7-dehydrocholesterol, which is converted to vitamin D after ultraviolet B radiation (MacLaughlin & Holick, 1985). Further, vitamin D nurture in older people may be compromised by their inadequate intake of fortified dairy products and their typically low exposure to sunlight. The decreases in calcium and vitamin D status result in a higher serum-intact parathyroid hormone concentration in the elderly (Eastell et al., 1991), which can be reversed by increasing the intake of one or both nutrients (Chapuy, Chapuy, & Meunier, 1987). This relationship may help to provide a useful index for optimal dietary intakes of these two nutrients (Krall, Sahyoun, Tannenbaum, Dallal, & Dawson-Hughes, 1989).

The adult body contains approximately 1200 g of calcium, approximately 99% of which is located in the skeleton. Optimal intakes of calcium and vitamin D can minimize the loss of skeletal minerals in older adults. While there is a lack of concordance in epidemiological studies associating calcium and vitamin D intake and fracture risk due to the limitations of observational research, clinical trials with daily supplements of these nutrients, usually in the range of 1000–1700 mg calcium and 400–800 IU vitamin D, have been able to significantly reduce the rate of age-related bone loss and secondary hyperparathyroidism and the incidence of fractures, especially of the hip (Chapuy et al., 1992; Heikinheimo et al., 1992; Aloia et al., 1994). In addition to calcium, other minerals including boron, copper, magnesium, manganese, and zinc appear to contribute to the maintenance of bone density with age (Saltman & Strause 1993; Nielsen 1990); of potential significance to the risk of osteoporosis, the dietary intake of several of these nutrients appears to be inadequate in older populations. It is always important to appreciate that falls may play as important a role in the risk of fracture as skeletal integrity. As weakness is a risk factor for falls, it is worth noting that age-associated loss of skeletal muscle may be related to the reduction in bone density seen in the elderly (Cohn et al., 1980).

B. Lean Body Mass and Muscle Strength

Between 25 and 75 years of age the lipid compartment expands from 14 to 38% of total body weight, while total body water (mainly extracellular water) and lean body mass decline. The loss of muscle mass is reflected by creatinine excretion rates decreasing from about 2000 mg/hr at age 20 to 1000 mg/hr at age 90 (Tzankoff & Norris, 1978). Direct regional assessments of the cross-sectional area of skeletal muscle by computed tomography indicate that muscle can account for 90% of area in active young men, but only 30% in frail elderly women (Fiatarone et al., 1991). This decline in lean body mass, termed sarcopenia, is accelerated after menopause and at advanced ages (Rosenberg, 1989). Sarcopenia is associated with an increase in intramuscular fat (Borkan, Hults, Gerzof, Robbins, & Silbert, 1983).

Cohn et al. (1980), differentiating muscle and nonmuscle mass via an assessment of total body potassium and nitrogen, determined that skeletal muscle loses protein with advancing age, while protein in nonmuscle tissue is maintained. Flynn, Nolph, Baker, Martin, and Krause (1989) suggested that there may also be a gender difference in the rate of body composition changes with age, as the most rapid loss of total body potassium occurs between 41 and 60 years in men but only after 60 years in women.

The impact of the age-related changes in lean body mass on nutritional status and physical fitness is substantial. Energy requirements have been suggested to diminish by about 100 cal per decade after age 45 as basal metabolism strongly reflects the lean, metabolizing component of body mass (Tzankoff & Norris, 1977). As energy intake is reduced with age due to a lower basal metabolic rate (and a more sedentary lifestyle), it becomes increasingly difficult for an older person to satisfy his or her micronutrient requirements through diet alone. With regard to micronutrients, Fiatarone et al. (1990) observed that inadequate intakes of vitamin D, magnesium, calcium, and zinc are strongly associated with sarcopenia.

Requirements for dietary protein are based largely on nitrogen balance studies rather than the maintenance of muscle mass. Protein provides about 10–20% of total energy intake in both young and older adults, despite the smaller energy intake characteristic of the latter group. While a number of reports have identified protein–calorie malnutrition as a major problem among the elderly, this status appears to be almost exclusive to elderly individuals with concomitant diseases associated with wasting. Among free-living older adults, median protein intakes tend to exceed RDA standards (Sahyoun, 1992), although biochemical markers for protein status, e.g., transferrin, total protein, and transthyretin in serum and plasma albumin, are generally noted to decline with advancing age after age 60 (Munro, 1992). Campbell, Crim, Dallal, Young, and Evans (1994a), by employing a new nitrogen balance study in elderly subjects and a recalculation of data from previous studies, have estimated the dietary protein requirement of healthy older men and women to be 0.91 ± 0.043 g kg^{-1} day^{-1}, a value that is higher than the intakes of 0.8 and 0.6 g kg^{-1} day^{-1} recommended by the RDA and the 1985 joint FDA/WHO/UNU Expert Consultation, respectively. They recommend that a safe protein allowance for the elderly requires an intake of 1.0–1.25 g kg^{-1} day^{-1} from a diet containing high-quality protein; similarly, Young

(1990) has suggested that protein requirements for older adults should be increased. That this higher requirement for protein in older adults occurs despite their decreased muscle mass appears to suggest a lower efficiency of dietary protein utilization. Interestingly, Meredith, Frontera, O'Reilly, and Evans (1992) found that providing elderly volunteers with a daily protein–energy supplement increased the size and mass of the midthigh muscle more than in nonsupplemented controls after a regimen of resistance training.

The functional significance of sarcopenia is also substantial, as preservation of the fat-free compartment is highly predictive of muscle function and mobility in the elderly (Fiatarone et al., 1991). Frontera, Hughes, Lutz, and Evans (1991) examined the isokinetic strength of the elbow and knee extensors and flexors in healthy older adults and observed that strength was significantly lower in those aged 65–78 years than in those aged 45–54 years. Adjusting the data for body composition revealed muscle mass as the major determinant of the age- and gender-related differences in muscle strength, independent of muscle location (upper vs lower extremities) and function (extension vs flexion). Thus, if muscle mass can be preserved into old age, it would be reasonable to expect that muscle strength could also be preserved. While the reduction in muscle mass with age appears to account for the quantitative loss of strength, Bruce, Newton, and Woledge (1989) note that qualitative changes in maximal force production may result from decrements in neural recruitment capacity. Fiatarone et al. (1990) have reported that resistance training can significantly restore muscle mass and strength even in very old people who have lost substantial amounts of both; the observation of inadequate intakes of several micronutrients associated with sarcopenia suggests that appropriate nutritional intervention may be synergistic with the resistance training. However, very modest micronutrient supplementation at approximately one-third of the RDA levels during such training does not appear to significantly enhance the response to training (Fiatarone et al., 1994). Moreover, in addition to a potentially greater requirement for protein with exercise, Campbell, Crim, Dallal, Young, and Evans (1994b) found that weight maintenance during resistance training by older adults was associated with an increased caloric requirement. Interestingly, Roberts et al. (1992) have suggested that the current RDA levels for those aged 50+ years not only may significantly underestimate usual energy requirements but, further, that the low levels of energy expenditure suggested by the RDA may favor increases in body fat mass.

The impact of sarcopenia extends beyond its contribution to weakness, risk of falls, and the inability to perform activities of daily living. The importance of muscle mass to the maintenance of basal metabolic rate, insulin sensitivity, and physical activity implicates sarcopenia as a risk factor in many of the leading chronic diseases common to older adults, including Type II diabetes, coronary artery disease, and hypertension.

III. Immune Function

A. Aging and Immunity

The age-related decline in lean tissue mass is not insignificantly composed of the losses in the immune system, which comprises 8% of total lean mass (Makinodan & Kay, 1980). Involution of the thymus, beginning at puberty and complete by middle age, may represent one of the earliest age-related decrements in the immune system, which correlates in part with other impairments in immunity through the life span (Hirokawa, 1992). Defects as diverse as dysfunction of T and B lymphocytes, elevated levels of circulating immune complexes, an increase in autoantibodies, and monoclonal gammopathies have been recognized as common to the aging process (Meydani & Blumberg, 1989). Alterations in intracellular calcium distribution, decreases in interleukin (IL)-2 production and IL-2 mRNA expression, and poor proliferative response to mitogens are some of the age-associated changes observed in lymphoid cells that are linked to the failure of the immune system with age (Miller, 1995).

Both T and B cells from older adults have defects in activation, particularly during the cell cycle events for differentiation (Thoman & Weigle, 1989). Shifts in the distribution of functionally distinct $CD4^+$ T-cell subsets with age, particularly the increased accumulation of memory T cells, by chronic antigenic stimulation have been reported; these memory T cells appear to be resistant to intracellular calcium, a condition that may lead to defects in signal transduction (Grossmann, Ledbetter, & Rabinovitch, 1990). In addition, alterations in T lymphocytes of protein phosphorylation pathways, cytokine production, and the number and function of membrane-bound receptors have also been closely associated with the decline in T-cell functions during aging (Rabinovitch, June, Grossmann, & Ledbetter, 1986; Fernandes & Venkatraman, 1993). Further, decreased lymphocyte reactivity in older adults is negatively correlated with an increased membrane microviscosity which may reflect a dysregulation of lipid homeostasis (Huber et al., 1991). Age-related T-cell defects may increase susceptibility to malignancies, infections, and the development of autoimmune diseases in the elderly (Schwab & Weksler, 1987).

B. Nutrition and Immune Responsiveness

Due to the dependence of immune responsiveness upon both macro- and miocronutrient adequacy, general assessments of nutritional status often include measures of total lymphocyte count, delayed-hypersensitivity skin test (DHST), mitogen-stimulated lymphocyte proliferation, and the stimulated elaboration of lymphocytic cytokines. Severe malnutrition or any one of several nutrient deficiency syndromes can compromise immune functions, which can be restored by provision of the appropriate nutrients (McMurray, 1984; Chandra, 1981; Cunningham-Rundles, 1993). However, as these severe nutritional states are relatively rare even among the older population, research has focused on whether enhancement of micronutrient status can prevent or retard the typical age-related declines in immune function.

Chandra, Joshi, Au, Woodford, and Chandra (1982) first examined the nutritional and immunological status of a group of apparently healthy elderly subjects without presenting underlying systemic disease; among those with clinical, hematological, and/or biochemical evidence of nutrient inadequacies, DHST and T-cell numbers (including CD4$^+$ subset) and response to mitogens were significantly reduced. Nutritional advice and supplementation sufficient to increase energy intake by approximately 500 kcal/day and to provide at least the RDA levels of micronutrients for 8 weeks improved each of these immune parameters and nutritional status as assessed by serum levels of albumin, prealbumin, transferrin, retinol-binding protein, zinc, and iron. Targeting nutritional advice and supplementation to the specific needs of his older patients, Chandra (1989) observed improvements in natural killer cell activity, mitogen-stimulated lymphocyte proliferation, and DHST, as well as higher antibody-forming cell responses and IL-2 production.

More general and longer term nutritional supplementation to free-living older adults has also resulted in improved immunological status. Bogden et al. (1990, 1994) administered One-a-Day type multivitamin–mineral supplements for 1 year in double-blind, placebo-controlled trials and found that the treatment significantly enhanced lymphocyte proliferative responses and/or DHST. Similarly, Chandra (1992), employing a multivitamin–mineral supplement containing moderately higher doses of vitamin E and β-carotene for 1 year, reported that the treatment significantly enhanced lymphocyte proliferative responses, IL-2 production, natural killer cell activity, and antibody responses to influenza vaccine. Importantly, Chandra (1992) also noted that those subjects using the supplement had 48% fewer days of infectious disease episodes and required 56% fewer days of antibiotic drug treatment from the placebo group.

The well-documented effects of various nutrients on maintenance of optimum immunity has led to clinical studies of single nutrients, particularly the antioxidants (Bendich & Chandra, 1990). For example, the administration of supplemental vitamin C to healthy older subjects has been found to enhance lymphocyte proliferative responses, DHST, serum IgG, IgM, and complement C3 levels (Kennes, Dumont, Brohee, Hubert, & Neve, 1983; Ziemlanski, Wartanowicz, & Kios, 1986). In their community-based survey, Goodwin and Garry (1983) found that older adults within the top 10% for plasma ascorbate concentration had significantly fewer anergic subjects as defined by DHST.

Several molecular and biochemical mechanisms of ascorbate-mediated immunostimulation have been proposed, including (a) modulation of intracellular cyclic nucleotide levels, (b) modulation of prostaglandin (PG) synthesis, (c) protection of 5'lipoxygenase, (d) enhancement of cytokine production, (e) antagonism of the immunosuppressive interactions of histamine and leukocytes, and (f) neutralization of phagocyte-derived autoreactive and immunosuppressive oxidants (Anderson, Smit, Joone, & Van Staden, 1990). Vitamin C appears to serve as the first-line plasma antioxidant in the defense against phagocyte-derived reactive oxidants; only when ascorbate is depleted does detectable free radical damage, measured by the appearance of lipid peroxides, ensue (Frei, Stocker, & Ames, 1988).

In placebo-controlled, double-blind trials with vitamin E in healthy older adults, S. N. Meydani et al. (1990) and M. Meydani et al. (1993b) have demonstrated significant improvements in DHST and/or lymphocyte proliferation, as well reductions in plasma lipid peroxides and the production of PGE_2 by peripheral blood mononuclear cells. Cannon et al. (1990) found that, in older men, vitamin E supplementation effectively restored several blunted acute phase immune responses, including increases in circulating neutrophils and creatine kinase, following an intense bout of eccentric exercise to levels comparable to those of young men; this enhancement in immune responsiveness, together with an inhibition of lipid peroxidation and pro-inflammatory cytokines IL-1 and IL-6, appears to be consistent with the concept that vitamin E provides protection against exercise-induced oxidative injury (Cannon et al., 1991; M. Meydani et al., 1993a). Ziemlanski, Wartanowicz, and Kios (1986) reported that vitamin E supplementation of institutionalized elderly women increased total serum protein, with the principal effect on α_2- and β_2-globulin fractions; significant increases in IgG and complement C3 levels were noted when vitamin C was combined with vitamin E. Penn et al. (1991) administered a combination of vitamins A, C, and E to hospitalized geriatric patients and reported improvements in cell-mediated immune function, as assessed by significant increases in the absolute number of T cells, T4 subsets, T4:T8 ratio, and mitogen-stimulated lymphocyte proliferation in the treated vs placebo group.

Vitamin E may exert its immunostimulatory effect in older adults by inhibiting PG synthesis and/or decreasing free radical formation. Vitamin E can affect both the lipoxygenase and cyclooxygenase pathways of arachidonic acid metabolism. Oxygen metabolites, especially hydrogen peroxide, produced by activated macrophages depress lymphocyte proliferation; α-tocopherol has been shown to decrease hydrogen peroxide formation by polymorphonuclear leukocytes (Blumberg, 1993).

After supplementing older subjects with β-carotene, Watson, Prabhala, Plezia, and Alberts (1991) found a dose-dependent increase in T-helper cells, natural killer cells, and peripheral blood mononuclear cells with IL-2 and transferrin receptors. Talbott, Miller, and Kerkvliet (1987) reported that supplementation of healthy elderly individuals with vitamin B_6 significantly increased lymphocyte proliferative responses to several mitogens and the percentage of T-helper cells. S. N. Meydani et al. (1991b), by employing a vitamin B_6 depletion–repletion protocol, showed that IL-2 production and mitogenic response to T- and B-cell mitogens are affected by changes in dietary vitamin B_6; supplementation with high doses of pyridoxine improved these responses beyond their baseline values in these healthy older adults.

The occurrence of low serum thymulin and other indirect evidence of a prevalent mild zinc deficiency in the elderly population have prompted some trials with zinc supplementation (Chandra et al., 1982; Chandra, 1984a; Bogden et al., 1988). Duchateau, Delepesse, Vrijens, and Collet (1981) examined the effect of zinc supplementation on immune responses of healthy institutionalized subjects over 70 years of age and observed an increase in DHST and the percent of circulating T cells, as well as improved serum IgG antibody formation against tetanus toxin. However, Chandra (1984b) has reported that excessive zinc supplementation impairs the immune responses.

Essential fatty acids and dietary fats

may affect immunity via altering cell membrane composition and fluidity, serum lipoproteins, or hormone status, although attention has been focused on their capacity to modulate cytokine and eicosanoid biosynthesis. The effects of supplementing the diet with $n - 3$ fatty acids in the form of fish oils have been investigated in healthy older adults, as well as in patients with inflammatory and autoimmune disorders. The reported antiinflammatory effects of fish oils are partly mediated by inhibiting the 5-lipoxygenase pathway in neutrophils and monocytes and inhibiting the leukotriene (LT) B_4-mediated function of neutrophils, while increasing the production of the less inflammatory LTB_5 (Kremer, Jubiz, & Michalek, 1987). Fish oil supplementation can also decrease the inducible production of IL-1 and tumor necrosis factor (Endres et al., 1989). These mechanisms may be partly responsible for the reported beneficial actions of fish oil treatment on arthritis, psoriasis, and ulcerative colitis (Simopoulos, 1991). S. N. Meydani et al. (1991a) found that fish oil supplementation was markedly more potent in reducing IL-1β, IL-6, and tumor necrosis factor in healthy older women than in younger women. However, the older women also experienced significant reductions in IL-2 and mitogenic responses, suggesting that the fish oil may be beneficial as part of an antiinflammatory regimen or in decreasing the severity of autoimmune disease, but may have untoward suppressive actions on cell-mediated immunity in older adults. Some data suggest that this effect on cell-mediated immunity may be reversed by increasing vitamin E status (Kremer et al., 1991).

IV. Vascular Function

The pathogenesis of atherosclerosis during aging is consistent with a "reaction to injury" hypothesis, whereby the endothelial cells lining the intima are exposed to repeated or continuing insults to their integrity (Ross, 1986). Such injury may be caused by chronic hypercholesterolemia, mechanical stress associated with hypertension, and elevated oxidative stress status associated with cigarette smoking. Indeed, the most significant reversible risk factors for atherosclerosis now include lowering cholesterol, treating hypertension, and smoking cessation, in addition to reducing obesity. The evidence for an association between diet, particularly fat intake and plasma lipids, and heart disease is well-established and directly relevant to the age-related changes in the vascular system. Contributions to this diet–vascular function relationship have come from studies of three B vitamins, vitamins B_6 and B_{12} and folic acid, and the antioxidants, vitamins C and E and β-carotene.

A. B Vitamins and Homocysteine

McCully (1991) has described several observations correlating arteriosclerotic lesions with elevations of blood homocysteine, a non-protein-forming sulfur amino acid derived from methionine metabolism with demonstrated atherogenic properties in animals. Patients with homocysteinuria caused by genetic defects, e.g., cystathionine synthetase deficiency, develop arteriosclerosis during childhood with many pathological features similar to those of the atherosclerotic lesions seen in older adult populations. Homocysteine concentrations are also regulated by several micronutrients (Fig. 1). Increased interest in this topic has been generated not only by growing evidence that homocysteine is an independent risk factor for vascular disease (Genest et al., 1990; Clark et al., 1991; Pancharuniti et al., 1994) but also because of the recognition that moderate homocysteinemia is fairly prevalent (at about 30% among older adults; Selhub, Jacques, Wilson, Rush, & Rosenberg, 1993) and, further, that it is reversible with nutri-

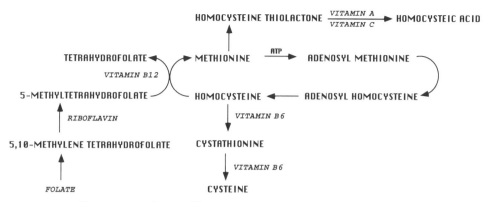

Figure 1. Regulation of homocysteine metabolism by micronutrients.

tional intervention (Ubbink, Hayward Vermaak, van der Merwe, & Becker, 1993). Inadequate B vitamin status has been associated with elevated homocysteine concentrations in approximately two-thirds of individuals with elevated homocysteine levels (Selhub, Jacques, Wilson, Rush, & Rosenberg, 1993).

The data associating homocysteine and vascular disease are derived primarily from retrospective studies of elevated fasting plasma homocysteine or abnormal methionine-loading test results in patients (Ureland, Refsum, & Brattstrom, 1992). The pooled prevalence of abnormal postload homocysteine concentrations for all vascular disease patients and controls from nine studies was 24 and 2%, respectively. Fasting homocysteine concentrations are consistently elevated among patients with all types of vascular disease and on average are 31% higher than concentrations among controls. Cross-sectional studies have demonstrated positive correlations between arterial stenosis based on ultrasound measurements and homocysteine concentrations (Rubba *et al.*, 1990; Clark *et al.*, 1992; Malinow, Nieto, Szklo, Chambless, & Bond, 1993). In a prospective analysis, Stampfer *et al.* (1992) found that the risk for myocardial infarction was 3.4 times greater among middle-aged and older male physicians with elevated baseline homocysteine con-

centrations, independent of other vascular disease risk factors. Interestingly, the lower risk of vascular disease among premenopausal vs postmenopausal women is reflected in their lower homocysteine levels and may be related to an estrogen-dependent activation of homocysteine catabolism via transamination (Boers, Smals, Trijbels, Leermakers, & Kloppenborg, 1983; Blom *et al.*, 1988). Conclusive evidence from intervention studies demonstrating that a lowering of plasma homocysteine by improving B vitamin status results in a reduction in thrombogenesis and vascular disease risk is not yet available.

B. Antioxidants and Oxidative Lipoprotein Modification

The oxidative modification of low-density lipoprotein (LDL) appears to play an important part in the process of atherosclerosis (Steinberg, 1991). Oxidized LDL is taken up more readily than native LDL by macrophages to create foam cells. Further, oxidized LDL is chemotactic for circulating monocytes, is cytotoxic to endothelial cells, inhibits the motility of tissue macrophages, and increases arterial vasoconstriction (Steinberg, Parthasarathy, Carew, Khoo, & Witztum, 1989). In addition, oxidized LDL has been identified in atherosclerotic lesions (Ylä-Herttuala *et al.*, 1989), and elevated titers of circulating autoantibodies to epitopes of oxidized LDL are present in patients with atherosclerosis (Salonen *et al.*, 1992). Greater concentrations of lipid peroxides are also noted in patients with atherosclerosis (Stringer, Görög, Freeman, & Kakkar, 1989). The susceptibility of LDL to oxidation has also been correlated with the severity of atherosclerosis (Regnström, Nilsson, Tornvall, Landou, & Hamsten, 1992).

Several laboratories have demonstrated that antioxidant nutrients can inhibit the oxidative modification of LDL when added *in vitro* (Esterbauer, Striegl, Puhl, & Rotheneder, 1988; Jialal & Grundy, 1991). Supplementation of healthy subjects with vitamin E or a combination of antioxidants, but not β-carotene alone, has been shown to be effective in decreasing the susceptibility of LDL to oxidation (Dieber-Rotheneder, Puhl, Waeg, Streigl, & Esterbauer, 1991; Abbey, Nestel, & Baghurst, 1993; Jialal & Grundy, 1993; Princen, van Poppel, Vogelezang, Buytenhek, & Kok, 1992).

Inverse correlations have been reported between plasma vitamin E and mortality from ischemic heart disease in cross-cultural epidemiology studies (Gey *et al.*, 1993a). Two large prospective diet studies have revealed a significant decreased risk of coronary heart disease associated with high intakes, particularly via supplements, of vitamin E (Stampfer *et al.*, 1993). Plasma vitamin E concentrations have also been found to be lower in newly diagnosed angina than in controls (Riemersma *et al.*, 1991). Consistent with these observations is the efficacy of vitamin E in decreasing the rate of restenosis among patients after angioplasty (DeMaio *et al.*, 1992). However, similar findings were not obtained when vitamin E measurements were made in previously collected and stored serum samples from patients with myocardial infarction and controls (Salonen *et al.*, 1985; Kok *et al.*, 1987); these

contrasting data may result from the general absence of supplement use in this population and/or the degradation of α-tocopherol in the stored samples.

An inverse association of β-carotene intake with coronary heart disease risk among current and former smokers has been observed (Rimm *et al.*, 1993), and serum β-carotene concentrations have been found to be inversely associated with myocardial infarction (Street, Comstock, Salkeld, Schüep, & Klag, 1991) and ischemic heart disease mortality (Gey *et al.*, 1993b). Preliminary findings in patients with stable angina suggest that β-carotene supplements may reduce the risk of cardiovascular complications (Gaziano, Manson, Ridker, Buring, & Hennekens, 1990). Consistent with this intervention trial, an inverse association of adipose tissue β-carotene, derived from normal dietary intake, and myocardial infarction was observed in a case control study (Kardinaal *et al.*, 1993). A limited number of reports suggest that very low intakes and poor status of vitamin C are associated with an increased risk of mortality from coronary causes (Gey, Brubacher, & Stähelin, 1987; Enstrom, Kanim, & Klein, 1992).

V. Visual Function

A. Cataract

Age-related cataract is the most common disorder of the crystalline lens and is characterized by the degeneration and atrophy of epithelium, water clefts in the cortex, lens fiber fragmentation, and deposits of crystals such as calcium and cholesterol. While amenable to treatment by surgical removal, age-related cataract is the leading cause of blindness and visual impairment in the world and a major contributor to functional impairment and morbidity in older adults (Stark, Sommer, & Smith, 1989). While ultraviolet (solar) radiation has been identified as a principal risk factor in age-related cataracts, other forms of radiation, aspirin use, smoking, and diarrhea and dehydration have also been suggested as possible causes of this condition.

Protein oxidation, e.g., via disulfide bond formation, and precipitation into water-insoluble aggregates represent a likely mechanism of senile cataract formation. Photooxidation of lens proteins may occur either indirectly through photosensitizers or directly through the absorption of radiation by the aromatic amino acids tryptophan and tyrosine (Taylor & Davies, 1987). The whole lens is capable of maintaining ascorbate and glutathione at millimolar concentrations, which is many times greater than that found in plasma, and also contains micromolar levels of tocopherol and carotenoids, which are compartmentalized in the membrane fraction. Thus, it is suggested that, over decades, ultraviolet photooxidative denaturation of the crystalline lens eventually overcomes age-associated declines in antioxidant and proteolytic defenses in the lens, resulting in protein precipitation and opacification (Taylor, Jacques, & Dorey, 1993).

Evidence has accumulated that suggests an important relationship between age-related cataract and nutritional status, particularly of the antioxidants (Jacques, Chylack, & Taylor, 1994). Most of the epidemiological investigations have found an association between the intake and/or status of vitamin C and the prevalence of cataract (Jacques & Chylack, 1991; Robertson, Donner, & Trevithick, 1989; Leske, Chylack, & Wu, 1991; Hankinson et al., 1992), although some found no relationship (Mohan et al., 1989; Italian–American Cataract Study Group, 1991). Vitamin E intake and/or status and cataract have also been inversely associated in several (Vitale et al., 1993; Robertson, Donner, & Trevithick, 1989; Leske, Chylack, & Wu, 1991), but not all reports (Mohan et al., 1989; Italian–American Cataract Study Group, 1991; Hankinson

et al., 1992). Carotenoids and vitamin A have also been inversely associated with cataract (Jacques & Chylack, 1991; Leske et al., 1991; Hankinson et al., 1992). From a prospective analysis of a large cohort, Seddon et al. (1994b) reported that middle-aged and older men who consumed multivitamin supplements tended to experience a decreased risk of cataract. In two prospective randomized clinical trials conducted in China, Sperduto et al. (1993) found that supplementation with a multivitamin preparation or a riboflavin–niacin formula significantly reduced the prevalence of nuclear cataract in older subjects relative to placebo controls; as a cofactor for glutathione reductase, riboflavin can serve to maintain the cellular pool of reduced glutathione, an important antioxidant in the lens.

B. Age-Related Macular Degeneration

Age-related macular degeneration (AMD) is the leading cause of irreversible blindness among older adults (Bressler, Bressler, & Fine, 1988). The more common atrophic (dry) form of AMD is characterized by the presence of drusen and atrophy of the retinal pigment epithelium. Signs of neovascular (wet) AMD include choroidal neovascularization, serous or hemorrhagic detachment of the retinal pigment epithelium, and disciform scarring. Although less prevalent, neovascular AMD is more likely to result in severe vision loss. The retina is rich in highly polyunsaturated fatty acids, particularly docosahexaenoic acid, and thus, is vulnerable to lipid peroxidation. This situation is compounded by exposure to light, high oxygen tension, and high concentrations of retinol (Mittag, 1984). The macula contains a full complement of antioxidant defenses and has been noted to be unusually rich in the carotenoids lutein and zeaxanthin, but the two most abundant carotenoids in human plasma, β-carotene and lycopene are absent (Schalch, 1992).

An evaluation of the data from the First National Health and Nutrition Examination Survey suggested that antioxidants may reduce the occurrence of AMD (Goldberg, Flowerdew, Smith, Brody, & Tso, 1988). Subsequently, West *et al.* (1994) found that high plasma α-tocopherol levels and an index combining plasma levels of ascorbate, α-tocopherol, and β-carotene, but not vitamin supplement use, indicated a protective effect for AMD. In contrast, the Eye Disease Case-Control Study Group (1993) found that high levels of plasma carotenoids, but not α-tocopherol, were associated with a reduced risk of AMD, although the antioxidants showed a statistically significant effect when expressed as a total antioxidant index. Seddon *et al.* (1994a) reported that increased intake of carotenoid-rich foods, particularly those containing lutein and zeaxanthin, is strongly correlated with a reduced risk of AMD. Two reports have failed to confirm a relationship between antioxidant status and AMD (Blumenkranz, Russell, Robey, Blumenkranz, & Penneys, 1986; Sanders, Haines, Wormald, Wright, & Obeid, 1993). Zinc plays a role in the metabolic function of several enzymes in the chorioretinal complex, including superoxide dismutase, catalase, and retinol dehydrogenase; in a small, prospective randomized trial, Newsome, Swartz, Leone, Elston, and Miller (1988) found that treatment with zinc supplements resulted in a limited, but positive effect on visual acuity in AMD patients.

VI. Cognitive Function

The effect of aging on cognitive function is beginning to be well-characterized (Albert & Moss, 1996). Age-related reductions in recall and speed of processing have been reported in healthy older people (Salthouse, 1991), while more dramatic changes in memory, orientation, judgment, and affect are noted in patients with dementias (Strub & Black, 1981). The central nervous system is exquisitely dependent upon its nutrient supply, and many studies have documented the neurological and behavioral effects of nutritional deficiency syndromes (Rosenberg & Miller, 1992; Rosenberg & Ronnenberg, 1994).

Several studies have suggested that mild or subclinical vitamin deficiencies in free-living populations play a role in the pathogenesis of declining neurocognitive function in aging. Goodwin, Goodwin, and Garry (1983) found that healthy elderly subjects who had low blood levels of some vitamins, particularly folate, vitamin B_{12}, vitamin C, and riboflavin, scored poorly on tests of memory and nonverbal abstract thinking. Tucker *et al.* (1990) observed significant correlations between poor indices of thiamin, riboflavin, and iron nutriture and impaired cognitive performance and electroencephalographic indices of neuropsychological function. Selhub *et al.* (1995) observed a significant inverse correlation between plasma homocysteine levels and carotid artery stenosis and suggested that low B vitamin status may be related to the risk of cerebrovascular disease, with its associated changes in cognitive function.

Bell *et al.* (1990a,b) have associated low or low to normal vitamin B_{12} and folate levels with neuropsychiatric disorders, particularly depression, in elderly patients and suggest that low B vitamin status might accentuate the effects of other causes of cognitive dysfunction. Levitt and Karlinsky (1992) reported a significant correlation between vitamin B_{12} status and performance on the Mini Mental Status Exam in patients with possible or probable Alzheimer's dementia, but not in patients with other dementias. Results from some case studies indicate that patients with coexisting dementia or neurological symptoms and clinical deficiencies of folate or vitamin B_{12} respond to supplementation with these vitamins (Martin, 1988). For example, Lindenbaum *et al.* (1988) reported that patients with a variety of neuropsychiatric disorders and biochemical evidence of cobalamin insufficiency (but no signs of anemia or macrocytosis) showed marked cognitive improvements upon parenteral administration of vitamin B_{12}; this treatment was also associated with a reduction of elevated levels of homocysteine and methylmalonic acid. Karnaze and Carmel (1987) suggest that up to 30% of elderly patients with dementia may present with low, but not necessarily deficient, vitamin B_{12} status.

Few controlled studies have tested whether cognitive or other changes can be reversed by B vitamin administration. Botez, Botez, and Maag (1984) tested the effect of folate supplementation in a placebo-controlled trial with folate-deficient patients presenting signs of mild depression and memory and concentration problems and reported that the treatment significantly improved neuropsychological test scores. Martin, Francis, Protetch, and Huff (1992) found that vitamin B_{12} supplementation of geriatric patients with signs of cognitive impairment and low serum cobalamin levels resulted in improvements on the Mattis Dementia Rating Scale if they had had symptoms for less than 1 year, but no improvements were seen in those with longer term impairments.

The fraction of age-related pathological cognitive and neurological disorders that may be responsive to nutritional intervention is not known. Similarly, the lack of studies directly addressing the role of nutrition in the pathogenesis of cognitive impairments in older adults allows no recommendations for prevention. Nonetheless, the apparent impact of vitamin status on the development of mental disorders, particularly those due to vascular disease, represents a potentially practical approach for health promotion (Hachinski, 1992).

VII. Conclusion

As emphasized here, several nutrients possess important roles beyond their classically recognized functions in preventing deficiency diseases and their biochemical action as coenzymes. Thus, vitamins and minerals have now been demonstrated to serve in "nonclassical" roles as biological regulators and modulators, such that they can act to maximize physiological function, promote health, and delay or prevent the onset of many prevalent chronic diseases in older adults (Sauberlich & Machlin, 1992). This information can now be utilized to employ dietary recommendations and specific nutrient interventions as adjuncts in the effort to promote successful aging. While the evidence associating the intake of certain nutrients with optimal function during the aging process is strong, knowledge about the mechanisms underlying these relationships is far from complete. For example, the bone remodeling response to vitamin D appears to be dependent upon common allelic variants in the gene encoding the vitamin D receptor (Morrison et al., 1994). Some of the benefits of vitamin E and β-carotene may derive from actions unrelated to their antioxidant properties, e.g., the modulation of intracellular signaling by vitamin E through protein kinase C (Azzi, Bartoli, Boscoboinik, Hensey, & Szewczyk, 1993) and the conversion of β-carotene to retinoic acid, which binds to the RAR and RXR families of nuclear receptor proteins (Mangelsdorf, Umesono, & Evans, 1994). The efficacy of supplementation in some patients with both B vitamin deficiency and cognitive disorders suggests an acute effect of B vitamin status independent of homocysteine involvement.

Determination of the impact of nutrition on physiological function and risk of chronic disease across the life span requires a full exploration not only of nutrient dose–response relationships, mechanisms of action, and the dynamic interactions between the essential nutrients and other dietary constituents but also of the behavioral and environmental factors that influence dietary patterns. Nonetheless, current dietary guidelines do not reflect nutrition-sensitive alterations in metabolism or body composition, with significant consequences for the aging process and risk of chronic disease.

References

Abbey, M., Nestel, P. J., & Baghurst, P. A. (1993). Antioxidant vitamins and low-density-lipoprotein oxidation. *American Journal of Clinical Nutrition, 58,* 525–532.

Albert, M. S., & Moss, M. (1996). Neuropsychological assessment of age-related cognitive decline: human and animal models. In E. Schneider & J. W. Rowe (Eds.), *Handbook of the Biology of Aging* (pp. 217–233). San Diego: Academic Press.

Aloia, J. F., Vaswani, A., Yeh, J. K., Ross, P., Flaster, E., & Dilmanian, A. (1994). Calcium supplementation with and without hormone replacement therapy to prevent postmenopausal bone loss. *Annals of Internal Medicine, 120,* 97–103.

Anderson, R., Smit, M. J., Joone, G. K., & Van Staden, A. M. (1990). Vitamin C and Cellular Immune Functions. *Annals of the New York Academy of Sciences, 587,* 34–48.

Ausman, L. M., & Russell, R. M. (1990). Nutrition and aging. In E. L. Schneider & J. W. Rowe (Eds.), *Handbook of the Biology of Aging* (pp. 384–406). San Diego, CA: Academic Press.

Azzi, A. M., Bartoli, G., Boscoboinik, D., Hensey, C., & Szewczyk, A. (1993). α-Tocopherol and protein kinase C regulation of intracellular signaling. In P. Lester & J. Fuchs (Eds.), *Vitamin E in Health and Disease* (pp. 371–384). New York: Marcell Dekker, Inc.

Barragry, J. M., France, M. W., Corless, D., Gupta, S. P., Switala, S., Boucher, B. J., & Cohen, R. D. (1978). Intestinal cholecalciferol absorption in the elderly and in younger adults. *Clinical Science, 55,* 213–220.

Bell, I. R., Edman, J. S., Marby, D. W., Satlin, A., Dreier, T., Liptzin, B., & Cole, J. O. (1990a). Vitamin B12 and folate status in acute neuropsychiatric inpatients: affective and cognitive characteristics of a vitamin nondeficient population. *Biological Psychiatry, 27,* 125–137.

Bell, I. R., Edman, J. S., Miller, J., Hebben, N., Linn, R. T., Ray, D., & Kayne, H. L. (1990b). Relationship of normal serum vitamin B-12 and folate levels to cognitive test performance in sub-types of geriatric major depression. *Journal of Geriatric Psychiatry and Neurology, 3,* 98–105.

Bendich, A., & Chandra, R. K. (Eds.) (1990). Micronutrients and immune functions. *Annals of the New York Academy of Sciences* (Vol. 587). New York: Academy of sciences.

Blom, H. J., Boers, G. H., van den Elzen, J. P., van Roessel, J. J., Trijbels, J. M., & Tangerman, A. (1988). Differences between premenopausal women and young men in the transamination pathway of methionine catabolism, and the protection against vascular disease. *Journal of Clinical Investigation, 18,* 633–638.

Blumberg, J. B. (1991). Considerations of the Recommended Dietary Allowances for older adults. *Clinics in Applied Nutrition, 1,* 9–18.

Blumberg, J. B. (1993). The Role of Vitamin E in Immunity During Aging. In M. Mino, H. Nakamura, A. T. Diplock, & H. J. Kayden (Eds.), *Vitamin E: Its Usefulness in Health and Disease* (pp. 219–229). Tokyo and Basel: Japan Scientific Societies Press and Karger, respectively.

Blumenkranz, M. S., Russell, S. R., Robey, M. G., Blumenkranz, R. K., & Penneys, N. (1986). *Ophthalmology, 96,* 552–558.

Boers, G. H., Smals, A. G., Trijbels, F. J., Leermakers, A. I., & Kloppenborg, P. W. (1983). Unique efficiency of methionine metabolism in premenopausal women may protect against vascular disease in the reproductive years. *European Journal of Clinical Investigation, 72,* 1971–1976.

Bogden, J. D., Oleske, J. M., Munves, M., Lavenhar, M. A., Bruening, K. S., Kemp, F. W., Holding, K. J., Kenny, T. N., & Lauria, D. B. (1988). Serum thymulin in zinc deficiency. *Journal of Clinical Investigation, 88,* 1202–1210.

Bogden, J. D., Oleske, J. M., Lavenhar, M. A., Munves, E. M., Kempt, F. W., Bruening, K. S., Holding, K. J., Denny, T. N., Guarino, M. A., & Holland, B. K. (1990). Effects of 1y supplementation with zinc and other micronutrients on cellular immunity in the elderly. *Journal of the American College of Nutrition, 9,* 214–225.

Bogden, J. D., Bendich, A., Kemp, F. W., Bruening, K. S., Skurnick, J. H., Denny, T., Baker, H., & Louria, D. B. (1994). Daily micronutrient supplements enhance delayed hypersensitivity skin test responses in older people. *American Journal of Clinical Nutrition, 60,* 437–447.

Borkan, G. A., Hults, D. E., Gerzof, S. G., Robbins, A. H., & Silbert, C. K. (1983). Age changes in body composition revealed by computed tomography. *Journal of Gerontology, 38,* 673–677.

Botez, M. I., Botez, T., & Maag, U. (1984). The Wechsler subtests in mild organic brain damage associated with folate deficiency. *Psychological Medicine, 14,* 431–437.

Bressler, M. H., Bressler, S. B., & Fine, S. L. (1988). Age-related macular degeneration—a major review. *Survey of Ophthalmology, 32,* 375–412.

Bruce, S., Newton, D., & Woledge, R. (1989). Effect of age on voluntary force and cross-sectional area of human adductor poilicis muscle. *Quarterly Journal of Experimental Physiology, 74,* 359–362.

Bullamore, J. R., Wilkinson, R., Gallagher, J. C., Nordin, B. E. C., & Marshall, D. H. (1970). Effects of age on calcium absorption. *Lancet, II,* 535–537.

Campbell, W. W., Crim, M. C., Dallal, G. E., Young, V. R., & Evans, W. J. (1994a). Increased protein requirements in the elderly: new data and retrospective reassessments. *American Journal of Clinical Nutrition, 60,* 501–509.

Campbell, W. W., Crim, M. C., Dallal, G. E., Young, V. R., & Evans, W. J. (1994b). Increased energy requirements and body composition changes with resistance training in older adults. *American Journal of Clinical Nutrition, 60,* 167–175.

Cannon, J. G., Orencole, S. F., Fielding, R. A., Meydani, M., Meydani, S. N., Fiatarone, M. A., Blumberg, J. B., & Evans, W. J. (1990). The Acute Phase Response in Exercise: Interaction of Age and Vitamin E on Neutrophils and Muscle Enzyme Release. *American Journal of Physiology, 259,* R1214–R1219.

Cannon, J. G., Meydani, S. N., Fielding, R. A., Fiatarone, M. A., Meydani, M., Farhangmehr, M., Orencole, S. F., Blumberg, J. B., & Evans, W. J. (1991). Acute Phase Response in Exercise. II. Associations between Vitamin E, Cytokines and Muscle Proteolysis. *American Journal of Physiology, 260,* R1235–R1240.

Chandra, R. K. (1981). Immunodeficiency in undernutrition and overnutrition. *Nutrition Reviews, 39,* 225–236.

Chandra, R. K. (1984a). Nutritional regulation of immunity at the extremes of life: in infants and in the elderly. In P. White (Ed.), *Malnutrition, Determinants and Consequences* (pp. 245–248). New York: Alan Liss.

Chandra, R. K. (1984b). Excessive intake of zinc impairs immune responses. *Journal of the American Medical Association, 252,* 1443–1446.

Chandra, R. K. (1989). Nutritional regulation of immunity and risk of infection in old age. *Immunology, 67,* 141–147.

Chandra, R. K. (1992). Effect of vitamin and trace-element supplementation on immune responses and infection in elderly subjects. *Lancet, 340,* 1124–1127.

Chandra, R. K., Joshi, P., Au, B., Woodford, G., & Chandra, S. (1982). Nutrition and immunocompetence of the elderly. Effect of short-term nutritional supplementation on cell-mediated immunity and lymphocyte subsets. *Nutrition Research, 2,* 223–232.

Chapuy, M. C., Chapuy, P., & Meunier, P. J. (1987). Calcium and vitamin D supplements: effects on calcium metabolism in elderly people. *American Journal of Clinical Nutrition, 46,* 324–328.

Chapuy, M. C., Arlot, M. E., Duboeuf, F., Brun, J., Crouzet, B., Arnaud, S., Delmas, P. D., & Meunier, P. J. (1992). Vitamin D_3 and calcium to prevent hip fractures in elderly women. *New England Journal of Medicine, 327,* 1637–1642.

Clark, R., Daly, L., Robinson, K., Naughten, E., Cahalane, S., Fowler, B., & Graham, I. (1991). Hyperhomocysteinemia: an independent risk factor for vascular disease. *New England Journal of Medicine, 324,* 1149–1155.

Clark, R., Fitzgerald, D., O'Brien, C., Roche, G., Parker, R. A., & Graham, I. (1992). Hyperhomocysteinemia: a risk factor for extracranial carotid artery atherosclerosis. *Irish Journal of Medical Science, 161,* 61–65.

Clemens, T. L., Zhou, W. Y., Myles, M., Endres, D., & Lindsay, R. (1986). Serum vitamin D_2 and vitamin D_3 metabolite concentrations and absorption of vitamin D_2 in elderly subjects. *Journal of Clinical Endocrinology, 63,* 656–660.

Cohn, S. H., Vartsky, D., Yasurura, S., Savitsky, A., Zanazi, I., Vaswani, A., & Ellis, K. J.

(1980). Compartmental body composition based on total body potassium and calcium. *American Journal of Physiology, 239,* E524–E530.

Committee on Diet and Health, Food and Nutrition Board. (1989). *Diet and Health: Implications for Reducing Chronic Disease Risk.* Commission on Life Sciences, National Research Council. Washington, DC: National Academy Press.

Cumlea, W. C., & Baumgartner, R. N. (1989). Status of anthropometry and body composition data in elderly subjects. *American Journal of Clinical Nutrition, 50,* 1158–1166.

Cunningham-Rundles, S. (1993). *Nutrient Modulation of the Immune Response.* New York: Marcel Dekker, Inc.

DeMaio, S. J., King, S. B., III, Lembo, N. J., Roubin, G. S., Hearn, J. A., Bhagavan, H. N., & Sgoutas, O. S. (1992). Vitamin E supplementation, plasma lipids and incidence of restenosis after percutaneous transluminal coronary angioplasty (PTCA). *Journal of the American College of Nutrition, 11,* 68–73.

Dieber-Rotheneder, M., Puhl, H., Waeg, G., Streigl, G., & Esterbauer, H. (1991). Effect of oral supplementation with D-alpha-tocopherol on the vitamin E content of human low density lipoproteins and resistance to oxidation. *Journal of Lipid Research, 32,* 1325–1332.

Duchateau, J., Delepesse, G., Vrijens, R., & Collet, H. (1981). Beneficial effects of oral zinc supplementation on the immune response of old people. *American Journal of Medicine, 70,* 1001–1004.

Eastell, R., Yergey, A. L., Vieira, N. E., Cedel, S. L., Kumar, R., & Riggs, B. L. (1991). Interrelationships among vitamin D metabolism, true calcium absorption, parathyroid function, and age in women: evidence of an age-related resistance to 1,25-dihydroxyvitamin D action. *Journal of Bone and Mineral Research, 6,* 125–132.

Ebeling, P. R., Sandgren, M. E., DiMagno, E. P., Lane, A. W., DeLuca, H. F., & Riggs, B. L. (1992). Evidence of an age-related decrease in intestinal responsiveness to vitamin D: relationship between serum 1,25-dihydroxyvitamin D_3 and intestinal vitamin D receptor concentration in normal women. *Journal of Clinical and Endocrinology Metabolism, 75,* 176–182.

Endres, S., Ghorbani, R., Kelley, V. E., Georgilis, K., Lonnemann, G., van der Meer, J. W. M., Cannon, J. G., Rogers, T. S., Klempner, M. S., Weber, P. C., Schaefer, E. J., Wolff, S. M., & Dinarello, C. A. (1989). The effect of dietary supplementation with n-3 polyunsaturated fatty acids on the synthesis of interleukin-1 and tumor necrosis factor by mononuclear cells. *New England Journal of Medicine, 320,* 265–271.

Enstrom, J. E., Kanim, L. E., & Klein, M. A. (1992). Vitamin C intake and mortality among a sample of the United States population. *Epidemiology, 3,* 194–202.

Esterbauer, H., Striegl, G., Puhl, H., & Rotheneder, M. (1988). Continuous monitoring of in vitro oxidation of human low density lipoprotein. *Free Radical Research Communications, 6,* 67–75.

Eye Disease Case-Control Study Group (1993). Antioxidant status and neovascular age-related macular degeneration. *Archives of Ophthalmology, 111,* 104–109.

Fernandes, G., & Venkatraman, J. T. (1993). Dietary restriction effection on immunological function and aging. In D. M. Klurfeld (Ed.), *Human Nutrition—A Comprehensive Treatise* (pp. 91–120). New York: Plenum Press.

Fiatarone, M. A., Marks, E. C., Ryan, N. D., Meredith, C. N., Lipsitz, L. A., & Evans, W. J. (1990). High-intensity strength training in nonagenarians. *Journal of the American Medical Association, 263,* 3029–3034.

Fiatarone, M. A., O'Neill, E. F., Ryan, N., Joseph, L., Roberts, S. B., Kehayias, J. J., Lipsitz, L. A., & Evans, W. J. (1991). Body composition and muscle function in the very old. *Medicine and Science in Sports and Exercise, 23,* S20.

Fiatarone, M. A., O'Neill, E. F., Ryan, N. D., Clements, K. M., Solares, G. R., Nelson, M. E., Roberts, S. B., Kehayias, J. J., Lipsitz, L. A., & Evans, W. J. (1994). *New England Journal of Medicine, 330,* 1769–1775.

Flynn, M. A., Nolph, G. B., Baker, A. S., Martin, W. M., & Krause, G. (1989). Total body potassium in aging humans: a longitudinal study. *American Journal of Clinical Nutrition, 50,* 713–717.

Frei, B., Stocker, R., & Ames, B. N. (1988). Antioxidant Defenses and Lipid Peroxidation in Human Blood Plasma. *Proceedings of the National Academy Sciences, 85,* 9748–9752.

Frontera, W. R., Hughes, V. A., Lutz, K. J., & Evans, W. J. (1991). A cross-sectional study of muscle strength and mass in 45- to 78-year-old men and women. *Journal of Applied Physiology, 71,* 644–650.

Gaziano, J. M., Manson, J. E., Ridker, P. M., Buring, J. E., & Hennekens, C. H. (1990). Beta-carotene therapy for chronic stable angina. *Circulation, 82,* 201.

Genest, J. J., Jr., McNamara, J. R., Salem, D. N., Wilson, P. W. F., Schaefer, E. J., & Malinow, M. R. (1990). Plasma homocyst(e)ine levels in men with premature coronary artery disease. *Journal of the American College of Cardiology, 16,* 1114–1119.

Gey, K. F., Brubacher, G. B., & Stähelin, H. B. (1987). Plasma levels of antioxidant vitamins in relation to ischemic heart disease and cancer. *American Journal of Clinical Nutrition, 45,* 1368–1377.

Gey, K. F., Moser, U. K., Jordan, P., Stähelin, H. B., Eichholzer, M., & Ludin, E. (1993a). Increased risk of cardiovascular disease at suboptimal plasma concentration of essential antioxidants: an epidemiological update with special attention to carotene and vitamin C. *American Journal of Clinical Nutrition, 57,* 787S–797S.

Gey, K. F., Stähelin, H. B., & Eichholzer, M. (1993b). Poor plasma status of carotene and vitamin C is associated with higher mortality from ischemic heart disease and stroke: Basel Prospective Study. *Clinical Investigation, 71,* 3–6.

Goldberg, J., Flowerdew, G., Smith, E., Brody, J. A., & Tso, M. O. M. (1988). Factors associated with age-related macular degeneration: an analysis of data from the First National Health and Nutrition Examination Survey. *American Journal of Epidemiology, 128,* 700–710.

Goodwin, J. S., & Garry, T. J. (1983). Relationship between Megadose Vitamin Supplementation and Immunological Function in a Healthy Elderly Population. *Clinical and Experimental Immunology, 51,* 647–653.

Goodwin, J. S., Goodwin, J. M., & Garry, P. J. (1983). Association between nutritional status and cognitive functioning in a healthy elderly population. *Journal of the American Medical Association, 249,* 2917–2921.

Grossmann, A., Ledbetter J. A., & Rabinovitch, P. S. (1990). Aging related deficiency in intracellular calcium response to anti-CD3 or concanavalin A in murine T-cell subsets. *Journal of Gerontology, 45,* B81–B86.

Hachinski, V. (1992). Preventable senility: a call for action against vascular dementia. *Lancet, 340,* 645–648.

Hankinson, S. E., Stampfer, M. J., Seddon, J. M., Colditz, G. A., Rosner, B., Speizer, F. E., & Willett, W. C. (1992). Nutrient intake and cataract extraction in women: a prospective study. *British Medical Journal, 305,* 335–339.

Heikinheimo, R. J., Inkovaara, J. A., Harju, E. J., Haavisto, M. V., Kaarela, R. H., Kataja, J. M., Hokko, A. M., Kolho, L. A., & Rajala, S. A. (1992). Annual injection of vitamin D and fractures of aged bones. *Calcification Tissue International, 51,* 105–110.

Hirokawa, K. (1992). Understanding the mechanism of the age-related decline in immune function. *Nutrition Reviews, 50,* 361–366.

Huber, L. A., Xu, Q., Jürgens, G., Böck, G., Bühler, E., Gey, F., Schönitzer, D., Traill, K. N., & Wick, G. (1991). Correlation of lymphocyte lipid composition, membrane microviscosity and mitogen response in the aged. *European Journal of Immunology, 21,* 2761–2765.

Italian–American Cataract Study Group (1991). Risk factors for age-related cortical, nuclear, and posterior subcapsular cataracts. *American Journal of Epidemiology, 133,* 541–553.

Jacques, P. F., & Chylack, L. T., Jr. (1991). Epidemiologic evidence of a role of the antioxidants vitamins and carotenoids in cataract prevention. *American Journal of Clinical Nutrition, 53,* 352S–355S.

Jacques, P. F., Chylack, L. T., Jr., & Taylor, A. (1994). Relationships between natural antioxidants and cataract formation. In B. Frei (Ed.), *Natural Antioxidants in Human Health and Disease* (pp. 515–533). San Diego: Academic Press.

Jialal, I., & Grundy, S. M. (1991). Preservation of the endogenous antioxidants in LDL by ascorbate but not probucol during oxidative modification. *Journal of Clinical Investigation, 87,* 597–601.

Jialal, I., & Grundy, S. M. (1993). Effect of combined supplementation with α-tocopherol, ascorbate, and beta carotene on low-density lipoprotein oxidation. *Circulation, 88,* 2780–2786.

Kardinaal, A. F. M., Kok, F. J., Ringstad, J., Gomez-Aracena, J., Mazanev, V. P., Kohlmeier, L., Martin, B. C., Aro, A., Kark, J. D., Delgado-Rodriguez, M., Riemersma, R. A., van't Veer, P., Huttunen, J. K., & Martin-Moreno, J. M. (1993). Antioxidants in adipose tissue and risk of myocardial infarction: the EURAMIC study. *Lancet, 341,* 1379–1384.

Karnaze, D. S., & Carmel, R. (1987). Low serum cobalamin levels in primary degenerative dementia. Do some patients harbor atypical cobalamin deficiency states? *Archives of Internal Medicine, 147,* 429–431.

Kennes, B., Dumont, I., Brohee, D., Hubert, C., & Neve, P. (1983). Effect of Vitamin C Supplementation on Cell-mediated Immunity in Old People. *Gerontology, 29,* 305–310.

Knox, T. A., Kassarjian, Z., Dawson-Hughes, B., Golner, B. B., Dallal, G. E., Arora, S., & Russell, R. M. (1991). Calcium absorption in elderly subjects on high- and low-fiber diets: effect of gastric acidity. *American Journal of Clinical Nutrition, 53,* 1480–1486.

Kok, F. J., de Bruijn, A. M., Vermeeren, R., Hofman, A., van Laar, A., de Bruin, M., Hermus, R. J., & Valkenburg, H. A. (1987). Serum selenium, vitamin antioxidants, and cardiovascular mortality: a 9-year follow-up study in the Netherlands. *American Journal of Clinical Nutrition, 45,* 462–468.

Krall, E. A., Sahyoun, N., Tannenbaum, S., Dallal, G. E., & Dawson-Hughes, B. (1989). Effect of vitamin D intake on seasonal variations in parathyroid hormone secretion in postmenopausal women. *New England Journal of Medicine, 321,* 1777–1783.

Kremer, J. M., Jubiz, W., & Michalek, A. (1987). Fish-oil fatty acid supplementation in active rheumatoid arthritis. *Annals of Internal Medicine, 106,* 497–503.

Kremer, J. R., Schoene, N., Dougless, L. W., Judd, J. T., Ballard-Barbash, R., Taylor, P. R., Bhagavan, N., & Nair, P. P. (1991). Increased vitamin E intake restores fish-oil-induced suppressed blastogenesis of mitogenic-stimulated T lymphocytes. *American Journal of Clinical Nutrition, 54,* 896–902.

Leske, M. C., Chylack, L. T., Jr., & Wu, S. (1991). The lens opacities case-control study: risk factors for cataract. *Archives of Ophthalmology, 109,* 244–251.

Levitt, A. J., & Karlinsky, H. (1992). Folate, vitamin B12 and cognitive impairment in patients with Alzheimer's disease. *Acta Psychiatrica Scandinavica, 86,* 301–305.

Lindenbaum, J., Healton, E. B., Savage, D. G., Brust, J. C., Garrett, T. J., Padell, E. R., Marcell, P. D., Stabler, S. P., & Allen, R. H. (1988). Neuropsychatric disorders caused by cobalamin deficiency in the absence of anemia or macrocytosis. *New England Journal of Medicine, 318,* 1720–1728.

MacLaughlin, J., & Holick, M. F. (1985). Aging decreases the capacity of human skin to produce vitamin D_3. *Journal of Clinical Investigation, 76,* 1536–1538.

Makinodan, T., & Kay, M. M. B. (1980). Age influences on the immune system. *Advances in Immunology, 29,* 287–295.

Malinow, M. R., Nieto, F. J., Szklo, M., Chambless, L. E., & Bond, G. (1993). Carotid artery intimal-wall thickening and plasma homocyst(e)ine in asymptomatic adults. The Atherosclerosis Risk in Communities Study. *Circulation, 87,* 1107–1113.

Mangelsdorf, D. J., Umesono, K., & Evans, R. M. (1994). The retinoid receptors. In M. B. Sporn, A. B. Roberts, & D. S. Goodman (Eds.), *The Retinoids. Biology, Chemistry, and Medicine* (pp. 319–349). New York: Raven Press.

Martin, D. C. (1988). B12 and folate deficiency dementia. *Clinics in Geriatric Medicine, 4,* 841–852.

Martin, D. C., Francis, J., Protetch, J., & Huff, F. H. (1992). Time dependency of cognitive recovery with cobalamin replacement: report of a pilot study. *Journal of the American Geriatric Society, 40,* 168–172.

McCully, K. S. (1991). Micronutrients, homocysteine metabolism, and atherosclerosis. In A. Bendich & C. E. Butterworth, Jr. (Eds.), *Micronutrients in Health and in Disease Prevention* (pp. 69–96). New York: Marcel Dekker, Inc.

McMurray, D. N. (1984). Cell-mediated immunity in nutritional deficiency. *Progress in Food and Nutrition Science, 8,* 193–228.

Meredith, C. N., Frontera, W. R., O'Reilly, K. P., & Evans, W. J. (1992). Body Composition in Elderly Men: Effect of Dietary Modification during Strength Training. *Journal of the American Geriatrics Society, 40,* 155–162.

Meydani, M., Evans, W., Handelman, G., Biddle, L., Fielding, R. A., Meydani, S. N., Burrill, J., Fiatarone, M. A., Blumberg, J. B., & Cannon, J. G. (1993a). Protective Effect of Vitamin E on Exercise-Induced Oxidative Damage in Young and Older Adults. *American Journal of Physiology, 264*, R992–R998.

Meydani, M., Meydani, S. N., Leka, L., Gong, J., & Blumberg, J. B. (1993b). Effect of Long-Term Vitamin E Supplementation on Lipid Peroxidation and Immune Response of Young and Old Subjects. *FASEB Journal, 7*, A415.

Meydani, S. N., & Blumberg, J. B. (1989). Nutrition and Immune Function in the Elderly. In H. Munro & D. Danforth (Eds.), *Human Nutrition: A Comprehensive Treatise* (pp. 61–87). New York: Plenum Press.

Meydani, S. N., Barklund, P. M., Liu, S., Meydani, M., Miller, R., Cannon, J. G., Morrow, F., Rocklin, R., & Blumberg, J. B. (1990). Vitamin E Supplementation Enhances Cell-Mediated Immunity in Healthy Elderly Subjects. *American Journal of Clinical Nutrition, 52*, 557–563.

Meydani, S. N., Endres, S., Woods, M. M., Goldin, B. R., Soo, C., Morrill-Labrode, A., Dinarello, C. A., & Gorbach, S. L. (1991a). Oral (n-3) fatty acid supplementation suppresses cytokine production and lymphocyte proliferation: comparison between young and older women. *Journal of Nutrition, 121*, 547–555.

Meydani, S. N., Ribaya-Mercado, J. D., Russell, R. M., Sahyoun, N., Morrow, F. D., & Gershoff, S. N. (1991b). Vitamin B-6 deficiency impairs interleukin-2 production and lymphocyte proliferation in elderly adults. *American Journal of Clinical Nutrition, 53*, 1275–1280.

Miller, R. (1995). Immunology. In E. L. Schneider & J. W. Rowe (Eds.), *Handbook of the Biology of Aging* (3rd ed.). San Diego: Academic Press, Inc.

Mittag, T. (1984). Role of oxygen radicals in ocular inflammation and cellular damage. *Experimental Eye Research, 39*, 759–769.

Mohan, M., Sperduto, R. D., Angra, S. K., Milton, R. C., Mathur, R. L., Underwood, B., Jaffery, N., & Pandya, C. B. (1989). India-US case-control study of age-related cataracts. *Archives of Ophthalmology, 107*, 670–676.

Morrison, N. A., Qi, J. C., Tokita, A., Kelly, P. J.,

Crofts, L., Nguyen, T. V., Sambrook, P. N., & Eisman, J. A. (1994). Prediction of bone density from vitamin D receptor alleles. *Nature, 367*, 284–287.

Munro, H. N. (1992). Protein. In S. C. Hartz, R., Russell, & I. H. Rosenberg (Eds.), *Nutrition in the Elderly: The Boston Nutritional Status Survey* (pp. 75–85). London, UK: Smith-Gordon & Co.

Munro, H. N., & Danford, D. E. (Eds.) (1989). *Nutrition, Aging, and the Elderly, Human Nutrition, A Comprehensive Treatise* (Vol. 6). New York: Plenum Press.

Munro, H., & Schlierf, G. (Eds.) (1992). *Nutrition of the Elderly*. New York: Raven Press.

Nelson, M. E., Meredith, C. N., Dawson-Hughes, B., & Evans, W. J. (1988). Hormone and bone mineral status in endurance-trained and sedentary postmenopausal women. *Journal of Clinical Endocrinology Metabolism, 64*, 927–933.

Nelson, M. E., Dilmanian, F. A., Dallal, G. E., & Evans, W. J. (1991). A one-year walking program and increased dietary calcium in postmenopausal women: Effects on bone. *American Journal of Clinical Nutrition, 53*, 1304–1311.

Newsome, D. A., Swartz, M., Leone, N. C., Elston, R. C., & Miller E. (1988). Oral zinc in macular degeneration. *Archives of Ophthalmology, 106*, 192–198.

Nielsen, F. H. (1990). Studies on the relationship between boron and magnesium which possibly affects the formation and maintenance of bones. *Magnesium Trace Elements, 9*, 61–69.

Nutrition Policy Board (1988). *The Surgeon General's Report on Nutrition and Health* (Public Health Service Publication No. 88–50210). Washington, DC: U.S. Dept. Health and Human Services.

Pancharuniti, N., Lewis, C. A., Sauberlich, H. E., Perkins, L. L., Go, R. C. P., Alvarez, J. O., Macaluso, M., Acton, R. T., Copeland, R. B., Cousins, A. L., Gore, T. B., Cornwell, P. E., & Roseman, J. M. (1994). Plasma homocyst(e)ine, folate, and vitamin B-12 concentrations and risk for early-onset coronary artery disease. *American Journal of Clinical Nutrition, 59*, 940–948.

Penn, N. D., Purkins, L. Kelleher, J., Heatley, R. V., Mascie-Taylor, B. H., & Belfield, P. W.

(1991). The effect of dietary supplementation with vitamins A, C and E on cell-mediated immune function in elderly long-stay patients: a randomized controlled trial. *Age and Ageing, 20*, 169–174.

Princen, H. M. G., van Poppel, G., Vogelezang, C., Buytenhek, R., & Kok, F. J. (1992). Supplementation with vitamin E but not β-carotene in vivo protects low density lipoprotein from lipid peroxidation in vitro: effect of cigarette smoking. *Arteriosclerosis and Thrombosis, 12*, 554–562.

Rabinovitch, P. S., June, C. H., Grossmann, A., & Ledbetter, J. A. (1986). Heterogeneity among T cells in intracellular free calcium responses after mitogen stimulation with PHA or anti-CD3. Simultaneous use of indo-1 and immunofluorescence with flow cytometry. *Journal of Immunology, 137*, 952–961.

Recker, R. R. (1985). Calcium absorption and achlorhydria. *New England Journal of Medicine, 313*, 70–73.

Regnström, J., Nilsson, J., Tornvall, P., Landou, C., & Hamsten, A. (1992). Susceptibility to low-density lipoprotein oxidation and coronary atherosclerosis in man. *Lancet, 339*, 1183–1186.

Riemersma, R. A., Wood, D. A., Macintyre, C. C. A., Elton, R. A., Gey, K. F., & Oliver, M. F. (1991). Risk of angina pectoris and plasma concentrations of vitamins A, C, and E and carotene. *Lancet, 337*, 1–5.

Rimm, E. B., Stampfer, M. J., Ascherio, A., Giovannucci, E., Colditz, G. A., & Willett, W. C. (1993). Vitamin E consumption and the risk of coronary heart disease in men. *New England Journal of Medicine, 328*, 1450–1456.

Roberts, S. B., Young, V. R., Fuss, P., Heyman, M. B., Fiatarone, M., Dallal, G. E., Cortiella, J., & Evans, W. J. (1992). What are the dietary energy needs of elderly adults? *International Journal of Obesity, 16*, 969–976.

Robertson, J. M., Donner, A. P., & Trevithick, J. R. (1989). Vitamin E intake and risk for cataracts in humans. *Annals of the New York Academy of Science, 570*, 372–382.

Rosenberg, I. H. (1989). Summary comments: Epidemiological and methodological problems in determining nutritional status of older persons. *American Journal of Clinical Nutrition, 50*, 1231–1233.

Rosenberg, I. H. (Ed.) (1995). *Nutritional Assessment of Elderly Populations* (Bristol-Myers Squibb/Mead Johnson Nutrition Symposia, Vol. 13). New York: Raven Press.

Rosenberg, I. H., & Miller, J. W. (1992). Nutritional factors in physical and cognitive functions of elderly people. *American Journal of Clinical Nutrition, 55*, 1237S–1243S.

Rosenberg, I. H., & Ronnenberg, A. (Eds.) (1994). *Vitamins and Brain Function.* Boston: Foundation for Nutritional Advancement.

Ross, R. (1986). The pathogenesis of atherosclerosis—an update. *New England Journal of Medicine, 314*, 488–492.

Rubba, P., Faccenda, F., Pauciullo, P., Carbone, L., Mancini, M., Strisciuglio, P., Carrozzo, R., Sartorio, R., del Giudice, E., & Andria, G. (1990). Early signs of vascular disease in homocystinuria: a noninvasive study by ultrasound methods in eight families with cystathionine-β-synthase deficiency. *Metabolism, 39*, 1191–1195.

Sahyoun, N. (1992). Nutrient intake by the NSS elderly population. In S. Hartz, I. H. Rosenberg, & R. M. Russell (Eds.), *Nutrition in the Elderly: The Boston Nutritional Status Survey* (pp. 31–44). London, UK: Smith-Gordon & Co.

Salonen, J. T., Salonen, R., Penttila, I., Herranen, J., Jauhianen, M., Kantiola, M., Lappetelainen, R., Maenpaa, P. H., Alfthan, G., & Puska, P. (1985). Serum fatty acids, apolipoproteins, selenium and vitamin antioxidants and the risk of death from coronary artery disease. *American Journal of Cardiology, 56*, 226–231.

Salonen, J. T., Ylä-Herttuala, S., Yamamoto, R., Butler, S., Korpela, H., Salonen, R., Nyyssonen, K., Palinski, W., & Witztum, J. L. (1992). Autoantibody against oxidised LDL and progression of carotid atherosclerosis. *Lancet, 339*, 883–887.

Salthouse, T. A. (1991). *Theoretical Perspectives on Cognitive Aging.* Hillsdale: Lawrence Erlbaum Associates.

Saltman, P. D., & Strause, L. G. (1993). The role of trace minerals in osteoporosis. *Journal of the American College of Nutrition, 12*, 384–389.

Sanders, T. A. B., Haines, A. P., Wormald, R., Wright, L. A., & Obeid, O. (1993). Essential fatty acids, plasma cholesterol, and fat-soluble vitamins in subjects with age-related maculopathy and matched control subjects. *American Journal of Clinical Nutrition, 57,* 428–433.

Sauberlich, H. E., & Machlin, L. J. (Eds.) (1992). Beyond Deficiency: New Views on the Function and Health Effects of Vitamins. *Annals of the New York Academy of Sciences, 669,* 1–404.

Schalch, W. (1992). Carotenoids in the retina—a review of their possible role in preventing or limiting damage caused by light and oxygen. In I. Emerit & B. Chance (Eds.), *Free Radicals and Aging* (pp. 280–298). Basel: Birkhäuser Verlag.

Schneider, E. L., & Brody, J. A. (1983). Aging, natural death, and the compression of morbidity: another view. *New England Journal of Medicine, 309,* 854–856.

Schneider, E. L., & Guralnik, J. M. (1990). The aging of America: impact on health care costs. *Journal of the American Medical Association, 263,* 2335–2340.

Schwab, R., & Weksler, M. E. (1987). Cell biology of the impaired proliferation of T cells from elderly humans. In E. A. Goidl (Ed.), *Aging and Immune Response: Cellular and Humoral Aspects* (pp. 67–80). New York: Dekker.

Seddon, J. M., Ajani, U. A., Sperduto, R. D., Hiller, R., Blair, H. N., Burton, T. C., Farber, M. D., Gragoudas, E. S., Haller, J., Miller, D. T., Yannuzzi, L. A., & Willett, W. (1994a). Dietary carotenoids, vitamins A, C, and E, and advanced age-related macular degeneration. *Journal of the American Medical Association, 272,* 1413–1420.

Seddon, J. M., Christen, W. G., Manson, J. E., LaMotte, F. S., Glynn, R. J., Buring, J. E., & Hennekens, C. H. (1994b). The use of vitamin supplements and the risk of cataract among US male physicians. *American Journal of Public Health, 84,* 788–792.

Selhub, J., Jacques, P. F., Wilson, P. W. F., Rush, D., & Rosenberg, I. H. (1993). Vitamin status and intake as primary determinant of homocysteinemia in the elderly. *Journal of the American Medical Association, 270,* 2693–2698.

Selhub, J., Jacques, P. F., Bostom, A. G., D'Agostino, R. B., Wilson, P. W. F., Belanger, A. J., O'Leary, D. H., Wolf, P. A., Schaefer, E. J., & Rosenberg, I. H. (1995). Association between plasma homocysteine concentrations and extracranial carotid-artery stenosis. *New England Journal of Medicine, 332,* 286–291.

Simopoulos, A. P. (1991). Omega-3 fatty acids in health and disease and in growth and development. *American Journal of Clinical Nutrition, 54,* 438–463.

Sperduto, R. D., Hu, T.-S., Milton, R. C., Zhao, J. L., Everett, D. F., Cheng, Q.-F., Blot, W. J., Bing, L., Taylor, P. R., Jun-Yao, L., & Guo, W.-D. (1993). The Linxian Cataract Studies: two nutrition intervention trials. *Archives of Opthalmology, 111,* 1246–1253.

Stampfer, M. J., Malinow, M. R., Willett, W. C., Newcomer, L. M., Upson, B., Ullmann, D., Tishler, P. V., & Hennekens, C. H. (1992). A prospective study of plasma homocyst(e)ine and risk of myocardial infarction in US physicians. *Journal of the American Medical Association, 268,* 877–881.

Stampfer, M. J., Hennekens, C. H., Manson, J. E., Colditz, G. A., Rosner, B., & Willett, W. C. (1993). Vitamin E consumption and the risk of coronary disease in women. *New England Journal of Medicine, 328,* 1444–1449.

Stark, W. J., Sommer, A., & Smith, R. E. (1989). Changing trends in intraocular lens implantation. *Archives of Ophthalmology, 107,* 1441–1444.

Steinberg, D. (1991). Antioxidants and atherosclerosis: a current assessment. *Circulation, 84,* 1420–1425.

Steinberg, D., Parthasarathy, S., Carew, T. E., Khoo, J. C., & Witztum, J. L. (1989). Beyond cholesterol: modifications of low-density lipoprotein that increase its atherogenicity. *New England Journal of Medicine, 320,* 915–924.

Street, D. A., Comstock, G. W., Salkeld, R. M., Schüep, W., & Klag, M. A. (1991). A population-based case-control study of the association of serum antioxidants and myocardial infarction. *American Journal of Epidemiology, 134,* 719–720.

Stringer, M. D., Görög, P. G., Freeman, A., & Kakkar, V. V. (1989). Lipid peroxides and atherosclerosis. *British Medical Journal, 298,* 281–284.

Strub, R. L., and Black, F. W. (1981). *Organic Brain Syndromes: An Introduction to Neurobehavioral Disorders.* Philadelphia: Davis.

Talbott, M. C., Miller, L. T., & Kerkvliet, N. (1987). Pyridoxine supplementation: effect of lymphocyte response in elderly persons.

American Journal of Clinical Nutrition, 46, 569–664.

Taylor, A., Davies, K. J. A. (1987). Protein oxidation and loss of protease activity may lead to cataract formation in the aged lens. *Free Radical Biology Medicine, 3,* 371–377.

Taylor, A., Jacques P. F., & Dorey, C. K. (1993). Oxidation and aging: impact on vision. In G. M. Williams (Ed.), *Antioxidants: Chemical, Physiological, Nutritional, and Toxicological Aspects* (pp. 349–371). Princeton: Princeton Science Publishers.

Thoman, M. L., & Weigle, W. O. (1989). The ceullular and subcellular bases of immunosenescence. *Advances in Immunology, 46,* 221–261.

Tsai, K.-S., Heath, H., III, Kumar, R., & Riggs, B. L. (1984). Impaired vitamin D metabolism with aging women. Possible role in pathogenesis of senile osteoporosis. *Journal of Clinical Investigation, 73,* 1668–1672.

Tucker, D. M., Penland, J. G., Sandstead, H. H., Milne, D. B., Heck, D. G., & Klevay, L. M. (1990). Nutrition status and brain function in aging. *American Journal of Clinical Nutrition, 52,* 93–102.

Tzankoff, S. P., & Norris, A. H. (1977). Effect of muscle mass decrease on age-related basal metabolic rate changes. *Journal of Applied Physiology, 43,* 100–110.

Tzankoff, S. P., & Norris, A. H. (1978). Longitudinal changes in basal metabolism in man. *Journal of Applied Physiology, 45,* 536–539.

Ubbink, J. B., Hayward Vermaak, W. J., van der Merwe, A., & Becker, P. J. (1993). Vitamin B-12, vitamin B-6, and folate nutritional status in men with hyperhomocysteinemia. *American Journal of Clinical Nutrition, 57,* 47–53.

Ueland, P. M., Refsum, H., & Brattstrom, L. (1992). Plasma homocysteine and cardiovascular disease. In R. B. Francis, Jr. (Ed.), *Atherosclerotic Cardiovascular Disease, Hemostasis, and Endothelial Function* (pp. 183–235). New York: Marcel Dekker, Inc.

Vitale, S., West, S., Hallfrisch, J., Alston, C., Wang, F., Moorman, C., Muller, D., Singh, V., & Taylor, H. R. (1993). Plasma antioxidants and risk of cortical and nuclear cataract. *Epidemiology, 4,* 195–203.

Watson, R. R., Prabhala, R. H., Plezia, P. M., & Alberts, D. S. (1991). Effect of β-carotene on lymphocyte subpopulations in elderly humans: evidence for a dose-response relationship. *American Journal of Clinical Nutrition, 53,* 90–94.

West, S., Vitale, S., Hallfrisch, J., Muñoz, B., Muller, D., Bressler, S., & Bressler, N. M. (1994). Are antioxidants or supplements protective for age-related macular degeneration? *Archives of Ophthalmology, 112,* 222–227.

Ylä-Herttuala, S., Palinski, W., Rosenfeld, M. E., Parthasarathy, S., Carew, T. E., Butler, S., Witztum, J. L., & Steinberg, D. (1989). Evidence for the presence of oxidatively modified low density lipoprotein in atherosclerotic lesions of rabbit and man. *Journal of Clinical Investigation, 84,* 1086–1095.

Young, V. (1990). Amino acids and protein in relation to the nutrition of elderly people. *Age and Ageing, 19,* 510–524.

Ziemlanski, S., Wartanowicz, M., & Kios, A. (1986). The Effects of Ascorbic Acid and Alpha-tocopherol Supplementation on Serum Proteins and Immunoglobulin Concentrations in the Elderly. *Nutrition International, 2,* 1–5.

Eighteen

Menopause and Its Consequences

Michele F. Bellantoni and Marc R. Blackman

I. Introduction

The female menopause is defined clinically as the cessation of menses for a period
of at least 12 months as a consequence of
irreversible ovarian failure. The changes
in reproductive hormone profiles related
to ovarian dysfunction are often gradual in
onset, with wide individual variation in
the frequency, intensity, pattern, and duration of associated clinical symptoms,
which may last from several months to
years. The most common pattern is one
of a transition over 2–7 years. The terms
perimenopause, climacteric, and menopausal transition are used to describe the
period of time when such changes are first
experienced until 12 months of amenorrhea have elapsed.

In the United States, the average age of
menopause is approximately 50 years with
a wide normal range of 40–60 years. As the
female life expectancy in this country is
currently 78 years, on the average, a woman in this country experiencing menopause still has more than one-third of her
life ahead of her. The development of cardiovascular disease, the leading cause of
death in U.S. women, is accelerated after
menopause. Likewise, menopause is often

associated with increased risk of osteoporosis, musculoskeletal impairment, and
urinary incontinence, all common conditions that predispose to frailty in older
women. Thus, the physiological changes
of menopause impact on the health and
quality of life of older women.

The cessation of female reproductive
function is not unique to people living in
industrial societies. Indeed, animals in
captivity often exhibit reproductive failure in both sexes later in life. In freely living animals, there are fewer postreproductive individuals. In marine mammals, for
example the life span of the females of a
few species extends beyond the reproductive years, presumably to permit a prolonged parental role including extended
lactation. Paleodemographic studies have
not provided clear data regarding the extent of postreproductive life expectancy in
preagricultural humans. It is evident that
adult women of hunter–gathering societies spent about 15 years of their lives in a
lactational amenorrhea state, in contrast
to women of modern industrial societies
who spend nearly 35 years in menstrual
cycling.

This chapter outlines the physiological
changes associated with menopause and

Handbook of the Biology of Aging, Fourth Edition
Copyright © 1996 Academic Press, Inc. All rights of reproduction in any form reserved.

how these alterations impact on selected disease states. The role of ovarian hormone replacement in preventing or attenuating menopause-related diseases is discussed.

II. Physiological Changes Associated with Menopause

A. Reproductive Hormone Axis

De novo oogenesis ceases by birth in the female mammal. Aging is associated with a progressive loss of ovarian follicles, the mechanisms for which remain ill-understood. In women, there appears to be an acceleration in follicular depletion beginning at age 35–40 years, which appears to be related to a critical number of about 25,000 follicles (Faddy *et al.*, 1992). It is estimated that menopause occurs when about 1000 follicles remain. Oral contraceptive use and high parity have been associated with a somewhat delayed onset of menopause; conversely, factors associated with accelerated follicular atresia include genetic predisposition, autoimmunity to ovarian components, cytotoxic drugs, ionizing radiation, cigarette smoking, pelvic infections, and malnutrition. Of note is that menopause in underdeveloped countries may occur more often before age 45 years (Gray, 1976).

Follicular development appears to involve an interaction between stromal and epithelial elements with a permissive role played by higher centers through the pituitary gland. Follicular artresia is associated with a decrease in granulosa cell production of the regulatory glycoprotein hormone, inhibin (Buckler *et al.*, 1991). This alters the gonadal–hypothalamic–pituitary feedback system, such that early in the menopausal transition there is an increase in follicular phase circulating levels of follicle-stimulating hormone (FSH). It is hypothesized that this higher tonic FSH level results in accelerated preovula-

tory follicular growth rates, increased estradiol secretion, and possibly an increased number of ovulations. The latter may account for the age-related higher rate of dizygotic twin gestations (Thatcher & Naftolin, 1991). This mild-to-moderate increase in circulating levels of FSH in the early and midfollicular phase has been documented in women over age 35 years, and more marked FSH elevations are typically seen in women over age 45 years, despite normal lutenizing hormone (LH) values, ovulatory levels of progesterone, and regular cycles. These endocrine changes correspond well with the documented decrease in fecundity after age 35 years and probably explain the utility of elevated basal FSH levels in predicting poor outcomes of *in vitro* fertilization cycles.

In addition to ovarian dysfunction, reproductive aging may also result from the effects of aging on the neural timekeeping mechanisms in the hypothalamic suprachiasmatic nuclei. Rodent studies suggest that the preovulatory and steroid-induced LH surges change in middle-aged rats in association with changes in the diurnal pattern of hypothalamic neurotransmitters such as norepinephrine, serotonin, and β-endorphin. These neurotransmitters in turn regulate the release of GnRH from the hypothalamus (Wise *et al.*, 1990). The role of the hypothalmus in human menopause may differ from that in the rodent, as the female rodent experiences hypogonadotropic hypogonadism, whereas women experience hypergonadotropic hypogonadism.

As the menopausal transition progresses, monthly follicular development and ovulation are impaired, resulting in erratic ovulation. Anovulatory cycles result in a rise and fall in estrogen levels in the absence of a significant rise in progesterone. Peak circulating levels of estradiol are reduced. Over time, no follicular maturation takes place, resulting in low steady state levels of both estradiol and progesterone.

At the completion of the menopausal

transition, the principal tissue responsible for the secretion of estrogens is adipose tissue. Estradiol is made from the peripheral conversion of estrone and testosterone. Estrone is made from the peripheral conversion of androstenedione and testosterone. Thus, obesity plays a major role in the amount of circulating estrogens after menopause.

Estrogens are metabolized via hydroxylation at one of three positions, resulting in compounds that have varying degrees of bioactivity. Ultimately these metabolites are excreted in the urine. Little is known about menopausal changes in the proportions of the different hydroxyestrogens and their roles in menopause-associated diseases such as osteoporosis and breast cancer.

In contrast to the marked dysfunction of the ovarian cortex with follicular atresia, the theca–interstitial cell component of the ovarian medulla remains active, albeit at a reduced rate. This site of androgen production undergoes atrophy as well, but to a lesser degree, resulting in reduced ovarian secretion of some, but not all, androgens. Androstenedione, the principal ovarian androgen, is reduced by about 50%, whereas testosterone production is only slightly diminished. The continued role of the ovarian medulla in the synthesis of androgens, which serve as precursors for estrogen synthesis in the peripheral adipose tissues, must be emphasized. Thus, ovariectomy may result in circulating levels of both estrogens and androgens below those of natural menopause (Longcope, 1974).

Under normal conditions, the adrenal gland is the principal source of dehydroepiandrosterone (DHEA) and DHEA sulfate. However, adrenal gland production of this androgen declines continually after age 30 years, independent of ovarian function.

In the postmenopausal state, small amounts of progesterone are made by the adrenal gland. However, adipose tissue does not synthesize progesterone as it does estrogens. This explains in part the increased incidence of endometrial cancer in obese postmenopausal women, who presumably have higher endogenous estrogen levels without progesterone.

After completion of the menopausal transition, the reduced levels of circulating sex steroids do not change further with aging. However, circulating levels of LH, and to a lesser extent FSH, are less elevated in older versus younger postmenopausal women, suggesting an age-related diminution in hypothalamic and/or pituitary gonadotropic function (Bellantoni et al., 1992).

Throughout a woman's reproductive life, there is a gradual reduction in the length of the menstrual cycle. Early in perimenopause, there is often a shortening of the follicular phase of the cycle by 2–3 days, resulting from increases in follicular growth rates due to the higher FSH levels. Later in the transition, most women experience irregularity in menstrual cycle length, reflecting increasingly erratic follicular development and anovulatory cycles, which may result in heavy bleeds from a proliferative endometrium.

B. Nonreproductive Neuroendocrine Axes

Menopausal changes in the reproductive hormone axis are associated with alterations in other endocrine functions.

Growth hormone (GH) is an important anabolic hormone that promotes increases in muscle and bone mass and decreases in body fat. Most of the peripheral tissue effects of GH are mediated by insulin-like growth factor I (IGF-I), which is produced in response to GH at various tissue sites. Studies of 24-hr secretion of GH, assessed by frequent sampling techniques, have shown variable reductions (15–70%) in most 24-hr GH secretory parameters in middle-aged (40–65 years) and older (>60 years) women. Moreover, the acute secretory response of GH to direct pituitary stimulation with GHRH is present, but significantly reduced, in healthy older women (Corpas *et al.*, 1993).

Circulating levels of IGF-I decrease with age in women and men, so that in subjects in the seventh decade, IGF-I values may fall to levels approximately 30–50% of that of persons in the third decade. The prevalence of low IGF-I serum concentrations increases progressively from 11 to 55% from the fourth to the ninth decades. Levels of IGF-binding protein-3, the major plasma IGF-I-binding protein, also decrease with advancing age in both women and men (Baxter & Martin, 1986). It seems likely that the decreases in GH and IGF-I release with aging are, at least in part, responsible for the reported reductions in IGFBP-3 levels. Taken together, the preceding observations suggest that age-related decreases in lean body mass and increases in fat are related, in part, to diminished activity of the GH–IGF-I axis (Corpas *et al.*, 1993).

Whereas pubertal increases in plasma estradiol are associated with increases in pulsatile GH, cross-sectional studies suggest that decreases in sex steroid levels may contribute directly to age-related decreases in GH and IGF-I. In women, adjustments for plasma estradiol values greatly diminish the apparent effects of both sex and age on 24-hr integrated GH levels (Ho *et al.*, 1987). However, estrogen replacement does not restore circulating GH and IGF-I to premenopausal levels, although sex steroids may modulate local production and paracrine/autocrine effects of IGF-I and IGF-binding proteins (Dawson-Hughes *et al.*, 1986). Taken together, the preceding data suggest that the menopausal transition is accompanied by a physiologically relevant decline in pituitary somatotropic function.

Currently, it is not possible to accurately measure GHRH or hypothalamic somatostatin in peripheral blood. The finding that intravenous infusion of arginine, a known inhibitor of somatostatin

secretion, potentiates GH responsivity to GHRH suggests that in humans, as in the rat, somatostatin tone is increased with age. Conversely, the finding that repetitive administration of GHRH to older women (Franchimont *et al.*, 1989) partly reverses their diminished GH responsiveness to GHRH suggests that there may also be a reduction with age in GHRH input to the pituitary. Moreover, administration of GHRH or GHRH analogues may represent an alternative, and perhaps more physiological, method of increasing subnormal GH and IGF-I levels in healthy older women.

In their review, Seeman and Robbins (1994) comment that there are insufficient human data to state whether there are gender-related differences in the hypothalamic–pituitary–adrenal (HPA) axis with aging. Nonetheless, several observations are suggestive. Thus, in one study plasma ACTH responses to an ovine CRH stimulation test were similar in healthy older women and men, whereas basal, peak, and nadir cortisol levels were all higher in older women (Greenspan *et al.*, 1993). In another investigation, the maximal plasma cortisol responsivity to injections of increasing doses of ACTH was reduced in old versus young men, whereas the slope of the dose–response curve was increased in old versus young women (Roberts *et al.*, 1990). In a third study, levels of cortisol, but not of ACTH, were higher in older women following hip fracture than in their healthy age-matched counterparts (Doncaster *et al.*, 1993). Studies in both endurance athletes (Heuser *et al.*, 1991) and depressed patients (von Bardeleben & Holsboer, 1991) have revealed age-related increases in cortisol responses to ovine CRH after pretreatment with dexamethasone, although gender differences in this phenomenon were not investigated. These and other observations suggest that, in humans, aging is associated with heterogeneous patterns of change in hypothalamic–pituitary function, including prolonged patterns of HPA response to challenge; the risk of decline in HPA resiliency with age is related to lifelong cumulative exposure to glucocorticoids.

In contrast to the minimal effects of aging on cortisol secretion, levels of the adrenal androgens, dehydroepiandrosterone (DHEA) and DHEA sulfate, diminish progressively from the third decade onward. Consequently, elderly people have plasma levels of adrenal androgens only one-fourth to one-third those of young adults (Orentreich et al., 1984). Studies in older, postmenopausal women versus younger, normally cycling women have revealed that the age-related reduction in DHEA results from a decrease in pulse amplitude and circadian amplitude, without changes in the timing or pulse frequency, of DHEA secretion (Liu et al., 1990). In addition, adrenal stimulation with exogenous or endogenous ACTH elicits markedly decreased DHEA responses in older subjects.

Epidemiological evidence suggests that there is an inverse relationship between DHEAS levels and the incidence of coronary artery disease in men (Barrett-Connor et al., 1986), but not in women (Barrett-Connor et al., 1987). In one study in which DHEA was administered to six healthy postmenopausal women for 4 weeks (Mortola & Yen, 1990), there were no changes in body weight or percent body fat, as measured by hydrodensitometry. The response of glucose to a 3-hr OGTT was unaltered and that of insulin was increased. Levels of total and HDL cholesterol were significantly reduced, and there were nonsignificant trends toward lower LDL cholesterol and triglyceride values.

Thyroid dysfunction is more prevalent in women than in men and is often temporally related to significant alterations in ovarian physiology, such as pregnancy and menopause. Two reports in which large numbers of apparently healthy community-dwelling subjects were investigated revealed age-related TSH elevations in as

many as 3% of men and 8% of women (Blackman et al., 1995). In one of the latter studies, individuals with thyrotropin (TSH) elevations also exhibited subnormal levels of peripheral thyroid hormones, suggesting that they had primary thyroid failure, presumably secondary to autoimmune thyroid disease. The effects of age on TRH-stimulated TSH secretion have also been examined in several studies. Thus, TSH responses to bolus intravenous injections of TRH have been reported to be decreased in women but not in men, decreased in men but not in women, and increased in both men and women (Blackman et al., 1995). Demographic and other population differences and variable control for certain potentially confounding variables may explain some of the discrepancies. The effects of postmenopausal estrogen and/or progestin replacement therapy on the hypothalamic–pituitary–thyroidal axis remain to be determined.

Baseline and TRH-stimulated serum concentrations of prolactin are about 30–50% greater in women than in men at all ages. Baseline serum prolactin levels have been reported to decrease in women beginning in the mid-to-late fifth decade, in temporal association with the estrogen-deficient state of menopause, in some, but not other studies (Blackman et al., 1995). In one investigation, no age-related differences in the frequency or amplitude of spontaneous prolactin secretion were observed in seven older (mean age 80 years) versus six younger (mean age 53 years) postmenopausal women (Rossmanith et al., 1992). To date, we are unaware of reports of the effects of TRH stimulation, or of dopaminergic agonists or antagonists, on prolactin secretion in postmenopausal women. The observation of an absolute and relative decrease in the proportion of PRL biological activity to immunoreactivity in sera from postmenopausal versus premenopausal women suggests that there is a qualitative, age-related alteration in the prolactin molecule (Maddox et al.,

1991). Prolactin secretion increases with postmenopausal estrogen therapy.

C. Body Composition

Although both caloric intake and energy expenditure decline with age, older people tend to weigh about 25% more than younger people and exhibit a decline in muscle and bone mass and a gain in fat mass relative to total body weight (Poehlman & Horton, 1990). Cross-sectional and longitudinal data from the Baltimore Longitudinal Study of Aging and other studies reveal age-related declines in muscle mass and strength (Fleg & Lakatta, 1988; Kallman et al., 1990), even after considering the confounding effects of physical inactivity, obesity, disease, and nutritional status. Reductions in ovarian and adrenal androgens and the GH–IGF-I axis associated with menopause may contribute to age-related decrements in muscle mass and function.

There is a propensity for redistribution of adipose tissue into the deep abdominal viscera associated with the menopausal transition. This body fat is metabolically distinct from subcutaneous fat and is associated with impairments in glucose, insulin, and lipoprotein metabolism and increased risks for diabetes mellitus and cardiovascular disease. Epidemiological studies suggest that these changes in body composition in women occur during the menopausal transition (Shimokata et al., 1989).

D. Metabolic Functions

Accompanying the above-mentioned changes in body composition are changes in metabolic function. Both cross-sectional and longitudinal studies of perimenopausal women suggest that the transition from premenopause to postmenopause is associated with a more atherogenic lipoprotein profile, including increases in total and LDL cholesterol, triglycerides, and apolipoproteins A-I and A-II (Kuller et al., 1990). HDL cholesterol changes are more controversial. These alterations in lipoprotein profiles appear to be independent of changes in total body weight, although little longitudinal data are available regarding the relationship between perimenopausal changes in the amount and distribution of body fat and changes in lipoprotein profiles.

Natural menopause has not been shown to affect blood pressure (Matthews et al., 1989) or plasma glucose and insulin levels either in the fasted state or following oral glucose administration (Busby et al., 1992). It is possible that more sophisticated measures of glucose and insulin metabolism, such as euglycemic or hyperglycemic glucose clamping techniques, might reveal changes associated with the menopausal transition.

E. Immune Function

Both animal and human studies support a modulatory role of female sex hormones in humoral and cellular immune function. Indeed, premenopausal women are predisposed to autoimmune disorders in terms of both earlier age of onset and more pronounced clinical severity than are observed in men. In contrast, aging in both women and men is associated with alterations in immune function predisposing them to malignancy and infection. It is hypothesized that age-related diseases such as osteoporosis and atherosclerosis may in part be caused by immune dysfunction. For example, there are data to support increases in the postmenopausal state in peripheral monocyte and macrophage production of proinflammatory cytokines such as interleukins, which in vitro increase bone resorption (Cannon & Dinarello, 1985).

III. Impact of Menopause on Specific Disease States

The multiple pathophysiological consequences and diseases of aging that are influenced by menopause vary with respect to their time of onset. The following are listed in temporal order of presentation following the hormonal changes of menopause.

A. Vasomotor Instability and Disturbances of Sleep

The single most common systemic symptom of perimenopause is episodic vasomotor instability, termed the hot flush. There is a range in severity, but the hot flush is most typically described as a sensation of warmth in the upper body and head, which when fully manifested includes visible perspiration. Physiological studies demonstrate elevations in core and skin temperature by 1–7°C and decreased skin resistance. One study reported a mean duration of 3.3 min (range 0.08–60 min) and a frequency of less than daily to 3 per hour (Tulandi & Samarthji, 1985). Longitudinal studies suggest that more than half of women experience hot flushes within the 2-year period surrounding their final menses. Typically, flushes continue for more than 1 year, but in about one-quarter to one-half of perimenopausal women, symptoms last for longer than 5 years. Thermoregulatory defects may alter sleep patterns and contribute to daytime fatigue and low productivity. The etiology of this disturbance in thermoregulatory function is uncertain. Early hypotheses suggested a causative role of LH and/or GnRH. However, neither pituitary resection, nor LH suppression through GnRH agonist administration, nor isolated GnRH deficiency states prevent thermoregulatory dysfunction (Judd, 1986). Currently, evidence favors a role for brain catecholamines and/or hypothalamic opioids. Supportive data include the finding that α-adrenergic blockade reduces hot flushes. Infusion with naloxone, an opioid antagonist, can produce a rise in LH in premenopausal women, with no such effect in estrogen-depletc women.

B. Genitourinary Tract Dysfunction

Uterine epithelium and smooth muscle atrophy after ovarian hormonal depletion. Uterine fibromyomata usually involute in the postmenopausal state. In addition, the lower genital tract, including the vaginal epithelium and the supporting subcutaneous soft tissue and musculature, is hormonally sensitive. With estrogen depletion, the predominant epithelial cell morphology is parabasal, with little mitotic activity and decreased protein synthesis and secretion of mucous. Vaginal pH is increased, resulting in increased susceptibility to both bacterial and mycotic infections. The vagina is less elastic and becomes shortened. Dyspareunia, or painful sexual intercourse, often accompanies these changes in vaginal mucous production. In contrast, the cervical epithelium is of squamous origin and is not hormonally sensitive. However, the endocervical mucous-producing cells are under hormonal control, and cervical stenosis at times complicates the clinical evaluation of postmenopausal vaginal bleeding with endometrial sampling.

The lower urinary tract, including the bladder trigone, urethral epithelium, and periurethral muscles, also contains estrogen-sensitive tissues and undergoes menopausal atrophy (Fantl et al., 1988). The urethra is shortened in length and thinned, exposing sensory nerves to urine flow. Periurethral and pelvic soft tissue and muscles are weakened both from estrogen deficiency and the mechanical stresses of vaginal childbirth. Prolapse of the urethrovesicular junction from the intraabdominal site to the pelvis may result. A constellation of voiding abnormalities can result even without infection, including dysuria, frequency, and urgency. Urinary continence may be affected by these anatomical and physiological changes in the lowerurinary tract. Inadequate pressure generated by the urethra and surrounding tissues, particularly during stresses such as a large volume of urine and increased intraabdominal pressure associated with coughing, may result in stress urinary incontinence. Lower sensory threshold to void has also been reported in postmenopausal women, adding a component of urge incontinence to stress-related symptoms.

C. Disorders of Affect and Cognition

In one longitudinal study, it was reported that all medical symptoms increased in the short term (McKinlay *et al.*, 1992), while in another study, an increase only in menopausal symptoms was found (Hunter *et al.*, 1986). Menopausal symptoms cannot be related simply to serum estradiol levels. Other variables such as stress, dissatisfaction with current life, perceived poor health, low self-esteem, anxiety about the future, and having few intimate friends have been implicated as risk factors for the development of medical symptoms during perimenopause (McKinlay *et al.*, 1992). Earlier menstrual symptoms and the mother's menopausal experience may predict the daughter's perimenopausal symptoms. Multiple causes of disordered sleep during the menopausal transition have been suggested, including vasomotor instability, depression, ill health, sedentary lifestyle, and difficulty coping prior to menopause.

Reports of the frequency and duration of psychological complaints during the menopausal transition are uncertain, although studies suggest that for a subset of women who experienced premenopausal depression there was an exacerbation of the depressed mood during the menopausal transition. Negative, stereotyped views of menopause and social stresses may contribute to perimenopausal changes in affect. Hormonal and psychological factors may be interrelated (Hällström & Samuelsson, 1985). Low levels of serum estradiol may be associated with reduced serotonin synthesis or reduced dopamine receptor sensitivity, contributing to depression. Hormone replacement has been shown to result in reductions in self-rated

distress, anxiety, and depression (Montgomery *et al.*, 1987). The importance of long-standing personality traits in the development of medical symptoms and psychosocial functioning during the menopausal transition has not been adequately assessed.

It is clear that sex hormones influence the fetal development of the brain, resulting in gender differences in patterns of intellectual function. On average, women have greater skills with regard to verbal fluency, perception, and manual precision tasks, while men perform better on spatial tasks and mathematical reasoning. Mechanisms for estrogenic effects on brain function are currently under investigation. Estrogen is known to reduce monoamine oxidase activity. Estrogen has also been shown to increase the activity of choline acetyltransferase, an enzyme that synthesizes the neurotransmitter, acetylcholine. Small clinical trials have shown significant cognitive improvement in elderly women during estrogen replacement therapy. There is a suggestion that estrogen deficiency may modulate the clinical manifestations of dementia (Barrett-Connor & Kritz-Silverstein, 1993). For example, one study demonstrated a faster deterioration of language in women versus men with Alzheimer's disease (Buckwalter *et al.*, 1993).

D. Cancer

During the follicular phase of a woman's menstrual cycle, the uterine endometrium in response to estrogen is proliferative with cells undergoing mitotic divisions. With the ovulatory production of progesterone by the corpus luteum, the endometrium is transformed into a secretory pattern with little cell division. In the absence of circulating progesterone in the menopausal state, unopposed estrogen can lead to endometrial hyperplasia, a premalignant condition, and possibly adenocarcinoma. For example, postmenopausal women at risk for endometrial cancer tend to be obese, with higher than normal circulating estrogen levels due to the peripheral conversion of androgens to estrogens in adipose tissue. Clearly, a second group of women at risk is those receiving unopposed estrogen replacement therapy (Whitehead & Fraser, 1987).

While estrogen and progesterone are trophic factors for breast tissue, their role in the transformation of benign to malignant cell growth is unproved (Staffa et al., 1992; Steinberg et al., 1991). However, epidemiological studies have shown that obese women are at increased risk of breast and colon cancers.

E. Osteoporosis

Menopause is associated with an accelerated loss of bone mass and an increase in fractures (Melton & Riggs, 1986). It is likely that bone loss begins before the cessation of menses (Sowers et al., 1992). The time course and magnitude of the perimenopausal bone loss appear to be variable. Rates of bone loss during the menopausal transition can be up to 4% per year and may last 10–15 years. It is estimated that one-third to one-half of all bone loss in women may be attributable to menopause (Riggs & Melton, 1992). The mechanisms for this bone loss are not fully understood. While estrogen receptors have been located on osteocytes (Komm et al., 1988), indirect effects of estrogen on bone also seem likely. Estrogen promotes the local production of growth factors such as IGF-I, as well as cytokines (Horowitz, 1993). Estrogens also influence circulating levels of other bone-related hormones, such as parathyroid hormone (Kotowicz et al., 1990) and growth hormone (Corpas et al., 1993).

F. Cardiovascular Disease

The incidence of peripheral vascular and coronary atherosclerosis in women increases with age. The relative contributions provided by age and by menopause to coronary artery disease and stroke risk are unknown. Epidemiological studies strongly suggest that estrogen therapy may prevent coronary artery disease in postmenopausal women (Stampfer et al., 1991). The mechanisms by which estrogen may influence the development or progression of CAD are incompletely understood. The beneficial effects were first related to favorable alterations in lipid levels (Walsh et al., 1991), and it has been estimated that 25–50% of the reduction in coronary artery disease can be attributed to estrogen effects on lipid profiles (Barrett-Connor & Bush, 1991). However, direct estrogenic effects on vascular structure and function are also thought to contribute to the prevention of atherosclerosis. Estrogen receptors have been demonstrated on arterial endothelial cells and myocytes (Lin et al., 1986). Studies suggest an estrogen-mediated inhibition of both endothelial hyperplasia and smooth muscle cell growth (Williams et al., 1990). Platelet activation is inhibited by estrogen. Together with effects on the levels of circulating clotting factors, estrogens are thought to modulate arterial blood flow. For example, postmenopausal women have higher levels of fibrinogen and factor VII (Fuster et al., 1992). Acute and chronic administration of estrogen in animals is associated with changes in coronary vasoreactivity. In vitro studies of normal arteries have demonstrated a direct vascular relaxant effect of estrogen (Williams et al., 1992).

IV. Overview of Hormone Replacement

A. Potential Benefits

There are multiple reasons for an individual woman to consider hormone replacement therapy during the perimenopausal transition and the postmenopausal state (Greendale & Judd, 1993). The most common clinical symptom of menopause for which women seek medical advice is thermoregulatory instability. Controlled trials show dose-related benefits of both estrogens and progestins in reducing the frequency and severity of symptoms, although there is a large placebo effect (Tulandi & Samarthji, 1985).

Vaginal dryness and dyspareunia are improved with both local and systemic estrogen. Recurrent infections of the lower urinary tract are reduced with estrogen therapy (Fantl et al., 1994). Clinical improvements in both stress and urge incontinence have been described with a combination of estrogen and phenylpropanolamine, an α-agonist that increases urethral sphincter pressure.

Estrogen replacement reduces the age-related increase in body fat in postmenopausal women and, in particular, reduces abdominal fat mass (Haarbo et al., 1991). The effect of estrogen replacement on muscle mass is controversial, although grip strength may be greater in women treated with estrogen replacement therapy than in their untreated counterparts (Cauley et al., 1987). While the effects of hormonal interventions in mood and affect show individual variation, one study of women undergoing surgical menopause suggested a reduction in depressed affect following intervention as compared with placebo (Sherwin, 1991).

There is well-documented evidence that estrogen replacement therapy results in the prevention of accelerated bone loss attributed to menopause and decreases the number of osteoporosis-related fractures (Ettinger et al., 1985; Nachtigall et al., 1979). The minimum fully effective dose of oral estrogens is 0.625 mg of conjugated equine estrogen, 1 mg of 17-β-estradiol orally, or 50–100 μg of estradiol transdermally per day (Belchetz, 1994). One study of daily low-dose estrogen, 0.3 mg of conjugated equine estrogen, combined with 2 g of calcium supplementation showed efficacy of this regimen to prevent short-term bone loss; however, this has not been confirmed in long-term studies. Given the well-documented efficacy of estrogen in

the prevention of osteoporosis, the routine use of perimenopausal hormone replacement is becoming common place. Epidemiological studies support a beneficial effect of estrogen-containing oral contraceptives on bone density in women prior to menopause (Kleerekoper et al., 1991). The earliest time in menopause in which to intervene with exogenous estrogens to achieve maximum osteoporosis prevention has not been determined. Also, strategies are under investigation to appropriately target estrogen replacement to those women with clinically significant rates of bone loss or reduced premenopausal bone density.

Controversy exists as to the maximum age or duration of menopause at which the initiation of estrogen remains of clinical utility. The beneficial effects of estrogens on bone have been demonstrated in patients up to age 70 years and in women with established osteoporosis; however, it appears that to achieve maximum benefit estrogen replacement must begin at least at the time of cessation of menses.

The optimum duration of estrogen treatment is difficult to determine, although several factors must be considered in the decision to stop estrogen treatment. First, accelerated bone loss occurs immediately following estrogen withdrawal (Christiansen & Christiansen, 1981). Data obtained from the Framingham Study (Felson et al., 1993) suggest that, for the long-term preservation of bone mineral density, women should take estrogen for at least 7 years after menopause and that even this duration of therapy may have little residual effect on bone density among women age 75 years and older.

From a public health perspective, the most compelling reason for the initiation and maintenance of long-term estrogen replacement therapy is the apparent protection against cardiovascular disease. The Nurses' Health Study (Stampfer et al., 1991) provided epidemiological evidence of a relative risk reduction of 0.5 for women who used estrogen replacement compared to nonusers. Other case control and cohort studies have supported a reduction in cardiovascular mortality of 0.33–0.65 associated with postmenopausal estrogen use (Barrett-Connor & Bush, 1991). The Postmenopausal Estrogen/Progestin Interventions Trial, the largest randomized, double-blind, placebo-controlled study, concluded that estrogen alone, or in combination with a progestin, improves lipoproteins and lowers fibrinogen levels without detectable effects on postchallenge insulin levels or blood pressure (Mebane-Sims et al., 1995). While unopposed estrogen was the optimal regimen for the elevation of HDL-C, the addition of cyclic micronized progesterone provided a similar increment in HDL-C. Although no clinical trials have been performed to demonstrate that increasing HDL-C or lowering LDL results in reductions in cardiovascular disease in women, observational studies suggest that HDL-C levels achieved by optimal hormone replacement are associated with 20–25% less cardiovascular disease (Bass et al., 1993).

B. Potential Adverse Effects

Frequent side effects of estrogens in older women include breast tenderness and bloating, both of which tend to peak by 6 weeks of therapy. The effects of postmenopausal estrogen replacement therapy on clotting factors are not clinically significant, unlike those of oral contraceptive treatments. However, women with previous clotting disorders, especially in the setting of elevated sex hormone levels such as pregnancy, are often counselled about the possibility of a recurrent clinical clotting event. A poorly studied potential side effect of long-term estrogen use is biliary stone formation resulting from lithogenic effects of estrogen on the liver.

The endometrial lining of the uterus proliferates in the presence of unopposed estrogen. Endometrial hyperplasia and ad-

enocarcinoma are long-term consequences of postmenopausal estrogen. However, when appropriate doses of exogenous progestins are added to estrogen, the risk of endometrial abnormalities is negated (Mebane-Sims et al., 1995). Progestins appear to enhance the effect of estrogen on bone; however, their effects on lipoprotein profiles is opposite that of estrogen. The type and dose of progestin greatly influence its metabolic effects on lipoproteins. Current clinical regimens optimize estrogen/progestin effects on lipids.

The most controversial aspect of estrogen replacement remains the potential increase in breast cancer risk resulting from prolonged estrogen use. To date, the majority of studies support no significant increase in breast cancer risk in women receiving postmenopausal estrogen therapy (Staffa et al., 1992). However, randomized, placebo-controlled studies with longitudinal data are needed to address this issue.

C. Current Clinical Guidelines

A practical approach is to begin hormonal therapy during the menopausal transition and to maintain therapy until the long-term prevention of osteoporosis is no longer an important aspect of health care or until a significant adverse event related to the therapy is experienced. Smokers, who metabolize exogenous estrogens more rapidly than nonsmokers, may require higher doses.

Studies suggest that low-dose daily progestin, such as medroxyprogesterone acetate at 2.5–5 mg daily added to daily estrogen, may improve medication compliance by preventing monthly vaginal bleeding (Mebane-Sims et al., 1995). However, a significant portion of women experience unpredictable bleeding in the first 6 months of this treatment. An alternative therapy that results in predictable monthly vaginal bleeding is sequential progestin, medroxyprogesterone acetate at 10 mg daily for 10–14 days at the beginning of each calendar month combined with daily estrogen. In the past, progestins were added to estrogen therapy even for women who had undergone hysterectomy under the assumption that progestins counterbalanced the effects of estrogen on breast tissue. It is now known that both estrogens and progestins stimulate breast tissue growth. This effect on the breast, combined with the dose-related adverse effect on cholesterol profiles, precludes the use of progestins in women who are no longer at risk of endometrial cancer due to hysterectomy (Belchetz, 1994).

For women who have proven breast cancer, estrogen and progestin therapy is contraindicated. The nonsteroidal antiestrogen, tamoxifen, which also possesses weak estrogenic agonist activity, is used in the treatment of breast cancer. Tamoxifen has been shown *in vitro* to inhibit bone resorption (Stewart & Stern, 1986) and in a small clinical trial (Love *et al.,* 1994) to increase bone density. Tamoxifen also improves the lipid profile, yet there are potential adverse effects of therapy such as thromboembolic disease and hepatic and endometrial tumors. Large-scale clinical trials are underway to assess the benefits versus the risks of this therapy for women who have contraindications to estrogen treatment.

D. Current Research Topics

Multiple areas of research regarding menopause and hormone replacement are currently being pursued. A major long-term longitudinal study of hormone replacement is underway to address the issues of cardiovascular protection and breast cancer risk. Additional basic research is needed to elucidate the mechanisms by which estrogens mediate their effects on target tissues such as bone, vasculature, and brain. Estrogenic analogues might be synthesized that mimic the beneficial effects of estrogen, but that minimize the growth of endometrial and breast tissues.

The ability to reverse age-related diseases through combined hormonal intervention is also under investigation. In particular, the potential benefits of exogenous agents to increase growth hormone secretion and/or action in combination with sex steroids are being studied. Adrenal androgen replacement is also of interest with regard to body composition and cardiovascular function. Studies are underway to assess the interactions among hormonal therapies, nutrition, and physical activity.

V. Summary

The clinical sequelae consequent to menopausal ovarian dysfunction occur over a prolonged period of time. The profound changes in reproductive hormones impact on other endocrine and metabolic systems and exert strong influences on multiple organ systems, including bones, cardiovascular system, immune function, and cognition. Moreover, menopause contributes to age-related diseases such as cardiovascular disease and osteoporosis. Hormonal intervention can negate the detrimental effects of menopause; however, more research is needed to achieve a better risk/benefit ratio of long-term hormonal replacement.

References

Barrett-Connor, E., & Bush, T. L. (1991). Estrogen and coronary heart disease in women. *Journal of the American Medical Association, 265,* 1861–1867.
Barrett-Connor, E., & Khaw, K. T. (1987). Absence of an inverse relation of dehydroepiandrosterone sulfate with cardiovascular mortality in postmenopausal women [letter]. *New England Journal of Medicine, 317,* 711.
Barrett-Connor, E., & Kritz-Silverstien, D. (1993). Estrogen replacement therapy and cognitive function in older women. *Journal of the American Medical Association, 269,* 2637–2641.

Barrett-Connor, E., Khaw, K. T., & Yen, S. S. (1986). A prospective study of dehydroepiandrosterone sulfate, mortality, and cardiovascular disease. *New England Journal of Medicine, 315*, 1519–1524.

Bass, K. M., Newschaffer, C. J., Klag, M. J., & Bush, T. L. (1993). Plasma lipoprotein levels as predictors of cardiovascular death in women. *Archives of Internal Medicine, 153*, 2209–2216.

Baxter, R. C., & Martin, J. L. (1986). Radioimmunoassay of growth hormone-dependent insulin-like growth factor binding protein in human plasma. *Journal of Clinical Investigation, 78*, 1504–1512.

Belchetz, P. E. (1994). Hormonal treatment of postmenopausal women. *New England Journal of Medicine, 330*, 1062–1071.

Bellantoni, M. F., Harman, S. M., Cullins, V. E., Engelhardt, S. M., & Blackman, M. R. (1992). Transdermal estradiol with oral progestin: biological and clinical effects in younger and older postmenopausal women. *Journal of Gerontology, 46*, M216–222.

Blackman, M. R., Elahi, D., & Harman, S. M. (1995). Endocrinology and Aging, In L. DeGroot (Ed.), *Endocrinology* (3rd ed., pp. 2702–2730). New York: Grune and Stratton.

Buckler, H. M., Evans, C. A., Mamtora, H., Burger, H. G., & Anderson, D. C. (1991). Gonadotropin, steroid, and inhibin levels in women with incipient ovarian failure during anovulatory and ovulatory rebound cycles. *Journal of Clinical Endocrinology and Metabolism, 72*, 116–124.

Buckwalter, J. G., Sobel, E., Dunn, M. E., Diz, M. M., & Henderson, V. W. (1993). Gender differences on a brief measure of cognitive functioning in Alzheimer's disease. *Archives of Neurology, 50*, 757–760.

Busby, M. J., Bellantoni, M. F., Tobin, J. D., Muller, D., Kafonek, S., Blackman, M. R., & Andres, R. (1992). Glucose tolerance in women: The effects of age, body composition, and sex hormones. *Journal of The American Geriatrics Society, 40*, 497–502.

Cannon, J. G., & Dinarello, C. A. (1985). Increased plasma interleukin-1 activity in women after ovulation. *Science, 227*, 1247–1249.

Cauley, J. A., Petrini, A. M., LaPorte, R. E., Sandler, R. B., Bayles, C. M., Robertson, R. J., & Slemenda, C. W. (1987). The decline in grip strength in the menopause: relationship to physical activity, estrogen use and anthropometric factors. *Journal of Chronic Diseases, 40*, 115–120.

Christiansen, C., & Christiansen, M. S. (1981). TransbØI IB. Bone mass in postmenopausal women after withdrawal of oestrogen/gestagen replacement therapy. *Lancet, 1*, 459–461.

Corpas, E., Harman, S. M., & Blackman, M. R. (1993). Human growth hormone and human aging. *Endocrine Reviews, 14*, 20–39.

Dawson-Hughes, B., Stern, D., & Goldman, J. (1986). Regulation of growth hormone and somatomedin-C in postmenopausal women: effect of physiological estrogen replacement. *Journal of Clinical Endocrinology and Metabolism, 63*, 424–432.

Doncaster, H. D., Barton, R. N., Horan, M. A., & Roberts, N. A. (1993). Factors influencing cortisol-adrenocorticotrophin relationships in elderly women with upper femur fractures. *Journal of Trauma, 34*, 49–55.

Ettinger, B., Genant, H. K., & Cann, C. E. (1985). Long-term estrogen replacement therapy prevents bone loss and fractures. *Annals of Internal Medicine, 102*, 319–324.

Faddy, M. J., Gosden, R. G., Gougeon, A., Richardson, S. J., & Nelson, J. F. (1992). Accelerated disappearance of ovarian follicles in mid-life—implications for forecasting menopause. *Human Reproduction, 7*, 1342–1346.

Fantl, J. A., Wyman, J. F., Anderson, R. L., Matt, D. W., & Bump, R. C. (1988). Postmenopausal urinary incontinence: Comparison between nonestrogen-supplemented and estrogen-supplemented women. *Obstetrics and Gynecology, 71*, 823–828.

Fantl, J. A., Cardoza, L., & McClish, D. K. (1994). Estrogen supplementation in the management of urinary incontinence in older women: A meta-analysis. *Obstetrics and Gynecology, 83*, 12–18.

Felson, D. T., Zhang, Y., Hannan, M. T., Kiel, D. P., Wilson, P. W. F., & Anderson, J. J. (1993). The effect of postmenopausal estrogen therapy on bone density in elderly women. *New England Journal of Medicine, 329*, 1141–1146.

Fleg, J. L., & Lakatta, E. G. (1988). Role of muscle loss in the age-associated reduction in VO2 max. *Journal of Applied Physiology, 65*, 1147–1151.

Franchimont, P., Urbain-Choffray, D., Lambelin, P., Fontaine, M. A., Frangin, G., &

Reginster, J. Y. (1989). Effects of repetitive administration of growth hormone-releasing hormone on growth hormone secretion, insulin-like growth factor I, and bone metabolism in postmenopausal women. *Acta Endocrinologica (Copenhagen), 120,* 121–128.

Fuster, V., Badimon, L., Badimon, J. J., Chesebro, J. H. (1992). The pathogenesis of coronary artery disease and the acute coronary syndromes (II). *New England Journal of Medicine, 326,* 310–318.

Gray, R. (1976). The menopause: epidemiological and demographic considerations. In R. J. Beard (Ed.), *The Menopause* (pp. 25–39). Lancaster: MTP Press.

Greendale, G. A., & Judd, H. L. (1993). The Menopause: Health implications and clinical management. *Journal of the American Geriatrics Society, 41,* 426–436.

Greenspan, S. L., Rowe, J. W., Maitland, L. A., McAloon-Dyke, M., & Elahi, D. (1993). The pituitary-adrenal glucocorticoid response is altered by gender and disease. *Journal of Gerontology, 48,* M72–M77.

Haarbo, J., Marslew, U., Gotfredsen, A., & Christiansen, C. (1991). Postmenopausal hormone replacement therapy prevents central distribution of body fat after menopause. *Metabolism, 40,* 1323–1326.

Hällström, T., & Samuelsson, S. (1985). Mental health in the climacteric: The longitudinal study of women in Gothenburg. *Acta Obstetrica Gynecologica Scandinavia, 130,* 13–18.

Heuser, I. J., Wark, H. J., Keul, J., & Holsboer, F. (1991). Hypothalamic-pituitary-adrenal axis function in elderly endurance athletes. *Journal of Clinical Endocrinology and Metabolism, 73,* 485–488.

Ho, K. Y., Evans, W. S., Blizzard, R. M., Veldhuis, J. D., Merriam, G. R., Somojlik, E., Furlanetto, R., Rogol, A. D., Kaiser, D. L., & Thorner, M. O. (1987). Effects of sex and age on 24-hour profile of growth hormone secretion in men: importance of endogenous estradiol concentrations. *Journal of Clinical Endocrinology and Metabolism, 64,* 51–58.

Horowitz, M. C. (1993). Cytokines and estrogen in bone: Anti-ostoporotic effects. *Science, 260,* 626–627.

Hunter, M., Battersby, R., & Whitehead, M. (1986). Relationships between psychological symptoms, somatic complaints and menopausal status. *Maturitas, 8,* 217–228.

Judd, H. L. (1986). The basis of menopausal vasomotor symptoms. In L. Mastroianni, Jr. & C. A. Paulsen (Eds.), *Aging, Reproduction and the Climacteric* (pp. 216). New York: Plenum Press.

Kallman, D. A., Plato, C., & Tobin, J. D. (1990). The role of muscle loss in the age-related decline of grip strength: cross-sectional and longitudinal perspectives. *Journal of Gerontology, 45,* M82–88.

Kleerekoper, M., Brienza, R. S., Schultz, L. R., & Johnson, C. C. (1991). Oral contraceptive use may protect against low bone mass. *Archives of Internal Medicine, 151,* 1971–1976.

Komm, B. S., Terpening, C. M., Benz, D. J., Kimberlie, A., Graeme, A. G., Korc, M., Greene, G. L., O'Malley, B., & Haussler, M. (1988). Estrogen binding, receptor RNA, and biologic response in osteoblast-like osteosarcoma cells. *Science, 241,* 81–84.

Kotowicz, M. A., Klee, G. G., Kao, P. C., O'Fallon, W. M., Hodgson, S. F., Cedel, S. L., Eriksen, E. F., Gonchoroff, D. G., Judd, H. L., & Riggs, B. L. (1990). Relationship between serum intact parathyroid hormone concentrations and bone remodeling in Type I osteoporosis: Evidence that skeletal sensitivity is increased. *Osteoporosis International, 1,* 14–22.

Kuller, L. H., Gutai, J. P., Meilahn, E., Mathews, K. A., & Plantinga, P. (1990). Relationship of endogenous sex steroid hormones to lipids and apoproteins in postmenopausal women. *Arteriosclerosis, 10,* 1058–1060.

Lin, A. L., Gonzalez, R., Carey, K. D., & Shain, S. A. (1986). Estradiol-17B affects estrogen receptor distribution and elevates progesterone receptor content on baboon aorta. *Atherosclerosis, 6,* 495–504.

Liu, C. H., Laughlin, G. A., Fischer, U. G., & Yen, S. S. (1990). Marked attentuation of ultradian and circadian rhythms of dehydroepiandrosterone in postmenopausal women: evidence for a reduced 17,20-desmolase enzymatic activity. *Journal of Clinical Endocrinology and Metabolism, 71,* 900–906.

Longcope, C. (1974). Steroid production in pre- and postmenopausal women. In R. B. Greenblatt, V. B. Mahesh, & P. G. McDonough (Eds.), *The Menopausal Syndrome* (pp. 6–11). New York: Medcom Press.

Love, R. R., Barden, H. S., Mazess, R. B., Epstein, S., & Chappell, R. J. (1994). Effect of tamoxifen on lumbar spine bone mineral density in postmenopausal women after 5 years. *Archives of Internal Medicine, 154,* 2585–2588.

Maddox, P. R., Jones, D. L., & Mansel, R. E. (1991). Basal prolactin and total lactogenic hormone levels by microbioassay and immunoassay in normal human sera. *Acta Endocrinologica (Copenhagen), 125,* 621–627.

Matthews, K. A., Meilahn, E., Kuller, L. H., Kelsey, S. F., Caggiula, A. W., & Wing, R. R. (1989). Menopause and risk factors for coronary heart disease. *New England Journal of Medicine, 321,* 641–646.

McKinlay, S. M., Brambilla, D. J., & Posner, J. G. (1992). The normal menopausal transition. *Maturitas, 14,* 103–115.

Mebane-Sims, I. L., & The Writing Group for the PEPI Trial (1995). Effects of estrogen or estrogen/progestin regimens on heart disease risk factors in postmenopausal women: The postmenopausal estrogen/progestin interventions (PEPI) trial. *Journal of the American Medical Association, 273,* 199–208.

Melton, L. J., III, & Riggs, B. L. (1986). Epidemiology and cost of osteoporotic fractures. In A. Vagenakis, P. Soucacos, & A. Avramides (Eds.), *2nd International Conference on Osteoporosis, Social and Clinical Aspects* (pp. 23–27). Milan: Masson Publishers.

Montgomery, J. C., Brincat, M., Tapp, A., Appleby, L., Versi, E., Fenwick, P. B. C., & Studd, J. W. W. (1987). Effect of oestrogen and testosterone implants on psychological disorders in the climacteric. *Lancet,* Feb 7, 297–299.

Mortola, J. F., & Yen, S. S. (1990). The effects of oral dehydroepiandrosterone on endocrine-metabolic parameters in postmenopausal women. *Journal of Clinical Endocrinology and Metabolism, 71,* 696–704.

Nachtigall, L. E., Nachtigall, R. H., Nachtigall, R. D., & Beckman, E. M. (1979). Estrogen replacement therapy I: a 10 year prospective study in the relationship to osteoporosis. *Obstetrics and Gynecology, 53,* 277–281.

Orentreich, N., Brind, J. L., Rizer, R. L., & Vogelman, J. H. (1984). Age changes and sex differences in serum dehydroepiandrosterone sulfate concentrations from puberty through adulthood. *Journal of Clinical Endocrinology and Metabolism, 59,* 551–555.

Poehlman, E. T., & Horton, E. S. (1990). Regulation of energy expenditure in aging humans. *Annual Review of Nutrition, 10,* 255–275.

Riggs, B. L., & Melton, L. J., III. (1992). The prevention and treatment of osteoporosis. *New England Journal of Medicine, 327,* 620–627.

Roberts, N. A., Barton, R. N., & Horan, M. A. (1990). Ageing and the sensitivity of the adrenal gland to physiological doses of ACTH in man. *Journal of Endocrinological Investigation, 126,* 507–513.

Rossmanith, W. G., Szilagyi, A., & Scherbaum, W. A. (1992). Episodic thyrotropin (TSH) and prolactin (PRL) secretion during aging in postmenopausal women. *Hormone Metabolism Research, 24,* 185–190.

Seeman, T. E., & Robbins, R. J. (1994). Aging and hypothalamic-pituitary-adrenal response to challenge in humans. *Endocrine Reviews, 15,* 233–260.

Sherwin, B. B. (1991). The impact of different doses of estrogen and progestin on mood and sexual behavior in postmenopausal women. *Journal of Clinical Endocrinology and Metabolism, 72,* 336–343.

Shimokata, H., Tobin, J. D., Muller, D. C., Elahi, D., Coon, P. J., & Andres, R. (1989). Studies in the distribution of body fat. I. Effects of age, sex, and obesity. *Journal of Gerontology, 44,* M67–M73.

Sowers, M. R., Clark, M. K., Hollis, B., Wallace, R. B., & Jannausch, M. (1992). Radial bone mineral density in pre- and perimenopausal women: A Prospective study of rates and risk factors for loss. *Journal of Bone and Mineral Research, 7,* 647–657.

Staffa, J. A., Newschaffer, C. J., Jones, J. K., & Miller, V. (1992). Progestins and breast cancer: An epidemiologic review. *Fertility and Sterility, 57,* 473–491.

Stampfer, M. J., Colditz, G. A., Willett, W. C., Manson, J. E., Rosner, B., Speizer, F. E., & Hennekens, C. H. (1991). Postmenopausal estrogen therapy and cardiovascular disease: Ten year follow-up from the Nurses' Health Study. *New England Journal of Medicine, 325,* 756–762.

Steinberg, K. K., Thacker, S. B., Smith, S. J., Stroup, D. F., Zack, M. M., Flanders, W. D., Berkelman, R. L. (1991). A meta-analysis of the effect of estrogen replacement therapy on the risk of breast cancer. *Journal of the American Medical Association, 265,* 1985–1990.

Stewart, P. J., & Stern, P. H. (1986). Effects of

the aintiestrogens tamoxifen and clomiphene on bone resorption in vitro. *Endocrinology, 118,* 125–131.

Thatcher, S. S., & Naftolin, F. (1991). The aging and aged ovary. *Seminars in Reproductive Endocrinology, 9,* 189–199.

Tulandi, T., & Samarthji, L. (1985). Menopausal hot flush. *Obstetrics and Gynecology Surveys, 40,* 553–563.

von Bardeleben, U., & Holsboer, F. (1991). Effect of age on the cortisol response to human corticotropin-releasing hormone in depressed patients pretreated with dexamethasone. *Biological Psychology, 29,* 1042–1050.

Walsh, B. W., Schiff, I., Rosner, B., Greenberg, L., Ravinkar, V., & Sacks, F. M. (1991). Effects of postmenopausal estrogen replacement on the concentrations and metabolism of plasma lipoproteins. *New England Journal of Medicine, 325,* 1196–1204.

Whitehead, M. I., & Fraser, D. (1987). Controversies concerning the safety of estrogen replacement therapy. *American Journal of Obstetrics and Gynecology, 156,* 1313–1322.

Williams, J. C., Adams, M. R., & Klopfenstein, H. S. (1990). Estrogen modulates responses of atherosclerotic coronary arteries. *Circulation, 81,* 1680–1687.

Williams, J. C., Adams, M. R., Herrington, D. M., & Clarkson, T. B. (1992). Short term administration of estrogen and vascular responses of atherosclerotic coronary arteries. *Journal of the American College of Cardiology, 20,* 452–457.

Wise, P. M., Scarbrough, K., Weiland, N. G., & Larson, G. H. (1990). Diurnal patterns of proopiomelanocortin gene expression in the arcuate nucleus of proestrous, ovariectomized, and steroid-treated rats: A possible role in cyclic luteinizing hormone secretion. *Molecular Endocrinology, 4,* 886–892.

Nineteen

Skeletal Integrity

Carolyn Murray, Marjorie Luckey, and Diane Meier

I. Introduction

Bone loss is a universal consequence of skeletal aging. Age-related osteoporosis combined with a heightened susceptibility to falls places the elderly at high risk for fractures, especially osteoporotic fractures of the hip, wrist, and spine. In 1990, an estimated 350,000 hip fractures occurred in North America alone, with over 1.6 million hip fractures occurring throughout the world. Direct medical costs of osteoporosis were estimated to be $5.2 billion in 1986 with $2.8 billion for in-patient care and $2.1 billion for nursing home care (Phillips et al., 1988). Marked demographic changes in the population over 65 years of age will greatly increase the number of hip fractures in the future. In Asia, South America, Africa, and the Middle East, the population over 65 is expected to increase from 190 million to more than 1 billion persons by 2050 (Cooper et al., 1992). Because of this increased life expectancy and the growing world population, estimates suggest that more than 6 million hip fractures will occur in 2050. More than two-thirds of these hip fractures will occur in Asia, Africa, Latin America, and the Middle East, with a doubling of the incidence

in North America to 750,000 hip fractures per year (Cooper et al., 1992).

Although the aging of the population accounts for the majority of the increases in hip fractures, there are also reports of age-adjusted increases in the incidence of hip fractures as well. In Malmo, Sweden, for example, the age-adjusted incidence of trochanteric fractures has more than doubled from 1951–1960 to 1983–1985 (Obrant, 1989). Similarly, the age-adjusted hip fracture incidence in Oxford, England, doubled between 1954–1958 and 1983 (Boyce, 1985). Other areas, including the northern United States, have not experienced age-adjusted increases in hip fracture incidence (Kanis et al., 1992; Melton et al., 1989). The reasons for marked geographic variations in hip fracture incidence are not known, but are well-documented (Melton, 1993). Hip fracture incidence in Europe is more than 6 times greater in the northern European countries than in southern Europe (Johnell, 1992). Within the United States, higher age-adjusted rates of hip fracture are found in the south than in the north (Jacobsen et al., 1990). The hip fracture incidence was higher in agricultural areas with a greater percentage of those over 65 years of age

Handbook of the Biology of Aging, Fourth Edition
Copyright © 1996 Academic Press, Inc. All rights of reproduction in any form reserved.

living below the poverty level. The etiology of this regional variation is unclear, but it does not appear to be related to smoking, alcohol, Scandinavian ancestry, weight, or requiring assistance in ambulation. Differences in calcium consumption, vitamin D status, falls, or physical activity that might account for this variability have not been evaluated.

Morbidity and mortality from hip fracture are the most serious sequelae of osteoporosis. A prospective cohort study of community-dwelling elders found that, of 120 persons with hip fractures, 22 died within 6 months and a marked decline in physical function persisted 6 months after the fracture among the survivors (Marottoli et al., 1992). Marked decreases in function were observed 6 months postfracture, with unassisted walking prevalence declining from 75 to 15%, stair climbing from 63 to 8%, and independence in transfers from 90 to 32%. Excess mortality rates after hip fracture have been estimated as 5% for patients under 65, 10% for those 65–79 years of age, and 20% for those over 80 (Cummings et al., 1989). However, a study found declining mortality rates in association with femoral neck fractures in men and women 80–84 years of age in England and Wales, West Germany, Northern Ireland, Sweden, Italy, and France (Heyse, 1993).

Although they are difficult to identify in the general population, vertebral fractures are common among osteoporotic persons. Prevalence rates of vertebral fractures among women in Rochester, Minnesota, ranged from 20.9% for those aged 70–74 years to 43.0% for those 85–89 years old (Melton et al., 1989). Although the majority of vertebral fractures never come to clinical attention, many individuals with spinal osteoporosis experience ongoing back pain that is related to both the number and the severity of the vertebral fractures (Ryan et al., 1994). Among 85 women with spinal osteoporosis referred to a specialty bone clinic, 63% had persistent

lumbar pain and 62% had persistent thoracic pain (Ryan et al., 1994). Estimates of lifetime risk of fracture for a 50-year-old white woman are 16% at the hip, 32% at the spine, and 15% at the wrist (Cummings et al., 1989).

II. Risk Factors for Fracture

The major risk factors for fracture are female gender, age, falls, and low bone density. Ninety to ninety-seven percent of hip fractures occur after a fall. Individuals fall more often as they age, with an annual incidence of 25% falling at age 70 and 35% falling over age 75 (Tinetti & Speechley, 1989). General risk factors for falls include lower limb dysfunction, visual impairment, use of an ambulatory aid, Parkinson's disease, stroke, and use of antidepressants, vasodilators, barbiturates, and benzodiazepines (Granek et al., 1987; Grisso et al., 1991). Characteristics that increase the likelihood of fracture from a fall include falls from greater heights (Granek et al., 1987), falls sideways or straight down landing on or near a hip, not falling on a hand or not breaking the fall, landing on a hard surface, and having weaker triceps (Nevitt & Cummings, 1993).

Efforts to prevent hip fractures, therefore, must focus not only on improving bone mass but also on decreasing the trauma associated with falls. Ten of twenty-eight nursing home wards in Denmark were randomized to receive external hip protectors for their residents. The hip fracture rate was significantly decreased in the treatment wards, with 3% hip fractures over 11 months compared to 7% in the control group (Lauritzen et al., 1993). Multiple risk factor interventions to decrease falls in community-dwelling elderly people have also been shown to be effective. In a study, 300 men and women aged 70 or older with at least one risk factor for falling were assigned to an intervention or usual care group (Tinetti *et al.*, 1994). The intervention group received risk factor modifications such as adjustments in medication to decrease sedative use, balance and strengthening exercise programs, alterations in the home environment such as installation of grab bars and handrails, and behavioral recommendations to improve postural hypotension. During 1 year of follow-up, 35% of the intervention group experienced falls compared to 47% of the usual care group ($p = 0.04$).

III. Bone Density as a Risk Factor for Fracture

The most powerful measurable risk factor for fracture in the elderly is bone mineral density (BMD). Low bone density at the radius, spine, calcaneus, or hip significantly increases the risk of hip fracture (Cummings *et al.*, 1993). For example, a 1 standard deviation decrease in bone mineral density at the femoral neck increases the risk of hip fracture 2.6 times, whereas a similar decrease in bone density at the lumbar spine increases the hip fracture risk 1.6 times. Low bone density measures also predict increased risk of fracture of the wrist, foot, humerus, rib, toe, leg, pelvis, hand, and clavicle with each standard deviation decrease in bone density, increasing the risk of nonspine fracture by 50–60% (Seeley, 1991). A 2 standard deviation decrease in bone mineral density at the lumbar spine predicts a 4.4 times increased risk of fracturing the spine over 5 years of follow-up (Ross *et al.*, 1991). Despite the increased risk of fracture with low bone density, considerable overlap in bone density exists between those who fracture and those who do not. However, bone density is a better predictor of fractures than other commonly accepted risk factors for diseases, such as serum cholesterol for coronary artery disease or blood pressure for stroke (Gordon, 1972; Hui *et al.*, 1988).

Risk factors for low bone density are well-described. A longitudinal study of 121 women followed for over 10 years found that lactation, oral contraceptive use, and dietary calcium intake above 1500 mg per day were associated with higher bone mass at menopause, but did not affect early postmenopausal bone loss rates. Increased weight protected against postmenopausal bone loss (Hansen *et al.*, 1991). The Study of Osteoporotic Fractures evaluated factors associated with appendicular bone mass in 9704 nonblack women over 65 years of age. Factors associated with low bone mass included gastric surgery, age, history of maternal fracture, smoking, and caffeine. Higher bone mass was associated with estrogen use, thiazide use, weight, greater muscle strength, and later age at menopause (Bauer *et al.*, 1993). Osteoporosis is more common among Caucasians and Asians than African Americans (Schnitzler, 1993). A study of family history of osteoporosis found that bone mineral density of the hip was lower in men with a family history of osteoporosis, whereas bone mineral density of the spine was associated with family history in women (Soroko *et al.*, 1994). The association between low BMD and family history was strongest for a history of paternal osteoporosis, although the positive predictive value of family history was only 22–33%.

Although a family history of osteoporosis has been considered a risk factor for years, investigators have relatively recently discovered genes encoding the vitamin D receptor, which may explain up to 75% of the genetic effect on bone density (Morrison *et al.*, 1994). In a study of 70 monozygotic and 54 dizygotic twins, dizygotic twins with the same genes for the vitamin D receptor were as similar to each other in their lumbar spine bone densities as monozygotic twins. Hip bone densities were less strongly predicted by the presence of identical genes for the vitamin D receptor, suggesting a stronger influence of environmental factors at the hip site. Additional studies of 311 women found that genotype was an independent predictor of bone mineral density at the lumbar spine and femoral neck after adjusting for height, weight, age, and years since menopause. Calculations suggest that variation in the gene for the vitamin D receptor accounts for a 8- to 10-year age difference in bone density (Morrison et al., 1994).

IV. Changes in Bone with Aging

Women experience rapid bone loss in the early postmenopausal period, which contributes significantly to the higher incidence of osteoporosis in women than in men. Significant bone loss continues into the ninth decade. It has been estimated that the 62% of bone loss experienced by a 70-year-old woman is attributable to loss from aging, as opposed to 38% from menopause (Nordin et al., 1990). Cross-sectional studies suggest that annual losses in women over age 65 range from 0.3 to 1.3%, depending on the site. Estimates of bone loss at the femoral neck have been fairly consistent in these studies, ranging from 0.68 to 0.82% per year (Steiger et al., 1992; Hannan et al., 1992). A longitudinal study of 85 women over 65 years of age identified similar rates of bone loss at the hip (Greenspan et al., 1994). Bone mineral density at the spine increased with age in this study, suggesting that changes in the spine with aging such as the development of osteophytes or vascular calcifications significantly alter the validity of spinal bone density measurements in the very old. Bone loss at the ultradistal radius in these studies was minimal at 0.16–0.30% per year.

Not only does bone density decrease with age, but age acts as a risk factor for fracture independent of declines in bone density. Each 10-year increment in age is associated with a 1.4–1.8 increased risk of vertebral fracture, after adjusting for bone mass and prior fracture (Ross et al., 1991). Similarly, Cummings et al. (1990) found that the risk for hip fracture increased by 2.09 times for each additional 10 years of age.

Although the susceptibility of the elderly to falls contributes to the effect of age on fracture risk, changes in bone quality not measurable by bone density may account for a portion of the fracture risk due to aging. Studies of changes in trabecular bone with aging show both a reduction in trabecular number and an increase in trabecular perforation (Schnitzler, 1993; Parfitt et al., 1983). In osteoporotic women with vertebral fractures, the trabecular perforations were significantly more frequent and mean trabecular bone volume was significantly lower than expected for age, but no difference in trabecular thickness was observed. Patients with hip fractures, however, did exhibit significantly reduced trabecular thickness (Parfitt et al., 1983). These findings suggest that the changes induced in bone architecture by estrogen deficiency and aging may differ. It has been postulated that the well-documented increase in osteoclastic activity and bone resorption at menopause may lead to trabecular perforations and loss of trabeculae (Manolagas & Jilka, 1995), whereas an age-related decrease in osteoblastic function could lead to progressive thinning of trabecular plates. Other investigators have found an increased number of healing microfractures with aging and an even greater number of microfractures in women with diffuse spinal osteoporosis (Vernon-Roberts & Pirie, 1973). The microfractures were located primarily in vertical trabeculae, while horizontal trabeculae disproportionately disappear with the development of osteoporosis.

Metabolic changes in bone are also seen with aging. Tetracycline-labeled bone biopsies have shown an age-related decline in mineral apposition rates with lengthened remodeling cycles (Recker et al., 1988). A defect in osteoblast recruitment or activity affecting mean bone formation rates is noted by Parfitt *et al.* (1983). Another study showed decreased activity of two metabolic enzymes, G6PD and 6PGD, in cortical bone osteoblasts in patients with osteoporotic hip fractures. The decreased metabolic activity was not evident with traumatic hip fractures (Dodds *et al.*, 1990).

The relationship between bone turnover, bone age, and fatigue damage remains unclear. One theory that lower bone turnover in elderly osteoporotic women could lead to increased bone age and increased fatigue damage in trabecular bone was not supported in a study comparing women with and without vertebral fractures. Although there was evidence of increased bone age, there was no increase in osteocyte death or fatigue damage. Decreased bone turnover and increased bone age may have a more significant effect on femur and hip fractures due to the increased portion of cortical bone (Parfitt, 1993).

The clinical utility of serum or urine biochemical markers of bone turnover has not been established. In research studies, the most sensitive markers available for the assessment of bone turnover in women with vertebral osteoporosis appear to be serum osteocalcin, a marker of bone formation, and urinary pyridinoline crosslinks, a marker of bone resorption (Delmas, 1993). Alternate markers of bone formation include bone-specific alkaline phosphatase and type 1 collagen peptides. Markers of bone resorption include plasma tartrate-resistant urinary hydroxyproline and urinary hydroxylysine glycosides.

V. Additional Risk Factors for Fracture

Additional risk factors for hip fractures in white women over 65 years of age were identified in a prospective cohort study of 9516 women. These risk factors include maternal history of hip fracture, previous fractures after 50 years of age, tallness at 25 years of age, history of hyperthyroidism, treatment with long-acting benzodiazepines or anticonvulsant medication, higher caffeine intake, spending less than 4 hr per day on their feet, inability to rise from a chair without using the upper extremities, tachycardia at rest, self-reported poor health, poor depth perception, and poor contrast sensitivity. Weight gain since the age of 25 years was protective against hip fracture (Cummings *et al.*, 1995). In a study of African-American women, risk factors for hip fracture included prior stroke, requiring aid in ambulation, greater than seven alcoholic drinks per day, and thinness. Postmenopausal estrogen use was protective (Grisso *et al.*, 1994).

The presence of prior fractures also increases the risk of fracture independent of low bone density. In the Hawaiian Osteoporosis Study, women with one vertebral fracture at baseline were 2.6–3.0 times more likely to fracture the spine again within 5 years after adjustment for low bone density. Two or more previous spine fractures increased the risk of recurrence to 7–9 times that in women without fracture (Ross *et al.*, 1991; Wasnich, 1993). Prior vertebral fracture significantly increases the risk of hip fractures to 1.8 times that expected, especially for intertrochanteric fractures (Kotowicz *et al.*, 1994).

The geometric properties of the hip may also play a role in hip fracture risk. Faulkner *et al.* (1993) established that an increase in hip axis length by 1 standard deviation raises the risk of femoral neck fracture by 1.9 times. The hip axis length is readily measured by dual energy X-ray absorptiometry (DEXA) as the distance from the greater trochanter to the inner pelvic brim (Faulkner *et al.*, 1994). A study suggests that the shorter femoral neck length in Japanese women may explain their lower risk of hip fracture, despite having lower bone mineral density at the hip than North American white women. The femoral neck length in American women was 5.6 cm, but only 4.4 cm in Japanese women (Nakamura et al., 1994).

VI. Ethnic Differences in Bone Metabolism

Higher bone mass and lower fracture incidence have been consistently reported for African-American women compared with women of European ancestry (Farmer et al., 1984; Solomon, 1979; Luckey et al., 1989). A study reported biochemical evidence of lower bone turnover rates in pre- and postmenopausal black women compared to white women. Pre- and postmenopausal black women had lower fasting urinary hydroxyproline and calcium excretions, lower 24-hr urinary calcium excretion, and lower serum osteocalcin levels, suggesting decreased bone turnover compared to whites (Meier et al., 1992). These findings were consistent with the results of direct histomorphometry, which also demonstrated lower bone turnover in both black men and women as compared to white men and women (Weinstein & Bell, 1988).

VII. Calcium, Vitamin D, and Parathyroid Hormone

Another risk factor for bone disease with aging is calcium malabsorption, which is commonly seen in the elderly. This finding may be due to vitamin D deficiency, low production of 1,25-dihydroxyvitamin D by the kidney, or intestinal resistance to 1,25-dihydroxyvitamin D (Eastell et al., 1991; Goldray et al., 1989; Petersen, 1983). Low 25-hydroxyvitamin D levels are found especially in the sick or institutionalized elderly. Decreased vitamin D levels in the elderly may be due to decreased intake of vitamin D, decreased

gastrointestinal absorption, decreased sunlight exposure, impaired synthesis of vitamin D in response to sunlight in aging skin, and impaired ability of the aging kidney to hydroxylate inactive 25-hydroxyvitamin D to the active 1,25-dihydroxyvitamin D metabolite. An age-related decline in the formation of 1,25-dihydroxyvitamin D in response to parathyroid hormone stimulation has been described (Silverberg et al., 1989; Tsai et al., 1984). A similar blunting in 1,25-dihydroxyvitamin D levels after infusion of parathyroid hormone fragments was seen in elderly patients with hip fracture as compared to elderly controls without hip fracture. A study showed that elderly subjects often have impaired calcitonin secretion, both at baseline and after calcium infusion (Quesada et al., 1994). Treatment with calcitriol corrected both the basal and stimulated calcitonin secretion to nearly the levels seen in young adults.

Parathyroid hormone levels appear to increase in response to the calcium malabsorption, leading to increased bone turnover as evidenced by increased serum osteocalcin, a biochemical marker of bone turnover. Parathyroid hormone levels have been reported to increase with age by as much as 35% (Eastell et al., 1991). Both 25-hydroxyvitamin D and calcium supplementation in the elderly has been reported to significantly decrease parathyroid hormone levels by approximately 15% (Lips et al., 1988; Francis et al., 1983; Kochersberger et al., 1991). Osteocalcin levels increase with age and correlate inversely with 25-hydroxyvitamin D levels. In one study of 195 women 70–101 years of age, the risk of hip fracture was increased 5.9 times in women with increased osteocalcin levels (Szulc et al., 1992). As part of a larger randomized trial, these 195 women were randomized to treatment with calcium and vitamin D or a placebo. Osteocalcin levels decreased in the treatment group but increased in the placebo group, suggesting that bone turnover declined with calcium and vitamin D supplementation.

Few studies have evaluated the long-term effectiveness of vitamin D supplementation in the elderly. The most important study randomly assigned 3270 ambulatory women with a mean age of 84 to receive 800 IU of vitamin D with 1200 mg of calcium or a placebo. The hip fracture rate in the intention to treat group declined by approximately one-third compared to the placebo group over 18 months of therapy (Chapuy et al., 1992). Other nonvertebral fractures decreased by 26% ($p < 0.001$). In a clinical trial in Finland, annual injections of ergocalciferol (150,000–300,000 IU) were assigned on the basis of month of birth and given to 341 men and women older than 75 years of age between 1985 and 1989. Fractures occurred in 16% of the treatment group and 21.8% of the untreated controls over a 7-year period of follow-up. Fractures of the upper extremities and ribs were significantly decreased; however, lower extremity fractures were not significantly decreased (9.1 versus 10.7%) (Heikinheimo et al., 1992). Vitamin D analogues such as 1,25-dihydroxy-vitamin D and 1α-hydroxyvitamin D have also been shown to decrease bone loss. However, hypercalcemia or hypercalciuria may occur unless calcium intake is restricted, and a rapid increase in bone loss had been noted upon cessation of therapy. Neither calcitriol or 1α-hydroxy-vitamin D has been proven to decrease hip fracture rate (Gallagher, 1993).

VIII. Cytokines

Cytokines, secreted in bone, regulate local bone resorption and formation. Interleukin 1 (IL-1) and interleukin 6 (IL-6) are very powerful stimulators of bone resorption by osteoclasts. Interleukin 1 activity, which is partially mediated by prostaglandins, appears to increase both the number of osteoclasts and their resorptive activity,

whereas interleukin 6 stimulates osteoclast formation (Mundy, 1993; Jilka et al., 1992). The effect of estradiol on bone may be mediated, at least in part, through IL-6 activity. IL-6 levels increase with ovariectomy or menopause, and the excretion of IL-6 by osteoblasts is inhibited by estradiol (Horowitz, 1993). Prostaglandin E and leukotrienes may mediate the bone destruction seen with chronic inflammatory conditions such as periodontal disease (Mundy, 1993).

Anabolic cytokines involved in bone turnover include insulin-like growth factor 2 (IGF-2), insulin-like growth factor 1 (IGF-1), and transforming growth factor β (TGF-β) with IGF-1 and TGF-β being most abundant in bone (Baylink et al., 1993). IGF-2 is fixed to the bone matrix by IGF-binding protein 5, which has a strong affinity for hydroxylapatite. TGF-β is fixed to a proteoglycan in bone. Baylink et al. hypothesize that the storage of these growth factors in bone may be a component of the coupling of bone resorption and formation. Interestingly, an age-related decline of IGF-1 in bone has been found in men and women, and in rats, ovariectomy causes a decrease of TGF-β in bone (Baylink et al., 1993). Knowledge of cytokines in bone opens a new avenue for the development of anabolic medications to treat postmenopausal osteoporosis. Early animal studies of IGF-1 and TGF-β have been promising. Infusion of IGF-1 in rats improved cortical and trabecular bone formation and increased bone mineral density of the spine, tail, and tibia (Spencer, 1991; Ammann, 1991). TGF-β stimulates local bone formation in areas of injection in rats (Joyce, 1990).

Studies of recombinant human growth hormone (rhGH), which increases levels of IGF-1, have, however, been disappointing. A randomized controlled trial of rhGH in 27 elderly women found that bone mineral at the lumbar spine and hip did not increase after 12 months of therapy, despite increased levels of IGF-1 (Holloway et al.,

1994). Furthermore, treatment was limited by the development of fluid retention and carpal tunnel syndrome. These authors hypothesized that even the decreases in body fat initially described with growth hormone may be related to fluid shifts in the body.

IX. Treatment of Osteoporosis

Despite promising animal studies of anabolic agents, the mainstay of osteoporosis treatment remains the antiresorptive agents: calcium, estrogen, calcitonin, and biphosphonates. Currently, estrogen is the treatment of choice for both the prevention and treatment of osteoporosis. Several epidemiological studies suggest that hormone replacement therapy reduces the risk of hip fracture by up to 50% (Naessen et al., 1990; Kanis & Pitt, 1992; Grady et al., 1992; Cauley et al., 1995). Current and former estrogen users appear to have decreased risks of cardiovascular mortality by 44 and 28%, respectively (Stampfer et al., 1991). Estrogen therapy in the very old (over age 75) remains controversial due to the lack of information regarding treatment in this age group. The Framingham study suggests that women not only need to take estrogen for at least 7 years to have a long-term bone effect, but that even 7 years of estrogen taken at an early age may not affect bone density among women over age 75 (Felson et al., 1993). Similarly, a prospective cohort study of women over age 65 showed that current estrogen use was protective against fractures, and prior estrogen use for greater than 10 years did not provide significant benefits for women over age 65 unless use was continued indefinitely into old age (Cauley et al., 1995). Studies have also shown that estrogen use over age 65 increases bone density in both oral and transdermal formulations (Marx et al., 1992; Lufkin et al., 1992). A significant decrease in vertebral fractures was seen with

transdermal estrogen replacement in a small randomized trial of 39 women over age 65 (Lufkin et al., 1992). Use of postmenopausal estrogens may, however, increase breast cancer risk especially after 15 years of estrogen use, but the magnitude of this effect varies between studies (Varma, 1992). Concern regrading the increased risk of breast cancer must be weighed against both the risk of osteoporosis and the protective effect of estrogens against cardiovascular disease.

Calcitonin provides an alternative antiresorptive agent for postmenopausal women, but is available in the United States only by injection. In one study vertebral fracture rate decreased by 60% in 32 women who received 100 IU of salmon calcitonin (IM) for 10 days of each month, while it increased by 30% over 24 months in 28 women receiving 500 mg of calcium alone (Rico et al., 1992). An epidemiological study in Europe found that calcitonin decreased the risk of hip fracture significantly by 31% (0.69; 0.51–0.92) after adjustment for other risk factors (Kanis et al., 1992). The effectiveness of calcitonin improved with increasing duration of treatment and was similar in older and younger women. A dose–response study randomly assigned 208 women with a bone mineral content in the distal forearm that was 30% below that of young normal women to receive either 50, 100, or 200 IU of intranasal salmon calcitonin or a placebo (Overgaard et al., 1992). A 1.0% increase in bone mineral content of the lumbar spine was noted with each 100 IU of calcitonin; however, no significant change in the forearm was seen. The incidence of new vertebral and peripheral fractures was significantly reduced by 63% (0.37; 0.14–0.95). Long-term side effects with calcitonin appear to be minimal, although the development of neutralizing antibodies can be seen with both salmon and human calcitonin (Reginster, 1993; Grauer et al., 1993).

Although calcium deficiency and calcium wasting syndromes have long been linked to the development of osteoporosis, the effectiveness of calcium supplementation in reducing bone loss and fracture remained unknown until recently. In 1990, Dawson-Hughes *et al.*, showed that women more than 5 years past menopause experienced significant decreases in rates of bone loss with calcium supplementation, particularly if their dietary calcium intake was low. Over 2 years of follow-up, women randomized to receive 500 mg of calcium rather than a placebo increased their bone density at the femoral neck (0.87 versus -2.11%) and wrist (1.05 versus -2.33%), and losses in lumbar spine density were reduced (-0.38 versus -2.85%). An Australian randomized trial later found that women at least 3 years past menopause with mean dietary calcium intakes of 750 mg also benefited from calcium supplementation (Reid *et al.*, 1993). In that study, 122 women were randomly assigned to either 1000 mg of calcium or a placebo for 2 years. Bone density at the lumbar spine increased significantly in the treatment group compared to the placebo group. Changes at the hip were not significantly different between groups except at Ward's triangle. As noted previously, a large randomized trial of 3270 elderly women receiving calcium and vitamin D or a placebo found significant declines in the intention to treat group of approximately 25–30% for both hip fractures and other nonvertebral fractures (Chapuy *et al.*, 1992).

Bisphosphonates, such as etidronate, alendronate, tiludronate, clodronate, and risedronate, act as antiresorptive agents through direct physicochemical binding to bone matrix and inhibition of osteoclast function and appear to protect against bone loss. The effect of bisphosphonates in preventing vertebral or hip fractures remains unknown. Initial studies of etidronate suggested a protective effect of etidronate for vertebral fractures in women with preexisting spinal compression fractures. However, methodological problems such as small sample size and short duration of study hampered definitive results (Watts *et al.*, 1990; Storm *et al.*, 1990). Several new, more potent bisphosphonates are being studied extensively to evaluate both fracture efficacy and safety of long-term use (Papapoulos, 1993; Rossini *et al.*, 1994).

X. Conclusion

One of the most important developments in the maintenance of musculoskeletal integrity in the elderly over the past several years is the establishment of bone densitometry as an important predictor of future fracture. This technology provides a tool to identify individuals at high risk for fracture, as well as individuals who may benefit most from preventive measures to decrease postmenopausal bone loss, and to follow the effectiveness of treatment regimens. The hip axis length may become an adjunct measure of fracture risk by utilizing bone densitometry images. The publication of a prospective study of hip fracture risk factors identified physical activity, health status, weight gain, use of benzodiazepines and anticonvulsants, prior fracture after 50 years of age, alterations in vision, and maternal history of hip fracture as significant contributors to an individual's risk of hip fracture.

The mainstay of both the prevention and treatment of osteoporosis remains the antiresorptive agents, including calcium, estrogen, calcitonin, and bisphosphonates. Although estrogen remains the drug of choice for the treatment and prevention of osteoporosis, use among women over age 75 remains controversial. Furthermore, there are unresolved clinical issues inhibiting estrogen use, including both the potential increase in breast cancer risk and the need for long-term therapy to maintain bone mass. The development of the bisphosphonate group of medications may significantly alter the treatment of osteoporosis over the next decade by providing a nonhormonal, oral alternative to estrogen. However, the long-term fracture studies utilizing bisphosphonates have not yet been published. The use of active analogues of 1,25-dihydroxyvitamin D such as calcitriol may prove beneficial, but long-term safety and effectiveness in preventing fracture must be established. Finally, new research on the role of cytokines in osteoporosis may lead to future therapy with bone-forming agents, a critical need for patients with established osteoporosis.

References

Ammann, P., Rizzoli, R., Muller, K., Slosman, D., Bonjour, J. P. (1993). IGF-1 and pamidronate increase bone mineral density in ovariectomized adult rats. *American Journal of Physiology, 265* (5Pt 1), E770–776.

Bauer, D. C., Browner, W. S., Cauley, J. A., Orwoll, E. S., Scott, J. C., Black, D. M., Tao, J. L., & Cummings, S. R. (1993). Factors associated with appendicular bone mass in older women. *Annals of Internal Medicine, 118,* 657–665.

Baylink, D. J., Finkelman, R. D., & Mohan, S. (1993). Growth factors to stimulate bone formation. *Journal of Bone Mineral Research, 8* (S2), 565–572.

Boyce, W. J., & Vessey, M. P. (1985). Rising incidence of fracture of the proximal femur. *Lancet, 1* (8421), 150–151.

Cauley, J. A., Seeley, D. G., Ensrud, K., Ettinger, B., Black, D., & Cummings, S. R. (1995). Estrogen replacement therapy and fractures in older women. *Annals of Internal Medicine, 122,* 9–16.

Chapuy, M. C., Arlot, M. E., Duboeuf, F., *et al.* (1992). Vitamin D3 and calcium to prevent hip fractures in elderly women. *New England Journal of Medicine, 327,* 1637–1642.

Cooper, C., Atkinson, E. J., O'Fallon, W. M., & Melton, L. J. (1992). Incidence of clinically diagnosed vertebral fractures: a population-based study in Rochester, Minnesota, 1985–1989. *Journal of Bone Mineral Research, 7* (2), 221–227.

Cummings, S. R., Black, D. M., & Rubin, S. M. (1989). Lifetime risks of hip, colles, or vertebral fracture and coronary heart disease among white postmenopausal women. *Archives of Internal Medicine, 149,* 2445–2448.

Cummings, S. R., Black, D. M., Nevitt, M. C., Browner, W. S., Cauley, J. A., Genant, H. K., Mascioli, S. R., Scott, J. C., Seeley, D. G., Steiger, P., & Vogt, T. M. (1990). Appendicular bone density and age predict hip fracture in women. *Journal of the American Medical Association, 263,* 665–668.

Cummings, S. R., Black, D. M., Nevitt, M. C., Browner, W., Cauley, J., Ensrud, K., Genant, H. K., Palermo, L., Scott, J., & Vogt, T. M. (1993). Bone density at various sites for prediction of hip fractures. *Lancet, 341,* 72–75.

Cummings, S. R., Nevitt, M. C., Browner, W. S., Stone, K., Fox, K. M., Ensrud, K. E., Cauley, J., Black, D., & Vogt, T. M. (1995). Risk factors for hip fracture in white women. *New England Journal of Medicine, 332,* 767–773.

Dawson-Hughes, B., Dallal, G. E., Krall, E. A., Sadowski, L., Sahyoun, N., & Tannenbaum, S. (1990). A controlled trial of the effect of calcium supplementation on bone density in postmenopausal women. *New England Journal of Medicine, 323,* 878–883.

Delmas, P. D. (1993). Biochemical markers of bone turnover. *Journal of Bone Mineral Research, 8* (S2), 549–555.

Dodds, R. A., Emery, R. J. H., Klenerman, L., Chayen, J., & Bitensky, L. (1990). Selective depression of metabolic activities in cortical osteoblasts at the site of femoral neck fractures. *Bone, 11,* 157–161.

Eastell, R., Yergey, A. L., Vieira, N. E., Cedel, S. L., Kumar, R., & Riggs, B. L. (1991). Interrelationship among vitamin D metabolism, true calcium absorption, parathyroid function, and age in women: evidence of an age-related intestinal resistance to 1,25-dihydroxyvitamin D action. *Journal of Bone Mineral Research, 6,* 125–129.

Farmer, M. E., White, L. R., & Brody, J. A. (1984). Race and sex differences in hip fracture incidence. *New England Journal of Medicine, 44,* 1374–1380.

Faulkner, K. G., Cummings, S. R., Black, D., Palermo, L., Gluer, C. C., & Genant, H. K. (1993). Simple measurement of femoral geometry predicts hip fracture: the study of osteoporotic fractures. *Journal of Bone Mineral Research, 8,* 1211–1217.

Faulkner, K. G., McClung, M., & Cummings, S. R. (1994). Automated evaluation of hip axis length for predicting hip fracture. *Journal of Bone Mineral Research*, 9, 1065–1070.

Felson, D. T., Zhang, Y., Hannan, M. T., Kiel, D. P., Wilson, P. W. F., & Anderson, J. J. (1993). The effect of postmenopausal estrogen therapy on bone density in elderly women. *New England Journal of Medicine*, 329, 1141–1146.

Francis, R. M., Peacock, M., Storer, J. H., Davies, A. E. J., Brown, W. B., & Nordin, B. E. C. (1983). Calcium malabsorption in the elderly: The effect of treatment with oral 25-hydroxyvitamin D3. *European Journal of Clinical Investigation*, 13, 391–396.

Gallagher, J. C. (1993). Prevention of bone loss in postmenopausal and senile osteoporosis with vitamin D analogues. *Osteo International* suppl. 1, S172–175.

Goldray, D., Mizrahi-Sasson, E., Merdler, C., Edelstein-Singer, M., Algoetti, A., Eisenberg, Z., Jaccard, N., & Weisman, Y. (1989). *Journal of the American Geriatric Society*, 37, 589–592.

Gordon, T., & Kannel, W. B. (1972). Predisposition to atherosclerosis in the head, heart, and legs. The Framingham study. *Journal of the American Medical Association*, 221 (7), 661–666.

Grady, D., Rubin, S. M., Petitti, D. B., *et al.* (1992). Hormone therapy to prevent disease and prolong life in postmenopausal women. *Annals of Internal Medicine*, 117, 1016–1037.

Granek, E., Baker, S. P., Abbey, H., Robinson, E., Myers, A. H., Samkoff, J. S., & Klein, L. E. (1987). Medications and diagnoses in relation to falls in a long-term care facility. *Journal of the American Geriatric Society*, 35, 503–511.

Grauer, A., Reinel, H. H., Lunghall, S., Lindh, E., Ziegler, R., & Raue, F. (1993). Formation of neutralizing antibodies after treatment with human calcitonin. *American Journal of Medicine*, 95, 439–442.

Greenspan, S. L., Maitland, L. A., Myers, E. R., Krasnow, M. B., & Kido, T. H. (1994). Femoral bone loss progresses with age: a longitudinal study in women over age 65. *Journal of Bone Mineral Research*, 9, 1959–1965.

Grisso, J. A., Kelsey, J. L., Strom, B. L., Chiu, G. Y., Maislin, G., O'Brien, L. A., Hoffman, S., & Kaplan, F. (1991). Risk factors for falls as a cause of hip fracture in women. *New England Journal of Medicine*, 324, 1326–1331.

Grisso, J. A., Kelsey, J. L., Strom, B. L., O'Brien, L. A. Maislin, G., LaPann, K., Samelson, L., & Hoffman, S. (1994). Risk factors for hip fracture in black women. *New England Journal of Medicine*, 330, 1555–1559.

Hannan, M. T., Felson, D. T., & Anderson, J. J. (1992). Bone mineral density in elderly men and women: results from the Framingham osteoporosis study. *Journal of Bone Mineral Research*, 7, 547–553.

Hansen, M. A., Overgaard, K., Riis, B. J., & Christiansen, C. (1991). Potential risk factors for development of postmenopausal osteoporosis—examined over a 12-year period. *Osteo International*, 1, 95–102.

Heikinheimo, R. J., Inkovaara, J. A., Harju, E. J., Haavisto, M. V., Kaarela, R. H., Kataja, J. M., Kokko, A. M., Kolho, L. A., & Rajala, S. A. (1992). Annual injection of vitamin D and fractures of aged bones. *Calcified Tissue International*, 51 (2), 105–110.

Heyse, S. P. (1993). Epidemiology of hip fractures in the elderly: a cross-national analysis of mortality rates for femoral neck fractures. *Osteo International*, Suppl. 1, S16–19.

Holloway, L., Butterfield, G., Hintz, R. L., Gesundheit, N., & Marcus R. (1994). Effects of recombinant human growth hormone on metabolic indices, body composition, and bone turnover in healthy elderly women. *Journal of Clinical and Endocrinology Metabolism*, 79, 470–479.

Horowitz, M. C. (1993). Cytokines and estrogen in bone: anti-osteoporotic effects. *Science*, 260, 626–627.

Hui, S. L., Slemenda, C. W., & Johnston, C. C. (1988). Age and bone mass as predictors of fracture in a prospective study. *Journal of Clinical Investigation*, 81, 1804–1809.

Jacobsen, S. J., Goldberg, J., Miles, T. P., Brody, J. A., Stiers, W., & Rimm, A. A. (1990). Regional variation in the incidence of hip fracture. *Journal of the American Medical Association*, 264, 500–513.

Jilka, R. L., Hangoc, G., Girasole, G., Passeri, G., Williams, D. C., Abrams, J. S., Boyce, B., Broxmeyer, H., & Manolagas, S. C. (1992). Increased osteoclast development after estrogen loss: mediation by interleukin-6. *Science*, 257, 88–91.

Johnell, O., Stenbeck, M., Rosen, M., Gulberg,

B., Kanis, J. A. (1993). Therapeutic strategies in the prevention of hip fracture with drugs affecting bone metabolism. *Bone, 14*, S85–S87.

Joyce, M. E., Roberts, A. B., Sporn, M. B., Bolander, M. E. (1990). Transforming growth factor-beta and the initiation of chondrogenesis and osteogenesis in the rat femur. *Journal of Cell Biology, 110* (6), 2195–2207.

Kanis, J. A., & Pitt, F. A. (1992). Epidemiology of osteoporosis. *Bone, 13*, S7–15.

Kanis, J. A., Johnell, O., Gullberg, B., Allander, E., Dilsen, G., Gennari, C., Lopes Vaz, A. A., Lyritis, G. P., Mauoli, G., Miravet, L., Passeri, M., Perez Cano, R., Rapado, A., & Ribot, C. (1992). Evidence for efficacy of drugs affecting bone metabolism in preventing hip fracture. *British Medical Journal, 305*, 1124–1128.

Kochersberger, G., Westlund, R., & Lyles, K. W. (1991). The metabolic effects of calcium supplementation in the elderly. *Journal of the American Geriatric Society, 39*, 192–196.

Kotowicz, M. A., Melton, L. J., Cooper, C., Atkinson, E. J., O'Fallon, W. M., & Riggs, B. L. (1994). Risk of hip fracture in women with vertebral fracture. *Journal of Bone Mineral Research, 9* (5), 599–605.

Lauritzen, J. B., Petersen, M. M., & Lund, B. (1993). Effect of external hip protectors on hip fractures. *Lancet, 341*, 11–13.

Lips, P., Wiersinga, A., van Ginkel, F. C., Jongen, M. J. M., Netelenbos, J. C., Hackeng, W. H. L., Delmas, P. D., & van der Vijgh, W. J. F. (1988). The effect of vitamin D supplementation on vitamin D status and parathyroid function in elderly subjects. *Journal of Clinical and Endocrinogy Metabolism, 67*, 644–649.

Luckey, M. M., Meier, D. E., Mandeli, J., DaCosta, M., & Goldsmith, S. J. (1989). Axial and appendicular bone density in white and black women: Evidence of racial differences in premenopausal bone homeostasis. *Journal of Clinical Endocrinology Metabolism, 69*, 762–770.

Lufkin, E. G., Wahner, H. W., & O'Fallon, W. M. (1992). Treatment of postmenopausal osteoporosis with transdermal estrogen. *Annals of Internal Medicine, 117*, 1–9.

Manolagas, S. C., & Jilka, R. L. (1995). Bone marrow, cytokines, and bone remodeling. *New England Journal of Medicine, 332*, 305–311.

Marottoli, R. A., Berkman, L. F., & Cooney, L. M. (1992). Decline in physical function following hip fracture. *Journal of the American Geriatric Society, 40*, 860–866.

Marx, C. W., Dailey, G. E., Cheney, C., Vint, V. C., & Muchmore, D. B. (1992). Do estrogens improve bone mineral density in osteoporotic women over age 65? *Journal of Bone Mineral Research, 7* (11), 1275–1279.

Meier, D. E., Luckey, M. M., Wallenstein, S., Lapinski, R. H., & Catherwood, B. (1992). Racial differences in pre- and postmenopausal bone homeostasis: association with bone density. *Journal of Bone Mineral Research, 7*, 1181–1189.

Melton, L. J. (1993). Hip fractures: a worldwide problem today and tomorrow. *Bone, 14*, S1–8.

Melton, L. J., Kan, S. H., Frye, M. A., Wahner, H. W., O'Fallon, W. M., & Riggs, B. L. (1989). Epidemiology of vertebral fractures in women. *American Journal of Epidemiology, 129*, 1000–1011.

Morrison, N. A., Qi, J. C., Tokita, A., Kelly, P. J., Crofts, L., Nguten, T. V., Sambrook, P. N., & Eisman, J. A. (1994). Prediction of bone density from vitamin D receptor alleles. *Nature, 367*, 284–287.

Mundy, G. R. (1993). Cytokines and growth factors in the regulation of bone remodeling. *Journal of Bone Mineral Research, 8* (S2), 505–510.

Naessen, T., Persson, I., Adami, H. O., Bergstrom, R., & Bergkvist, L. (1990). Hormone replacement therapy and the risk for first hip fracture: a prospective, population based cohort study. *Annals of Internal Medicine, 113*, 95–103.

Nakamura, T., Turner, C. H., Yoshikawa, T., Slemenda, C. W., Peacock, M., Burr, D. B., Mizuno, Y., Orimo, H., Ouchi, Y., & Johnston, C. C. (1994). Do variations in hip geometry explain differences in hip fracture risk between Japanese and White Americans? *Journal of Bone Mineral Research, 9*, 1071–1076.

Nevitt, M. C., & Cummings, S. R. (1993). Type of fall and risk of hip and wrist fractures: the study of osteoporotic fractures. *Journal of the American Geriatric Society, 41*, 1226–1234.

Nordin, B. E. C., Need, A. G., Chatterton, B. E., Horowitz, M., & Morris, H. A. (1990). The relative contributions of age and years since menopause to postmenopausal bone loss.

Journal of Clinical Endocrinology Metabolism, 70, 83–88.

Obrant, K. (1989). Increasing age-adjusted risk of fragility fractures: a sign of increasing osteoporosis in successive generations? *Calcified Tissue International, 44,* 157–167.

Overgaard, K., Hansen, M. A., Jensen, S. B., & Christiansen, C. (1992). Effect of salcatonin given intranasally on bone mass and fracture rates in established osteoporosis: a dose-response study. *British Medical Journal, 305,* 556–561.

Papapoulos, S. E. (1993). The role of bisphosphonates in the prevention and treatment of osteoporosis. *American Journal of Medicine, 95* (S5A), 48–52.

Parfitt, A. M. (1993). Bone age, mineral density, and fatigue damage. *Calcified Tissue International, 53* (Suppl. 1), S82–S86.

Parfitt, A. M., Mathews, C. H. E., Villanueva, A. R., Kleerekoper, M., Frame, B., & Rao, D. S. (1983). Relationships between surface, volume, and thickness of iliac trabecular bone in aging and in osteoporosis. *Journal of Clinical Investigation, 72,* 1396–1409.

Petersen, M. M., Briggs, R. S., Ashby, M. A., Reid, R. I., Hall, M. R., Wood, P. J., & Clayton, B. E. (1983). Parathyroid hormone and 25-hydroxyvitamin D concentrations in sick and normal elderly people. *British Medical Journal, 287.*

Phillips, S., Fox, N., Jacobs, J., & Wright, W. E. (1988). The direct medical costs of osteoporosis for American women aged 45 and older, 1986. *Bone, 9,* 271–279.

Quesada, J. M., Mateo, A., Jans, I., Rodriguez, M., & Bouillon, R. (1994). Calcitriol corrects deficient calcitonin secretion in the vitamin D-deficient elderly. *Journal of Bone Mineral Research, 9,* 53–57.

Recker, R. R., Kimmel, D. B., Parfitt, A. M., Davies, K. M., Keshawarz, N., & Hinders, S. (1988). Static and tetracycline-based bone histomorphometric data from 34 normal postmenopausal females. *Journal of Bone Mineral Research, 3,* 133–144.

Reginster, J. Y. (1993). Calcitonin for prevention and treatment of osteoporosis. *American Journal of Medicine, 95* (S5A), 44S–47S.

Reid, I. R., Ames, R. W., Evans, M. C., Gamble, G. D., & Sharpe, S. J. (1993). Effect of calcium supplementation on bone loss in postmenopausal women. *New England Journal of Medicine, 328,* 460–464.

Rico, H., Hernandez, E. R., Revilla, M., & Gomez-Castresana, F. (1992). Salmon calcitonin reduces vertebral fracture rate in postmenopausal crush fracture syndrome. *Bone Mineral, 16,* 131–138.

Ross, P. D., Davis, J. W., Epstein, R. S., & Wasnich, R. D. (1991). Pre-existing fractures and bone mass predict vertebral fracture incidence in women. *Annals of Internal Medicine, 114,* 919–923.

Rossini, M., Gatti, D., Zamberlan, N., Braga, V., Dorizzi, R., & Adam, S. (1994). Long term effects of a treatment course with oral alendronate of postmenopausal osteoporosis. *Journal of Bone Mineral Research, 9,* 1833–1837.

Ryan, P. J., Blake, G., Herd, R., & Fogelman, I. (1994). A clinical profile of back pain and disability in patients with spinal osteoporosis. *Bone, 15,* 27–30.

Schnitzler, C. M. (1993). Bone quality: a determinant for certain risk factors for bone fragility. *Calcified Tissue International, 53* (S1), S27–31.

Seeley, D. G., Browner, W. S., Nevitt, M. C., Genant, H. K., Scott, J. C., Cummings, S. R. (1991). Which fractures are associated with low appendicular bone mass in elderly women? *Annals of Internal Medicine, 115,* 837–842.

Silverberg, A. J., Shane, E., De la Cruz, L., Segre, G. V., Clemens, T. L., & Bilezikian, J. P. (1989). Abnormalities in parathyroid hormone secretion and 1,25-dihydroxyvitamin D3 formation in women with osteoporosis. *New England Journal of Medicine, 320,* 277–281.

Solomon, L. (1979). Bone density in aging caucasian and African populations. *Lancet, 3,* 1326–1329.

Soroko, S. B., Barrett-Connor, E., Edelstein, S. L., & Kritz-Silverstein, D. (1994). Family history of osteoporosis and bone mineral density at the axial skeleton: the Rancho Bernardo study. *Journal of Bone Mineral Research, 9,* 761–769.

Spencer, E. M., Liu, C. C., Si, E. C., Howard, G. A. (1991). In vivo actions of insulin-like growth factor-I (IGF-I) on bone formation and resorption in rats. *Bone, 12* (1), 21–26.

Stampfer, M. J., Colditz, G. A., Willett, W. C., Manson, J. E., Rosner, B., Speizer, F. E., & Hennekens, C. H. (1991). Postmenopausal estrogen therapy and cardiovascular disease:

ten year followup from the Nurses' Health study. *New England Journal of Medicine, 325,* 756–762.

Steiger, P., Cummings, S. R., Black, D. M., Spencer, N. E., & Genant, H. K. (1992). Age related decrements in bone mineral density in women over 65. *Journal of Bone Mineral Research, 7,* 625–632.

Storm, T., Thamsborg, G., Steiniche, T., Genant, H. K., & Sonensen, O. H. (1990). Effect of intermittent cyclical etidronate therapy on bone mass and fracture rate in women with postmenopausal osteoporosis. *New England Journal of Medicine, 322,* 1265–1271.

Szulc, P., Chapuy, M. C., Meunier, P. J., & Delmas, P. D. (1992). Serum undercarboxylated osteocalcin is a marker of the risk of hip fracture in elderly women. *Journal of Clinical Investigation, 91,* 1769–1774.

Tinetti, M. E., & Speechley, M. (1989). Prevention of falls among the elderly. *New England Journal of Medicine, 329,* 1055–1059.

Tinetti, M. E., Baker, D. I., McAvay, G., Claus, E. B., Garrett, P., Gottschalk, M., Koch, M. L., Trainor, K., & Horwitz, R. I. (1994). A multifactorial intervention to reduce the risk of falling among elderly people living in the community. *New England Journal of Medicine, 331,* 821–827.

Tsai, K. S., Heath, H., Kumar, R., & Riggs, B. L. (1984). Impaired vitamin D metabolism with aging in women: possible role in pathogenesis of senile osteoporosis. *Journal of Clinical Investigation, 73,* 1668–1672.

Varma, T. R. (1992). Sex steroids and cancer in older women. *Drugs and Aging, 2,* 174–195.

Vernon-Roberts, B., & Pirie, C. J. (1973). Healing trabecular microfractures in the bodies of lumbar vertebrae. *Annals of the Rheumatic Diseases, 32,* 406–412.

Wasnich, R. (1993). Bone mass measurement: prediction of risk. *American Journal of Medicine, 95,* S6–S10.

Watts, N. B., Harris, S. T., Genant, H. K., *et al.* (1990). Intermittent cyclical etidronate treatment of postmenopausal osteoporosis. *New England Journal of Medicine, 323,* 73–79.

Weinstein, R. S., & Bell, N. H. (1988). Diminished rates of bone formation in normal black adults. *New England Journal of Medicine, 319,* 1698–1701.

Author Index

Numbers in italics refer to the pages on which the complete references are listed

Subject Index

WIDENER UNIVERSITY
WOLFGRAM
LIBRARY
CHESTER, PA.